Diagnostic Assessment and Treatment of Peripheral Nerve Tumors

Fernando Guedes
Eric L. Zager • Debora Garozzo
Lukas Rasulic • Mariano Socolovsky
Editors

Diagnostic Assessment and Treatment of Peripheral Nerve Tumors

Springer

Editors
Fernando Guedes
WFNS Peripheral Nerve Surgery Committee
Division of Neurosurgery
Department of Surgery
Gaffrée e Guinle University Hospital (HUGG)
School of Medicine
Federal University of Rio de Janeiro State (UNIRIO)
Rio de Janeiro
RJ
Brazil

Debora Garozzo
WFNS Peripheral Nerve Surgery Committee
Department of Neurosurgery
Mediclinic Parkview Hospital
Dubai
UAE

Mariano Socolovsky
WFNS Peripheral Nerve Surgery Committee
Peripheral Nerve & Brachial Plexus Surgery Program
Department of Neurosurgery
University of Buenos Aires
School of Medicine
Buenos Aires
Argentina

Eric L. Zager
WFNS Peripheral Nerve Surgery Committee
Department of Neurosurgery
University of Pennsylvania
Perelman School of Medicine
Philadelphia, PA
USA

Lukas Rasulic
WFNS Peripheral Nerve Surgery Committee
Faculty of Medicine University of Belgrade
Clinic for Neurosurgery, University Clinical Center of Serbia
Department of Peripheral Nerve Surgery, Functional Neurosurgery and Pain Management Surgery
Belgrade
Serbia

ISBN 978-3-030-77632-9 ISBN 978-3-030-77633-6 (eBook)
https://doi.org/10.1007/978-3-030-77633-6

This Springer imprint is published by the registered company Springer Nature Switzerland AG
The registered company address is: Gewerbestrasse 11, 6330 Cham, Switzerland

Dr. Fernando Guedes:

I dedicate this book to my lovely wife Elizabeth and our dear son Thiago.
I'd like to thank my dear fellow coeditors and also my dear colleagues from many parts of the world who contributed with their expertise in several chapters.
I cannot forget to thank the people in Springer, particularly Ms. Niveka Somasundaram, for the incredible support they gave us throughout this project.
To all patients suffering from peripheral nerve tumors: that they may benefit from this work.

Dr. Eric L. Zager:

I dedicate this book to my loving family:
To my parents, Daniel and Florence, and my sister, Robin, all of blessed memory.
To my wonderful wife, Marirosa, for her love and support.
To my fabulous children, Camila, David, and Daniel.
To my mentors in nerve surgery, Professors David Kline and Alan Hudson.
And to my larger family of colleagues, residents, students, and especially to my patients and their families.

Dr. Debora Garozzo:

To the everlasting memory of Lauris Muischneek and to what we were for each other.

Dr. Lukas Rasulic:

I dedicate this book to my driving force, my family: my wife Katarina, our daughter Milica, and our son Mihailo;
my parents: my father Grujica and my mother Dusanka;
my sister Katarina;
my mentor, Prof. Dr. Miroslav Samardzic, and my associates;
and last but not the least, my patients with peripheral nerve disorders.

Dr. Mariano Socolovsky:

I dedicate this book to the wonderful team I have the honor to work with: Gilda di Masi, Danilo Battaglia, Verónica Brandolin, Gonzalo Bonilla, Karina Barillaro, Ana Lovaglio, Daniela Binaghi, and Rafael Barousse.

Foreword

It is a great pleasure and honor to write the Foreword for this book on peripheral nerve tumors, written and edited by distinguished colleagues and dear friends from the WFNS Peripheral Nerve Surgery Committee.

The activity of the WFNS PNS Committee has been outstanding over the past few years. A continuous effort from the group of devoted neurosurgeons, with their compassionate endeavors in the preservation of peripheral nerve surgery within neurosurgery, once again led to the most comprehensive book on peripheral nerve tumors to date.

These lesions (accounting for only about 1% of all soft tissue tumors) demand a dedicated and meticulous approach. With the era of "life-saving," functional or even extremity sacrifice having passed, contemporary approaches to peripheral nerve tumors include basic principles, a deep understanding of pathophysiology and pathomorphology, as well as modern surgical techniques and tricks. With the development of chemotherapeutics and radiation-oncology, with targeted therapies taking their rightful place, we now have all the best tools at our disposal, and this book is here to guide new generations of neurosurgeons and peripheral nerve surgeons. The book is also aimed at all physicians dealing with these complex lesions, however with the emphasis on young neurosurgeons, as well as those expected to solve the most demanding cases.

This book will help in educating general neurosurgeons and beyond. On the other hand, it should inspire experts to expand knowledge and to improve patient outcomes. The field of peripheral nerve surgery is considered one of the less represented areas in any average neurosurgical department worldwide. I am confident that this book will raise awareness about the importance of this field and contribute to its visibility and increasing interest.

I would like to congratulate the editors of this book, Fernando Guedes, Mariano Socolovsky, Lukas Rasulic, Eric L. Zager, and Debora Garozzo, as well as all chapter authors for publishing a very useful book to support all surgeons involved in the diagnostic assessment and treatment of peripheral nerve tumors.

Franco Servadei
Department of Neurosurgery, Humanitas
University and Research Hospital Milano, Milan, Italy
WFNS, Milan, Italy
Italian Society of Neurosurgery (SINCh), Milan,Italy

Foreword

What a pleasure it is to be asked to write a foreword for this book on peripheral nerve tumors. One of the great challenges and sometimes the joy of working with surgical nerve lesions are managing patients with nerve tumors. The editors Fernando Guedes (Brazil), Eric L. Zager (USA), Debora Garozzo (Italy and UAE), Lukas Rasulic (Serbia), and Mariano Socolovsky (Argentina) as well as 30 chapters from North, Central, and South America, Europe, India, and UAE have created a fascinating compendium covering epidemiology, genetics, pathology, clinical assessment, neurophysiology, ultrasound, MRI, biopsy, surgical resection, intraoperative monitoring, complications, pain management, radiotherapy and chemotherapy, neurofibromatosis, schwannomatosis, and malignancies, and I imagine a number of other tumor types in addition to the most common benign neural sheath tumors, schwannomas, neurofibromas, and others such as perineuriomas—localized hypertrophic neuropathy (LHN), hemangiomas, ganglion cysts, desmoids, triton tumors, and more. The different loci of tumors such as the brachial and pelvic plexus are also delineated. You will enjoy both consulting and reading this new and up-to-date book on peripheral nerve tumors.

As a minor historic addendum—when we began to operate on nerve tumors in the late 60s, 70s, and 80s, we already had experience with operative recordings of CNAPs (Compound Nerve Action Potentials) for injured nerves in continuity. It became evident that what was very important was to expose both the proximal and distal poles of schwannomas and neurofibromas because there were fascicles or groups of fibers entering and leaving both poles (more in neurofibromas than schwannomas) and when entering fascicles were stimulated proximally and recordings done on exiting fascicles distally, the traces were flat on these rather globular tumors. By comparison, fascicles or groups of fibers more superficial in the capsule or pseudocapsule conducted an NAP as did the nerve as a whole even when fascicles or fiber groups entering and leaving the mass of the tumor were sectioned. Histological examination of the entering and leaving fascicles or fibers from the tumor mass itself showed a rudimentary array of immature poorly developed, small axons in a very disorganized background. As one Ochsner pathologist commented—the entering and exiting fascicles had an embryonic appearance. This was also confirmed by Masson, Bodian, and Luxol fast blue as well as HandE stains in our own neurohistology laboratory at LSUHSC NS (Louisiana State University Health Sciences Center, Department of Neurosurgery).

These observations were made not only on sporadic neurofibromas but those associated with neurofibromatosis.

- Donner TR, Voorhies RM, Kline DG. Neural sheath tumors of major nerves. J Neurosurg. 1994;81:362–73
- Kim DH, Hudson AR, Kline DG. Surgical techniques for nerve tumors. In Atlas of peripheral nerve surgery. 2nd Ed. Philadelphia: Saunders-Elsevier; 2013. p. 235–40.
- Kline DG, Hudson AR, Kim DH. Benign neural sheath tumors. In Atlas of peripheral nerve surgery. Philadelphia: Saunders-Elsevier; 2001. p. 190–6.

David G. Kline
LSUHSC-NS
New Orleans, LA, USA

Preface

We are pleased to present this text **Diagnostic Assessment and Treatment of Peripheral Nerve Tumors** to the medical community. This work was conceived by the Peripheral Nerve Surgery Committee of the World Federation of Neurosurgical Societies and follows upon the previous text **Manual of Peripheral Nerve Surgery: From the Basics to Complex Procedures**, which was published in 2018. We are very fortunate to have received superb contributions from many of the leading nerve surgeons in the world, along with our colleagues in neuroradiology, neuropathology, and neurology. Peripheral nerve tumors comprise a fascinating group of heterogeneous lesions that challenge our diagnostic and therapeutic capabilities. Our management of these lesions has progressed substantially in recent decades through the pioneering efforts of our colleagues in many disciplines, but many controversies and challenges remain. No longer do we accept the routine sacrifice of functional nerve fascicles when resecting benign nerve sheath tumors. However, even the most experienced and skillful nerve surgeons do inadvertently injure nerves occasionally when removing certain difficult lesions, even when benign. Recognizing and dealing with potentially malignant lesions is even more challenging, and we have not even reached uniform agreement as to when a biopsy is mandatory prior to tumor resection. Imaging has improved substantially for these tumors, but is still incapable of reliably diagnosing malignancy in many cases without a tissue diagnosis. Once a malignant lesion is diagnosed, there is still major controversy regarding optimal management in terms of the type and timing of adjuvant therapy and reconstructive options.

In this text, we present first the general principles of clinical and surgical approaches to nerve tumors. This section includes chapters on epidemiology, genetics and pathology of nerve tumors, the clinical and radiological assessment of these patients, indications and techniques for biopsy, the fundamental aspects of surgical technique along with intraoperative neurophysiological monitoring, and recognition and management of the inevitable and unfortunate complications which accompany any surgical endeavors. We also discuss the indications for adjuvant therapy of malignant tumors. The second and third parts of this book include chapters that deal with specific tumor types and locations in the body in both the general population and in specific genetic disorders.

Our goal here is to provide a readable collection of chapters that cover this fascinating topic comprehensively for both the generalist and the specialist, with contemporary and classic references for further reading. Our target audience is broad and includes neurosurgeons, neurologists, hand surgeons in orthopedic and plastic surgery, surgical oncologists, radiation therapists, physiatrists, physical and occupational therapists, and even vascular and general surgeons who often collaborate and provide operative exposure for us. We wish to thank our authors for their expertise and eloquence, and our publisher for their support in this endeavor. Most importantly, we wish to thank our patients for their trust and confidence that we are constantly striving to improve our care for their neurological disorders.

Rio de Janeiro, Brazil — Fernando Guedes
Philadelphia, PA, USA — Eric L. Zager
Dubai, UAE — Debora Garozzo
Belgrade, Serbia — Lukas Rasulic
Buenos Aires, Argentina — Mariano Socolovsky

Contents

Part I

General Clinical and Surgical Principles in Peripheral Nerve Tumors

1 Epidemiology of Peripheral Nerve Sheath Tumors

Andrew S. Jack, Charlotte J. Huie, and Line G. Jacques

The first description of what was likely a peripheral nerve tumor was published by Cheselden in 1741 [1]. Since that time, not only has management of peripheral nerve tumors obviously changed dramatically, but so has their reported epidemiology (as summarized in Table 1.1). With the advent of newer and more readily accessible imaging modalities such as magnetic resonance imaging (MRI) and MR neurography, reported peripheral nerve tumor incidence has increased substantially. Peripheral nerve tumors can be subdivided into nerve sheath and non-nerve sheath tumors. As their name implies, peripheral nerve sheath tumors (PNSTs) are tumors arising from cells surrounding an axon or nerve fascicle(s), which may include, for example, Schwann cells, fibroblasts, and histiocytic or macrophage-like cells, among others. They can also be further subdivided into benign or malignant. In this chapter, we will compare and contrast the different epidemiological characteristics of the most frequently encountered PNST—both benign (schwannomas, neurofibromas, perineuriomas, granular cell tumors, ganglioneuromas) and malignant (malignant granular cell tumors and malignant peripheral nerve sheath tumors) alike. By understanding the respective epidemiology of these rare tumors, a better appreciation for their clinical burden will hopefully prevail.

A. S. Jack (✉)
Division of Neurosurgery, University of Alberta, Edmonton, AB, Canada
e-mail: asjack@ualberta.ca

C. J. Huie · L. G. Jacques
Department of Neurosurgery, University of California San Francisco (UCSF), San Francisco, CA, USA
e-mail: Line.Jacques@ucsf.edu

1.1 Schwannomas

Schwannomas are a benign PNST originating from Schwann cells encasing and insulating nerve fibers. They are the most common benign PNST, a category that also includes neurofibromas (NF), perineuriomas, and granular cell tumors (to be discussed elsewhere). However, they can be quite heterogeneous in nature with respect to their reported epidemiology, including incidence and/or prevalence, location, and natural history, among others. Values and statistics for the aforementioned tumor characteristics will also vary substantially depending on the context in which they are being discussed. More specifically, reported values will vary depending on whether they are occurring sporadically or in association with a genetic syndrome (e.g., neurofibromatosis 1 versus 2 (NF-1 and NF-2, respectively), schwannomatosis, or Carney's complex).

How the incidence and prevalence of schwannomas are qualified (the context or circumstance in which they are being described) will ultimately dictate how common or uncommon they are reported to be. Because schwannomas can potentially arise from any nerve throughout the body (or anywhere Schwann cells may be found for

F. Guedes et al. (eds.), *Diagnostic Assessment and Treatment of Peripheral Nerve Tumors*,
https://doi.org/10.1007/978-3-030-77633-6_1

Table 1.1 Summary table of the epidemiological characteristics of peripheral nerve sheath tumors

	Schwannoma	Neurofibroma	Peri-neurioma	Granular cell tumor	Ganglio-neuroma	MPNST	Malignant granular cell tumor
Incidence	20/million/year [127]	5% of soft tissue tumors [70, 115]	1% of nerve sheath tumors [80, 89, 93, 145]	0.5% of soft tissue tumors [128]	1/million/year [21, 44]	1/100,000/year general population vs 1/3500/year NF-1 [12, 13, 26, 27, 61, 74, 86, 101]	1–3% of granular cell tumors [128, 141]
Age (years)	20–50	20–30	Intraneural: adolescence to adulthood Extraneural: adulthood	30–50	Childhood	30–50 (mean 41 vs 28 in NF-1)	30–50
Sex	Females = Males	Females = Males	No clear sex predilection	Females > Males	No clear sex predilection	No clear sex predilection	Females > Males
Location	Central: intracranial, intraspinal, intracerebral and/or intramedullary Peripheral	Anywhere: any nerve	Intraneural: lower > upper extremities Extraneural: trunk or extremities	Anywhere: commonly head and neck	Anywhere: neural crest cell derivatives	Superficial (cutaneous) or deep (plexiform)	Lower extremity, nuchal region, chest wall, gastrointestinal tract, head, and neck
Classification	Conventional Ancient Cellular Plexiform Melanotic Intermediate Epithelioid	Dermal: localized or diffuse Intraneural localized Plexiform Atypical Massive soft-tissue type	Intraneural Extraneural	Benign Atypical Malignant	Neuroblastic tumor: ganglioneuroma, ganglioneuroblastoma, ganglioneurobalstoma intermixed, neuroblastoma	Low grade High grade	Low grade High Grade

that matter), most reports will classify schwannomas in context of their histology or based on their location. For example, schwannomas are often categorized as being peripheral (occurring predominantly in the head and neck area or flexor aspects of the extremities) or central (affecting the cranial nerves or spinal nerve rootlets and/or roots). Their prevalence is also often described on the basis of location, intracranial, intraspinal, intracerebral, and/or intramedullary, or in the context of other soft tissue or nerve sheath tumors. These schwannoma qualifiers will then determine and affect the specific values reported. For example, schwannomas are reported to be the most common benign PNST (as high as 80% in some reports) [2–4]; however, they only account for 8% of all soft tissue tumors [1]. They have also been reported to represent 33% of primary spinal tumors [5–8], 8–10% of primary brain tumors [9–12], and 5.8% of foot and ankle peripheral nerve tumors [13]. Moreover, the matter of tumor symptomatology (asymptomatic or incidental diagnosis versus diagnosis based on symptomatic investigations) and how the tumors are being diagnosed (cadaveric study versus radiological cross-sectional study) will also greatly affect the prevalence reported. For example, in earlier studies using cadaveric dissection for diagnosis, the prevalence of vestibular schwannomas (VS, incidental) was reported to be 0–2.4% [10, 14–17]. However, with the increasing use of MRI, other studies have found the VS prevalence to be 0.02–0.07% [16, 18–20].

In a similar vein, the incidence that is reported with respect to these tumors can also vary substantially depending on how it is defined (the context of the reported incidence). For example, in one prospective epidemiological database from Denmark, the incidence of diagnosed VS was reported to have increased from 8/million/year at its inception to more recently 20/million/year [21]. The rapid increase in the incidence of VS is likely related to increasing awareness of these tumors and improved diagnostic investigations such as audiological testing and MRI techniques. In keeping with this latter value, other studies have found an incidence for VS to be between 0.01 and 0.1% [16, 22–25]. Other studies have characterized the incidence of schwannomas based on location and tissue of origin or age. For example, in a radiological study examining the most common soft tissue tumors of the upper extremity, Hoglund et al. found 5% of benign soft tissue tumors in their series to be schwannomas [26]. In keeping with their prevalence and incidence, gender and age peaks may also vary based on the schwannoma location. Although it is generally accepted that schwannomas generally affect adults more than children (usually occurring in patients between 20 and 50 years of age) [21, 27–31], whether or not a sex predilection exists for schwannomas remains controversial. Some studies state no difference in tumor incidence between males and females [2, 10, 16, 27, 28, 30, 32–35], while others state females are more affected [1].

The natural history of schwannomas with respect to their growth rate is an important element to consider when trying to determine the best patient management strategy. This can oftentimes be difficult as the reported growth rate for these tumors is very heterogeneous depending on the study (likely related to the heterogeneity in methods used for tumor size and growth measurements, the presence of extrinsic factors affecting tumor growth, as well as the tumor biology and histological subtype itself). For example, sporadic growth rates have been said to vary from 1–2 mm/year up to 17 mm/year. In their review, Paldor et al. found an average growth rate of approximately 1 mm/year; however, it can be 3 mm/year in those tumors demonstrating growth at early follow-up [34]. Furthermore, approximately one-third of newly diagnosed sporadic VS had grown within 1–3 years and 50% after 5 years of follow-up. And finally, factors determined to increase growth rate or predict tumor growth included hormonal therapy (specifically, erythropoietin), hemorrhagic or cystic tumor features, and early demonstrated growth on follow-up. Age, sex, location, symptomatic status, and size, however, did not predict growth. In another study examining schwannomas of other cranial nerves, growth rate was again noted to be quite variable (0.7 mm–2.6 mm/year, average 1.4 mm/year) [36, 37]. Although many of these extrinsic factors may influence schwannoma growth patterns, as mentioned above, perhaps a more likely explanation for the varied growth rates reported is that different histological subtypes (as shown in Fig. 1.1) of schwannomas [38] (subcategorized as cellular, conventional, intermediate, ancient, melanotic (1% of PNST) [39], plexiform (5% of schwannomas) [40], epithelioid) simply have different genotypes. The specific genetic or epigenetic mutations and factors will then result in similar phenotypic tumors potentially behaving much differently. For example, cellular schwannomas (approximately 20–30% of retroperitoneal schwannomas) which are still considered a benign PNST have been shown to have a higher growth rate and rate of recurrence compared to other subtypes [38, 41–43]. Although beyond the scope of this chapter, the advent of more targeted therapies has led to more and more research being done investigating these specific molecular mechanisms that may be responsible for different schwannoma growth characteristics [23, 44, 45]. The latter is highlighted when considering schwannomas in the context of genetic diseases and syndromes such as NF-1, NF-2, Carney's complex, or schwannomatosis. Although discussed here are mainly sporadic schwannoma characteristics, their occurrence in diseases such as those just mentioned will ultimately lead to different epidemiological and behavioral characteristics (to be discussed in later chapters).

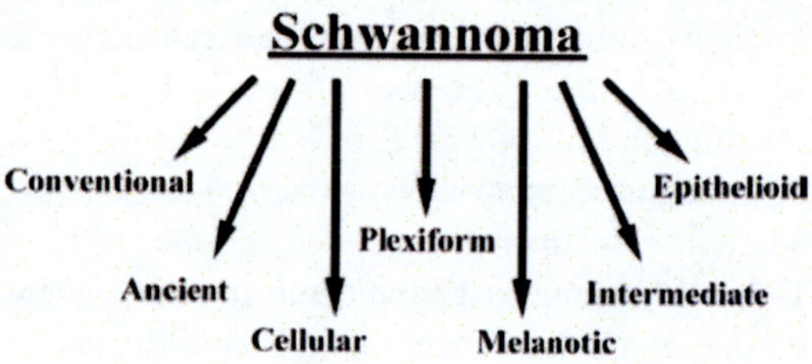

Fig. 1.1 Histological classification of schwannomas

1.2 Neurofibromas

Neurofibromas are benign PNSTs originating from Schwann cells, with admixed fibroblasts, perineurial cells, hematopoietic cells, and nerve fascicles also being seen on histopathological section [46, 47]. They are the second most common type of benign PNST after schwannomas with a reported prevalence of 10–24% of all isolated nerve tumors and making up 5% of all soft tissue tumors [32, 48]. These can be classified as solitary (or sporadic, not occurring in the context of NF-1 and existing as a solitary nodule emanating from a single peripheral nerve) or plexiform (seen almost exclusively in the context of NF-1 in which multiple neoplastic tumors from individual nerves or nerve fascicles coalesce into a plexiform-like "bag of worms"). As shown in Fig. 1.2a, neurofibromas can be subclassified based on location and gross pathology: dermal/cutaneous (which can then also be subcategorized as localized dermal neurofibromas which are more common than their counterpart, diffuse

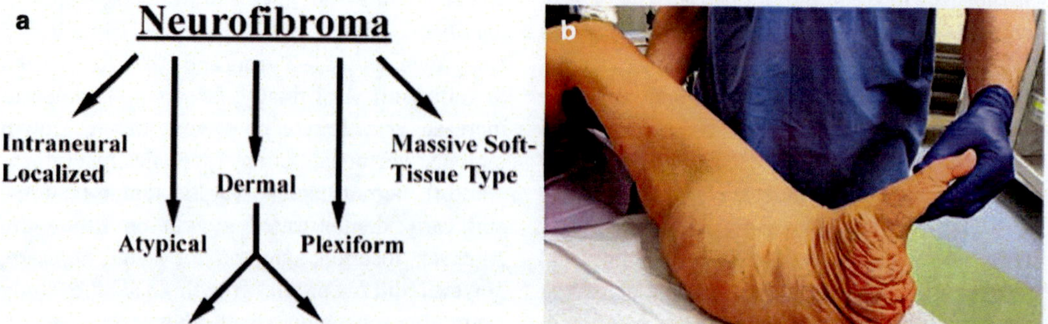

Fig. 1.2 Classification of neurofibromas (a) and photograph of a patient with a massive soft tissue-type neurofibroma (b)

dermal neurofibromas), intraneural localized (in which a localized intraneural neurofibroma of the cranial, spinal, or autonomic nerves is seen), plexiform (multiple nerve or fascicular neurofibromas coalescing as described above), and massive soft tissue-type (least common subtype, exclusively seen in NF-1 in which extensive soft tissue expansion is seen with an underlying enlarged nerve) [49]. The localized dermal neurofibromas (most common subtype) make up approximately 90% of dermal neurofibromas, whereas the other 10% are diffuse in nature. Furthermore, 90% of both localized and diffuse neurofibromas are seen sporadically or as a solitary tumor versus 10% occurring in the context of NF-1 [48, 49]. The distinction between localized and diffuse dermal neurofibromas is a gross histopathological one: although both are considered unencapsulated, the localized neurofibroma is a relatively circumscribed fusiform-like outgrowth, whereas the diffuse neurofibroma is a less commonly seen, plaque-like infiltrative outgrowth, less circumscribed and less delimited from its surrounding tissues. As mentioned previously, plexiform neurofibromas are almost exclusively seen in the context of NF-1 with some considering this to be pathognomonic for NF-1 [27, 29, 30] (with few reports detailing this subtype as occurring sporadically or representing a mosaic NF-1 lesion as seen in cases of segmental-type NF-1) [46].

In contrast to schwannomas, neurofibromas tend to affect a slightly younger population. These tumors will usually occur in patients between 20 and 30 years of age [3, 32, 33], although similar to schwannomas, ambiguity persists regarding specific tumor sex predilection. Some studies suggest a sporadic neurofibroma male predominance (male to female ratio as high as 8.7) [3, 33], while others suggest no sex predilection exists [30, 46] or even a female preponderance [1, 50, 51]. Even in the context of neurofibromatosis, this ambiguity exists with reports of there being either no sex predilection [1] or males being more commonly affected [30]. Furthermore, unlike schwannomas, neurofibromas have a more widespread anatomic distribution (depending on the subtype)—a full comparison/contrast of the two tumors can be seen in Table 1.1. Dermal neurofibromas can arise essentially from any nerve and are more randomly distributed over the surface of the body, whereas plexiform neurofibromas tend to be located more proximally in the upper (supraclavicular plexus 55%, major nerve trunks 45%) and lower (pelvic plexus and major nerve trunks) extremities [1, 3, 33, 52].

The natural history and malignant potential of neurofibromas are going to vary substantially depending on whether solitary or syndromic varieties are considered. Dermal neurofibromas have almost no malignant potential (the localized subtype having essentially no potential for malignancy and the diffuse subtype having a very low malignant proclivity). They are both generally considered slow-growing, benign tumors (though rarely have been reported to exhibit more rapid growth). Interestingly, in the context of NF-1, dermal neurofibromas tend to grow during adolescence, as well as during pregnancy, suggesting a hormonal influence on their growth rate [49]. Intraneural neurofibromas are the second most common type of neurofibroma and may also be sporadic or NF-1 associated. Although this type of neurofibroma can display malignant transformation (usually in the setting of NF-1), it is more rarely seen than in plexiform neurofibromas or massive soft tissue neurofibromas (an example of which is shown in Fig. 1.2b) where it is commonly seen (both tumor types being virtually pathognomonic for NF-1) [49, 53]. Although malignant transformation is rare in the setting of sporadic or solitary plexiform neurofibromas, it has been reported to occur in upward of 15% of plexiform neurofibromas associated with NF-1—the highest potential for malignant transformation among the neurofibroma subtypes [49]. Furthermore, most of these plexiform neurofibromas tend to grow in early childhood, whereas such growth in adulthood should raise suspicion for malignancy [53, 54]. Although detailed studies outlining the natural history of radiation-induced neurofibromas (or other PNSTs such as schwannomas) are lacking [55, 56], local growth in a previously irradiated PNST should also prompt workup for malignancy. More recently, a nodular "atypical neurofibroma" has been described associated with plexiform neurofibromas and is believed to represent a precursor for tumor transformation into a malignant peripheral nerve sheath tumor (MPNST). These nodules display more rapid growth rates and have high uptake on fluorodeoxyglucose positron emission tomography (FDG-PET) compared to low uptake in conventional plexiform tumor areas [53, 57, 58]. Although not all of these "atypical neurofibromas" will transform into a MPNST [59, 60], their accumulation of genetic aberrations leading to divergent imaging characteristics represents, among others, clinical and radiographic cues, a tangible way of helping distinguish malignant transformation prompting more aggressive therapy. As more molecular and genomic research is done to help to better classify these tumors, so too will the natural history of them change and more targeted therapeutics emerge.

1.3 Perineurioma

Perineuriomas, as implied by their name, are a peripheral nerve sheath tumor originating from perineurial cells surrounding nerve fascicles. They are classically described on histopathological sections as having characteristic hypercellular and enlarged nerve fascicles with abundant neoplastic, perineurial spindle cells arranged in pseudo-onion bulb whorls. These tumors are subclassified as either intraneural (IPN, also called localized hypertrophic neuropathy and associated with a nerve) or extraneural (EPN, also called soft tissue perineurioma). In the case of EPNs, the collection of perineurial cells are not usually associated with a nerve and are seemingly the more common of the two types [61–63]. Moreover, there are several different EPN variants, including intestinal, reticular, sclerosing, and plexiform [64–69]. Perineuriomas have also been described in the context of hybrid peripheral nerve sheath tumors such as perineurioma/schwannoma and perineurioma/neurofibroma (also reported is the hybrid combination of schwannoma/neurofibroma) [70].

Although these tumors are frequently underrecognized and thus likely underreported, perineuriomas are still rare tumors making up only 1% of all nerve sheath tumors [62, 71–73]. However, a shift in clinical practice has more recently occurred which may lead to an increase in their reported incidence and/or prevalence. Pathological confirmation was once believed to be required for diagnosis, although many now diagnose these PNSTs based on their clinical and radiological features which are believed to be sufficient and obviate the need for biopsy [73]. IPNs occur most frequently in adolescent to young adult patients, with no predilection for either sex [61]. They typically occur in the lower extremities (sciatic, femoral, common peroneal, tibial nerves) more commonly than the trunk or upper extremities (median, ulnar, radial nerves) [74, 75] with almost no reports of cranial nerve involvement [61]. In contrast, EPNs may occur in the subcutaneous soft tissue of the extremities or trunk [61, 62], although other less common perineurioma variants such as sclerosing perineuriomas have also been described in the hands of mainly male patients, as well as in visceral locations [61, 62, 66, 68, 76–80]. Furthermore, although reported as being more common in females (female to male ratio as high as 4:1), other studies have failed to observe this sex predilection of EPNs [61, 62].

Perineuriomas are generally considered to be low-grade, benign PNSTs with reports of low-grade malignant perineuriomas, atypical perineuriomas, or low-grade MPNSTs with perineurial differentiation being the exception (making up approximately 4% of MPNSTs) [63, 81–86]. However, despite being a benign tumor with a static or slowly progressive growth pattern, they are generally considered to have a natural history with a poor functional outcome [74]. This is because the slow-growing tumor affects predominantly motor nerves and commonly presents as a painless, motor mononeuropathy with little sensory involvement (although multiple nerves/nerve fascicles may be involved in up to one-sixth of cases) [74, 87]. Perineuriomas grow to envelop and diffusely enlarge the fusiform nerve fascicles while maintaining gross fascicular architecture giving the lesion a honeycomb-like appearance [74, 88]. There is little overall morbidity associated with them because they are usually benign; however, they can also continue to slowly progress imparting neurologic deficit and inexorably leading to complete loss of nerve function. As such, many favor surgical excision with end-end repair of the parent nerve [74, 87, 89]. Others, on the other hand, believe optimal treatment consists of internal neurolysis and decompression in an attempt to preserve what function remains [90]. In addition to this, controversy persists with respect to optimal timing of surgical intervention with a balance being required between imparting a new or worsened neurologic deficit from surgical resection and ongoing and potentially irreversible deterioration of distal nerve sheaths and long-standing denervation atrophy [71, 91, 92].

1.4 Ganglioneuromas

Ganglioneuromas are a neuroblastic tumor variant which also include neuroblastomas, ganglioneuroblastomas, and ganglioneuroblastoma-intermixed. Neuroblastic tumor classification has been established according to the International Neuroblastoma Pathology Classification (INPC) with these tumors best being thought of as existing on a histological spectrum. Where these tumors are on this spectrum and how these tumors are then classified as per the INPC are dependent on the relative presence of neural and Schwann-type cells (with ganglioneuromas being Schwann cell predominant and neuroblastomas being neural cell predominant) [93]. Neuroblastic tumors arise from neural crest cells and can also display varying degrees of differentiation—although likely not entirely accurate, ganglioneuromas are thought to represent the differentiated form and neuroblastomas the undifferentiated [94, 95].

Because neuroblastic tumors (including ganglioneuromas) arise from neural crest cells, these tumors can be found throughout the body (neural crest cell derivatives including, e.g., the adrenal medulla, neuronal cells of the autonomic nervous system, Schwann cells, melanocytes, neuroendocrine cells, and head and neck mesenchymal cells, among others) [95]. Although neuroblastic tumors account for 15% of all childhood neoplasms seen in the first 4 years of life [95], ganglioneuromas specifically are much more rare (reported incidence of 1 per million or approximately 600 new cases reported per year) [96, 97]. They can occur both sporadically and in association with certain genetic syndromes such as Turner syndrome [98], Hirschsprung's disease [99], and NF-1 [100]. In their retrospective study of childhood ganglioneuromas, De Bernardi et al. found that the median age of diagnosis was 79 months (or approximately 6.5 years old) with no sex predilection [101]. Ganglioneuromas are thus predominantly childhood tumors that are typically benign in nature. However, few have reported cases of late malignant transformation [101]. As for most tumors, when considering the natural history of ganglioneuromas and thus the optimum treatment for these tumors, it is important to distinguish them from other neuroblastic tumors due to differences in their clinical course. For example, depending on symptomatology, treatment for ganglioneuromas may include observation or surgical resection (with good overall prognosis reported, including for subtotal resections as gross total resection may not be feasible due to unacceptably high morbidity) [102].

1.5 Granular Cell Tumors and Malignant Granular Cell Tumors

First described in 1926 by the Russian pathologist Abrikossoff [103], granular cell tumors are rare soft tissue tumors initially thought to originate from Schwann cells. However, their cellular origin remains somewhat controversial with other proposed candidates including monocyte-histiocyte-macrophage cells, neuroendocrine cells, fibroblastic cells, myoblast/myofibroblastic cells, as well as undifferentiated mesenchymal and endomesenchymal cells [104]. More recently, the expression of S-100 protein has supported the notion of granular cell tumors originating from Schwann cells.

The overall incidence of granular cell tumors is quite low, accounting for 0.5% of soft tissue tumors [105]. They are typically benign soft tissue tumors, though rarely they can be malignant (approximately 3% of granular cell tumors) [105, 106]. Peak incidence occurs between the ages of 30 and 50 years old for both the benign (range 17–59 and median 36.5 years old) and malignant subtypes, and although reported to occur at any age, by far the majority occur in adults (98% cases) [107–109]. More specifically, they are most commonly seen in dark-skinned, middle-aged females [104, 110]. Tumors typically present as solitary nodules and arise on the tongue in about 40% of patients [111]; however, they can also be found on the skin and in the subcutaneous and soft tissue, thyroid, mediastinum, respiratory tract, gastrointestinal tract, pancreaticobiliary system, genitourinary system, and central/peripheral nervous systems [104].

In 1998, Fanburg-Smith et al. proposed criteria to classify granular cell tumors as being benign, atypical, or malignant [109]. Establishing malignancy was based on three or more of the following histological criteria being present: (1) necrosis, (2) spindling, (3) vesicular nuclei with large nuclei, (4) increased mitotic activity (>2 mitoses/10 high-power fields at 200× magnification), (5) high nuclear to cytoplasmic ratio (N/C), and (6) pleomorphism [109]. The natural history and prognostic factors will then obviously be affected by factors such as grading of these tumors and whether they are sporadic versus syndromic in nature (e.g., in the context of LEOPARD syndrome, a rare autosomal dominant disease caused by PTPN11 mutation), among others [110]. Benign tumors usually present as solitary, slow-growing lesions [112], though they can be multifocal in up to 25% of the cases [110]. Treatment of these benign tumors then involves surgical excision with local recurrence being quite unusual. Malignant granular cell tumors, however, behave much differently. They will commonly metastasize to lymph nodes, lungs, and bone [112] and have a reported mortality as high as 40% [113]. Poor prognostic factors for these rarer tumors include elevated Ki-67 values (>10%), p53 immunoreactivity, older patient age, increased tumor size, as well as local recurrence and metastases [109].

1.6 Malignant Peripheral Nerve Sheath Tumors

As evident by their name, MPNSTs are a neoplastic and malignant sarcoma originating from the peripheral nervous system or peripheral nerve sheath cells (predominantly Schwann cells and perineural fibroblasts) [114–117]. This includes tumors previously described as malignant neuroma, neurogenic sarcoma, malignant neurilemmoma, neurofibrosarcoma, and malignant schwannoma [116, 118, 119]. These tumors typically arise in the context of NF-1, although they may also arise sporadically, either de novo or from malignant transformation of a preexisting benign tumor (>80% of MPNSTs originate from preexisting plexiform neurofibromas) [120].

In keeping with their first description in 1909 by Francis Harbitz [121], the majority of MPNSTs arise from malignant transformation from preexisting benign tumors (predominantly neurofibromas and very rarely schwannomas). Although rare, malignant transformation from cutaneous or dermal type neurofibromas may occur (classified as cutaneous conventional or spindle cell MPNST (CC-MPNST) and cutaneous epithelioid MPNST (CE-MPNST)) [117]. CC- and CE-MPNSTs represent 2% and 5% of all MPNSTs, respectively, and affect slightly more males than females. Unlike other forms of MPNSTs, these latter two types occur less frequently in association with NF-1 and are more superficial making them more amenable to radical surgical excision [117, 122–125]. More commonly, MPNSTs develop from plexiform neurofibromas which represent the highest risk of malignant transformation with massive soft tissue neurofibromas also being at high risk for malignancy (though because this last subtype of tumor is also the least common, their clinical burden remains low) [49].

The latter two tumor subtypes are almost exclusively seen in the context of NF-1 which represents a significant risk factor for MPNST development and accounts for approximately 50% of all MPNSTs [49, 116, 120, 126, 127]. Although up to 50% of all NF-1 patients will develop a plexiform neurofibroma, only approximately 8–13% of these will undergo malignant transformation [49, 116, 120, 128–130]. The other 50% of MPNSTs develop sporadically in patients without a known genetic predisposition, for example, at the site of previous radiation treatment (another known risk factor for MPNST development and representing 10–13% of MPNSTs) [49, 117, 131–133]. The occurrence of MPNSTs in the general population is thus relatively rare. The reported incidence for MPNSTs in the general population is approximately 1/100,000/year (compared to the much higher incidence of 1/3500/year in NF-1 patients), and these make up only 2–5% of all soft tissue sarcomas [49, 114–116, 134–137].

Although MPNSTs may present in a broad age range of patients, the majority of sporadic MPNSTs present in middle-aged patients between 30 and 50 years old (mean age 41) with no clear sex predilection [115, 117, 136]. In patients with NF-1, MPNSTs usually develop at a substantially younger age (mean age 28), at times developing during childhood and adolescence. Again, ambiguity exists regarding which sex is affected more [115, 117, 136].

Untreated, MPNSTs are an ultimately fatal diagnosis. Even with treatment, reported survival rates are dismal. These may vary somewhat, however, depending on the specific type of MPNST, grade of MPNST, and stage, among other factors. For example, the relative influence of certain MPNST prognostic factors such as the association of NF-1 or radiation-induced MPNSTs on outcome is controversial [49, 116, 128, 131, 132, 136–139]. Regardless, most agree that the diagnosis of MPNST carries a grim prognosis with poor overall survival rates, the strongest predictor of which is likely complete surgical resection with wide negative margins [81, 115, 118, 136, 138, 140–143]. Unfortunately, this is not always feasible especially in the setting of high-grade MPNSTs which have a reported 5-year overall survival of 20–50% and overall mortality of 75% [49, 115, 132, 133, 136, 138–140, 144–146]. In many cases, these tumors will metastasize (30–60%, commonly to the lungs) [81, 136, 147–149], and even with optimal treatment, the incidence of recurrence can be as high as 65% [136]. However, these figures likely do not hold true for low-grade MPNSTs or "atypical neurofibromas." In a study specifically examining low-grade MPNSTs and atypical neurofibromas, Bernthal et al. found no evidence of metastatic disease nor disease-specific death in the setting of positive surgical margins post-resection in 78% of cases. Furthermore, although local recurrence occurred in 16.7% of cases with positive surgical margins, none of these patients developed metastatic disease, died of their disease, and were able to undergo re-resection when clinically indicated with little morbidity. This study suggests that for "atypical neurofibromas" and low-grade MPNSTs, radical tumor resection with negative oncological margins which can harbor increased morbidity may not be necessary [150]. As discussed in the neurofibroma section of this chapter, an "atypical neurofibroma" has been described as being a precursor lesion to MPNSTs from the malignant transformation of a plexiform neurofibroma. These lesions have been reported to be more nodular in appearance and may display more aggressive behavior compared to more benign neurofibromas [53, 57–59]. These "atypical neurofibromas" can oftentimes be difficult to distinguish from low-grade MPNSTs. These different grades of tumors may exist as a continuum and not distinct entities and, as demonstrated by Bernthal et al., may carry a different prognosis necessitating a different surgical approach than their higher-grade counterparts [150]. This diagnostic dilemma and controversy have led to the formation of MPNST consortiums and consensus statements/guidelines to better classify these tumors in the hope of improving diagnostic accuracy and guiding MPNST research going forward [53].

Acknowledgments None.
Funding disclosure: None.

Conflict of Interest The authors have nothing to disclose, nor conflicts of interest related to this article, and the contents of this manuscript have not been previously published.

References

1. Kim DH, Friedman AH, Kitagawa RS, Kiline DG. Management of peripheral nerve tumors. In: Filler AG, Kline DG, Zager EL, editors. Youmans neurological surgery. 6th ed. Philadelphia, PA: Elsevier Saunders; 2011. p. 3264.
2. Chick G, Alnot JY, Silbermann-Hoffman O. Benign solitary tumors of the peripheral nerves. Rev Chir Orthop Reparatrice Appar Mot. 2000;86(8):825–34.
3. Chick G, Hollevoet N, Victor J, Bianchi S. The role of imaging in isolated benign peripheral nerve tumors: a practical review for surgeons. Hand Surg Rehabil. 2016;35(5):320–9.
4. Sandberg K, Nilsson J, Soe Nielsen N, Dahlin LB. Tumours of peripheral nerves in the upper extremity: a 22-year epidemiological study. Scand J Plast Reconstr Surg Hand Surg. 2009;43(1):43–9.
5. Jenkins AL 3rd, Ahuja A, Oliff AH, Sobotka S. Spinal schwannoma presenting due to torsion and hemorrhage: case report and review of literature. Spine J. 2015;15(8):e1–4.
6. Jinnai T, Koyama T. Clinical characteristics of spinal nerve sheath tumors: analysis of 149 cases. Neurosurgery. 2005;56(3):510–5; discussion –5.
7. Nittner K, Venkins P, Bruyn G. Meningiomas, neuromas, neurofibromas, and hourglass tumors. New York, NY: Elsevier; 1976.
8. Seppala MT, Haltia MJ, Sankila RJ, Jaaskelainen JE, Heiskanen O. Long-term outcome after removal of spinal schwannoma: a clinicopathological study of 187 cases. J Neurosurg. 1995;83(4):621–6.
9. Bruni P, Esposito S, Greco R, Oddi G. Solitary intracerebral schwannoma in von Recklinghausen's disease. Surg Neurol. 1984;22(4):360–4.
10. Schmidt RF, Boghani Z, Choudhry OJ, Eloy JA, Jyung RW, Liu JK. Incidental vestibular schwannomas: a review of prevalence, growth rate, and management challenges. Neurosurg Focus. 2012;33(3):E4.
11. Scott WW, Koral K, Margraf LR, Klesse L, Sacco DJ, Weprin BE. Intracerebral schwannomas: a rare disease with varying natural history. J Neurosurg Pediatr. 2013;12(1):6–12.
12. Komminoth R, Sokic P, Florange W, Komminoth J, Hartleyb H. Intracerebellar schwannoma. Neurochirurgie. 1977;23(1):81–8.
13. Tladi MJ, Saragas NP, Ferrao PN, Strydom A. Schwannoma and neurofibroma of the posterior tibial nerve presenting as tarsal tunnel syndrome: review of the literature with two case reports. Foot (Edinb). 2017;32:22–6.
14. Karjalainen S, Nuutinen J, Neittaanmaki H, Naukkarinen A, Asikainen R. The incidence of acoustic neuroma in autopsy material. Arch Otorhinolaryngol. 1984;240(1):91–3.
15. Leonard JR, Talbot ML. Asymptomatic acoustic neurilemoma. Arch Otolaryngol. 1970;91(2):117–24.
16. Lin D, Hegarty JL, Fischbein NJ, Jackler RK. The prevalence of "incidental" acoustic neuroma. Arch Otolaryngol Head Neck Surg. 2005;131(3):241–4.
17. Stewart TJ, Liland J, Schuknecht HF. Occult schwannomas of the vestibular nerve. Arch Otolaryngol. 1975;101(2):91–5.
18. Anderson TD, Loevner LA, Bigelow DC, Mirza N. Prevalence of unsuspected acoustic neuroma found by magnetic resonance imaging. Otolaryngol Head Neck Surg. 2000;122(5):643–6.
19. Selesnick SH, Jackler RK. Atypical hearing loss in acoustic neuroma patients. Laryngoscope. 1993;103(4 Pt 1):437–41.
20. Selesnick SH, Jackler RK, Pitts LW. The changing clinical presentation of acoustic tumors in the MRI era. Laryngoscope. 1993;103(4 Pt 1):431–6.
21. Stangerup SE, Caye-Thomasen P. Epidemiology and natural history of vestibular schwannomas. Otolaryngol Clin N Am. 2012;45(2):257–68, vii
22. Evans DG, Moran A, King A, Saeed S, Gurusinghe N, Ramsden R. Incidence of vestibular schwannoma and neurofibromatosis 2 in the north west of England over a 10-year period: higher incidence than previously thought. Otol Neurotol. 2005;26(1):93–7.
23. Hilton DA, Hanemann CO. Schwannomas and their pathogenesis. Brain Pathol. 2014;24(3):205–20.
24. Propp JM, McCarthy BJ, Davis FG, Preston-Martin S. Descriptive epidemiology of vestibular schwannomas. Neuro-Oncology. 2006;8(1):1–11.
25. Tos M, Stangerup SE, Caye-Thomasen P, Tos T, Thomsen J. What is the real incidence of vestibular schwannoma? Arch Otolaryngol Head Neck Surg. 2004;130(2):216–20.
26. Hoglund M, Muren C, Engkvist O. Ultrasound characteristics of five common soft-tissue tumours in the hand and forearm. Acta Radiol. 1997;38(3):348–54.
27. Enzinger F, Weiss S. Soft tissue tumours. St. Louis: Mosby; 1988.
28. Jenkins SA. Solitary tumours of peripheral nerve trunks. J Bone Joint Surg Br. 1952;34-B(3):401–11.
29. Resnick D, Niwayama G. Diagnosis of bone and joint disorders. 2nd ed. Philadelphia: Saunders; 1988.
30. Stull MA, Moser RP Jr, Kransdorf MJ, Bogumill GP, Nelson MC. Magnetic resonance appearance of peripheral nerve sheath tumors. Skelet Radiol. 1991;20(1):9–14.
31. Mariottini A, Carangelo B, Peri G, Tacchini D, Mourmouras V, Muya M, et al. Schwannoma of median nerve at the elbow. Case report and short review of the literature. G Chir. 2011;32(1/2):55–8.

32. Kehoe NJ, Reid RP, Semple JC. Solitary benign peripheral-nerve tumours. Review of 32 years' experience. J Bone Joint Surg Br. 1995;77(3):497–500.
33. Kim DH, Murovic JA, Tiel RL, Kline DG. Operative outcomes of 546 Louisiana State University health sciences center peripheral nerve tumors. Neurosurg Clin N Am. 2004;15(2):177–92.
34. Paldor I, Chen AS, Kaye AH. Growth rate of vestibular schwannoma. J Clin Neurosci. 2016;32:1–8.
35. Woertler K. Tumors and tumor-like lesions of peripheral nerves. Semin Musculoskelet Radiol. 2010;14(5):547–58.
36. Perez R, Chen JM, Nedzelski JM. Intratemporal facial nerve schwannoma: a management dilemma. Otol Neurotol. 2005;26(1):121–6.
37. Xu F, Pan S, Alonso F, Dekker SE, Bambakidis NC. Intracranial facial nerve schwannomas: current management and review of literature. World Neurosurg. 2017;100:444–9.
38. Hirose T, Ishizawa K, Sakaki M, Fujii Y. Retroperitoneal schwannoma is characterized by a high incidence of cellular type and GFAP-immunoreactivity. Pathol Int. 2012;62(7):456–62.
39. Bakan S, Kayadibi Y, Ersen E, Vatankulu B, Ustundag N, Hasiloglu ZI. Primary psammomatous melanotic schwannoma of the spine. Ann Thorac Surg. 2015;99(6):e141–3.
40. Terasaki K, Mera Y, Uchimiya H, Katahira Y, Kanzaki T. Plexiform schwannoma. Clin Exp Dermatol. 2003;28(4):372–4.
41. Fletcher CD, Davies SE, McKee PH. Cellular schwannoma: a distinct pseudosarcomatous entity. Histopathology. 1987;11(1):21–35.
42. Lodding P, Kindblom LG, Angervall L, Stenman G. Cellular schwannoma. A clinicopathologic study of 29 cases. Virchows Arch A Pathol Anat Histopathol. 1990;416(3):237–48.
43. White W, Shiu MH, Rosenblum MK, Erlandson RA, Woodruff JM. Cellular schwannoma. A clinicopathologic study of 57 patients and 58 tumors. Cancer. 1990;66(6):1266–75.
44. de Vries M, van der Mey AG, Hogendoorn PC. Tumor biology of vestibular schwannoma: a review of experimental data on the determinants of tumor genesis and growth characteristics. Otol Neurotol. 2015;36(7):1128–36.
45. Roman-Naranjo P, Gallego-Martinez A, Lopez Escamez JA. Genetics of vestibular syndromes. Curr Opin Neurol. 2018;31(1):105–10.
46. Huang W, Chong WS. Facial plexiform neurofibroma: is it truly just skin deep? BMJ Case Rep. 2013;2013:bcr2013200716.
47. Martinez AP, Fritchie KJ. Update on peripheral nerve sheath tumors. Surg Pathol Clin. 2019;12(1):1–19.
48. Sakata A, Hirokawa Y, Kuwahara R, Hamada A, Kuroda M, Araki N, et al. Solitary oropharyngeal neurofibroma: MR appearance with pathologic correlation and review of the literature. Clin Imaging. 2013;37(3):554–7.
49. Longo JF, Weber SM, Turner-Ivey BP, Carroll SL. Recent advances in the diagnosis and pathogenesis of neurofibromatosis type 1 (NF1)-associated peripheral nervous system neoplasms. Adv Anat Pathol. 2018;25(5):353–68.
50. Jokinen CH, Argenyi ZB. Atypical neurofibroma of the skin and subcutaneous tissue: clinicopathologic analysis of 11 cases. J Cutan Pathol. 2010;37(1):35–42.
51. Mesbah Ardakani N, Yap F, Wood BA. Cutaneous atypical neurofibroma: a case report and review of literature. Am J Dermatopathol. 2018;40(11):864–7.
52. Kubiena H, Entner T, Schmidt M, Frey M. Peripheral neural sheath tumors (PNST)—what a radiologist should know. Eur J Radiol. 2013;82(1):51–5.
53. Miettinen MM, Antonescu CR, Fletcher CDM, Kim A, Lazar AJ, Quezado MM, et al. Histopathologic evaluation of atypical neurofibromatous tumors and their transformation into malignant peripheral nerve sheath tumor in patients with neurofibromatosis 1-a consensus overview. Hum Pathol. 2017;67:1–10.
54. Dombi E, Solomon J, Gillespie AJ, Fox E, Balis FM, Patronas N, et al. NF1 plexiform neurofibroma growth rate by volumetric MRI: relationship to age and body weight. Neurology. 2007;68(9):643–7.
55. Yamanaka R, Hayano A. Radiation-induced malignant peripheral nerve sheath tumors: a systematic review. World Neurosurg. 2017;105:961–70 e8.
56. Yamanaka R, Hayano A. Radiation-induced schwannomas and neurofibromas: a systematic review. World Neurosurg. 2017;104:713–22.
57. Beert E, Brems H, Daniels B, De Wever I, Van Calenbergh F, Schoenaers J, et al. Atypical neurofibromas in neurofibromatosis type 1 are premalignant tumors. Genes Chromosomes Cancer. 2011;50(12):1021–32.
58. Meany H, Dombi E, Reynolds J, Whatley M, Kurwa A, Tsokos M, et al. 18-fluorodeoxyglucose-positron emission tomography (FDG-PET) evaluation of nodular lesions in patients with neurofibromatosis type 1 and plexiform neurofibromas (PN) or malignant peripheral nerve sheath tumors (MPNST). Pediatr Blood Cancer. 2013;60(1):59–64.
59. Evans DGR, Salvador H, Chang VY, Erez A, Voss SD, Druker H, et al. Cancer and central nervous system tumor surveillance in pediatric neurofibromatosis 2 and related disorders. Clin Cancer Res. 2017;23(12):e54–61.
60. Evans DGR, Salvador H, Chang VY, Erez A, Voss SD, Schneider KW, et al. Cancer and central nervous system tumor surveillance in pediatric neurofibromatosis 1. Clin Cancer Res. 2017;23(12):e46–53.
61. Kleihues P, Louis DN, Scheithauer BW, Rorke LB, Reifenberger G, Burger PC, et al. The WHO classification of tumors of the nervous system. J Neuropathol Exp Neurol. 2002;61(3):215–25; discussion 26-9.
62. Macarenco RS, Ellinger F, Oliveira AM. Perineurioma: a distinctive and underrecognized peripheral nerve sheath neoplasm. Arch Pathol Lab Med. 2007;131(4):625–36.

63. Suster D, Plaza JA, Shen R. Low-grade malignant perineurioma (perineurial sarcoma) of soft tissue: a potential diagnostic pitfall on fine needle aspiration. Ann Diagn Pathol. 2005;9(4):197–201.
64. Cimino-Mathews AM. Peripheral nerve sheath tumors. Surg Pathol Clin. 2011;4(3):761–82.
65. Fetsch JF, Miettinen M. Sclerosing perineurioma: a clinicopathologic study of 19 cases of a distinctive soft tissue lesion with a predilection for the fingers and palms of young adults. Am J Surg Pathol. 1997;21(12):1433–42.
66. Gomes da Silva W, Martinez MM, Miranda AM, Silva RB, da Silveira HM, de Almeida OP, et al. Oral perineurioma: clinicopathologic features from two cases and review of literature. Oral Surg Oral Med Oral Pathol Oral Radiol. 2017;123(3):e91–e8.
67. Graadt van Roggen JF, McMenamin ME, Belchis DA, Nielsen GP, Rosenberg AE, Fletcher CD. Reticular perineurioma: a distinctive variant of soft tissue perineurioma. Am J Surg Pathol. 2001;25(4):485–93.
68. Hornick JL, Fletcher CD. Intestinal perineuriomas: clinicopathologic definition of a new anatomic subset in a series of 10 cases. Am J Surg Pathol. 2005;29(7):859–65.
69. Mentzel T, Kutzner H. Reticular and plexiform perineurioma: clinicopathological and immunohistochemical analysis of two cases and review of perineurial neoplasms of skin and soft tissues. Virchows Arch. 2005;447(4):677–82.
70. Ud Din N, Ahmad Z, Abdul-Ghafar J, Ahmed R. Hybrid peripheral nerve sheath tumors: report of five cases and detailed review of literature. BMC Cancer. 2017;17(1):349.
71. Lee HY, Manasseh RG, Edis RH, Page R, Keith-Rokosh J, Walsh P, et al. Intraneural perineurioma. J Clin Neurosci. 2009;16(12):1633–6.
72. Mauermann ML, Amrami KK, Kuntz NL, Spinner RJ, Dyck PJ, Bosch EP, et al. Longitudinal study of intraneural perineurioma—a benign, focal hypertrophic neuropathy of youth. Brain. 2009;132(Pt 8):2265–76.
73. Wilson TJ, Howe BM, Stewart SA, Spinner RJ, Amrami KK. Clinicoradiological features of intraneural perineuriomas obviate the need for tissue diagnosis. J Neurosurg. 2018;129(4):1034–40.
74. Ahlawat S, Chhabra A, Blakely J. Magnetic resonance neurography of peripheral nerve tumors and tumorlike conditions. Neuroimaging Clin N Am. 2014;24(1):171–92.
75. Prasad NK, Tubbs RS, Amrami KK, Dyck PJB, Mauermann ML, Giannini C, et al. Can intraneural perineuriomas occur intradurally? An anatomic perspective. Neurosurgery. 2017;80(2):226–34.
76. Giannini C, Scheithauer BW, Jenkins RB, Erlandson RA, Perry A, Borell TJ, et al. Soft-tissue perineurioma. Evidence for an abnormality of chromosome 22, criteria for diagnosis, and review of the literature. Am J Surg Pathol. 1997;21(2):164–73.
77. Val-Bernal JF, Hernando M, Garijo MF, Villa P. Renal perineurioma in childhood. Gen Diagn Pathol. 1997;143(1):75–81.
78. Hornick JL, Fletcher CD. Soft tissue perineurioma: clinicopathologic analysis of 81 cases including those with atypical histologic features. Am J Surg Pathol. 2005;29(7):845–58.
79. Pina-Oviedo S, Ortiz-Hidalgo C. The normal and neoplastic perineurium: a review. Adv Anat Pathol. 2008;15(3):147–64.
80. van Wyk AC, van Zyl H, Rigby J. Colonic perineurioma (benign fibroblastic polyp): case report and review of the literature. Diagn Pathol. 2018;13(1):16.
81. Wong WW, Hirose T, Scheithauer BW, Schild SE, Gunderson LL. Malignant peripheral nerve sheath tumor: analysis of treatment outcome. Int J Radiat Oncol Biol Phys. 1998;42(2):351–60.
82. Hirose T, Scheithauer BW, Sano T. Perineurial malignant peripheral nerve sheath tumor (MPNST): a clinicopathologic, immunohistochemical, and ultrastructural study of seven cases. Am J Surg Pathol. 1998;22(11):1368–78.
83. Hirose T, Sumitomo M, Kudo E, Hasegawa T, Teramae T, Murase M, et al. Malignant peripheral nerve sheath tumor (MPNST) showing perineurial cell differentiation. Am J Surg Pathol. 1989;13(7):613–20.
84. Karaki S, Mochida J, Lee YH, Nishimura K, Tsutsumi Y. Low-grade malignant perineurioma of the paravertebral column, transforming into a high-grade malignancy. Pathol Int. 1999;49(9):820–5.
85. Rekhi B. Perineurial malignant peripheral nerve sheath tumor in the setting of multiple soft tissue perineuriomas: a rare presentation of an uncommon tumor. J Cancer Res Ther. 2013;9(1):131–4.
86. Rosenberg AS, Langee CL, Stevens GL, Morgan MB. Malignant peripheral nerve sheath tumor with perineurial differentiation: "malignant perineurioma". J Cutan Pathol. 2002;29(6):362–7.
87. Abreu E, Aubert S, Wavreille G, Gheno R, Canella C, Cotten A. Peripheral tumor and tumor-like neurogenic lesions. Eur J Radiol. 2013;82(1):38–50.
88. Lacour-Petit MC, Lozeron P, Ducreux D. MRI of peripheral nerve lesions of the lower limbs. Neuroradiology. 2003;45(3):166–70.
89. Gruen JP, Mitchell W, Kline DG. Resection and graft repair for localized hypertrophic neuropathy. Neurosurgery. 1998;43(1):78–83.
90. Emory TS, Scheithauer BW, Hirose T, Wood M, Onofrio BM, Jenkins RB. Intraneural perineurioma. A clonal neoplasm associated with abnormalities of chromosome 22. Am J Clin Pathol. 1995;103(6):696–704.
91. Cortes W, Cheng J, Matloub HS. Intraneural perineurioma of the radial nerve in a child. J Hand Surg Am. 2005;30(4):820–5.
92. Isaac S, Athanasou NA, Pike M, Burge PD. Radial nerve palsy owing to localized hypertrophic neuropathy (intraneural perineurioma) in early childhood. J Child Neurol. 2004;19(1):71–5.
93. Shimada H, Ambros IM, Dehner LP, Hata J, Joshi VV, Roald B, et al. The international neuroblastoma pathology classification (the Shimada system). Cancer. 1999;86(2):364–72.

94. Decarolis B, Simon T, Krug B, Leuschner I, Vokuhl C, Kaatsch P, et al. Treatment and outcome of Ganglioneuroma and Ganglioneuroblastoma intermixed. BMC Cancer. 2016;16:542.
95. Shimada H, Ambros IM, Dehner LP, Hata J, Joshi VV, Roald B. Terminology and morphologic criteria of neuroblastic tumors: recommendations by the international neuroblastoma pathology committee. Cancer. 1999;86(2):349–63.
96. Dabrowska-Thing A, Rogowski W, Pacho R, Nawrocka-Laskus E, Nitek Z. Retroperitoneal ganglioneuroma mimicking a kidney tumor. Case report. Pol J Radiol. 2017;82:283–6.
97. Goodman MT. Sympathetic nervous system tumors. In: Gurney JG, editor. Cancer incidence and survival among children and adolescents: United States SEER Program. Bethesda: National Cancer Institute; 1995. p. 65–72.
98. Blatt J, Olshan AF, Lee PA, Ross JL. Neuroblastoma and related tumors in Turner's syndrome. J Pediatr. 1997;131(5):666–70.
99. Shahar E, Shinawi M. Neurocristopathies presenting with neurologic abnormalities associated with Hirschsprung's disease. Pediatr Neurol. 2003;28(5):385–91.
100. The I, Murthy AE, Hannigan GE, Jacoby LB, Menon AG, Gusella JF, et al. Neurofibromatosis type 1 gene mutations in neuroblastoma. Nat Genet. 1993;3(1):62–6.
101. De Bernardi B, Gambini C, Haupt R, Granata C, Rizzo A, Conte M, et al. Retrospective study of childhood ganglioneuroma. J Clin Oncol. 2008;26(10):1710–6.
102. Alexander N, Sullivan K, Shaikh F, Irwin MS. Characteristics and management of ganglioneuroma and ganglioneuroblastoma-intermixed in children and adolescents. Pediatr Blood Cancer. 2018;65(5):e26964.
103. Abrikossoff A. Uber Myome, ausgehend von der quergestreiften wilkuerlichen muskulatur. Virchows Arch Pathol Anat. 1926;260:215–33.
104. Machado I, Cruz J, Lavernia J, Llombart-Bosch A. Solitary, multiple, benign, atypical, or malignant: the "granular cell tumor" puzzle. Virchows Arch. 2016;468(5):527–38.
105. Stemm M, Suster D, Wakely PE Jr, Suster S. Typical and atypical granular cell tumors of soft tissue: a clinicopathologic study of 50 patients. Am J Clin Pathol. 2017;148(2):161–6.
106. Vaughan V, Ferringer T. Granular cell tumor. Cutis. 2014;94(6):275, 9-80.
107. Cui Y, Tong SS, Zhang YH, Li HT. Granular cell tumor: a report of three cases and review of literature. Cancer Biomark. 2018;23(2):173–8.
108. Bitar M. Granular cell tumor: case report. J Saudi Soc Dermatol Dermatol Surg. 2011;15:25–7.
109. Fanburg-Smith JC, Meis-Kindblom JM, Fante R, Kindblom LG. Malignant granular cell tumor of soft tissue: diagnostic criteria and clinicopathologic correlation. Am J Surg Pathol. 1998;22(7):779–94.
110. Vaughan VB. Granular cell tumor. In: Ferringer TM, editor. Cutis; 2014. p. 279–280.
111. Gayen T, Das A, Shome K, Bandyopadhyay D, Das D, Saha A. Granular cell tumor: an uncommon benign neoplasm. Indian J Dermatol. 2015;60(3):322.
112. Mirza FN, Tuggle CT, Zogg CK, Mirza HN, Narayan D. Epidemiology of malignant cutaneous granular cell tumors: A US population-based cohort analysis using the Surveillance, Epidemiology, and End Results (SEER) database. J Am Acad Dermatol. 2018;78(3):490–7.e1.
113. Singh VA, Gunasagaran J, Pailoor J. Granular cell tumour: malignant or benign? Singap Med J. 2015;56(9):513–7.
114. Ducatman BS, Scheithauer BW, Piepgras DG, Reiman HM. Malignant peripheral nerve sheath tumors in childhood. J Neuro-Oncol. 1984;2(3):241–8.
115. Ducatman BS, Scheithauer BW, Piepgras DG, Reiman HM, Ilstrup DM. Malignant peripheral nerve sheath tumors. A clinicopathologic study of 120 cases. Cancer. 1986;57(10):2006–21.
116. Kolberg M, Holand M, Agesen TH, Brekke HR, Liestol K, Hall KS, et al. Survival meta-analyses for >1800 malignant peripheral nerve sheath tumor patients with and without neurofibromatosis type 1. Neuro-Oncology. 2013;15(2):135–47.
117. Luzar B, Falconieri G. Cutaneous malignant peripheral nerve sheath tumor. Surg Pathol Clin. 2017;10(2):337–43.
118. Ferner RE, Gutmann DH. International consensus statement on malignant peripheral nerve sheath tumors in neurofibromatosis. Cancer Res. 2002;62(5):1573–7.
119. Perrin RG, Guha A. Malignant peripheral nerve sheath tumors. Neurosurg Clin N Am. 2004;15(2):203–16.
120. Staedtke V, Bai RY, Blakeley JO. Cancer of the peripheral nerve in neurofibromatosis type 1. Neurotherapeutics. 2017;14(2):298–306.
121. Harbitz F. Multiple neurofibromatosis (von Recklinhausen's disease). Arch Surg. 1909;22:258–81.
122. Feng CJ, Ma H, Liao WC. Superficial or cutaneous malignant peripheral nerve sheath tumor—clinical experience at Taipei veterans general hospital. Ann Plast Surg. 2015;74(Suppl 2):S85–8.
123. Inoue T, Kuwashiro M, Misago N, Narisawa Y. Superficial malignant peripheral nerve sheath tumor arising from diffuse neurofibroma in a neurofibromatosis type 1 patient. J Dermatol. 2014;41(7):631–3.
124. Jo VY, Fletcher CD. Epithelioid malignant peripheral nerve sheath tumor: clinicopathologic analysis of 63 cases. Am J Surg Pathol. 2015;39(5):673–82.
125. Luzar B, Shanesmith R, Ramakrishnan R, Fisher C, Calonje E. Cutaneous epithelioid malignant peripheral nerve sheath tumour: a clinicopathological analysis of 11 cases. Histopathology. 2016;68(2):286–96.
126. Carroll SL. Molecular mechanisms promoting the pathogenesis of Schwann cell neoplasms. Acta Neuropathol. 2012;123(3):321–48.

127. Mautner VF, Asuagbor FA, Dombi E, Funsterer C, Kluwe L, Wenzel R, et al. Assessment of benign tumor burden by whole-body MRI in patients with neurofibromatosis 1. Neuro-Oncology. 2008;10(4):593–8.
128. Evans DG, Baser ME, McGaughran J, Sharif S, Howard E, Moran A. Malignant peripheral nerve sheath tumours in neurofibromatosis 1. J Med Genet. 2002;39(5):311–4.
129. McCaughan JA, Holloway SM, Davidson R, Lam WW. Further evidence of the increased risk for malignant peripheral nerve sheath tumour from a Scottish cohort of patients with neurofibromatosis type 1. J Med Genet. 2007;44(7):463–6.
130. Pasmant E, Sabbagh A, Spurlock G, Laurendeau I, Grillo E, Hamel MJ, et al. NF1 microdeletions in neurofibromatosis type 1: from genotype to phenotype. Hum Mutat. 2010;31(6):E1506–18.
131. LaFemina J, Qin LX, Moraco NH, Antonescu CR, Fields RC, Crago AM, et al. Oncologic outcomes of sporadic, neurofibromatosis-associated, and radiation-induced malignant peripheral nerve sheath tumors. Ann Surg Oncol. 2013;20(1):66–72.
132. Stucky CC, Johnson KN, Gray RJ, Pockaj BA, Ocal IT, Rose PS, et al. Malignant peripheral nerve sheath tumors (MPNST): the Mayo Clinic experience. Ann Surg Oncol. 2012;19(3):878–85.
133. Zou C, Smith KD, Liu J, Lahat G, Myers S, Wang WL, et al. Clinical, pathological, and molecular variables predictive of malignant peripheral nerve sheath tumor outcome. Ann Surg. 2009;249(6):1014–22.
134. Bradtmoller M, Hartmann C, Zietsch J, Jaschke S, Mautner VF, Kurtz A, et al. Impaired Pten expression in human malignant peripheral nerve sheath tumours. PLoS One. 2012;7(11):e47595.
135. Brennan MF, Antonescu CR, Moraco N, Singer S. Lessons learned from the study of 10,000 patients with soft tissue sarcoma. Ann Surg. 2014;260(3):416–21; discussion 21-2
136. James AW, Shurell E, Singh A, Dry SM, Eilber FC. Malignant peripheral nerve sheath tumor. Surg Oncol Clin N Am. 2016;25(4):789–802.
137. Ng VY, Scharschmidt TJ, Mayerson JL, Fisher JL. Incidence and survival in sarcoma in the United States: a focus on musculoskeletal lesions. Anticancer Res. 2013;33(6):2597–604.
138. Porter DE, Prasad V, Foster L, Dall GF, Birch R, Grimer RJ. Survival in malignant peripheral nerve sheath tumours: a comparison between sporadic and neurofibromatosis type 1-associated tumours. Sarcoma. 2009;2009:756395.
139. Watson KL, Al Sannaa GA, Kivlin CM, Ingram DR, Landers SM, Roland CL, et al. Patterns of recurrence and survival in sporadic, neurofibromatosis type 1-associated, and radiation-associated malignant peripheral nerve sheath tumors. J Neurosurg. 2017;126(1):319–29.
140. Anghileri M, Miceli R, Fiore M, Mariani L, Ferrari A, Mussi C, et al. Malignant peripheral nerve sheath tumors: prognostic factors and survival in a series of patients treated at a single institution. Cancer. 2006;107(5):1065–74.
141. Kar M, Deo SV, Shukla NK, Malik A, DattaGupta S, Mohanti BK, et al. Malignant peripheral nerve sheath tumors (MPNST)—clinicopathological study and treatment outcome of twenty-four cases. World J Surg Oncol. 2006;4:55.
142. Longhi A, Errani C, Magagnoli G, Alberghini M, Gambarotti M, Mercuri M, et al. High grade malignant peripheral nerve sheath tumors: outcome of 62 patients with localized disease and review of the literature. J Chemother. 2010;22(6):413–8.
143. Gronchi A, Casali PG, Mariani L, Miceli R, Fiore M, Lo Vullo S, et al. Status of surgical margins and prognosis in adult soft tissue sarcomas of the extremities: a series of patients treated at a single institution. J Clin Oncol. 2005;23(1):96–104.
144. Lin CT, Huang TW, Nieh S, Lee SC. Treatment of a malignant peripheral nerve sheath tumor. Onkologie. 2009;32(8–9):503–5.
145. Fan Q, Yang J, Wang G. Clinical and molecular prognostic predictors of malignant peripheral nerve sheath tumor. Clin Transl Oncol. 2014;16(2):191–9.
146. Valentin T, Le Cesne A, Ray-Coquard I, Italiano A, Decanter G, Bompas E, et al. Management and prognosis of malignant peripheral nerve sheath tumors: the experience of the French sarcoma group (GSF-GETO). Eur J Cancer. 2016;56:77–84.
147. Goertz O, Langer S, Uthoff D, Ring A, Stricker I, Tannapfel A, et al. Diagnosis, treatment and survival of 65 patients with malignant peripheral nerve sheath tumors. Anticancer Res. 2014;34(2):777–83.
148. Hruban RH, Shiu MH, Senie RT, Woodruff JM. Malignant peripheral nerve sheath tumors of the buttock and lower extremity. A study of 43 cases. Cancer. 1990;66(6):1253–65.
149. Kourea HP, Bilsky MH, Leung DH, Lewis JJ, Woodruff JM. Subdiaphragmatic and intrathoracic paraspinal malignant peripheral nerve sheath tumors: a clinicopathologic study of 25 patients and 26 tumors. Cancer. 1998;82(11):2191–203.
150. Bernthal NM, Putnam A, Jones KB, Viskochil D, Randall RL. The effect of surgical margins on outcomes for low grade MPNSTs and atypical neurofibroma. J Surg Oncol. 2014;110(7):813–6.

2 Genetics of Nerve Tumors

Kimberly Harbaugh, Neel T. Patel, and Elias Rizk

Abbreviations

MPNST	Malignant peripheral nerve sheath tumor
NF1	Neurofibromatosis type 1
NF2	Neurofibromatosis type 2
SCHW	Schwannomatosis

2.1 Introduction

Due to their intimate association with neural structures, nerve tumors can cause significant pain, disfigurement, and neurologic deficit. More aggressive lesions can lead to metastasis and death. In recent years, there have been significant advances made in genetic sequencing techniques, animal modeling, and patient registry studies that have shed some light on the genes and pathways associated with the development of nerve tumors [1–3] (Fig. 2.1). Understanding the genetic factors that contribute to the development and growth of these tumors is important. The information obtained may assist in making an accurate clinical diagnosis and aid in family planning [4]. Ideally, it will also guide the development and selection of targeted treatment options for individual patients and families [5, 6]. This chapter will review some of the genetic concepts related to nerve tumors and the disorders associated with them.

2.2 Nerve Sheath Tumors

Nerve sheath tumors are typically benign lesions that arise from and within cranial, spinal, and peripheral nerves. Neurofibroma and schwannoma are the most common types and may occur sporadically as isolated lesions or in conjunction with neurofibromatosis type 1 (NF1) for neurofibromas, or neurofibromatosis type 2 (NF2) and schwannomatosis (SCHW) for schwannomas. The sarcomatous variant of the peripheral nerve sheath tumor is a malignant peripheral nerve sheath tumor (MPNST) that may also occur sporadically or in association with NF1. An additional type of nerve sheath tumor not associated with these genetic conditions is the perineurioma that may occur as an intraneural or soft tissue variant. The genetic considerations associated with these lesions will be discussed.

K. Harbaugh (✉) · N. T. Patel · E. Rizk
Department of Neurosurgery,
Penn State Health, Hershey, PA, USA
e-mail: ksh15@psu.edu,
kharbaugh@pennstatehealth.psu.edu

F. Guedes et al. (eds.), *Diagnostic Assessment and Treatment of Peripheral Nerve Tumors*,
https://doi.org/10.1007/978-3-030-77633-6_2

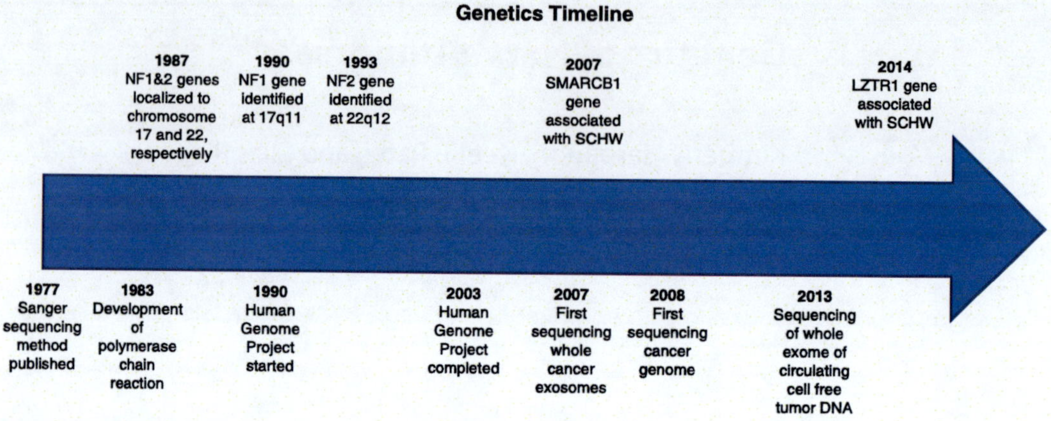

Fig. 2.1 Timeline of some of the genetic events related to peripheral nerve sheath tumors and genetic sequencing [adapted from Morganti [7]]

2.3 NF1 and Neurofibromas

NF1 is a condition also known as von Recklinghausen's disease associated with multiple neurofibromas, gliomas, café au lait lesions, and bony anomalies. It has a prevalence of approximately 1 in 3500 [1, 8]. Nearly half of the cases are spontaneous new mutations with no known family history, while the others are inherited from an affected parent in an autosomal dominant fashion. It arises as a result of mutations/variations in the NF1 gene [9, 10].

2.4 NF1 Gene

The NF1 gene was initially localized to chromosome 17 in 1987 and subsequently identified by positional cloning at chromosome 17q11.2 in 1990 [1, 11–13]. The gene is large at 350 kbp with 61 exons [12–14]. The NF1 gene product, neurofibromin, is a ubiquitous GTPase-activating protein that in its normal state inactivates RAS signaling and serves as a tumor suppressor [15]. Inactivation of neurofibromin leads to increased RAS signaling and tumor formation via loss of cellular growth control, increased cellular proliferation, and decreased apoptosis [8, 10, 15]. More than 2600 mutations of the gene have been described, 80% of which are inactivating variants [14]. For the most part, there is no clear association between the various mutations and a phenotypic presentation. Even within families, the phenotypic expression can vary significantly suggesting the role of other genetic, epigenetic, or environmental factors contributing to the ultimate phenotype expressed. One exception to this rule is a known phenotype associated with NF1 whole gene deletion also referred to as microdeletion. Patients with this variant typically have, among other things, dysmorphic facial features, macrocephaly, cognitive delays, increased tumor burden, and a higher tendency to develop MPNST [6, 8, 9, 16].

Most patients with NF1 can be diagnosed clinically based on standard criteria consisting of two or more of the following: six or more café au lait macules; two or more neurofibromas or one plexiform neurofibroma; inguinal or axillary freckling; optic pathway glioma; two or more Lisch nodules; a characteristic bony lesion—sphenoid dysplasia or long bone cortical thinning; and a first-degree relative with NF1 [10]. Genetic testing may play a role in some cases. Successful identification of the NF1 mutation can be made in approximately 95% of classical NF1 cases [14]. In patients with a de novo mutation, this may be helpful.

Segmental (localized) or generalized mosaic variants of the NF1 gene may occur in up to 10%

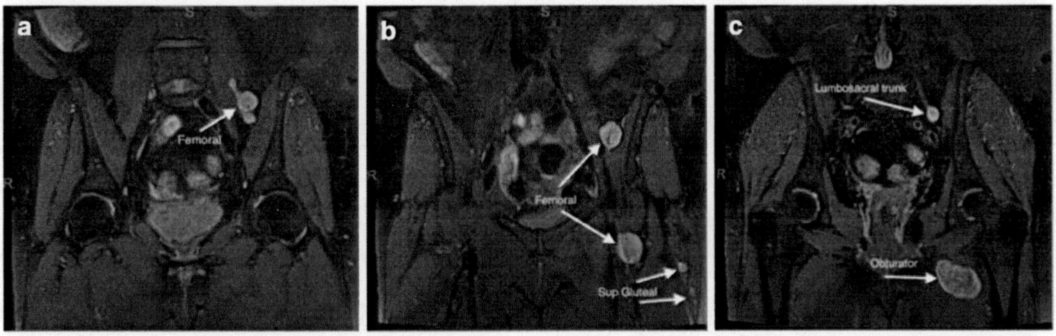

Fig. 2.2 Coronal proton density magnetic resonance imaging of a patient with mosaic NF1 localized to the left pelvis demonstrating multiple tumors involving the femoral nerve (**a, b**), superior gluteal nerve in the tensor fascia lata (**b**), and lumbosacral trunk and obturator nerve (**c**)

of cases [17]. In this situation, the genetic variant occurs after the zygote is created so that some of the patient's cells harbor the mutation, while others do not (Fig. 2.2). Transmission to offspring in that setting can vary from 0 to 50% as opposed to the 50% in non-mosaic cases and is dependent on the degree to which the gametes are involved with the mutation. In purely somatic mosaicism, the risk of transmission to offspring is zero. In rare cases, in patients with pure gonadal mosaicism, the genetic anomaly affects the gametes but not the somatic cells so that the parent has no stigmata of NF1, and yet there is a 50% chance of transmitting the gene to offspring. The diagnosis in a mosaic parent may not become obvious until two or more offspring are subsequently found to have NF1. Genetic testing of serum blood samples in mosaic cases is usually negative [18]. The anomalous gene may be detected in fibroblasts of a café au lait macule or tumors in these patients [19].

2.5 Neurofibromas

Anomalies in the NF1 gene are felt to play a role in the development of many sporadic and NF1-associated neurofibromas. Neurofibromas are unencapsulated tumors with Schwann cell-derived spindle cells with wavy nuclei in a background of fibromyxoid stroma containing axons as well as fibroblasts, perineurial cells, mast cells, and lymphocytes [20, 21]. They may occur sporadically or in association with NF1. The tumors may be dermal, subcutaneous, or deep in location and nodular, diffuse, or plexiform. The latter tumor type is characteristically found in patients with NF1 [9, 21]. In sporadic cases, neurofibromas are typically nodular with a very benign appearance. In NF1, the lesions may be benign or may be more variable with increased cellularity, atypia, and mitoses. As patients with NF1 have a 10% lifetime risk of developing a malignant peripheral nerve sheath tumor, often within a plexiform neurofibroma, the variable features seen in these neurofibromas can be concerning for early malignant degeneration [10]. Some NF1-associated neurofibromas, however, may have features concerning for malignancy but behave benignly without recurrence or metastasis despite simple resection without wide margins and avoidance of adjuvant therapy [23].

Recognizing the variable nature of these lesions, a consensus meeting was organized, and a grading scale was introduced that included a new category of atypical neurofibromatous neoplasm with uncertain biological potential (ANNUBP) [22]. In addition to abnormalities in the NF1 gene, these atypical lesions harbor anomalies of cyclin-dependent kinase inhibitor 2A/B (CDKN2A/B) genes located on chromosome 9 that code for tumor suppressor cell cycle regulator proteins p16 and p14 and p15 [8, 22, 23]. CDKN2A/B anomalies are also seen in MPNST and melanoma [24]. Interestingly, there have been reports of patients with multiple benign neurofibromas and the CDKN2A anomalies without NF1 anomalies [25, 26]. Alternatively, somatic mutations in the NF1 gene may be found in tumors not typically associated with neurofibromatosis such as melanoma and lung and bladder cancer, but those tumors have genetic mutations other than NF1 as well [14]. These findings highlight the fact that tumor formation and malignant degeneration are dependent on the interplay of multiple factors.

2.6 Malignant Peripheral Nerve Sheath Tumors

MPNSTs are sarcomatous lesions arising from Schwann cell lineage. They account for 4% of soft tissue sarcomas [27]. They occur in the setting of NF1 in 40–50%, sporadically in 40–47%, or following radiation exposure in 10%. Rarely, they may be seen in patients with NF2 or SCHW. The lesions tend to be aggressive with a disease-free survival rate between 34 and 60% [9]. Outcomes of MPNST seem to be worse in patients with NF1 than in patients with sporadic MPNST [10]. NF1 loss has been uniformly noted in NF1-related MPNSTs and in 72% of sporadic and radiation-associated MPNSTs [9]. The loss of CDKN2A has been reported in approximately half of MPNSTs. In addition to NF1 and CDKN2A/B mutations, MPNSTs often have mutations in TP53 located on chromosome 17p13.1 whose gene product p53 is involved in cell division [24]. These mutations may occur in up to 75% of MPNSTs, and commonly the mutation or loss occurs in only one copy [9]. Mutations in the BRAF gene have been noted in some sporadic and NF1-associated MPNSTs. The gene is a proto-oncogene located at chromosome 7q34 and is normally involved in the regulation of cellular proliferation and differentiation [28].

Loss-of-function mutations in genes that encode for protein components of the polycomb repressive complex 2 (PRC2) have been reported in approximately 85% of MPNSTs [8, 29]. The anomalous genes include suppressor of zeste 12 homolog gene (SUZ12) at chromosome 17q11.2 and embryonic ectoderm development (EED) gene at chromosome 11q14.2 [9, 23, 30]. PRC2 is a mediator of transcription with histone methyltransferase activity that trimethylates histone H3 on lysine 27 (H3K27me3). This histone is part of the nucleosome, the basic DNA complex unit composed of a strand of DNA wrapped around an eight-histone complex with two each of four separate histones. When H3K27 is trimethylated, the chromatin is in the compact state. This epigenetic change leading to decreased methylation translates to increased transcription. Intact H3K27me3 methylation and normal PRC2 status are almost universally seen in benign and atypical neurofibromas suggesting that mutations in the PRC2 genes may be the drivers in progression to malignancy. Proteomic data also suggest that PRC2 loss promotes tumor immune evasion [31].

Decreased H3K27me3 staining may help differentiate benign neurofibromas and ANNUBP from MPNST in some cases; however, it is not specific to MPNST as it can be seen in other tumors including synovial sarcoma and melanoma. Complete loss is more common in MPNST, whereas the other tumors typically demonstrate partial loss [29, 32, 33].

Interestingly, SUZ12 is often lost in patients with the NF1 microdeletion syndrome discussed above in which the entire NF1 gene is deleted. Given the SUZ12 gene location near the NF1 gene, this is not surprising, and its loss may contribute to the increased risk of malignancy seen in these patients [8, 16].

In some MPNSTs, the catalytic component of PRC2, enhancer of zeste homolog 2 (EZH2), is overexpressed [8, 30]. The exact mechanism by which the overexpression can drive tumor progression is not clear but may be independent of the methyltransferase activity [8]. PRC2 has been shown to silence genes that regulate cell differentiation and adhesion, cell cycle checkpoints, and DNA repair [34].

In addition to the genetic mutations noted above, MPNST chromosomal analysis via karyotyping or array comparative genomic hybridization (aCGH) demonstrates highly variable structural and/or numerical anomalies. Somatic copy number alterations (SCNAs) have been noted in essentially all of the chromosomes in various reports, and gains are typically more common than losses [6].

Extensive genome rearrangement is also seen with multiple fusion genes [9]. Losses of chromosome 9p21 corresponding to the CDKN2A tumor suppressor region are among the most common SCNAs reported but are not universal [6, 24, 35]. Overall, there is not a characteristic pattern of chromosomal abnormalities specific to MPNST or one that differentiates sporadic MPNST from those in NF1 patients [6, 36].

2.7 NF2 and Schwannomas

Whereas NF1 leads to the development of multiple neurofibromas, NF2 patients are predisposed to the development of the other common peripheral nerve sheath tumor type, schwannoma. In its classic presentation, NF2 patients harbor bilateral vestibular schwannomas, but they may also develop schwannomas in spinal, peripheral, and other cranial nerves. They may have intradermal schwannomas, an entity that seems to be unique to the NF2 population. Their presence can help lead to the diagnosis of NF2 and distinguish it from the other schwannoma predisposing conditions, SCHW [37]. In addition to schwannoma formation, patients are predisposed to the development of multiple meningiomas, spinal ependymomas that typically behave in an indolent fashion, and ocular anomalies such as lens opacities and peripheral neuropathy.

NF2 is caused by a mutation in the NF2 gene. It is less common than NF1 by a factor of 10 with a birth incidence of approximately 1 in 33,000 [10, 38, 39]. Like NF1, it is an autosomal dominant condition, but 50–60% of the patients have new mutations with no prior family history. In the de novo group, mosaicism is common, and based on recent evidence, it is estimated to account for approximately 60% of the cases, much higher than the 25–30% previously estimated rates [40]. This is important because, in patients with a family history or germline mutation, the subsequent transmission is 50%. In patients who are NF2 mosaics, however, the transmission may be 5% or less [37].

2.8 NF2 Gene

The NF2 gene is a tumor suppressor gene comprised of 110 kb with 17 exons [37]. It was initially localized to chromosome 22 in 1987 and subsequently identified at chr22q12.2 in 1993 [10, 41]. The primary gene product of NF2 is merlin (moesin, ezrin, radixin-like protein), with a structure resembling that of the members of the 4.1 family of cytoskeletal proteins that link the cytoskeleton to membrane-associated proteins. It is highly expressed in adults in Schwann and meningeal cells, nerves, and lenses [37]. It is involved in cell contact inhibition and is involved in transcriptional pathways in the cell nucleus resulting in growth suppression [10, 37, 38].

Correlation between the mutation type of the NF2 gene and phenotypic severity has been seen with truncating mutations of exons 2–13 resulting in a more severe presentation with earlier onset and increased tumor burden [37, 42]. More severe NF2 phenotype (earlier onset of symptoms, higher tumor burden, earlier death) is also seen in patients with nonsense or frameshift mutations, while larger deletions have a less severe clinical course. It is not clear that these correlations are strong enough, however, to predict an expected course for any individual patient [10]. In patients with a mosaic form of NF2 mutation, the presentation is often later and less severe. A delay in the development of vestibular schwannomas in mosaic patients may make it difficult to differentiate NF2 from SCHW, the other condition that predisposes patients to the development of multiple schwannomas.

2.9 Schwannomatosis

SCHW is a condition or several related conditions that predispose patients to the development of multiple spinal and peripheral nerve schwannomas and less commonly cranial nerve schwannomas. Approximately 15% of cases are familial, transmitted in an autosomal dominant fashion but with variable penetrance. The remaining 85% of cases are sporadic. The true prevalence of the disorder has yet to be determined. It was initially felt to be as common as NF2, but subsequent studies suggest that its prevalence and birth incidence are less than half that of NF2 [10, 43]. Chronic pain both generalized and in association with schwannomas also seems to be common in patients with SCHW [44].

When initially described, the presence of a vestibular schwannoma excluded patients from a diagnosis of SCHW [45]. Since then, a number of rare cases of unilateral vestibular schwannoma have been reported in patients with SCHW. Patients with SCHW may also have intracranial meningiomas, which are again less common than is seen in patients with NF2. Spinal ependymomas and intradermal schwannomas appear to be exclusive to NF2 [37, 43].

Assessment for germline NF2 mutations can be helpful to identify patients with this disorder, but an absence of an NF2 mutation does not exclude the possibility of NF2 mosaicism. A subset of patients initially thought to have SCHW have subsequently been found to be NF2 mosaics [40]. Identical NF2 mutations in separate schwannomas in a patient without a germline NF2 mutation are consistent with NF2 mosaicism.

Unlike the case in NF1 and NF2 in which anomalies of a single gene account for all cases, two separate gene anomalies have been associated with the development of SCHW, SMARCB1, and LZTR1. Additional patients have been noted without these mutations suggesting that other as yet unidentified gene anomalies or epigenetic factors may also play a role [43, 46].

2.10 SMARCB1

A germline anomaly in the SMARCB1 gene as a causal factor in the development of SCHW was reported in 2007. Anomalies in this gene account for approximately 50% of familial and 10% of sporadic SCHW cases [46]. The gene is located at chromosome 22q11.23, centromeric to the NF2 gene [43, 47, 48], and has 9 exons over 50 kb [49]. The current nomenclature, SMARCB1, is derived from SWI/SNF-related matrix-associated, actin-dependent regulator of chromatin, subfamily B member 1, but the gene has also been referred to as SNF5, INI1, and BAF47 [49]. It is expressed in all nucleated cells and acts as a tumor suppressor gene influencing cell transcription, cell cycle regulation, and cell differentiation [47, 48].

In addition to its association with SCHW, abnormal SMARCB1 expression has been identified in numerous tumors. Some, including malignant rhabdoid tumors, and atypical teratoid/rhabdoid tumors demonstrate a complete loss of SMARCB1 expression. In others, such as synovial sarcomas, there is reduced expression [47, 48]. In familial SCHW patients, there is a germline missense or splice-site non-truncating mutation usually at either end of the SMARCB1 gene. As a result, these patients are thought to have altered but not complete loss of protein activity and retain the ability to control cell cycle function [47, 49]. Although typically benign, rare cases of MPNST have been reported in patients with SMARCB1 SCHW. Additionally, when meningiomas occur in SCHW patients, they typically occur in patients with SMARCB1 anomalies [37, 46].

2.11 LZTR1

The association of leucine-zipper-like transcriptional regulator 1 (LZTR1) gene mutations and SCHW was initially reported in 2014 [50]. LZTR1 is located at chromosome 22q11.2, 8.7 Mb pairs centromeric to the NF2 gene and 2.8 Mb pairs centromeric to the SMARCB1 gene [46]. It is ubiquitously expressed in human tissues and localizes to the Golgi apparatus [50]. It is a tumor suppressor with involvement in chromatin conformation and cell cycle regulation [10, 37]. More recent data suggests that LZTR1 is also involved in polyubiquitination of proteins involved in the RAS-MAPK signaling pathway [51, 52]. Polyubiquitination, the process of bonding the ubiquitin molecule to the protein to inactivate it and tag it for destruction, results in decreased downstream signal transduction. As a result, LZTR1 has been labeled as a "Ras killer protein" [51].

LZTR1 mutations are noted in approximately 21–29% of familial and 21–24% of sporadic SCHW cases [43, 53]. Phenotypic expression is variable. In the original report, the fathers of two presumed sporadic patients were found to harbor the familial LZTR1 mutation. Both were asymptomatic, and neither had any known tumors although they had not been imaged [50].

Meningiomas have not yet been reported in SCHW patients with the LZTR1 mutation; however, cranial nerve schwannomas are seen in up to 20% of LZTR1 SCHW patients with trigeminal schwannoma being the most common [43]. Unilateral vestibular schwannomas may be present in 7% of these patients. This can make it difficult at times to differentiate sporadic SCHW from sporadic NF2 especially in mosaic NF2 patients who might not demonstrate the features unique to NF2 such as spinal ependymomas, intradermal schwannoma, and ocular anomalies. As a result, exclusion of the LZTR1 germline mutation is now recommended prior to making the NF2 diagnosis in these sporadic patients with unilateral vestibular schwannoma and two additional non-intradermal schwannomas [4]. Further complicating this issue is the finding in one report of two patients who lacked a germline NF2 mutation and had identical NF2 mutations in separate tumors which would typically be diagnostic for NF2 mosaicism but harbored a germline LZTR1 mutation suggesting a LZTR1 SCHW diagnosis [54].

LZTR1 mutations have been recently reported in association with some cases of Noonan syndrome where autosomal dominant and nondominant forms have been reported [52]. Biallelic mutations of LZTR1 in some cases of glioblastoma multiforme (GBM) have also been identified and were noted even before the association of LZTR1 and SCHW was reported [50]. Interestingly, a recent report noted GBM in the first-degree relatives, a father and a sister of two unrelated SCHW patients. Both SCHW patients harbored germline mutations in LZTR1 which were also present in the GBM samples of the relatives [55].

2.12 Schwannomas

Schwannomas are well-encapsulated lesions with spindle cells of Schwann cell origin. In addition to hyalinized vessels and degenerative changes, they have two distinct cellular patterns, Antoni A and Antoni B areas. Antoni A areas contain compact cells with palisading nuclei. Antoni B regions are microcystic, hypocellular areas with abundant collagen and macrophages. These tumors also stain positively for S100 protein [20, 21]. The majority of these tumors occur sporadically as solitary lesions. As noted above, they are also a hallmark of NF2 and SCHW. Not surprisingly, the genes responsible for these conditions play a role in schwannoma development.

The gene most consistently associated with the development of schwannomas is the NF2 gene. Abnormalities of the NF2 gene are found in the majority of schwannomas whether they occur sporadically or in association with NF2 or SCHW [41, 56]. NF2 patients harbor a germline NF2 mutation, and in the tumors, the second copy of NF2 is silenced either through mutation or loss of heterozygosity. In SCHW patients, there is a germline mutation of SMARCB1 or LZTR1. Additional mutations must then occur to lead to the inactivation of both NF2 alleles. This has been described as a three-step/four- or five-hit model of tumorigenesis. Given the proximity of the SMARCB1 and LZTR1 genes to the NF2 gene on chromosome 22, when the loss of heterozygosity occurs, the large deleted segment often involves not only NF2 but SMARCB1 and in some cases LZTR1. So, for SCHW tumors, the initial step/hit is the germline anomaly. The second step is the LOH of chromosome 22 with loss of NF2 and the remaining wild-type SMARCB1 or LZTR1, resulting in hits 2 and 3. The third step results in the mutation of the remaining NF2 wild-type copy leading to the fourth hit. As SMARCB1 is located between NF2 and LZTR1, loss of heterozygosity events that result in the deletion of NF2 and LZTR1 would be expected to also result in the loss of SMARCB1 to give the fifth hit [46]. In sporadic schwannomas, silencing of the NF2 gene is also seen in many of the tumors due to mutations and/or LOH [57, 58].

SMARCB1 and LZTR1 play a role in the development of schwannomas in patients carrying the SMARCB1 or LZTR1 germline anomaly, respectively. SMARCB1 likely plays a role in other schwannomas as well. Mosaic tumor staining of SMARCB1 has been noted in 93% of familial SCHW, 83% of NF2, and 55% of sporadic SCHW-associated cases. Interestingly, only 5% of sporadic solitary schwannomas have mosaic staining. In the remainder, normal diffuse staining is seen. This suggests that the pathway to schwannoma formation may be different in sporadic cases than in syndromic cases [59, 60]. The LZTR1 protein staining is normal in most tumors but may be decreased or absent in LZTR1-associated SCHW tumors depending on the type of mutation [61]. This along with the fact that there are a number of unaffected parents of LZTR1 patients who harbor the LZTR1 germline anomaly makes it difficult to determine the exact role of this gene in tumor formation [50, 54]. As noted previously, many tumors harbor a LOH of chr22 with a gene segment deletion that includes NF2, SMARCB1, and in some cases LZTR1. For this reason, determining the exact role of the individual gene anomalies in schwannoma formation is difficult [10].

In a subset of schwannomas occurring sporadically or in association with NF2 or SCHW, there is either no NF2 anomaly or a mutation or LOH of only one NF2 allele [41, 46]. It is not clear in those cases whether other unidentified genes may be involved in tumor formation or if epigenetic factors may be contributing to functional silencing of the NF2 gene either through DNA methylation or as a result of microRNA deregulation in the tumors [41, 46, 56, 58]. In a study that analyzed global gene expression in sporadic vestibular schwannomas, the upregulation of pathways related to viral infections was noted suggesting a possible viral etiology for the development and growth of some schwannomas [58, 62].

2.13 Perineuriomas

These tumors are comprised of cells with perineurial differentiation and elongated bipolar cytoplasmic processes often arranged in a whorl or storiform pattern. They may be intraneural or found in the soft tissues typically with no clear nerve association. The soft tissue lesions are usually well-circumscribed and may have a capsule. They are often located in the subcutaneous tissues but may be located in deep soft tissues or within organs. The intraneural lesions cause focal expansion of one or more fascicles of a nerve and are restricted to the boundaries of the nerve [62]. They have a classic pseudo-onion bulb appearance on cross sections due to perineurial cell proliferation that concentrically surrounds individual nerve fibers and endoneurial capillaries [20, 21].

Various chromosomal abnormalities have been demonstrated in intraneural and extraneural soft tissue perineuriomas including chromosome 13 deletion, chromosome 22 monosomy, or deletion of the 22q11-13.1 regions, deletions and point mutations of the NF2 gene on 22q12, as well as chromosome 10 rearrangements and deletions [62]. More recent genomic analyses of intraneural and extraneural soft tissue perineuriomas with whole-exome sequencing, copy number variation analysis, and high-resolution single-nucleotide polymorphism (SNP) array have found similar anomalies [63, 64].

Analysis of a group of intraneural perineuriomas identified chromosome 22q deletions and more importantly noted mutations in the TRAF7 gene in 62.5% and large deletions/duplications in 12.5%. No abnormalities were found in 25%. The TRAF7 gene is located on chromosome 16p, and its protein is a tumor necrosis factor receptor protein involved in cell signal transduction. Mutations in this gene have also been noted in meningiomas [63].

In an extraneural soft tissue perineurioma series, 13/14 cases had 2 or more chromosomal abnormalities (up to 7). Nine of the 14 tumors had deletions in either chromosome 22q (and its NF2 locus) or chromosome 17q (and the NF1 locus), and 1 had both. Chromosome 2 deletions were noted in five and chromosome 6 deletions in four. No mutations involving the TRAF7 gene were noted [64].

2.14 Conclusions

Peripheral nerve sheath tumors may develop sporadically or in association with a variety of inherited syndromes. Both benign and malignant tumors have a widely variable spectrum of growth and associated morbidity and mortality. Continued advances in the understanding of the genetic and molecular makeup are essential in the treatment and development of novel and targeted therapies for these devastating disorders.

References

1. Gottfried ON, Viskochil DH, Fults DW, Couldwell WT. Molecular, genetic, and cellular pathogenesis of neurofibromas and surgical implications. Neurosurgery. 2006;58(1):1–16.
2. Heather JM, Chain B. The sequence of sequencers: the history of sequencing DNA. Genomics [Internet]. 2016;107(1):1–8. https://doi.org/10.1016/j.ygeno.2015.11.003.
3. Mertens F, Dal Cin P, de Wever I, Fletcher CDM, Mandahl N, Mitelman F, et al. Cytogenetic characterization of peripheral nerve sheath tumours: a report of the CHAMP study group. J Pathol. 2000;190(1):31–8.
4. Smith MJ, Bowers NL, Bulman M, Gokhale C, Wallace AJ, King AT, et al. Revisiting neurofibromatosis type 2 diagnostic criteria to exclude LZTR1-related schwannomatosis. Neurology. 2017;88(1):87–92.
5. Peacock JD, Pridgeon MG, Tovar EA, Essenburg CJ, Bowman M, Madaj Z, et al. Genomic status of MET potentiates sensitivity to MET and MEK inhibition in NF1-related malignant peripheral nerve sheath tumors. Cancer Res. 2018;78(13):3672–87.
6. Pemov A, Li H, Presley W, Wallace MR, Miller DT. Genetics of human malignant peripheral nerve sheath tumors. Neuro-Oncol Adv. 2019;2(Suppl 1):1–12.
7. Morganti S, Tarantino P, Ferraro E, D'Amico P, Duso BA, Curigliano G. Next generation sequencing (NGS): a revolutionary technology in pharmacogenomics and personalized medicine in cancer. In: Advances in experimental medicine and biology; 2019.
8. Korfhage J, Lombard DB. Malignant peripheral nerve sheath tumors: from epigenome to bedside. Mol Cancer Res. 2019;17(7):1417–28.
9. Longo JF, Weber SM, Turner-Ivey BP, Carroll SL. Recent advances in the diagnosis and pathogenesis of neurofibromatosis type 1 (NF1)-associated peripheral nervous system neoplasms. Adv Anat Pathol. 2018;25(5):353–68.
10. Plotkin SR, Wick A. Neurofibromatosis and Schwannomatosis. Semin Neurol. 2018;38(1):73–85.
11. Lothe RA, Slettan A, Seater G, Brogger A, Borresen AL, Nesland JM. Alterations at chromosome 17 loci in peripheral nerve sheath tumors. J Neuropathol Exp Neurol. 1995;54(1):65–73.
12. Cawthon RM, Weiss R, Xu G, Viskochil D, Culver M, Stevens J, et al. A major segment of the neurofibromatosis type 1 gene: cDNA sequence, genomic structure, and point mutations. Cell. 1990;62(1):193–201.
13. Wallace MR, Marchuk DA, Andersen LB, Letcher R, Odeh HM, Saulino AM, et al. Type 1 neurofibromatosis gene: Identification of a large transcript disrupted in three NF1 patients. Science. 1990;249(4965):181–6.
14. Philpott C, Tovell H, Frayling IM, Cooper DN, Upadhyaya M. The NF1 somatic mutational landscape in sporadic human cancers. Hum Genomics. 2017;11(1):1–20.
15. Cichowski K, Jacks T. NF1 tumor suppressor gene function. Cell. 2001;104(4):593–604.
16. Kehrer-Sawatzki H, Mautner VF, Cooper DN. Emerging genotype–phenotype relationships in patients with large NF1 deletions. Hum Genet. 2017;136(4):349–76.
17. Foulkes WD, Real FX. Many mosaic mutations. Curr Oncol. 2013;20(2):85–7.
18. Hom GL, Moodley S, Rothner AD, Moodley M. The clinical Spectrum of mosaic neurofibromatosis in children and adolescents. J Child Neurol. 2020;35(3):242–6.
19. Ruggieri M. Mosaic (segmental) neurofibromatosis type 1 (NF1) and type 2 (NF2): no longer neurofibromatosis type 5 (NF5) [3]. Am J Med Genet. 2001;101:178–80.
20. Mertens F, Lothe RA. Nervous system: peripheral nerve sheath tumors. Atlas Genet Cytogenet Oncol Haematol. 2001;5(3):211–2.
21. Rodriguez FJ, Folpe AL, Giannini C, Perry A. Pathology of peripheral nerve sheath tumors: diagnostic overview and update on selected diagnostic problems. Acta Neuropathol. 2012;123(3):295–319.
22. Miettinen MM, Antonescu CR, Fletcher CDM, Kim A, Lazar AJ, Quezado MM, et al. Histopathologic evaluation of atypical neurofibromatous tumors and their transformation into malignant peripheral nerve sheath tumor in patients with neurofibromatosis 1—a consensus overview. Hum Pathol. 2017;67:1–10.
23. Fisher MJ, Belzberg AJ, de Blank P, de Raedt T, Elefteriou F, Ferner RE, et al. 2016 children's tumor foundation conference on neurofibromatosis type 1, neurofibromatosis type 2, and schwannomatosis. Am J Med Genet A. 2018;176(5):1258–69.
24. Berner JM, Sørlie T, Mertens F, Henriksen J, Sæter G, Mandahl N, et al. Chromosome band 9p21 is frequently altered in malignant peripheral nerve sheath tumors: studies of CDKN2A and other genes of the pRB pathway. Genes Chromosomes Cancer. 1999;26(2):151–60.
25. Vanneste R, Smith E, Graham G. Multiple neurofibromas as the presenting feature of familial atypical multiple malignant melanoma (FAMMM) syndrome. Am J Med Genet A. 2013;161(6):1425–31.
26. Baker MJ, Goldstein AM, Gordon PL, Harbaugh KS, Mackley HB, Glantz MJ, et al. An interstitial deletion within 9p21.3 and extending beyond CDKN2A predisposes to melanoma, neural system tumours and possible haematological malignancies. J Med Genet. 2016;53(11):721–7.
27. Widemann BC, Italiano A. Biology and management of undifferentiated pleomorphic sarcoma, myxofi-

brosarcoma, and malignant peripheral nerve sheath tumors: state of the art and perspectives. J Clin Oncol. 2018;36(2):160–7.
28. Gutmann DH. BRAFV600E mutation in sporadic and neurofibromatosis type 1-related malignant peripheral nerve sheath tumors. Neuro-Oncology. 2013;16(3):466–7.
29. Martinez AP, Fritchie KJ. Update on peripheral nerve sheath tumors. Surg Pathol Clin. 2019;12:1–19.
30. Pemov A, Hansen NF, Sindiri S, Patidar R, Higham CS, Dombi E, et al. Low mutation burden and frequent loss of CDKN2A/B and SMARCA2, but not PRC2, define premalignant neurofibromatosis type 1–associated atypical neurofibromas. Neuro-Oncology. 2019;21(8):981–92.
31. Wojcik JB, Marchione DM, Sidoli S, Djedid A, Lisby A, Majewski J, et al. Epigenomic reordering induced by polycomb loss drives oncogenesis but leads to therapeutic vulnerabilities in malignant peripheral nerve sheath tumors. Cancer Res. 2019;79(13):3205–19.
32. Asano N, Yoshida A, Ichikawa H, Mori T, Nakamura M, Kawai A, et al. Immunohistochemistry for trimethylated H3K27 in the diagnosis of malignant peripheral nerve sheath tumours. Histopathology. 2017;70(3):385–93.
33. Mito JK, Qian X, Doyle LA, Hornick JL, Jo VY. Role of histone H3K27 trimethylation loss as a marker for malignant peripheral nerve sheath tumor in fine-needle aspiration and small biopsy specimens. Am J Clin Pathol. 2017;148:179–89.
34. Moritz LE, Trievel RC. Structure, mechanism, and regulation of polycomb-repressive complex 2. J Biol Chem. 2017;293(36):13805–14.
35. Schmidt H, Würl P, Taubert H, Meye A, Bache M, Holzhausen HJ, et al. Genomic imbalances of 7p and 17q in malignant peripheral nerve sheath tumors are clinically relevant. Genes Chromosomes Cancer. 1999;25(3):205–11.
36. Fletcher CDM, Cin PD, de Wever I, Mandahl N, Mertens F, Mitelman F, et al. Correlation between clinicopathological features and karyotype in spindle cell sarcomas: a report of 130 cases from the CHAMP study group. Am J Pathol. 1999;154(6):1841–7.
37. Evans DGR, Salvador H, Chang VY, Erez A, Voss SD, Druker H, et al. Cancer and central nervous system tumor surveillance in pediatric neurofibromatosis 2 and related disorders. Clin Cancer Res. 2017;23(12):e54–61.
38. Karajannis MA, Ferner RE. Neurofibromatosis-related tumors: emerging biology and therapies. Curr Opin Pediatr. 2015;27(1):26–33.
39. Hexter A, Jones A, Joe H, Heap L, Smith MJ, Wallace AJ, et al. Clinical and molecular predictors of mortality in neurofibromatosis 2: a UK national analysis of 1192 patients. J Med Genet. 2015;52(10):699–705.
40. Evans DG, Hartley CL, Smith PT, King AT, Bowers NL, Tobi S, et al. Incidence of mosaicism in 1055 de novo NF2 cases: much higher than previous estimates with high utility of next-generation sequencing. Genet Med [Internet]. 2019;22(1):53–9. https://doi.org/10.1038/s41436-019-0598-7.
41. Hadfield KD, Smith MJ, Urquhart JE, Wallace AJ, Bowers NL, King AT, et al. Rates of loss of heterozygosity and mitotic recombination in NF2 schwannomas, sporadic vestibular schwannomas and schwannomatosis schwannomas. Oncogene. 2010;29(47):6216–21.
42. Halliday D, Emmanouil B, Pretorius P, MacKeith S, Painter S, Tomkins H, et al. Genetic severity score predicts clinical phenotype in NF2. J Med Genet. 2017;54(10):657–64.
43. Evans DG, Bowers NL, Tobi S, Hartley C, Wallace AJ, King AT, et al. Schwannomatosis: a genetic and epidemiological study. J Neurol Neurosurg Psychiatry. 2018;89:1215–9.
44. Alaidarous A, Parfait B, Ferkal S, Cohen J, Wolkenstein P, Mazereeuw-Hautier J. Segmental schwannomatosis: characteristics in 12 patients. Orphanet J Rare Dis. 2019;14(1):1–8.
45. Jacoby LB, MacCollin M, Barone R, Ramesh V, Gusella JF. Frequency and distribution of NF2 mutations in schwannomas. Genes Chromosomes Cancer. 1996;17(1):45–55.
46. Kehrer-Sawatzki H, Farschtschi S, Mautner VF, Cooper DN. The molecular pathogenesis of schwannomatosis, a paradigm for the co-involvement of multiple tumour suppressor genes in tumorigenesis. Hum Genet. 2017;136(2):129–48.
47. Kohashi K, Oda Y. Oncogenic roles of SMARCB1/INI1 and its deficient tumors. Cancer Sci. 2017;108(4):547–52.
48. Pawel BR. SMARCB1-deficient tumors of childhood: a practical guide. Pediatr Dev Pathol. 2018;21(1):6–28.
49. Kalimuthu SN, Chetty R. Gene of the month: SMARCB1. J Clin Pathol. 2016;69(6):484–9.
50. Piotrowski A, Xie J, Liu YF, Poplawski AB, Gomes AR, Madanecki P, et al. Germline loss-of-function mutations in LZTR1 predispose to an inherited disorder of multiple schwannomas. Nat Genet. 2014;46(2):182–7.
51. Abe T, Umeki I, Ichiro KS, Ichi IS, Niihori T, Aoki Y. LZTR1 facilitates polyubiquitination and degradation of RAS-GTPases. Cell Death Differ [Internet]. 2019;27(3):1023–35. https://doi.org/10.1038/s41418-019-0395-5.
52. Motta M, Fidan M, Bellacchio E, Pantaleoni F, Schneider-Heieck K, Coppola S, et al. Dominant Noonan syndrome-causing LZTR1 mutations specifically affect the Kelch domain substrate-recognition surface and enhance RAS-MAPK signaling. Hum Mol Genet. 2019;28(6):1007–22.
53. Justin T, Jordan M, Miriam J, Smith P, James A, Walker P, Serkan Erdin P, Michael E, Talkowski P, Vanessa L, Merker B, et al. Pain correlates with germline mutation in schwannomatosis. Medicine [Internet]. 2018;5(2018):1–6. Available from: http://arxiv.org/abs/1303.3997

54. Kehrer-Sawatzki H, Kluwe L, Friedrich RE, Summerer A, Schäfer E, Wahlländer U, et al. Phenotypic and genotypic overlap between mosaic NF2 and schwannomatosis in patients with multiple non-intradermal schwannomas. Human Genet [Internet]. 2018;137(6–7):543–52. https://doi.org/10.1007/s00439-018-1909-9.
55. Deiller C, Van-Gils J, Zordan C, Tinat J, Loiseau H, Fabre T, et al. Coexistence of schwannomatosis and glioblastoma in two families. Eur J Med Genet [Internet]. 2019;62(8):103680. https://doi.org/10.1016/j.ejmg.2019.103680.
56. Agnihotri S, Jalali S, Wilson MR, Danesh A, Li M, Klironomos G, et al. The genomic landscape of schwannoma. Nat Genet. 2016;48(11):1339–48.
57. de Carvalho RM, de Castro Sant' Anna C, Pinto GR, EHA P, Tuji FM, do Nascimento Borges B, et al. Frequency of the loss of heterozygosity of the NF2 gene in sporadic spinal schwannomas. Anticancer Res. 2018;38(4):2149–54.
58. Sass H, Cayé-Thomasen P. Contemporary molecular biology of sporadic vestibular schwannomas: a systematic review and clinical implications. J Int Adv Otol. 2018;14(2):322–9.
59. Patil S, Perry A, MacCollin M, Dong S, Betensky RA, Yeh TH, et al. Immunohistochemical analysis supports a role for INI1/SMARCB1 in hereditary forms of schwannomas, but not in solitary, sporadic schwannomas. Brain Pathol. 2008;18(4):517–9.
60. Caltabiano R, Magro G, Polizzi A, Praticó AD, Ortensi A, D'Orazi V, et al. A mosaic pattern of INI1/SMARCB1 protein expression distinguishes Schwannomatosis and NF2-associated peripheral schwannomas from solitary peripheral schwannomas and NF2-associated vestibular schwannomas. Childs Nerv Syst. 2017;33(6):933–40.
61. Paganini I, Chang VY, Capone GL, Vitte J, Benelli M, Barbetti L, et al. Expanding the mutational spectrum of LZTR1 in schwannomatosis. Eur J Human Genet [Internet]. 2015;23(7):963–8. https://doi.org/10.1038/ejhg.2014.220.
62. Macarenco RS, Ellinger F, Oliveira AM. Perineurioma: a distinctive and underrecognized peripheral nerve sheath neoplasm. Arch Pathol Lab Med. 2007;131(4):625–36.
63. Klein CJ, Wu Y, Jentoft ME, Mcr G, Spinner RJ, Dyck PJB, et al. Genomic analysis reveals frequent TRAF7 mutations in intraneural perineuriomas. Ann Neurol. 2017;81(2):316–21.
64. Carter JM, Wu Y, Blessing MM, Folpe AL, Thorland EC, Spinner RJ, et al. Recurrent genomic alterations in soft tissue perineuriomas. Am J Surg Pathol. 2018;42(12):1708–14.

3 Pathological Basis for Classification (Cytomolecular Aspects)

Gustavo Sevlever

The peripheral nervous system is a complex structure that includes neural tissue outside the central nervous system. It comprises somatic and autonomic nerves, receptors, and supporting structures. The axons are gradually coated with Schwann cells, originated from the neural crest, a highly migratory group of cells that arise from and lie lateral to the neural tube below the embryo's ectoderm.

The nerve fascicles are delimited by the epineurum, and each in turn is surrounded by a well-defined sheath known as the perineurium, arranged by layers of connective tissue, and multilayered, concentrically arranged flattened cells (Fig. 3.1). The perineurium, a histological continuum with the pia arachnoid of the central nervous system, is the principal component of the so-called blood-nerve barrier [1] and represents the principal diffusion barrier for the peripheral nerve. The perineurial cell is of mesodermal origin, and its phenotype is somehow similar to the cells of the pia arachnoid (S-100 protein negative, epithelial membrane antigen [EMA], GLUT1, and claudin-1 positive).

Tumors originating from the peripheral nerves exhibit some peculiar characteristics with some specificity within their taxonomic category: soft tissue tumors [2]. On the one hand, the extensive anatomical "capillary" distribution of the peripheral nervous system implies the potential presence of neoplasms in almost any location. On the other hand, concerning its histogenesis, most cells originate in the neural crest, while most of the soft tissue tumors derive from the mesoderm. The neoplastic transformation reflects the constituent cellular components, that is, the Schwann and perineurial cells. When these tumors grow inside a membrane formed by the perineurium, they have a true capsule, unlike most of the soft tissue tumors that seem to be encapsulated by the compression of adjacent tissues.

Another rather specific issue is the malignant transformation that is an eventual possibility in benign nerve sheath tumors. Some patients with neurofibromatosis 1 may develop sarcomas in a molecular defined pathway.

As usual in surgical pathology, peripheral nerve proliferative lesions are divided into non-neoplastic tumors (such as traumatic neuroma), benign tumors (such as schwannomas, neurofibromas, and perineuriomas), and malignant tumors, which are designated, as a whole, as malignant peripheral nerve sheath tumors (MPNSTs). These lesions may overlap and coexist with each other; nevertheless, their natural history is quite different.

In this chapter, we will discuss the classical histological types of the schwannomas and the neurofibromas originated in the cell types present in the peripheral nerve (Table 3.1).

G. Sevlever (✉)
Departamento de Neuropatología, Fleni, Buenos Aires, Argentina
e-mail: gsevlever@fleni.org.ar

F. Guedes et al. (eds.), *Diagnostic Assessment and Treatment of Peripheral Nerve Tumors*,
https://doi.org/10.1007/978-3-030-77633-6_3

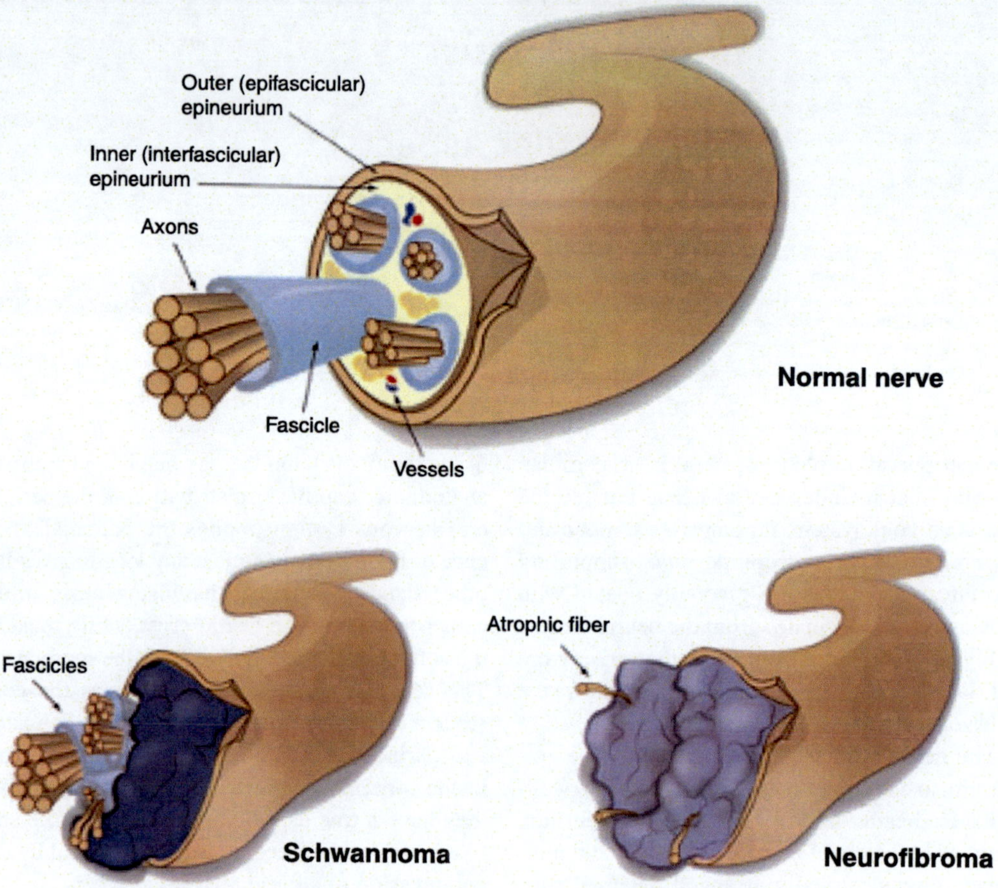

Fig. 3.1 Distribution of cellular elements in normal nerve, schwannoma, and neurofibroma

Table 3.1 Comparison of schwannoma and neurofibroma [3]

Schwannoma		Neurofibroma
Age	20–50 year	20–40 year.; younger in NF1
Common locations	Head and neck; flexor portion of extremities; retroperitoneum and mediastinum	Cutaneous nerves; deep locations in NF1
Encapsulation	Usually	Usually not
Growth patterns	Encapsulated tumor with Antoni A and B areas; plexiform type uncommon	Localized, diffuse, and plexiform patterns
Associated syndromes	Most lesions sporadic; some NF2 and schwannomatosis	Most lesions sporadic; some NF1
S-100 and SOX10 immunostain	Strong and uniform	Variable staining of cells
Malignant transformation	Exceptionally rare	Rare in sporadic cases but occurs in 2–3% of NF1 patients

3.1 Schwannomas (Neurilemmomas)

Schwannomas, formerly known as neurilemmomas (a term introduced by Stout in 1935), are common benign peripheral nerve sheath tumors composed of a relatively uniform population of cells showing schwannian differentiation [4].

Most of the cases (90%) are sporadic. In comparison, 3% are related to type 2 neurofibromatosis (caused by a germline mutation in the NF2 gene located on 22q12, which encodes merlin, also known as schwannomin), 2% in those with schwannomatosis, and 5% in association with multiple meningiomas in patients with or without NF2 [5].

Many distinct variants have been described, with a wide range of histologic appearances: ancient schwannoma [6], plexiform schwannoma [7], cellular schwannoma [8, 9], melanotic schwannoma [10], gastric schwannoma [11, 12], microcystic/reticular schwannoma [13], and epithelioid schwannoma [14, 15].

One defining characteristic of this oncotype is its tangential growth (Fig. 3.1). This feature is essential to understand that, until certain point, nerve conduction and function may be preserved.

This feature has surgical implications. The nerve of origin often can be macroscopically observed laterally, in the periphery (Figs. 3.2 and 3.3), related to the capsule but without penetrating the tumor. On the cut section, these tumors have a pink, white, or yellow appearance (Fig. 3.3). Larger tumors are more prone to manifest secondary degenerative changes such as cystification and calcification.

The characteristic histological image is a combination of two different patterns, Antoni A and B areas (Figs. 3.4, 3.5, and 3.6). The Antoni A zones, which may be predominant, are pretty cellular and compact, with spindle cells often organized in a palisading structure or in an organ-

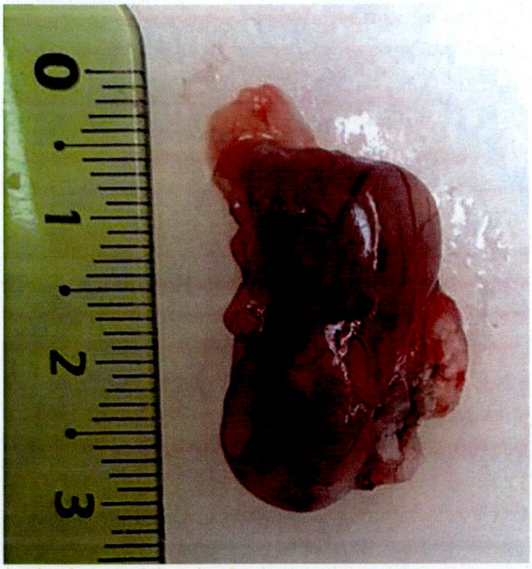

Fig. 3.2 Macroscopic view of a schwannoma. Note the tumor's capsule

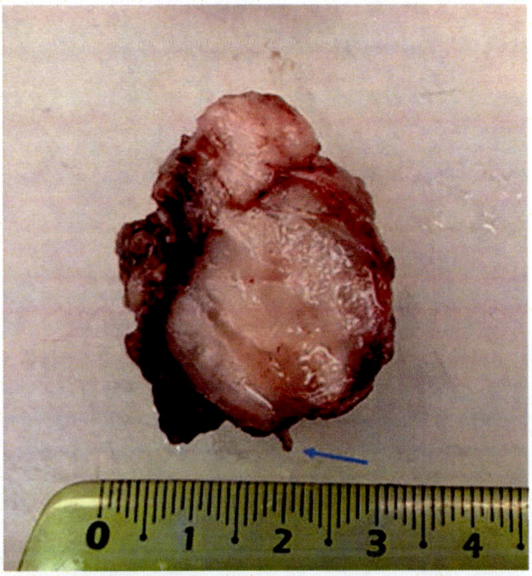

Fig. 3.3 Cut view of the same tumor. Arrow shows the peripheral nerve remnant

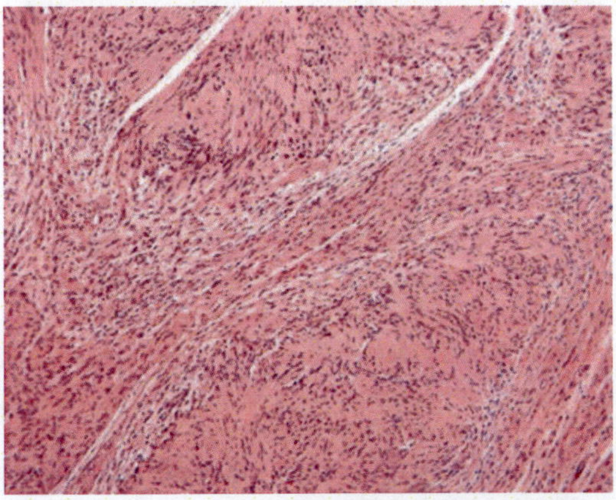

Fig. 3.4 Schwannoma: Antoni A areas and Verocay bodies. HE 400×

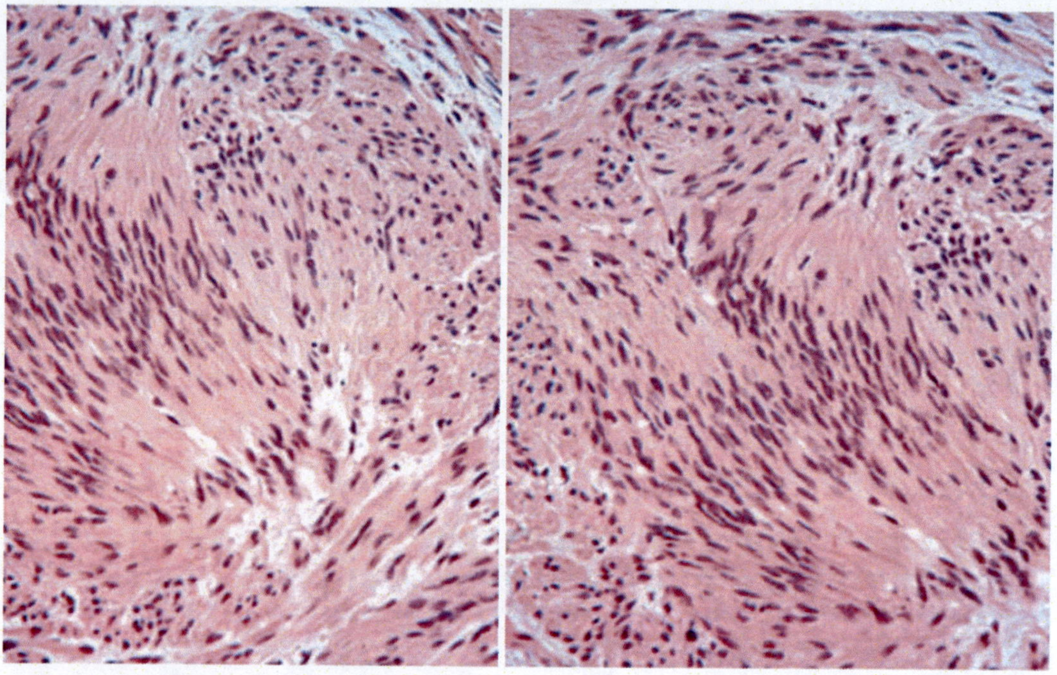

Fig. 3.5 Verocay bodies in Antoni A area. HE 400×

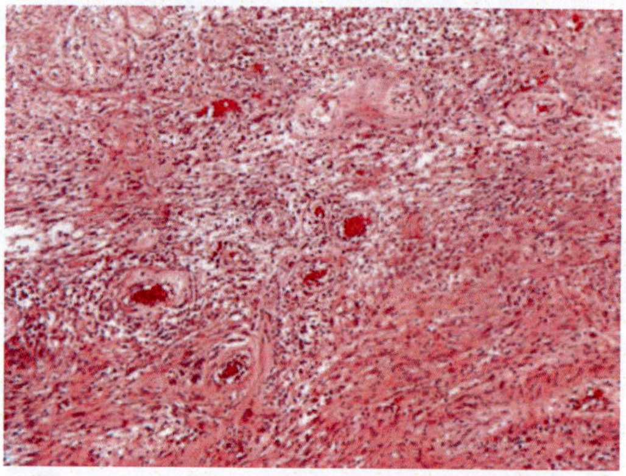

Fig. 3.6 Schwannoma: Antoni B areas. HE 200×

oid arrangement. The nuclei are ovoid with indistinct cytoplasmic borders. Verocay bodies are shaped by compact rows of well-aligned nuclei separated by fibrillary cell processes (Fig. 3.5).

In contrast, Antoni B zones are characterized by abundant edematous fluid that generates cystic spaces in a loosely textured matrix separating the tumor cells (Fig. 3.6). Both Antoni A and B tend to intermingle to varying degrees.

A unique diagnostic feature is the large vessels, which are characteristic of schwannomas and may exhibit luminal thrombosis and thicken fibrotic walls. They are more evident in the paucicellular Antoni B areas.

Ancient schwannoma is the name Ackerman and Taylor applied in 1951 [16] to define tumors with "*an intermingling of … the neurofibroma and the neurilemoma. We do not feel that such intermingling should be unexpected because of the common ancestry of both these tumors. For want of a better name, they were designated as ancient neurilemomas.*"

Curiously enough, this original description is more appropriate for the entity that we now call hybrid benign peripheral nerve sheath tumors. Nevertheless, time, habit, and medical literature stand out the "atypical," mostly nuclear changes that may be worrisome, raising the differential diagnoses with other sarcomatous entities. It is a general belief that these changes usually, as initially described, coexist with other degenerative ones as hyalinization, calcification, and hemorrhage, with the mentioned severe nuclear atypia.

The word "ancient" suggested by Ackerman and Taylor can be added to the diagnostic schwannoma to indicate that the histological findings are degenerative in nature and are not worrisome. These can be seen focally in "normal" schwannomas, as the result of long-term tumor growth and aging. Large numbers of siderophages and histiocytes usually infiltrate the tumor itself. These lesions behave as ordinary schwannomas; therefore, the nuclear atypia might be dismissed as a degenerative change. They have been described in a variety of organs and locations [17–20].

Figure 3.6 discloses degenerative changes and rare isolated cells with bizarre hyperchromatic nuclei with no clinical significance. Mitoses are rare.

The presence of "bona fide" epithelioid areas is a well-known histological component in schwannomas, although much less frequent than in neurofibroma and MPNST [21]. A predominance of these areas qualifies the tumor as benign epithelioid schwannoma. Curiously enough, almost 50% of these lesions showed loss of INI1 expression [22]. These lesions can rarely evolve into epithelioid MPNST, a pathway usually heralded by some striking cytologic atypia. Some schwannomas have been described that may even contain a glandular component [23] (benign glandular schwannomas).

Occasionally, some tumors disclose high cellularity, mitotic activity, and the presence of bone destruction. This histologic picture has been described as "cellular schwannoma" [24, 25]. Cellular schwannoma shares a similar age group as classic schwannoma but tends to develop in deep structures. Microscopically, Antoni A areas dominate the histologic picture, but small amounts of Antoni B may be present, usually not exceeding 10% of the lesion [3]. Mitotic activity may be observed but usually is low (<4 mitoses/10 high-power field) [9]. Focal areas of necrosis are seen in up to 10% of cases. Some discussion related to its true biological behavior is enriched by several extensive studies with adequate follow-up confirming their benignancy [9, 26]. More than 100 cases have been reported, fewer than 5% of patients had developed recurrences, and none had developed metastatic disease (Fig. 3.7).

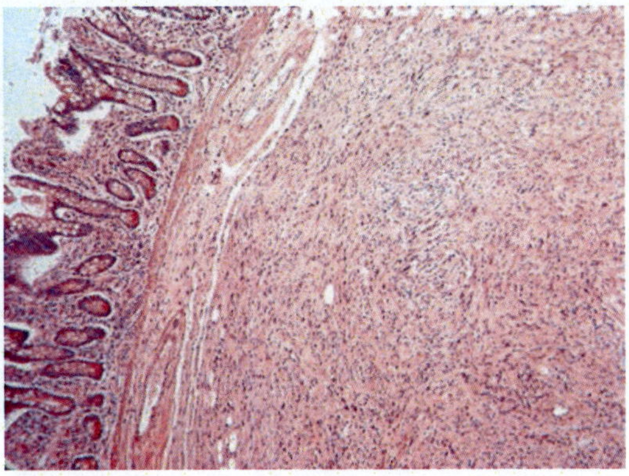

Fig. 3.7 Gastrointestinal schwannoma. HE 200×

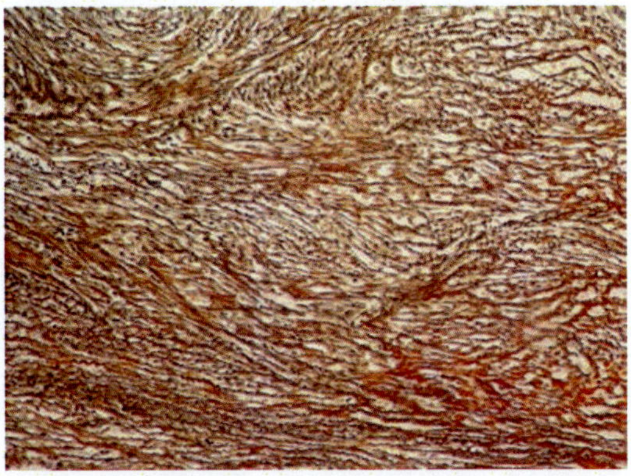

Fig. 3.8 Schwannoma: dense reticulin stain. HE 200×

3.2 Ancillary Techniques and Immunohistochemistry

A reticulin stain is most useful in diagnosis (Fig. 3.8). In a schwannoma, each cell is surrounded by basement membrane material, resulting in a dense array of reticulin fibers commonly presenting in parallel, slightly wavy bundles. When applied to this tumor, the silver impregnation method will outline the characteristic reticulin pattern for a quick diagnosis even, as described long ago, on frozen sections [27, 28].

The classical immunostain for schwannomas is S-100 protein, strongly expressed by most cells in a schwannoma (Fig. 3.9). It is problematic to support this diagnosis in the context of a negative stain for S-100. Neurofibroma cells, on the contrary, have variable staining. Sox10, a member of the sex-determining region Y-related HMG box family, is a neural crest stem cell marker. Nuclear staining for SOX10 has proved to be another excellent marker for schwannomas and is also expressed in the Schwann cell component of neurofibromas. In soft tissue neoplasms, Sox10 is significantly more specific than S-100 for peripheral nerve sheath tumors and should be used in place of or with S-100 for diagnostic purposes [29].

CD57 and glial fibrillary acidic protein (GFAP) are also present in these tumors, although their role is less relevant.

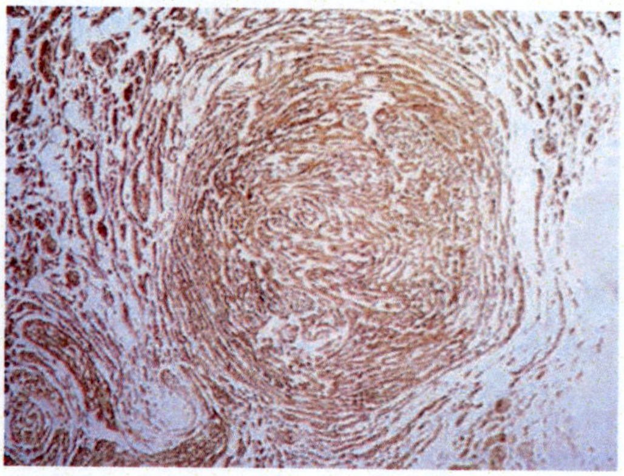

Fig. 3.9 Schwannoma: immunostaining for S-100. 200×

3.3 Neurofibroma

Neurofibromas are peripheral nerve sheath tumors with several clinicopathologic and anatomic variants, namely, localized cutaneous neurofibroma, diffuse cutaneous neurofibroma, localized intraneural neurofibroma, soft tissue neurofibroma, visceral neurofibroma, and plexiform neurofibromas (PN). PN involves multiple nerve fascicles, has complex shapes, grows more rapidly in young children, and can cause substantial morbidity, including pain and functional impairment [30].

Neurofibromas may assume one of the three growth patterns: localized, diffuse, and plexiform. The localized form is seen most often as a superficial, solitary tumor in healthy individuals. Diffuse and plexiform neurofibromas have a close association with neurofibromatosis 1 (NF1), the latter almost pathognomonic of the disease [20].

PN can transform to malignant peripheral nerve sheath tumors (MPNSTs), aggressive sarcomas associated with poor prognosis. The gross, microscopic, and immunophenotype features of neurofibroma, and its natural history, are distinct from those of schwannoma (Tables 3.1 and 3.2). In some instances, the differential diagnosis may be challenging, or in isolated cases, features of both lesions may coexist. The gross appearance of neurofibroma varies a great deal from lesion to lesion. As a rule, the tumors are not encapsulated and have a softer consistency than schwannoma. The more superficial tumors appear as small, soft, pedunculated nodules.

The histology of neurofibromas comprises a varied and combined proliferation of the elements usually present in a peripheral nerve: axons, Schwann cells, usually the predominant cellular element, fibroblasts, and sometimes perineurial cells, customarily in the plexiform type. Nuclei are very characteristic: significantly elongated, with a wavy, serpentine configuration and pointed ends [32] (Figs. 3.10, 3.11 and 3.12).

The stroma concentrates a definite network of collagen fibers combining the major types [33].

Other striking histological features are the prominent mucinous changes in the stroma that may result in a mistaken diagnosis of myxoma or even myxoid liposarcoma [34] and mast cells.

The typical histological attributes of schwannomas (capsule, Verocay bodies, fibrotic vessels, and Antoni A areas) are classically absent in neurofibromas.

As expected, the Schwann cells' component is immunoreactive for SOX10 and S-100 protein and surrounded by basement membrane components.

A small proportion (between 5% and 20%) of patients with type 1 neurofibromatosis develop MPNST.

Table 3.2 Pathologic and immunophenotypic features useful in the differential diagnosis of Schwann cell neoplasms [31]

	Neurofibroma	Schwannoma	MPNST
Cytology			
Nuclear size	+	++	+++
Nuclear hyperchromasia	+	++	+++
Wavy nuclei	+++	+	++
Histology			
"Shredded carrot"-type collagen	+++	–	–/+
Capsule	–	+++	–
Hyalinized vessels	–/+	+++	–
Fascicular growth pattern	–/+	++	+++
Mitotic activity	–/+	–/+	+++
Necrosis	–	–/+	+++
IHC marker			
S-100	++/+++	+++	+/++
Collagen IV	++/+++	+++	+/++
EMA	+	- (capsular)	- (except MPNST with perineurial diff)
CD34	+++	+++	++
Neurofilament protein	++	+ (rare intratumoral axons)	
Podoplanin	+	++	+
Calretinin	+	+++	NA
SOX10	+++	+++	+/++

+, ++, +++ Mean intensity of immunohistochemical reaction

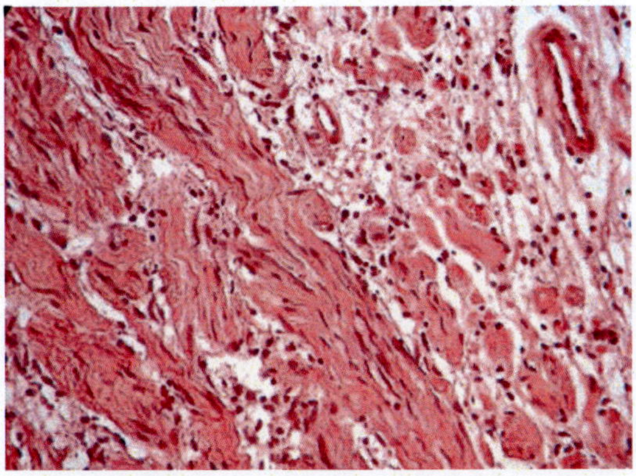

Fig. 3.10 Neurofibroma,interlacing bundles of elongated cells with wavy nuclei. The cells are intimately associated with wire-like strands of collagen

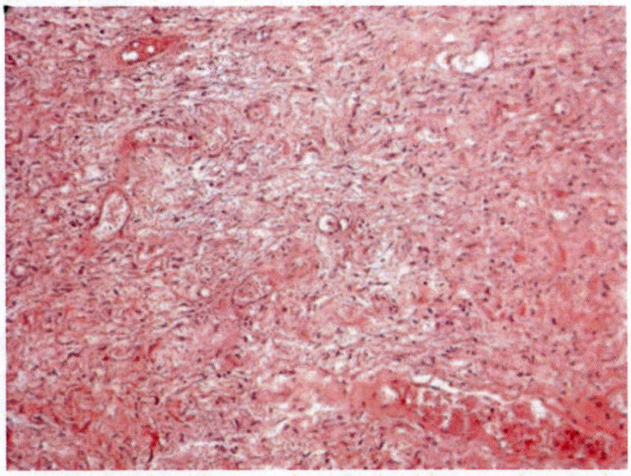

Fig. 3.11 Neurofibroma. Mucinous changes in the tumoral stroma. HE 200×

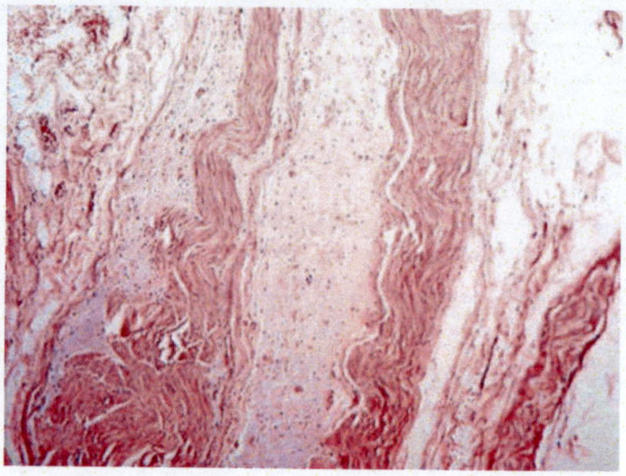

Fig. 3.12 Intraneural neurofibroma in a NF1 patient. HE 200×

Table 3.3 WHO classification on CNS tumors [31]

	WHO Code
Schwannomas	9560/0
Cellular schwannoma	9560/0
Plexiform schwannoma	9560/0
Melanotic schwannoma	9560/1
Neurofibroma	9540/0
Atypical neurofibroma	9540/0
Plexiform neurofibroma	9550/0
Perineurioma	9571/0
Hybrid nerve sheath tumors	
Malignant peripheral nerve sheath tumor	9540/3
Epithelioid MPNST	9540/3
MPNST with perineurial differentiation	9540/3

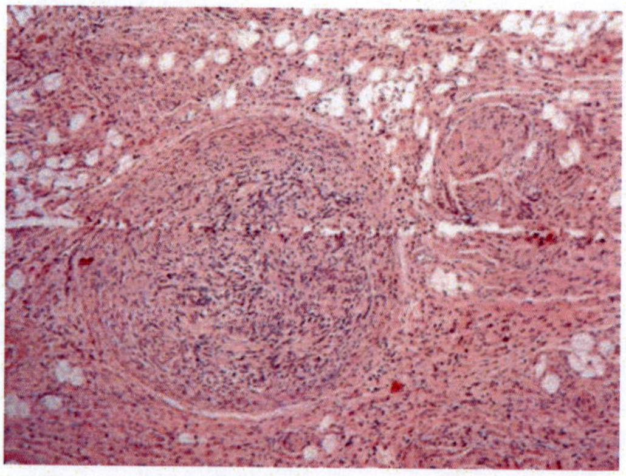

Fig. 3.13 Hybrid peripheral nerve sheath tumors. HE 200×

3.4 Hybrid Peripheral Nerve Sheath Tumors

Hybrid peripheral nerve sheath tumors (PNSTs) are benign peripheral nerve sheath tumors, which show combined features of more than one type of benign PNSTs, i.e., neurofibroma, schwannoma, and perineurioma. It was described initially by Feany [35] as tumors with predominant features of neurofibroma with distinct, often nodular regions of classical schwannomatous differentiation (Fig. 3.13). This concept was later expanded, describing further combinations; the most common types are schwannoma/perineurioma, which usually occurs sporadically, and neurofibroma/schwannoma, which is typically associated with neurofibromatosis (NF) type 1 or 2 or with schwannomatosis [36, 37].

These tumors have been recognized for some time but were only recently included officially in the fourth edition of the World Health Organization (WHO) Classification of Tumors of Soft tissue and Bone and the revised fourth edition of the WHO Classification of Tumors of the Central Nervous System (Table 3.3) published in 2013 and 2016, respectively [31, 38]. They are generally recognized as a benign entity. Nevertheless, those associated with NF1 carry a risk of malignant transformation to MPNSTs [39].

In a methylation-based classification study of a large cohort (171 cases) of benign and malignant peripheral nerve sheath tumors that included 7 hybrid neurofibroma/schwannoma, they clustered mostly as schwannomas, but some cases clustered as atypical neurofibromas. Moreover, four cases exhibit 22q loss, while three showed retained 22q [40].

3.5 Perineurioma

Perineurioma is a soft tissue tumor composed of cells resembling normal perineurium [39]. It was initially described by Lazarus and Trombetta [41] in 1978 based on ultrastructural findings. Histological diagnosis is complex, due to the inability to diagnose the lesion by light microscopy alone. More recently, the incorporation of

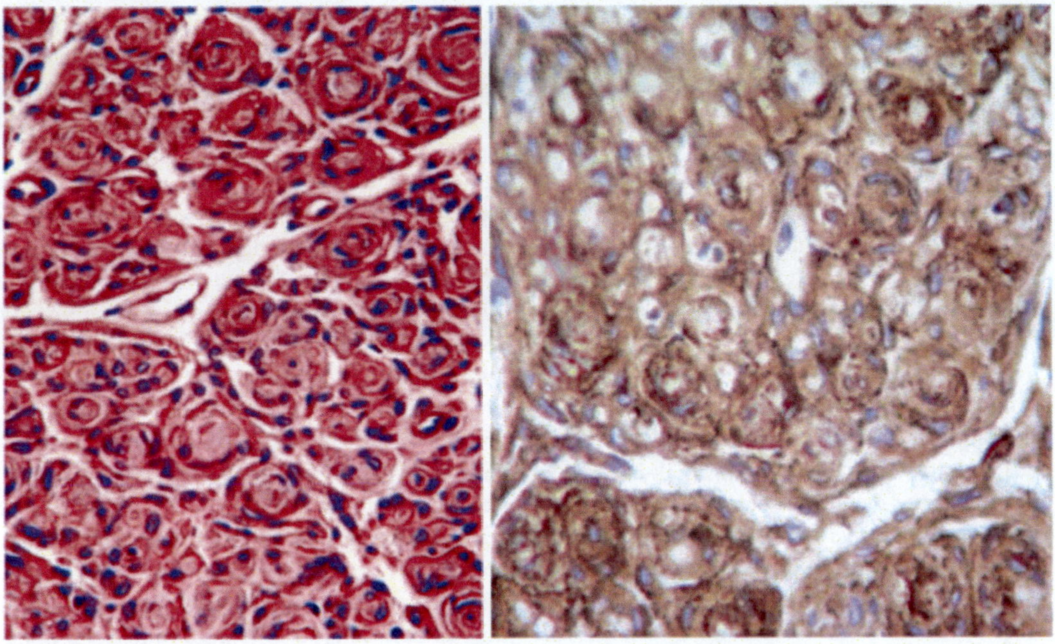

Fig. 3.14 Perineurioma: the entire nerve is expanded by the formation of tiny "onion bulbs" consisting of concentric layers of perineurial cells ensheathing a central axon and Schwann cell. HE (14a) and immunostaining for EMA (14b)

immunohistochemical markers related to perineurial differentiation has resulted in a more restricted and consistent diagnosis. They are still much less common than neurofibromas and schwannomas. On cross section of the intraneural type, the entire nerve is expanded by forming tiny "onion bulbs" consisting of concentric layers of perineurial cells ensheathing a central axon and Schwann cell (Fig. 3.14). Because of these lesions' highly organized nature, the general impression is that of a reactive or reparative process. There are principally three forms of perineurioma: intraneural, extraneural (soft tissue), and sclerosing. By definition, all benign perineuriomas are EMA positive and S-100 protein/SOX10 negative, an immunophenotype that mirrors the normal perineurial cell. Besides, the majority of perineuriomas also express claudin-1 (tight junction-associated protein) and GLUT1 (human erythrocyte glucose transporter), barrier function proteins present in normal perineurial cells [4].

With immunostains for EMA and S-100 protein, the striking preponderance of perineurial cells becomes readily apparent. EMA highlights the ensheathing perineurial cells, leaving the central portion of the onion bulb devoid of staining (Fig. 3.14). With S-100 protein and neurofilament protein immunostains, highlighting Schwann cells and axons, a reverse staining pattern is noted.

Perineurioma is a benign tumor. Most perineuriomas possess little or no atypia and no mitotic activity. However, some (<20%) may show atypical features, even some mitotic activity (up to 13 figures/30 high-power field), scattered pleomorphic cells, and/or hypercellular foci. Perineuriomas with these atypical features do not differ from typical cases [42].

3.6 Malignant Changes

As previously described, the malignant change is a relatively well-known phenomenon related to NF1.

Nevertheless, there are some transitional entities that deserve a short paragraph.

Atypical neurofibroma (ANF) is a recently described entity, reported as a precursor lesion for MPNST [43]. It consists of morphologically defined lesions with increased cellularity, cytological atypia, and pronounced fascicular growth patterns without the widespread atypia and fascicular growth, mitotic activity, and necrosis seen in MPNST [44, 45]. A deletion at 9p21.3, which includes gene CDKN2A/2B, was identified in 15/16 (94%) ANF and in 16/23 (70%) high-grade MPNST but not in PN [32]. This makes early detection and management of ANF a possible strategy to prevent MPNST.

Nevertheless, the problem of defining the histopathological spectrum of the transition from a benign plexiform neurofibroma to an MPNST is most relevant in patients with NF1. Especially complex is the distinction between neurofibroma with atypia (reactive or degenerative) and early transformation into MPNST. The spectrum of changes from plexiform neurofibroma to high-grade MPNST includes challenging lesions. The recent consensus about the "atypical neurofibromatous neoplasms" is a contribution to refining the diagnosis of these ambiguous neoplasms. As the authors stated, "We have therefore recommended a new category designated as 'atypical neurofibromatous neoplasm of uncertain biologic potential' for the tumors that show some worrisome features of malignant transformation, but histologically fall short of MPNST." The proposed histological definition is neurofibromatous tumors with nuclear atypia, hypercellularity, variable loss of neurofibroma architecture (e.g., herringbone or storiform-fascicular growth and/or loss of CD34-positive network), and/or mitotic activity beyond isolated mitotic figures (>1/50 high-power fields [HPFs] and <3/10 HPFs) should be designated as having uncertain malignant potential when at least two of these features are present [46].

3.7 Malignant Peripheral Nerve Sheath Tumor

The lifetime incidence of developing MPNST in patients with NF1 is 8%–15.8% compared with an incidence of 0.001% in the general population [47–49]. Each NF1 patient has an estimated 8–13% cumulative risk of developing a MPNST. This risk is even two or three times higher in patients with an NF1 microdeletion than patients with an intragenic NF1 mutation [50].

In NF1, MPNSTs occur at a younger age, and the majority arise in preexisting PN [51, 52]. They can present with enlarging mass, pain, and neurological deficit, but these symptoms often overlap and are difficult to distinguish from benign PN. The prognosis for MPNST in individuals with NF1 is poor, with a 5-year overall survival of 35%–50%. To date, complete surgical resection with wide negative margins is the only curative treatment, making early detection important.

This name, MPNST, is the currently preferred term for the neoplasm, after several controversies, also known over the years as malignant schwannoma, neurogenic sarcoma, and neurofibrosarcoma. Approximately half of these tumors arise de novo and the other half from neurofibromas as part of type 1 neurofibromatosis. Some arise in areas of previous irradiation typically after a latent period of at least 10 years [53].

MPNST histological diagnosis is a difficult task, with eventual errors diagnosing MPNST as some other type of soft tissue sarcoma. The clinicopathological correlation may be helpful in this context. Two features may bring this diagnosis as a primary option: (a) spindle cell tumor in a patient with NF1 and (b) a clearly defined anatomical relationship with a major nerve or continuity with a neurofibroma.

Most MPNSTs resemble adult-type fibrosarcomas in their overall organization, with certain modifications. Unlike the symmetrically spindle cells of adult-type fibrosarcoma, they have irregular contours (Fig. 3.15). In profile, the nuclei are wavy, buckled, or comma-shaped, whereas when viewed en face, they are asymmetrically oval. The cytoplasm is lightly stained and usually indistinct. The cells can range from spindle in shape to fusiform or even rounded [4].

Histological features are not entirely specific. They comprise fascicles of alternating cellularity, whorls, palisades or rosette-like arrangements, perineural/intraneural spread when associated with nerve, subendothelial accentuation of tumor cells, and large areas of geographic-like necrosis [54, 55].

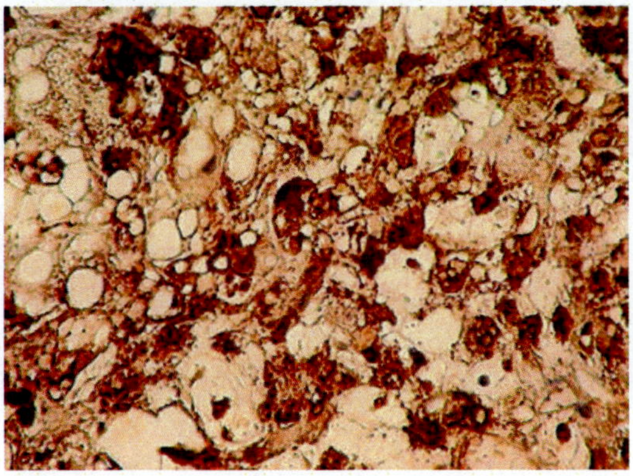

Fig. 3.15 Malignant nerve sheath tumor. Immunostaining for S-100. 400×

MPNST may disclose divergent differentiation [56] in the form of bone, cartilage, or skeletal muscle [57], a combination that has been referred to as malignant Triton tumor [58], smooth muscle [59], angiosarcoma [60], perineurial differentiation, and even glands [61]. The finding of heterologous elements in a monomorphic spindle cell sarcoma should suggest the diagnosis of MPNST [3].

Immunostaining of MPNST lacks a diagnostic immunophenotype. The majority of these tumors stain for S-100 protein, in a focal pattern [62]. SOX10, the other schwannian marker, is positive even in those S-100 negative [63]. CD34 and EMA, when present, may represent the immunomarker of perineurial differentiation.

Recently, the loss of histone H3K27 trimethylation by immunostaining has been described as a highly specific, not particularly sensitive marker of MPNST [64].

The protein product of the NF1 gene, neurofibromin, discloses the loss of expression in 88% of NF1-associated and 43% of sporadic MPNST [65] and in malignant triton tumors [66] but not in a large number of other tested sarcomas, except for rare myxofibrosarcomas, pleomorphic liposarcomas, leiomyosarcomas, and undifferentiated pleomorphic sarcomas [54]. This lack of expression helps in the differential diagnosis of MPNST from cellular schwannoma, which shows retained expression [67], but is not useful in the differential diagnoses of MPNST from spindle cell/desmoplastic melanoma, which frequently harbors NF1 mutations and is neurofibromin negative in up to 70% of cases [68].

MPNST grading is a hard task. Standardized evaluation is lacking at present. It becomes a common practice to divide these tumors into low grade (15% approximately) and high grade (85% approximately). The high-grade definition includes cytologic atypia, mitotic activity (>5 per 10 high-power fields), and hypercellularity with or without necrosis.

Furthermore, standard recognized grading schemes may be utilized as the French FNCLCC grading system [69].

3.8 Next Roads to be Traveled

Several molecular approaches are emerging, analyzing the neoplastic biology of nerve sheath tumors and defining biomarkers and treatment targets.

MicroRNAs (miRNAs) are a class of small non-protein-coding RNAs of approximately 19–26 nucleotides in length that function in post-transcriptional gene regulation. Azadeh Amirnasr et al. investigated the role of these molecules as biomarkers and molecular and found that plexiform neurofibromas can be distinguished from MPNST by their microRNA expression profile [70]. Other areas of research are related to the molecular identification of therapy targets [71].

Integrating of all the different data from diverse sources is one of the main challenges of the translational understanding of neoplasia. The recent creation of The Genomics of Malignant Peripheral Nerve Sheath Tumor (GeM) Consortium [72] as an international collaboration focusing on the multi-omics analysis of malignant peripheral nerve sheath is a welcome contribution to this task. Greater availability of molecular techniques also provides an opportunity to refine morphologic diagnoses and is likely to play an increasingly important role in the immediate future.

Hopefully, our knowledge will improve our actual classification systems, including and defining biomarkers and treatment targets.

References

1. Weerasuriya A, Mizisin AP. The blood-nerve barrier: structure and functional significance. Methods Mol Biol. 2011;686:149–73. https://doi.org/10.1007/978-1-60761-938-3_6.
2. Meyer A, Billings SD. What's new in nerve sheath tumors. Virchows Arch. 2020;476(1):65–80. https://doi.org/10.1007/s00428-019-02671-0.
3. Goldblum J, Weiss S, Folpe AL. Enzinger and Weiss's soft tissue tumors. 7th ed. Elsevier. Published Date: 11th November 2019.
4. Hornick, Jason L. Practical soft tissue pathology: a diagnostic approach E-book (pattern recognition) (p. 119). Elsevier Health Sciences.
5. Antinheimo J, Sankila R, Carpén O, et al. Population-based analysis of sporadic and type 2 neurofibromatosis-associated meningiomas and schwannomas. Neurology. 2000;54(1):71–6.
6. Dahl I. Ancient neurilemmoma (schwannoma). Acta Pathol Microbiol Scand A. 1977;85:812–8.
7. Agaram NP, Prakash S, Antonescu CR. Deep-seated plexiform schwannoma: a pathologic study of 16 cases and comparative analysis with the superficial variety. Am J Surg Pathol. 2005;29:1042–8.
8. Fletcher CD, Davies SE, McKee PH. Cellular schwannoma: a distinct pseudosarcomatous entity. Histopathology. 1987;11:21–35.
9. White W, Shiu MH, Rosenblum MK, et al. Cellular schwannoma. A clinicopathologic study of 57 patients and 58 tumors. Cancer. 1990;66:1266–75.
10. Killeen RM, Davy CL, Bauserman SC. Melanocytic schwannoma. Cancer. 1988;62:174–83.
11. Daimaru Y, Kido H, Hashimoto H, et al. Benign schwannoma of the gastrointestinal tract: a clinicopathologic and immunohistochemical study. Hum Pathol. 1988;19:257–64; 207.
12. Hou YY, Tan YS, Xu JF, et al. Schwannoma of the gastrointestinal tract: a clinicopathological, immunohistochemical and ultrastructural study of 33 cases. Histopathology. 2006;48:536–45.
13. Liegl B, Bennett MW, Fletcher CD. Microcystic/reticular schwannoma: a distinct variant with predilection for visceral locations. Am J Surg Pathol. 2008;32:1080–7.
14. Kindblom LG, Meis-Kindblom JM, Havel G, et al. Benign epithelioid schwannoma. Am J Surg Pathol. 1998;22:762–70.
15. Laskin WB, Fetsch JF, Lasota J, et al. Benign epithelioid peripheral nerve sheath tumors of the soft tissues: clinicopathologic spectrum of 33 cases. Am J Surg Pathol. 2005;29:39–51.
16. ACKERMAN LV, TAYLOR FH. Neurogenous tumors within the thorax; a clinicopathological evaluation of forty-eight cases. Cancer. 1951;4(4):669–91. https://doi.org/10.1002/1097-0142(195107)4:4<669::aid-cncr2820040405>3.0.co;2-b.
17. de Bakker JK, Witteveen E, van den Bergh J, Daams F. Ancient schwannoma of the gallbladder. ACG Case Rep J. 2020;7(2):e00330. Published 2020 Feb 28. https://doi.org/10.14309/crj.0000000000000330.
18. Yaslikaya S, Kizilay A, Şamdanci E. Endoscopic Transoral resection of Tongue Base ancient schwannoma. J Craniofac Surg. 2020;31(4):e409–11. https://doi.org/10.1097/SCS.0000000000006416.
19. Ho CF, Wu PW, Lee TJ, Huang CC. "Ancient" schwannoma of the submandibular gland: A case report and literature review. Medicine (Baltimore). 2017;96(51):e9134. https://doi.org/10.1097/MD.0000000000009134.
20. Bindra R, Gupta S, Gupta N, Asotra S, Sharma A. Ancient schwannoma of the neck mimicking soft tissue sarcoma. J Cancer Res Ther. 2010;6(2):234–5. https://doi.org/10.4103/0973-1482.65234.
21. Laskin WB, Fetsch JF, Lasota J, Miettinen M. Benign epithelioid peripheral nerve sheath tumors of the soft tissues: clinicopathologic spectrum of 33 cases. Am J Surg Pathol. 2005;29(1):39–51.
22. Jo VY, Fletcher CDM. SMARCB1/INI1 loss in epithelioid schwannoma: a clinicopathologic and immunohistochemical study of 65 cases. Am J Surg Pathol. 2017;41(8):1013–22.
23. Chuang S-T, Wang HL. An unusual case of glandular schwannoma. Hum Pathol. 2007;38(4):673–7.
24. Woodruff JM, Godwin TA, Erlandson RA, et al. Cellular schwannoma: a variety of schwannoma sometimes mistaken for a malignant tumor. Am J Surg Pathol. 1981;5(8):733–44.
25. Casadei GP, Scheithauer BW, Hirose T, et al. Cellular schwannoma: a clinicopathologic, DNA flow cytometric, and proliferation marker study of 70 patients. Cancer. 1995;75(5):1109–19.
26. Lodding P, Kindblom LG, Angervall L, et al. Cellular schwannoma: a clinicopathologic study of 29 cases. Virchows Arch. 1990;416(3):237–48.
27. Kepes JJ, Morantz RA, England AM. Reticulin stain in differentiating astrocytomas from neurilemmomas on frozen sections. Technical note. J Neurosurg. 1979;51(1):124–5. https://doi.org/10.3171/jns.1979.51.1.0124.
28. Kudo M, Mikami T, Maeda Y. Reticulin fiber staining of crush preparations for the rapid differentiation between schwannomas and meningiomas. Acta Cytol. 1991;35(5):521–3.
29. Karamchandani JR, Nielsen TO, van de Rijn M, West RB. Sox10 and S100 in the diagnosis of soft-tissue neoplasms. Appl Immunohistochem Mol Morphol. 2012;20(5):445–50. https://doi.org/10.1097/pai.0b013e318244ff4b.
30. Higham CS, Dombi E, Rogiers A, et al. The characteristics of 76 atypical neurofibromas as precursors to neurofibromatosis 1 associated malignant peripheral nerve sheath tumors. Neuro-Oncology. 2018;20(6):818–25. https://doi.org/10.1093/neuonc/noy013.
31. Hornick JL, Michal M. Hybrid nerve sheath tumors. In: Fletcher CDM, Bridge JA, Hogendoorn PCW, Mertens F, editors. WHO classification of tumors of soft tissue and bone. 4th ed. Lyon: IARC; 2013.

32. Goldblum JR, Lamps LW, McKenney J, Myers JL. Rosai and Ackerman's surgical pathology—2 volume set. 11th ed. Elsevier.
33. Chanoki M, Ishii M, Fukai K, et al. Immunohistochemical localization of type I, III, IV, V, and VI collagens and laminin in neurofibroma and neurofibrosarcoma. Am J Dermatopathol. 1991;13(4):365–73.
34. Megahed M. Histopathological variants of neurofibroma. A study of 114 lesions. Am J Dermatopathol. 1994;16(5):486–95.
35. Feany MB, Anthony DC, Fletcher CD. Nerve sheath tumours with hybrid features of neurofibroma and schwannoma: a conceptual challenge. Histopathology. 1998;32:405–10.
36. Harder A, Wesemann M, Hagel C, Schittenhelm J, Fischer S, et al. Hybrid neurofibroma/schwannoma is overrepresented among schwannomatosis and neurofibromatosis patients. Am J Surg Pathol. 2012;36:702–9.
37. Ud Din N, Ahmad Z, Abdul-Ghafar J, Ahmed R. Hybrid peripheral nerve sheath tumors: report of five cases and detailed review of literature. BMC Cancer. 2017;17(1):349. Published 2017 May 19. https://doi.org/10.1186/s12885-017-3350-1.
38. Antonescu CR, Stemmer-Rachamimov AO, Perry A. Hybrid nerve sheath tumors. In: Louis DN, Ohgaki H, Wiestler OD, Cavenec WK, Ellison DW, et al., editors. WHO classification of tumors of the central nervous system revised. 4th ed. Lyon: IARC; 2016. p. 224–5.
39. Kacerovska D, Michal M, Kuroda N, Tanaka A, Sima R, Denisjuk N, Kreuzberg B, Ricarova R, Kazakov DV. Hybrid peripheral nerve sheath tumors, including a malignant variant in type 1 neurofibromatosis. Am J Dermatopathol. 2013 Aug;35(6):641–9. https://doi.org/10.1097/DAD.0b013e31827e2917. PMID: 23676318
40. Röhrich M, Koelsche C, Schrimpf D, Capper D, Sahm F, Kratz A, Reuss J, Hovestadt V, Jones DT, Bewerunge-Hudler M, Becker A, Weis J, Mawrin C, Mittelbronn M, Perry A, Mautner VF, Mechtersheimer G, Hartmann C, Okuducu AF, Arp M, Seiz-Rosenhagen M, Hänggi D, Heim S, Paulus W, Schittenhelm J, Ahmadi R, Herold-Mende C, Unterberg A, Pfister SM, von Deimling A, Reuss DE. Methylation-based classification of benign and malignant peripheral nerve sheath tumors. Acta Neuropathol. 2016 Jun;131(6):877–87. https://doi.org/10.1007/s00401-016-1540-6. Epub 2016 Feb 8. PMID: 26857854
41. Lazarus SS, Trombetta LD. Ultrastructural identification of a benign perineurial cell tumor. Cancer. 1978;41(5):1823–9.
42. Hornick JL, Fletcher CD. Soft tissue perineurioma: clinicopathologic analysis of 81 cases including those with atypical histologic features. Am J Surg Pathol. 2005;29(7):845–58.
43. Beert E, Brems H, Daniëls B, et al. Atypical neurofibromas in neurofibromatosis type 1 are premalignant tumors. Genes Chromosomes Cancer. 2011;50(12):1021–32.
44. Rodriguez FJ, Folpe AL, Giannini C, Perry A. Pathology of peripheral nerve sheath tumors: diagnostic overview and update on selected diagnostic problems. Acta Neuropathol. 2012;123(3):295–319.
45. Bernthal NM, Jones KB, Monument MJ, Liu T, Viskochil D, Randall RL. Lost in translation: ambiguity in nerve sheath tumor nomenclature and its resultant treatment effect. Cancers (Basel). 2013;5(2):519–28.
46. Miettinen MM, Antonescu CR, Fletcher CDM, et al. Histopathologic evaluation of atypical neurofibromatous tumors and their transformation into malignant peripheral nerve sheath tumor in patients with neurofibromatosis 1-a consensus overview. Hum Pathol. 2017;67:1–10. https://doi.org/10.1016/j.humpath.2017.05.010.
47. Evans DG, Baser ME, McGaughran J, Sharif S, Howard E, Moran A. Malignant peripheral nerve sheath tumours in neurofibromatosis 1. J Med Genet. 2002;39(5):311–4.
48. Ferner RE, Gutmann DH. International consensus statement on malignant peripheral nerve sheath tumors in neurofibromatosis. Cancer Res. 2002;62(5):1573–7.
49. Uusitalo E, Rantanen M, Kallionpää RA, et al. Distinctive cancer associations in patients with neurofibromatosis type 1. J Clin Oncol. 2016;34(17):1978–86.
50. De Raedt T, Brems H, Wolkenstein P, et al. Elevated risk for MPNST in NF1 microdeletion patients. Am J Hum Genet. 2003;72(5):1288–92. https://doi.org/10.1086/374821.
51. King AA, Debaun MR, Riccardi VM, Gutmann DH. Malignant peripheral nerve sheath tumors in neurofibromatosis 1. Am J Med Genet. 2000;93(5):388–92.
52. Zhou H, Coffin CM, Perkins SL, Tripp SR, Liew M, Viskochil DH. Malignant peripheral nerve sheath tumor: a comparison of grade, immunophenotype, and cell cycle/growth activation marker expression in sporadic and neurofibromatosis 1-related lesions. Am J Surg Pathol. 2003;27(10):1337–45.
53. Ducatman BS, Scheithauer BW, Piepgras DG, et al. Malignant peripheral nerve sheath tumors. A clinicopathologic study of 120 cases. Cancer. 1986;57(10):2006–21.
54. Hruban RH, Shiu MH, Senie RT, Woodruff JM. Malignant peripheral nerve sheath tumors of the buttock and lower extremity. A study of 43 cases. Cancer. 1990;66:1253–65.
55. Scheithauer BW, Woodruff JM, Erlandson RA. Tumors of the peripheral nervous system. Washington, DC: Armed Forces Institute of Pathology; 1997.
56. Ducatman BS, Scheithauer BW. Malignant peripheral nerve sheath tumors with divergent differentiation. Cancer. 1984;54:1049–57.
57. Rose DS, Wilkins MJ, Birch R, Evans DJ. Malignant peripheral nerve sheath tumour with rhabdomyoblastic and glandular differentiation: immunohistochemical features. Histopathology. 1992;21:287–90.

58. Woodruff JM, Perino G. Non-germ-cell or teratomatous malignant tumors showing additional rhabdomyoblastic differentiation, with emphasis on the malignant triton tumor. Semin Diagn Pathol. 1994;11:69–81.
59. Rodriguez FJ, Scheithauer BW, Abell-Aleff PC, Elamin E, Erlandson RA. Low grade malignant peripheral nerve sheath tumor with smooth muscle differentiation. Acta Neuropathol. 2007;113:705–9.
60. Brown RW, Tornos C, Evans HL. Angiosarcoma arising from malignant schwannoma in a patient with neurofibromatosis. Cancer. 1992;70:1141–4.
61. Woodruff JM, Christensen WN. Glandular peripheral nerve sheath tumors. Cancer. 1993;72:3618–28.
62. Weiss SW, Langloss JM, Enzinger FM. Value of S-100 protein in the diagnosis of soft tissue tumors with particular reference to benign and malignant Schwann cell tumors. Lab Investig. 1983;49(3):299–308.
63. Nonaka D, Chiriboga L, Rubin BP. Sox10: a pan-schwannian and melanocytic marker. Am J Surg Pathol. 2008;32(9):1291–8.
64. Schaefer IM, Fletcher CD, Hornick JL. Loss of H3K27 trimethylation distinguishes malignant peripheral nerve sheath tumors from histologic mimics. Mod Pathol. 2016;29(1):4–13.
65. Reuss DE, Habel A, Hagenlocher C, et al. Neurofibromin specific antibody differentiates malignant peripheral nerve sheath tumors (MPNST) from other spindle cell neoplasms. Acta Neuropathol. 2014;127(4):565–72.
66. Röhrich M, Koelsche C, Schrimpf D, et al. Methylation-based classification of benign and malignant peripheral nerve sheath tumors. Acta Neuropathol. 2016;131(6):877–87. https://doi.org/10.1007/s00401-016-1540-6.
67. Pekmezci M, Reuss DE, Hirbe AC, et al. Morphologic and immunohistochemical features of malignant peripheral nerve sheath tumors and cellular schwannomas. Mod Pathol. 2015;28(2):187–200.
68. Kadokura A, Frydenlund N, Leone DA, et al. Neurofibromin protein loss in desmoplastic melanoma subtypes: implicating NF1 allelic loss as a distinct genetic driver? Hum Pathol. 2016;53:82–90.
69. Coindre JM. Grading of soft tissue sarcomas: review and update. Arch Pathol Lab Med. 2006;130:1448–53.
70. Amirnasr A, Verdijk RM, van Kuijk PF, et al. Deregulated microRNAs in neurofibromatosis type 1 derived malignant peripheral nerve sheath tumors. Sci Rep. 2020;10(1):2927. Published 2020 Feb 19. https://doi.org/10.1038/s41598-020-59789-4.
71. Binobaid L, Masternak MM. Molecular targets for NF1-associated malignant peripheral nerve sheath tumor. Rep Pract Oncol Radiother. 2020;25(4):556–61. https://doi.org/10.1016/j.rpor.2020.04.010.
72. Miller DT, Cortés-Ciriano I, Pillay N, et al. Genomics of MPNST (GeM) Consortium: Rationale and Study Design for Multi-Omic Characterization of NF1-Associated and Sporadic MPNSTs. Genes (Basel). 2020;11(4):387. Published 2020 Apr 2. https://doi.org/10.3390/genes11040387.

4 Clinical Assessment

Thomas Kretschmer, Christian Heinen, and Jakob Kraschl

Clinical assessment aims at:

1. Taking the specific history, evaluating clinical sensorimotor nerve status, and scrutinizing the presence and characteristics of associated pain
2. Discerning nerve tumor from other masses
3. Raising suspicion for or excluding potential malignancy
4. Systematically accumulating, interpreting, and analyzing findings in order to trigger next steps

Basically this is either surgery or follow-up.

There are only a few but important points in the clinical assessment of peripheral nerve tumors. In essence, taking the patient's history is focused on first subjective detection of mass, changes ever since, and observed speed of growth, as well as neurological deficits and presence of pain (Table 4.1).

Clinical assessment is mainly directed toward the identification that a growing mass possibly originates from neural elements in order to prevent treatment led by principles of sarcoma surgery, which would imply excision with tumor-free margins at the cost of function. Clinical presentation will also guide clinical decision, as it may be indicative of malignancy or not.

Table 4.1 Different aspects important for taking history in nerve tumor patients

Family history	Known NF1, genetic disorder?
Specific history of disease	Onset, mass discovered when, observed growth rate, neurological deficit noticed?
Medical history	Previous surgery elsewhere (reports), previous imaging, multiple surgeries in NF?
Pain history	Painful, progressive pain, spontaneous/resting pain vs discomfort/tenderness during touch/activity, pain suggestive of MPNST, inflammation or lymphomatosis of nerve? If the pain is radiating, the location of radiation may provide information on the likely nerve of origin

Most peripheral nerve tumors (PNT) are benign and can be extirpated with maintained function. So it is pivotal to have knowledge of the few clinical clues that point toward potential malignancy, which is relatively rare. To date, resting pain is still the clinical sign of highest significance when it comes to suspicion of malignancy in nerve tumors [1, 2]. Although the size of the lesion may not always be accurately measured during clinical assessment, a nerve tumor larger than 5 cm per se is suspicious of malignancy until proven otherwise [3].

T. Kretschmer (✉) · J. Kraschl
Department of Neurosurgery and Neurorestoration, Klinikum Klagenfurt, Klagenfurt, Austria
e-mail: Thomas.kretschmer@kabeg.at

C. Heinen
Center of Neuro-, Spine- and Nerve Surgery, Christliches Krankenhaus Quakenbrück, Quakenbrück, Germany

F. Guedes et al. (eds.), *Diagnostic Assessment and Treatment of Peripheral Nerve Tumors*,
https://doi.org/10.1007/978-3-030-77633-6_4

Regarding the importance and detailed technique of examination of single nerves or the plexus, we refer to the abundant text material available elsewhere [4], as it also applies to the examination of the parent nerve harboring the growth in question. It is necessary to rule out or document hypesthesia or motor loss attributable to the parent nerve. Apart from being locally tender, circumscribed hypesthesia and a motor deficit would be more unusual for a moderate-sized (e.g., 1–2 cm) benign peripheral nerve sheath tumor (PNST) of a peripheral nerve (not in the plexus). Tenderness to touch and electrifying dysesthesia, however, are also frequent signs of benign nerve tumor. These signs are more prominent when the growth lies within a tight compartment, close to joints, or is in a location where clothing directly compresses the nerve mass (e.g., ankle region, tibial nerve close to tarsal tunnel and rim of shoes, or popliteal fossa and tight pants, axilla and weight training, buttocks/sciatic nerve and rowing, etc.). Other important clinical aspects are directly related to imaging, and are not really discernible from clinical assessment, as they go hand in hand. This is why we will also give a more general outline on them. For elaboration on further imaging details, we refer to the distinct and in-depth chapters following.

4.1 Physical Examination and Case Presentation

On examination, benign PNSTs are typically mobile. A positive Tinel sign, elicited while tapping on the mass with electrifying paresthesias along the course of the parent nerve, is common. A fixed mass indicates a more aggressive growth pattern. The general terms of any clinical exam with regard to nerve apply: inspection, palpation, evaluation of passive joint mobility, and motor, sensory, and reflex exam are necessary parts of the clinical assessment. These are adjusted to the location. Considering topographical anatomy enables us to focus the exam. A systematic approach using the classic tests as in any other nerve lesion is of importance. It is recommended to always compare with the non-affected side.

Key Points

The typical presentation of a benign PNST is a slowly growing mass causing pain or paresthesia on contact. Spontaneous pain is the exception and should raise concern about malignancy. A neurological deficit as a first symptom is rare (2–5%); if it is present in conjunction with tumor size >5 cm or rapid growth, malignant transformation should be suspected [3].

The typical presentation of a benign PNST is either an asymptomatic palpable mass or a mass causing discomfort from paresthesias to pain on contact. If located along the extremities, which is frequent, a globular firm mass can be palpated and can usually be moved transversely but not longitudinally. Sometimes a Hoffman-Tinel sign can be elicited. If located close to flexor creases, patients notice discomfort when the lesion has grown (e.g., a tibial nerve PNST in the popliteal fossa). Not infrequently, the lesions can be seen bulging under the skin on bare inspection. Upper extremity nerves and brachial plexus are more frequently affected than lower extremity nerves [5]. Patients often know about a small palpable mass and have noted a slow growth over some years. Most of the cases are benign and do not present with sensorimotor deficits. A true and worsening motor deficit in conjunction with a nerve mass is a red flag and should heighten the awareness for a malignancy, a perineurioma, an inflammatory process, or rarely a desmoid tumor. Lymphoma in nerve can be excruciatingly painful and grows within days. Physicians not accustomed to the PNST entity sometimes diagnose lipoma, if imaging has yet not been performed. Lipoma, however, is usually softer and more amorphous and does not necessarily present in the course of larger nerves. A rare differential diagnosis is "cat-scratch disease" which can present as an extremely painful small mass with high homogeneous signal intensity on MRI (bacterial infection by *Bartonella henselae* that can result in a painful nodule). Coincidentally, it can be located close to nerves (e.g., ulnar or median in the proximity of the elbow flexor crease). Another is glomus tumor (also extremely painful to touch, although in the millimeter range, with a blueish appearance). Intraneural ganglion, another differential diagnosis, is frequently located in the peroneal nerve at the fibular head or on the ulnar nerve in proximity to the loge de Guyon (Guyon's canal). Intraneural ganglia in contrast can lead to rather acute and severe motor loss.

4.2 Atypical Case Presentation and Red Flags

Pain at rest and a quickly growing mass with new onset of neurological deficit related to the nerve affected are absolute red flags that suggest malignant transformation. If malignancy needs to be ruled out, a more extensive workup is necessary. Apart from the basic MRI with and without contrast, FDG-PET is recommended to detect or rule out potential hot spots within the lesion. Metastasis or spread to the thorax and abdomen needs to be ruled out as well. As progression and growth in such cases can be fast, it is important to schedule imaging and potential surgery in a timely fashion. Usually such patients undergo biopsy first, but only if a malignancy is suspected. Overall strategy, surgical approach, and preoperative counseling in such cases are different. All possible scenarios need to be discussed with the patient beforehand [6].

Key Points
If red flags for malignancy are present, more extensive MR imaging is mandatory. FDG-PET should be considered prior to surgical planning. "Hot spots" within the lesion have a high sensitivity for malignant change within a nerve mass [7, 8].

4.3 Assessment and Further Imaging

A peripheral nerve sheath tumor (PNST) is suspected when the clinical presentation of a palpable firm moveable globular mass in the course of a peripheral nerve depicts a fusiform shape on imaging. If fusiform in shape, and along a peripheral nerve, the primary differential diagnosis includes schwannoma and neurofibroma. These are the most frequently encountered types of PNST, which all account for approximately 10% of soft tissue tumors [5].

If a patient presents with a mass suspicious of a nerve tumor, imaging is the next and mandatory step. If not located in deep planes (e.g., sciatic nerve in gluteal region), ultrasound imaging is an excellent and fast screening tool (see Chap. 6). MRI should confirm the diagnosis and is the imaging modality of choice. An infiltrative growth or process needs to be ruled out. Surgery for suspected nerve tumors should not be planned without prior MR imaging (see Chap. 7). Sporadic PNST needs to be differentiated from sarcoma or PNST associated with a genetic disorder such as neurofibromatosis (NF) 1 or 2 or schwannomatosis. The incidence of a sporadic PNST is 2 in 100,000, whereas it reaches 100% in patients with NF 1 or 2 or schwannomatosis (also called NF 3). It is crucial to monitor NF patients on a regular basis for new lesions and growth, as PNST has a higher preponderance for malignant transformation in NF 1 patients, with a 10% lifetime risk to develop a malignant PNST [9]. This is in contrast to malignancy occurring in sporadic PNST, with an incidence of only 0.001%.

4.4 Imaging: MRI, High-Frequency Nerve Ultrasound (HFNUS), and FDG-PET

4.4.1 MRI

Contrast-enhanced MRI is the gold standard for imaging evaluation. PNSTs have distinct borders and are isointense to slightly hypointense relative to the skeletal muscle. They depict strong and homogeneous contrast uptake. On T2, the lesion is hyperintense. Several radiological signs are described; however, these are not always present. One is the target sign (T2: central T2 hypointensity encircled by T2 hyperintensity), and another is the split fat sign (T1: thin rim of fat signal around lesion).

4.4.2 HFNUS

This enables highly efficient (cheap and fast) continuous imaging of the nerves of the extremities, as well as on the trunk, neck, and axilla. This makes it a perfect screening tool. As tumors to be evaluated are usually in the centimeter range, older machines with scanheads of medium emitting frequency around 7.5 MHz can also be used for a preliminary exam. The current generation of HFNUS uses scanheads of up to 22 MHz, enabling a tissue resolution in the sub-mm range for the price of limited depth penetration. A scanner from 8 to 12 MHz is a good compromise for screening purposes. With such US scanners, imaging nerves in variable tissue depths reaching up to >10 cm is possible. Neurosonographically nerve tumors appear as very well-defined ovoid (fusiform) to round masses localized to a peripheral nerve with an echo-rich rim. To differentiate from an extraneural lesion (e.g., lymph node), the hallmark of the nerve tumor is its origin within a nerve trunk.

4.4.2.1 Schwannomas

In relation to the nerve trunk, schwannomas are thought to be located more eccentrically to the longitudinal axis. They are "echo-poor" and show homogeneous echotexture and a distinct "echo-rich" border. However, heterogeneous echotexture with cystic parts (e.g., cellular schwannoma, compared to vestibular schwannoma), necrosis and calcifications (e.g., "ancient schwannoma"), and hypervascularity on color-duplex mode are possible and are not necessarily a sign of malignancy [10].

4.4.2.2 Neurofibromas

They are thought to be more prone to central positioning with regard to the long axis of the parent nerve. Echogenicity is higher as compared to schwannoma, and they are relatively more inhomogeneous, with no or minor vascularization [11]. The target sign is described more frequently.

4.5 Decision-Making and Differential Diagnosis

In the end, the clinical evaluation can only be seen in conjunction with imaging. The synopsis of both should lead to decision-making with regard to surgery vs follow-up. Indications for surgery are controversially discussed, if benign tumors are small and non-tender.

To distinguish nerve tumor from other forms of "nerve growth" is a domain of imaging, as described above (inflammation, metastasis, hypertrophic nerve changes, peripheral neuropathy, perineurioma, lymphomatosis, glomus tumor, intraneural cyst). The exception might be the plexiform neurofibroma involving a major nerve, which is palpable like a "bag of worms," or cutaneous plexiform neurofibromas which are completely distinct, involve the whole skin, and cover a broad area not related to a major parent nerve (they unfortunately just bear a very similar name but are completely distinct lesions) and also metastasis, whenever history gives clues.

Plexiform neurofibromas which typically appear in NF 1 (von Recklinghausen disease) spread along one or more parent nerves and create a more dysmorphous mass of heterogeneous echogenicity with unclear margins and abolished inner nerve architecture. From the ultrasound aspect, these sometimes need to be differentiated from hypertrophic nerve changes (e.g., as in Charcot-Marie-Tooth disease type 1) and some autoimmune neuropathies (chronic inflammatory demyelinating polyneuropathy, multifocal motor neuropathy, and the like). Other nerve masses that need to be differentiated are perineuriomas and hamartomas (neural fibrolipomatosis) and intraneural angiomas. Intraneural ganglia are easy to diagnose on ultrasound and MRI.

Questions and Pearls

- Clinical history, family history, and a thorough physical examination, including whole-body skin inspection, are crucial.

- NF1, NF2, and schwannomatosis have to be ruled out or confirmed.
- The main clinical feature of a PNST is a palpable mass or a deeper lying mass visualized on imaging within the course of a nerve.
- If a PNST is suspected, MR imaging is mandatory, but high-resolution ultrasound can help in screening and surgical planning.
- Spontaneous pain, rapid growth, size >5 cm, and a fixed mass should raise concern about malignancy.

References

1. Furniss D, Swan MC, Moritz DG, Lim J, Khanna T, Way BLM, et al. A 10-year review of benign and malignant peripheral nerve sheath tumors in a single center: clinical and radiographic features can help to differentiate benign from malignant lesions. Plast Reconstr Sur. 2008;121(2):529–33.
2. Valeyrie-Allanore L, Ismaili N, Bastuji-Garin S, Zeller J, Wechsler J, Revuz J, Wolkenstein P. Symptoms associated with malignancy of peripheral nerve sheath tumours: a retrospective study of 69 patients with neurofibromatosis 1. Br J Dermatol. 2005;153(1):79–82.
3. Donner TR, Voorhies RM, Kline DG. Neural sheath tumors of major nerves. J Neurosurg. 1994;81:362–73.
4. König R, et al. Diagnoseverfahren. In: Kretschmer T, Antoniadis G, Assmus H, editors. Nervenchirurgie. Berlin, Heidelberg: Springer; 2014.
5. Knight DMA, Birch R, Pringle J. Benign solitary schwannomas: a review of 234 cases. J Bone Joint Surg. 2007;89(3):382–7.
6. Heinen C, Kretschmer T, Weis J. Nerventumoren. In: Kretschmer T, Antoniadis G, Assmus H, editors. Nervenchirurgie. Berlin, Heidelberg: Springer; 2014.
7. Higham CS, Dombi E, Rogiers A, Bhaumik S, Pans S, Connor SEJ, et al. The characteristics of 76 atypical neurofibromas as precursors to neurofibromatosis 1 associated malignant peripheral nerve sheath tumors. Neuro-Oncology. 2018;20(6):818–25.
8. Ferner RE, Gutmann DH. International consensus statement on malignant peripheral nerve sheath tumors in neurofibromatosis. Cancer Res. 2002;62(5):1573–7.
9. Baehring JM, Betensky RA, Batchelor TT. Malignant peripheral nerve sheath tumor: the clinical spectrum and outcome of treatment. Neurology. 2003;61:696–8.
10. Lin, Martel. Cross-sectional imaging of peripheral nerve sheath tumors: characteristic signs on CT, MR imaging, and sonography. AJR Am J Roentgenol. 2001;176(1):75–82.
11. Thai WC, Chiu HJ, Chou YH, Wang HK, Sy C, Chang CY. D. Differentiation between schwannomas and neurofibromas in the extremities and superficial body: the role of high-resolution and color Doppler ultrasonography. J Ultrasound Med. 2008;27:161–6.

5 Preoperative Neurophysiological Evaluation

Ricardo de Amoreira Gepp and Ênio Comerlato

5.1 Introduction

Peripheral nerve tumors have a variety of histological types and have a varied clinical picture. Despite this diversity, preoperative evaluation is based on the clinical complaint presented by the patient, physical examination, and complementary exams. The tumor shape and histology, especially whether it is benign or malignant, in addition to the affected nerve, is an important factor to define the patient's symptomatology. In the evaluation through examinations, radiology is of most importance to determine the diagnostic hypothesis, the shape of the lesion, the tissue invasion adjacent to the tumor, and the characteristics suggestive of the presence or absence of tumor malignancy. The evolution of complementary exams has allowed a better definition of the biological nature of nerve injury before surgical excision. Despite all this information possible with radiology, imaging studies still do not provide any evaluation regarding the neurological function of the affected nerve and the interference that the tumor causes. Preoperative neurophysiological evaluation is one of the ways we can assess the integrity and functionality of the nerve and its fascicles [1].

Peripheral nerve diseases present heterogeneous presentations and may involve more motor fibers and in other cases sensory fibers, but in the cases of tumors, the involvement is general and nonspecific. Another important function of the neurophysiological study is to analyze diseases of the nerve itself that may also be affecting the patient [1]. An example would be the patient with a nerve neoplasm and the presence of diabetic polyneuropathy. A not so rare situation is the association between spinal disease and peripheral nerve damage such as tumors. Shenai and colleagues reported a case of a patient with a median nerve schwannoma and the presence of C7 radiculopathy [2]. In these cases, careful examination may show clues that lead to the correct diagnosis [2].

In patients with malignant tumors undergoing radiotherapy or chemotherapy, neurophysiological examination may determine alteration of nerve function by polyneuropathy following chemotherapy or axonal injury. This data may be very important in differentiating between the progression of cancer disease and the neuropathy that may occur due to the use of chemotherapy, as some more neurotoxic agents such as vincristine cause more changes in neurophysiological examination [1, 3].

Another situation where neurophysiological study may be relevant occurs when tumors coexist with a differential diagnosis of compressive syndromes. Patients with clinical signs

R. de Amoreira Gepp (✉)
Neurosurgery Department - Sarah Network of Rehabilitation Hospitals, Brasilia, Federal District, Brazil
e-mail: rgepp@sarah.br

Ê. Comerlato
Neurophysiology Department - Sarah Network of Rehabilitation Hospitals, Brasilia, Federal District, Brazil

F. Guedes et al. (eds.), *Diagnostic Assessment and Treatment of Peripheral Nerve Tumors*, https://doi.org/10.1007/978-3-030-77633-6_5

suggestive of carpal tunnel and tarsal tunnel syndrome but who actually have a tumor can be diagnosed when a similar symptom occurs but the electrophysiological findings do not confirm. In these cases, the radiological examination confirms and locates the tumor. Moussa and colleagues described a case of tarsal tunnel syndrome that was caused by peripheral nerve lymphoma [4]. Tladi and colleagues described two cases of patients with schwannoma and neurofibroma who had a clinical presentation suggestive of tarsal tunnel syndrome [5]. Radiological examination was fundamental for the diagnosis, but the neurophysiological study showed atypical alterations in relation to the compressive syndrome, and thus the diagnosis of the tumors was made.

In this chapter, we will review the neurophysiological study and its implications for the treatment of peripheral nerve tumors and adjacent tumors with peripheral nerve involvement.

5.2 Principles of Peripheral Neurophysiological Examination

Perioperative evaluation of patients with peripheral nerve tumor consists of the study of sensory conduction, evaluation of motor conduction, and electromyography. In sensory conduction studies, the sensory nerve (SNAP) and compound motor action potentials (CMAP) are evaluated. Potential latencies, amplitudes, and duration are evaluated. Electromyography analyzes the potentials of motor units (MUPs) that are captured during voluntary muscle contraction.

In the perioperative evaluation, we can observe the following situations when facing a tumor lesion:

(a) Absence of electrophysiological abnormality in the presence of a tumor (case 2 below).
(b) Focal change in conduction velocity: Tumors in their early stage may affect only the myelin sheath due to local compression, thus translating an important element in cases with early diagnosis.
(c) Focal conduction block: This occurs due to increased demyelination area caused by tumor growth. Block is characterized by the dramatic loss of amplitude of the compound motor action potential (CMAP) or compound nerve action potential (CNAP) by the tumor area. Demyelinating changes can be more easily identified in the distal portions of the nerves. In case 2, with a proximal sciatic nerve tumor, it was not possible to identify the focal nerve lesion in the vicinity of the tumor due to the difficulty in performing proximal and distal nerve conduction analysis of the lesion (Sensory? and Motor? Table—case 2).
(d) Amplitude reduction: Axonal degeneration is a natural consequence of chronic focal compression. (See example case 1—study of sensory and motor table.) Thus, in the early stages of the lesions, we have the SNAP amplitude reduction (Fig. 5.1 case). It is estimated that in order to reduce SNAP amplitude, a loss of at least one third of the myelin fibers should occur. Thus, the reduction of SNAP is the characteristic finding of peripheral nerve injuries. The reduction in the

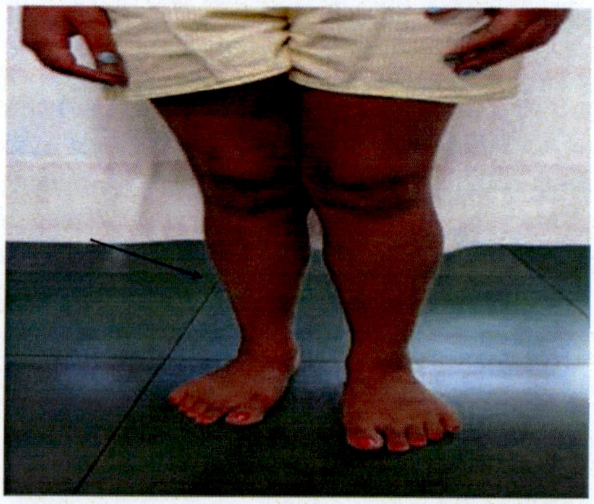

Fig. 5.1 Clinical examination at admission. The child complained of pain and worsening gait performance. It is observed that there was significant atrophy of the anterior tibial muscle (arrow)

amplitude of the CMAP can already be observed when there is a large axonal loss due to the muscle fiber reinnervation process, through the budding of unaffected motor units, observed during electromyography, due to the increase of MUAP (Fig. 5.3—case 1: peroneus longus muscle).

(e) Absence of CMAP and SNAP: It occurs when there has been a complete Wallerian degeneration of all fibers in the tumor-affected nerve (Fig. 5.1—case 1), an advanced lesion, with little chance of reinnervation. In this situation, we observed in the electromyography the presence of spontaneous muscle activity, characterized by the presence of fibrillations and positive sharp waves (Fig. 5.1—case 1). In complete lesions, it is not possible to study the distal nerve conduction to the lesion.

5.3 Specific Tumors and Neurophysiology

Peripheral nerve tumors are divided into malignant and benign. Malignant lesions derive in 50% of patients with neurofibromatosis, which may lead to nonspecific changes in neurophysiological response due to various lesions present, including within the spinal canal. In these cases, the neurophysiological study ends up being nonspecific and not useful for patient follow-up.

Benign tumors are much more frequent, and among them are schwannomas and neurofibromas. Despite this higher frequency, neurophysiological changes are not often described in these tumors; case reports or series are rare. The neurophysiological study ends up being little used, and when it is effective, it is because in the initial evaluation of the case, the diagnosis of the tumor had not yet been established. One exception is perineurioma. It is a rare tumor of the peripheral nervous system composed of layers of perineurial cells that surround the axons and Schwann cells and may have intraneural and extraneural changes [6]. Neurophysiological tests show alterations in sensory conduction and less frequently alterations in motor conduction [6]. These studies are important to differentiate from other nerve changes mainly because in the initial cases, perineurioma may be confused with other neuropathies. In these patients with perineurioma, sensory conduction velocity tends to have a greater drop, motor conduction velocity is less affected in the initial cases, and there is no repercussion on needle electromyography. The association with the radiological study is important for the diagnosis and localization of the tumor, remembering that sometimes the perineurioma can be extensive.

Another interesting situation occurs in neurofibromatosis. It is an autosomal dominant disease with tumor formation throughout the body [7]. There is diffuse pain in these patients, and the cause is not always due to the presence of tumors. Specifically, in type 2 neurofibromatosis (NF2), there may be a neuropathy that causes pain and neurological deficit and is unrelated to tumors. It is important in the face of a diagnosis of pain and sensory changes in NF2 to think about the possibility of this neuropathy. In NF1, this situation is rarer, but it can occur as well [8]. Especially in these cases, the neurophysiological study may be useful to differentiate tumor-related symptoms from NF neuropathy. Electroneuromyography should be performed on the other limbs not affected by symptoms to diagnose neuropathy [8, 9].

5.4 Case 1: Nerve Tumor—Primary Synovial Cell Sarcoma

Female patient, 12 years and 6 months, complaining of shock pain in the knee and radiation to the toes. She had progressive loss of right leg muscle strength for 1.5 years. On physical examination, she had decreased sensitivity in the space between the first and second toes. Tinel sign was positive in the popliteal fossa and fibular head region. There was also evidence of anterior tibialis muscle atrophy (Fig. 5.1) and zero-degree muscle strength for dorsiflexion of the foot.

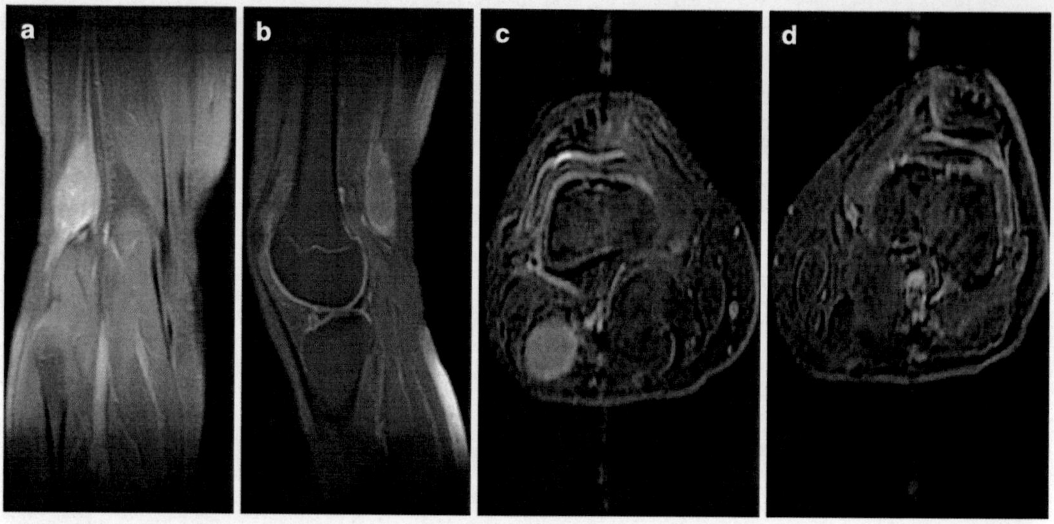

Fig. 5.2 (**a**) MR image demonstrating in the coronal plane the presence of an expansive lesion with contrast uptake in the fibular nerve territory. (**b**) Sagittal image showing the same lesion and its posterior positioning. (**c** and **d**) In the axial section, we see the tumor posterior from de knee

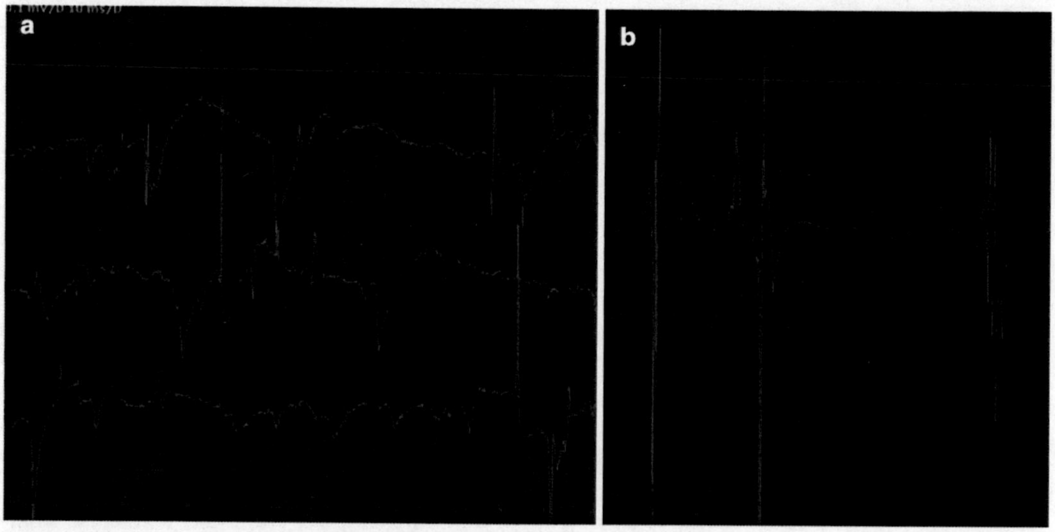

Fig. 5.3 Electromyography. (**a**) EMG showing signs of right anterior tibialis muscle denervation and peroneus longus muscle reinnervation. (**b**) Lack of recruitment of MUAP in the anterior tibial muscle

The complementary exams performed were the neurophysiological evaluation and the imaging study. Magnetic resonance imaging at 1.5 Tesla demonstrated the presence of a spindle-like expansive lesion, measuring the largest cranio-caudal diameter 50 mm and the largest transverse diameter 25 mm. The lesion originated from the common fibular (peroneal) nerve from its emergence (Fig. 5.2). Electromyography showed signs of right anterior tibialis muscle denervation and peroneus longus muscle reinnervation (Fig. 5.3). Recruitment failure of motor unit action potentials (MUAP) in the anterior tibialis muscle (Table 5.1). The patient was referred to surgery.

Table 5.1 MNCS

	Lat		Amp		CV		F-M lat	
Nerve	ms	Ref. Dev	mV	Ref. Dev	m/s	Ref. Dev	ms	Ref. Dev
Peroneus motor left								
Ankle—EDB	3.00	−2.1	3.0	−1.25			38.0	
Below knee—Ankle	10.4		3.3		45.9			
Fibular head—Below knee	11.6		3.7		50.0			
Peroneus motor right								
Ankle—EDB	–	–	–	–				
Fibular head—Tibial anterior	–		–	–				
Tibialis motor left								
Ankle—Abd hal	3.63		12.0				34.5	
Tibialis motor right								
Ankle—Abd hal	3.00		10.5				35.5	

Table 5.2 Sensory nerve conduction study (SNCS)

	Lat		Amp		CV	
Nerve	ms	Ref. Dev	uV	Ref. Dev	m/s	Ref. Dev
Peroneus profundus sensory left						
Stim 1—Rec 1	1.79		8.3		55.9	
Peroneus profundus sensory right						
Stim 1—Rec 1	–		–			
Peroneus superfic sensory left						
Calf—Med., dor., cutan.	1.20		23.7		83.3	
Peroneus superfic sensory right						
Calf—Med., dor., cutan.	1.49		11.4		73.8	
Saphenous sensory left						
Tibia—Malleolus medial	1.85		6.2		54.1	
Saphenous sensory right						
Tibia—Malleolus medial	1.56		8.9		70.5	
Sural sensory left						
Leg—Lat. Malleolus	2.35		13.6		46.8	
Sural sensory right						
Leg—Lat. Malleolus	1.58		20.3		67.7	

5.4.1 Electrophysiological Evaluation

Motor nerve conduction studies (MNCS): Unexcitable right deep fibular (peroneal) nerve

Sensory nerve conduction studies (SNCS)

Peroneus profundus nerve Unexcitable.

Peroneus superficialis nerve with low amplitude of SNAP (Table 5.2).

5.5 Case 2: Desmoid Tumor

A 14-year-old female patient complained of numbness in the left lower limb for 1 year without limitation of physical activities. Pain was not so frequent. Clinical examination showed decreased sensitivity in the common fibular (peroneal) nerve territory. There was no atrophy, and muscle strength and gait were normal.

Imaging was performed with 3 Tesla magnetic resonance imaging. The study demonstrated a heterogeneous expansive lesion in the deep soft tissues of the gluteus and posterior region of the left proximal thigh, inseparable from and displacing the left sciatic nerve after the emergence of this nerve through the sciatic foramen. The lesion was located between the quadratus femoral muscle and gluteus maximus muscle and in apparent contact in the proximal portion with the piriformis muscle fibers, where the limits are less defined. The tumor measures about 14.0 × 5.6 × 4.4 cm (in longitudinal, transverse, and anteroposterior diameters). After administration of intravenous contrast, intense and irregular heterogeneous enhancement is observed (Fig. 5.4). The EMG was performed and showed:

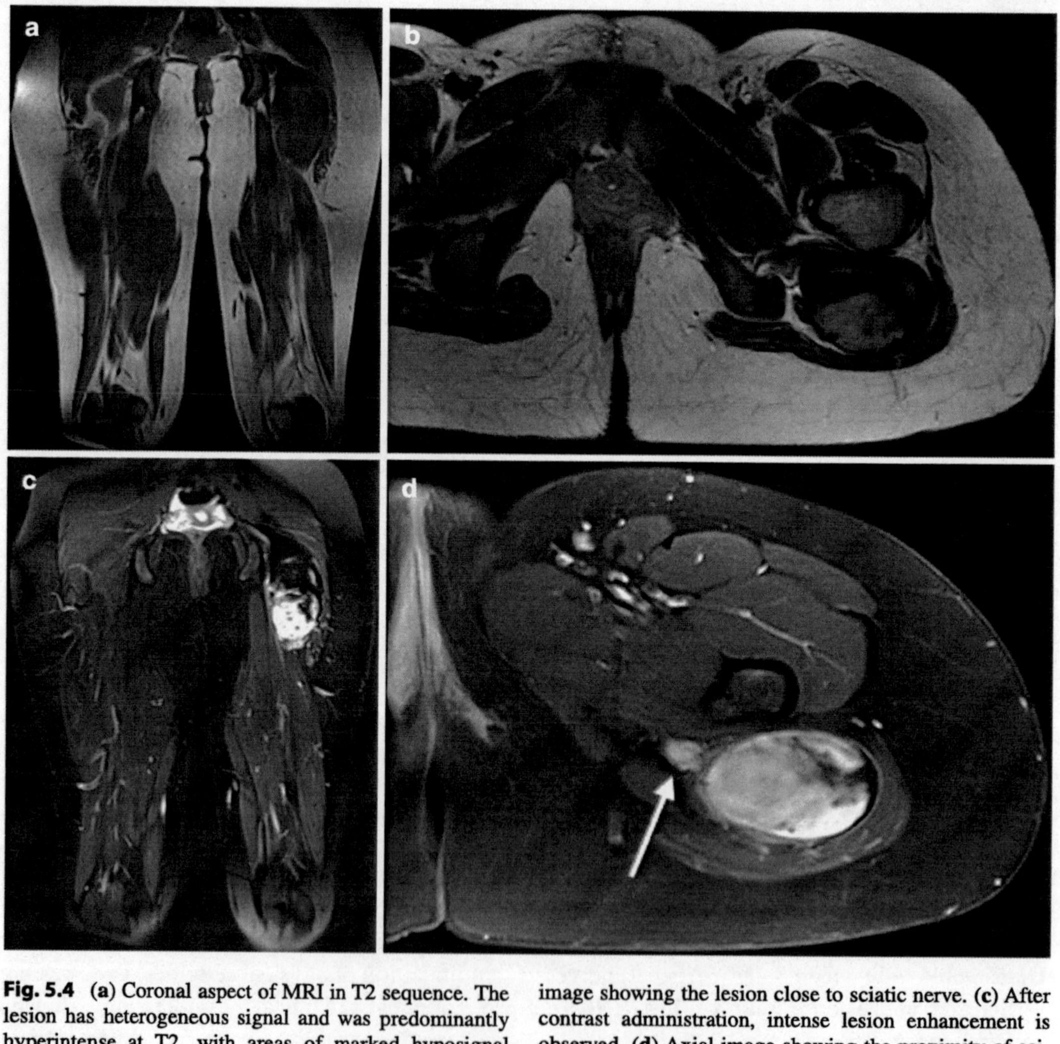

Fig. 5.4 (**a**) Coronal aspect of MRI in T2 sequence. The lesion has heterogeneous signal and was predominantly hyperintense at T2, with areas of marked hyposignal mainly in the proximal and peripheral portion. (**b**) Axial image showing the lesion close to sciatic nerve. (**c**) After contrast administration, intense lesion enhancement is observed. (**d**) Axial image showing the proximity of sciatic nerve (arrow) to tumor

Anterior tibialis muscle EMG and gastrocnemius EMG with:

- Physiological insertion activity.
- Electric silence at rest.
- Voluntary contraction and motor unit potentials with normal morphology and recruitment in the sampled muscles.

The EMG was very important to demonstrate that despite the tumor location close to the nerve, there was no impairment of sciatic nerve neurological function. This fact influenced the operative strategy. The tumor was operated and surgical resection was performed. The diagnosis was a desmoid tumor. Postoperatively, the patient maintained normal neurological function.

5.5.1 Electrophysiological Study

Sensory Conduction Study

Saphenous nerves, suralis nerves, and deep and superficial fibular (peroneal) nerves were normal.

Sensory nerve conduction studies

SNCS						
Nerve	Lat		Amp		CV	
	Ms	Ref. dev	uV	Ref. dev	m/s	Ref. dev
Peroneus profundus sensory left						
Stim 1—Rec 1	2.13		6.7		65.7	
Peroneus profundus sensory right						
Stim 1—Rec 1	2.13		5.5		65.7	
Peroneus superfic sensory left						
Calf—Med., dor., cutan.	1.44		13.1		69.4	
Peroneus superfic sensory right						
Calf—Med., dor., cutan.	1.54		16.0		61.7	
Saphenous sensory left						
Tibia—Med. Malleolus	1.96		4.9		56.1	
Saphenous sensory right						
Tibia—Med. Malleolus	1.74		7.4		63.2	
Suralis sensory left						
Mid. Lower leg—Lat. Malleolus	1.88		42.2		58.5	
Suralis sensory right						
Mid. Lower leg—Lat. Malleolus	1.44		47.8		62.5	

Motor Nerve Conduction Studies

Tibial and peroneal nerves were normal.

Motor nerve conduction studies

MNCS								
Nerve	Lat		Amp		CV		F-M Lat	
	Ms	Ref. dev	mV	Ref. dev	m/s	Ref. dev	Ms	Ref. dev
Peroneus motor left								
Ankle—EDB	**3.02**	−2.1	2.8	−1.33			38.1	
Bl. Knee–ankle	8.60		2.7		57.3			
Peroneus motor right								
Ankle—EDB	**2.35**	−3.0	5.3	−0.32			38.1	
Bl. Knee–ankle	8.42		4.7		54.4			
Tibialis motor left								
Ankle—Abd hal	3.64		18.7				35.5	
Tibialis motor right								
Ankle—Abd hal	3.50		23.3				35.0	

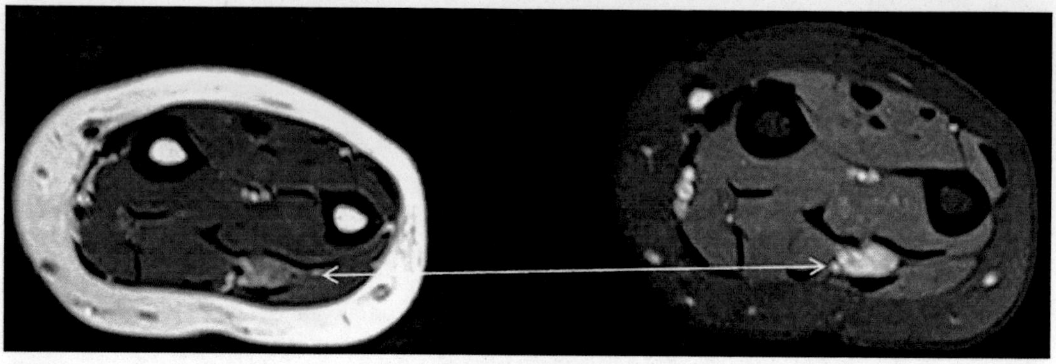

Fig. 5.5 The tumor could be identified (arrow) on T2 axial section and on T1 axial image with contrast enhancement

5.6 Case 3

A 15-year-old girl complained of decreased sensation and loss of strength in the left hand. There was minor numbness in the left hand. Pain was infrequent. She reported that some activities, such as playing guitar and piano, could not be performed. The fifth and fourth fingers were weaker too. There was no Tinel sign at the wrist.

Physical Examination.

No deformity in the left hand. Severe atrophy of the first interdigital space and interosseous muscles of the left hand.

Muscle Strength: Palmar interosseous grade 3 and only the last interosseous had grade 1. Handgrip strength was assessed with a dynamometer, and left hand weakness was identified. Graduated at 123 kilogram force (Kgf) and 22.3 (Kgf) in the right hand.

The EMG was performed, and the result showed impairment of ulnar nerve function, but was unable to show the specific etiology. The MRI was performed and showed a perineurioma below the elbow (Fig. 5.5). The EMG was important to show us the severity of the lesion and the necessity to investigate further with MRI.

5.7 Conclusion

Preoperative neurophysiological study has limited utility for the specific diagnosis of peripheral nerve tumor. References are few in the databases and reported experiences only in a few isolated cases. The neurophysiological test may be useful in the prior indication of an imaging examination, may assist in the relative measurement of nerve damage by the tumor, may assist in differential diagnosis, and may determine peripheral nerve involvement in adjacent non-primary nerve tumors. The presence of abnormalities in EMGs should also raise a red flag for the possibility of MPNST.

References

1. Crone C, Krarup C. Neurophysiological approach to disorders of peripheral nerve. Handb Clin Neurol. 2013;115:81–114.
2. Shenai MB, Menezes G, Falconer D, Leiphart J. Presentation and treatment of a combined median nerve schwannoma and a C7 Discogenic radiculopathy. Cureus. 2018;10(7):e3009.
3. Krarup C, Crone C. Neurophysiological studies in malignant disease with particular reference to involvement of peripheral nerves. J Neurol. 2002;249(6):651–61.

4. Moussa A, Chakhachiro Z, Sawaya RA. Posterior Tibial nerve lymphoma presenting as tarsal tunnel syndrome: a case report. J Foot Ankle Surg. 2018;57(1):167–9.
5. Tladi MJ, Saragas NP, Ferrao PN, Strydom A. Schwannoma and neurofibroma of the posterior tibial nerve presenting as tarsal tunnel syndrome: review of the literature with two case reports. Foot (Edinb). 2017;32:22–6.
6. McMillan HJ, Torres C, Michaud J, Ying Y, Boyd KU, Bourque PR. Diagnosis and outcome of childhood perineurioma. Childs Nerv Syst. 2016;32(8):1555–60.
7. Ferner RE, Shaw A, Evans DG, McAleer D, Halliday D, Parry A, et al. Longitudinal evaluation of quality of life in 288 patients with neurofibromatosis 2. J Neurol. 2014;261(5):963–9.
8. Ferner RE, Hughes RA, Hall SM, Upadhyaya M, Johnson MR. Neurofibromatous neuropathy in neurofibromatosis 1 (NF1). J Med Genet. 2004;41(11):837–41.
9. James AW, Shurell E, Singh A, Dry SM, Eilber FC. Malignant peripheral nerve sheath tumor. Surg Oncol Clin N Am. 2016;25(4):789–802.

6 Ultrasound Imaging

Maria Teresa Pedro and Ralph Werner König

6.1 Introduction

At present, the diagnostic work-up of PNT and tumor-like lesions remains challenging [1–3]: Magnetic resonance imaging (MRI) is the most frequently applied imaging modality, and magnetic resonance neurography (MRN) is considered as a "gold standard" for PNT [4]. But significant restrictions remain, e.g., secure tissue differentiation between PNT and inflammatory nerve pathologies and even more significant between benign and malignant entities is still not possible [2, 5]. Therefore, complementary diagnostic imaging modalities including ultrasound [6] and 18F-FDG PET or PET/MRI [7] are valuable adjuncts in the diagnostic process of patients with PNT.

Ultrasound is distinguished by its high availability and flexibility in the preoperative work-up and its unique attainability inside the OR, e.g., for approach planning. The ongoing development of transducer technology and digital image processing allows for a constantly improving tissue differentiation and offers higher image definition. Primary high-frequency linear array transducers of 15–20 MHz are used for peripheral nerve ultrasound. Due to the limited tissue penetration of high-frequency ultrasound, particularly superficially located soft tissue tumors of the extremities and neck are suitable for ultrasound examination. In some instances, intraoperative use after nerve dissection with direct application of the transducer to the affected nerve segment may be helpful [8]. Ultrasound classifications for PNT based on morphological B-scan sonography and contrast-enhanced ultrasound (CEUS) exist [6] (Table 6.1).

M. T. Pedro (✉) · R. W. König
Peripheral Nerve Surgery Unit,
Department of Neurosurgery at the University of Ulm, School of Medicine, Ulm, Germany
e-mail: maria-teresa.pedro@uni-ulm.de

6.2 Frequent Benign PNT (Schwannoma and Neurofibroma)

Schwannomas are benign peripheral nerve tumors arising from one fascicle, displacing the remaining fascicles. In HRNS, schwannomas appear hypoechoic, spindle-shaped in length, and homogeneous. Tumor margins are well defined [9]. The mass itself reveals no visible fascicular structure and lies usually eccentrically displacing the rest of the non-affected nerve fascicles. Especially in ancient schwannomas, cystic hypoechoic formations or calcifications can occur (Fig. 6.1) [10]. As a rule, vascularization is moderate in CCDS and SMI, and CEUS shows no enhancement uptake during the different dynamic phases (Fig. 6.2a, b) [11].

F. Guedes et al. (eds.), *Diagnostic Assessment and Treatment of Peripheral Nerve Tumors*,
https://doi.org/10.1007/978-3-030-77633-6_6

Table 6.1 Overview of HRNS characteristics of PNT

Tumor	Echotexture	Architecture of PNT	Vascularization
Schwannoma	Hypoechoic	Tumor mass reveals no fascicular structure	None or low
Neurofibroma	Hypo- to isoechoic, "target sign"	Tumor mass reveals no fascicular structure	None or low
Plexiform neurofibroma	Hypo- to isoechoic	Tumor masses merging into each other and revealing no fascicular structure	Low or moderate
Perineurioma	Hypoechoic enlarged fascicles	Fascicular structure preserved in tumor	None or low
MPNST	Heterogeneous irregular, cystic, satellite formation	Tumor mass reveals no fascicular structure	Moderate or high
Lymphoma	Hypo- to hyperechoic giant fascicles	Fascicular structure preserved in tumor	Low or moderate

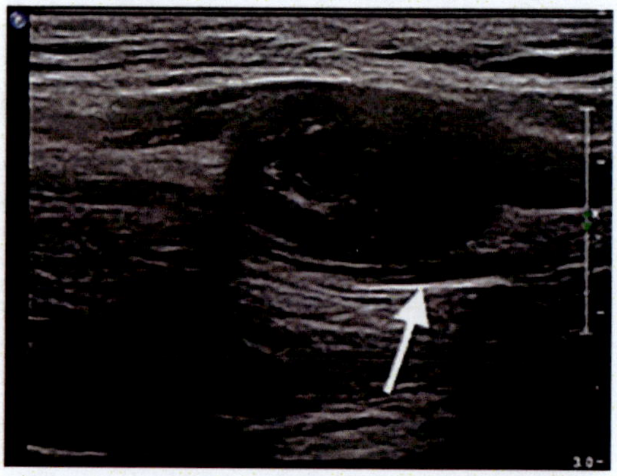

Fig. 6.1 Longitudinal HRNS scan of a schwannoma of the right median nerve. The hypoechoic tumor mass displaces non-affected fascicles aside (white arrow)

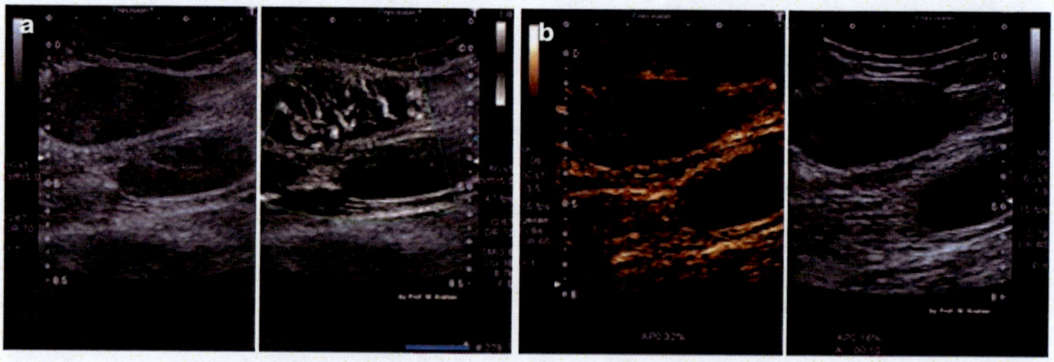

Fig. 6.2 (**a, b**) Two schwannomas arising out of the cutaneous femoris posterior nerve of the right thigh; on the left side, (**a**) SMI shows a moderate vascularization of the upper tumor, and on the right side, (**b**) CEUS reveals no perfusion pattern during the different dynamic phases

Neurofibromas as well belong to the group of benign peripheral nerve tumors but arise out of two or more fascicles. Compared to schwannomas, they can reveal a rather heterogeneous echotexture (target sign) with a hypoechoic outer and hyperechoic central zone in HRNS. The target sign was first described as a distinctive feature of neurofibromas in MRI with a hyperintense peripheral and hypointense core zone in T2-weighted images [12, 13]. Suh et al. described its imaging-histologic correlation with a dense fibro-collagenous core and abundant myxoid material with high fluid content in the outer tumor zone [12]. Comparable to schwannomas, vascularization of neurofibromas is normally low [14]. The tumor mass usually lies centrically enclosing all fascicles. Nonetheless, a secure ultrasound differentiation between both entities is often challenging.

Plexiform neurofibromas on the other hand consist of multiple tumor formations. Their echotexture is hypo- to isoechoic, and their vascularization is moderate (Fig. 6.3). The multiple round tumor masses are oval and merge into each other. They occur in patients with neurofibromatosis type 1 (NF1) [15], and by the time a malignant transformation is highly probable, this entity should be regularly controlled via ultrasound or other imaging modalities, such as MRN and 18F-FDG PET.

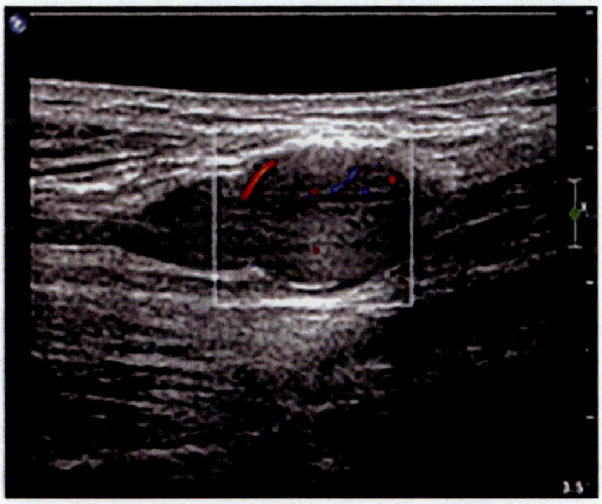

Fig. 6.3 Longitudinal HRNS scan of the right tibial nerve showing a plexiform neurofibroma. The tumor is hypoechoic and reveals minor vascularization in CCDS

6.3 Rare Benign PNT (Perineurioma)

Intraneural perineuriomas are slow-growing benign neoplasms of peripheral nerves leading to painless motor deficits. These formations can spread along the affected nerve and reveal a longitudinal hypoechoic fascicular enlargement (Fig. 6.4a) [6]. Fascicular architecture is preserved and definable but abnormally thickened [16]. Vascularization is absent or low. As a differential diagnosis with similar ultrasound characteristics, amyloidoma or demyelinating diseases, like Lewis-Sumner syndrome (LSS) (Fig. 6.4b), have to be considered [6, 17]. Especially in LSS, the clinical presentation of multifocal appearance and mixed motor and sensory symptoms may help for accurate diagnosis.

6.4 Malignant PNT (MPNST and Lymphoma)

In general, *MPNST* are rare malignant nerve tumors with a prevalence of 0.001%. In NF1 patients, MPNST have a significantly higher occurrence (up to 0.1%). Lifetime risk of NF1 patients to develop a malignant tumor is estimated to be as high as 8–13% [18]. MPNST usually arise out of plexiform neurofibromas. They can grow rapidly and may lead to immense neurological deterioration and severe pain. In HRNS, the tumor mass is inhomogeneous hypo- to isoechoic. Cystic components can occur. Round hypoechoic satellites can be detected lying on the main tumor mass, and its margins are usually unclear (Fig. 6.5). Vascularization is usually higher compared to benign PNT, and CEUS can reveal a rapid time to peak perfusion pattern [6].

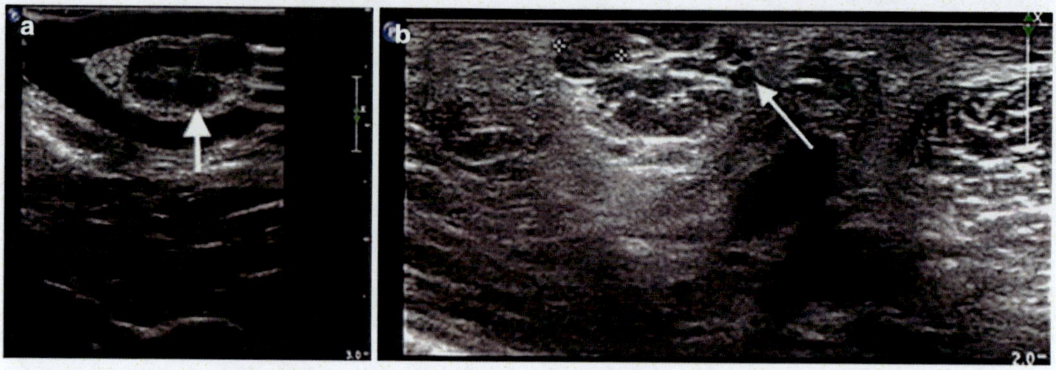

Fig. 6.4 (a, b) On the left side, intraoperative axial HRNS scan of the left sciatic nerve in a child showing thickened swollen hypoechoic fascicles (**a**). Histopathological examination resulted in perineurioma. On the right side, intraoperative axial HRNS scan of the left sciatic nerve depicting small hypoechoic fascicles (white arrow) next to thickened large hypoechoic fascicles (white crosses) (**b**). Nerve biopsy resulted in Lewis-Sumner syndrome

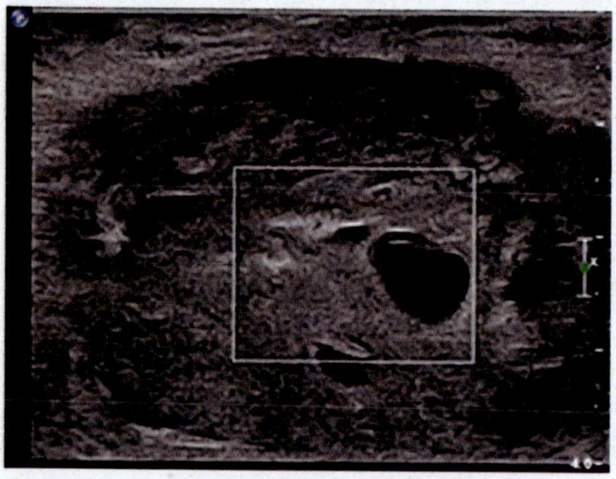

Fig. 6.5 Axial HRNS scan of the left sciatic nerve of a NF1 patient. The tumor mass is inhomogeneous cystic and necrotic. Fascicles are not definable. Tumor margins are irregular. Typical image of a MPNST

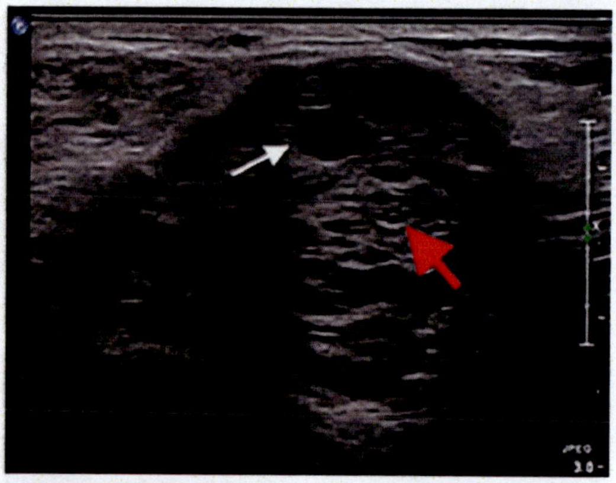

Fig. 6.6 Axial HRNS scan of the left tibial nerve showing large hypoechoic fascicles (white arrow) lying next to smaller fascicle groups (red arrow). Biopsy revealed B-cell lymphoma

Lymphomas of peripheral nerves are extremely rare. In our small sample group of only two patients, HRNS depicted extremely thickened and hypo- to hyperechoic fascicles, but their fascicular structure was preserved. Not all fascicles had the same size; some neighboring fascicles had a normal cross-sectional area (Fig. 6.6) [6]

6.5 Ultrasound-Guided Tumor Biopsy

According to the fourth edition of the 2013 WHO Classification of Tumors of Soft Tissue and Bone [23], PNT were reallocated to that group. The European Society for Medical Oncology (ESMO) guidelines recommend histological diagnosis from biopsy specimen (preferably core needle, excisional, and open biopsies are considered as an option in selected cases) as a standard approach [19] in suspected soft tissue sarcomas. Biopsy should be considered especially in the presence of certain "red flag criteria" for malignancy, such as pain, size (over 5 cm in diameter), rapid growth, or deep location. But there are certain risk factors for diagnostic failure [20]. The diagnostic work-up or treatment of benign PNT is responsible for up to 10% of iatrogenic nerve injuries in larger series [21, 22]. Therefore, according to our opinion, in suspected benign PNT, image-guided core needle biopsies should not be performed. In the rare cases of suspected malignancy, e.g., patients with raised red flags or NF1 patients, ultrasound-guided biopsy under nerve stimulation for preservation of motor function should be preferred. In case of deep lesions, which are not visualized by ultrasound, CT- or MRI-guided biopsy or even incisional biopsy can be performed. According to our experience, diagnostic accuracy of incisional biopsies can be even further enhanced with use of fluorescence-based microscopic visualization [24].

References

1. Murphey MD, Smith WS, Smith SE, et al. Imaging of musculoskeletal neurogenic tumors: radiologic-pathologic correlation. Radiographics. 1999;19:1253–80.
2. Karsy M, Guan J, Ravindra VM, et al. Diagnostic quality of magnetic resonance imaging interpretation for peripheral nerve sheath tumors: can malignancy be determined? J Neurol Surg Part A Cent Eur Neurosurg. 2016;77:495–504.
3. Chhabra A, Madhuranthakam AJ, Andreisek G. Magnetic resonance neurography: current perspectives and literature review. Eur Radiol. 2017;28:698–707.
4. Kransdorf MJ, Murphey MD. Radiologic evaluation of soft-tissue masses: a current perspective. AJR Am J Roentgenol. 2000;175(3):575–87.
5. Matsumine A, Kusuzaki K, Nakamura T, et al. Differentiation between neurofibromas and malignant peripheral nerve sheath tumors in neurofibromatosis 1 evaluated by MRI. J Cancer Res Clin Oncol. 2009;135:891–900.
6. Pedro MT, Antonidias G, Scheuerle A, et al. Intraoperative high-resolution ultrasound and contrast-enhanced ultrasound of peripheral nerve tumors and tumorlike lesions. Neurosurg Focus. 2015;39(3):E5.
7. Broski SM, Johnason GB, Howe BM, et al. Evaluation of (18)F-FDG PET and MRI in differentiation benign and malignant peripheral nerve sheath tumors. Skelet Radiol. 2016;45(8):1097–105.
8. Koenig RW, Schmidt T, Heinen CP, et al. Intraoperative high-resolution ultrasound: a new technique in the management of peripheral nerve disorders. J Neurosurg. 2011;114(2):514–21.
9. Lin J, Martel W. Cross-sectional imaging of peripheral nerve sheath tumors. Am J Roentgenol. 2001;176:75–82.
10. Kele H. Nervensonographie. In: Kretschmer T, Antoniadis G, Assmus H, editors. Nervenchirurgie. Berlin, Heidelberg: Springer; 2014. p. 37–49.
11. Kloth C, Eissler A, Schmidberger J, et al. Quantitative analysis of superb microvascular imaging in comparison with colour-coded doppler sonography for the preoperative evaluation of vascularisation of schwannoma. J Neurol Surg A Cent Eur Neurosurg. 2020;81:213–9. (Epub ahead of print).
12. Suh JS, Abenoza P, Galloway HR, et al. Peripheral (extracranial) nerve tumors: correlation of MR imaging and histologic findings. Radiology. 1992;183:341.
13. Varma DGK, Moulopoulos A, Sara AS, et al. MR imaging of extracranial nerve sheath tumors. J Comput Assist Tomogr. 1992;16:448.
14. Winter N, Rattay TW, Axer H, et al. Ultrasound assessment of peripheral nerve pathology in neurofibromatosis type 1 and 2. Clin Neurophysiol. 2017;128(5):702–6.
15. Riccardi VM. Von Recklinghausen neurofibromatosis. New Engl J Med. 1981;305:1617–27.
16. Salvalaggio A, Cacciavillani M, Coraci D, et al. Nerve ultrasound and 3D-MR neurography suggestive of intraneural perineurioma. Neurology. 2016;86(12):1169–70.
17. Koenig RW, Coburger J, Pedro MT. Intraoperative findings in peripheral nerve pathologies. In: Prada F, Solbiati L, Martegani A, DiMeco F, editors. Intraoperative ultrasound (IOUS) in neurosurgery. Cham, Switzerland: Springer; 2016. p. 71–9.
18. Evans DGR. Malignant peripheral nerve sheath tumours in neurofibromatosis 1. J Med Genet. 2002;39:311–4.
19. Casali PG, Bielack S, Abecassis N, et al. Bone sarcomas: ESMO-PaedCan-EURACAN Clinical Practice Guidelines for diagnosis, treatment and follow-up. Ann Oncol. 2018;29(Suppl 4):iv79–95.

20. Yoon MA, Chung HW, Chee CG, et al. Risk factors for diagnostic failure of ultrasound-guided core needle biopsy of soft-tissue tumors based on World Health Organization classification category and biologic potential. AJR Am J Roentgenol. 2019;31:1–9.
21. Rasulic L, Savic A, Vitosevic F, et al. Iatrogenic peripheral nerve injuries-surgical treatment and outcome: 10 years' experience. World Neurosurg. 2017;103:841–51.
22. Dengler NF, Antoniadis G, Grolik B, et al. Mechanisms, treatment, and patient outcome of iatrogenic injury to the brachial plexus-a retrospective single-center study. World Neurosurg. 2017;107:868–76.
23. Fletcher CD, Hogendoorn P, Mertens F, et al. WHO classification of tumours of soft tissue and bone. 4th ed. Lyon, France: IARC Press; 2013.
24. Pedro MT, Eissler A, Scheuerle A, et al. Sodium fluorescein as intraoperative visualization tool during peripheral nerve biopsies. World Neurosurg. 2020;133:e513–21. (Epub ahead of print).

7 Magnetic Resonance Neurography

Daniela Binaghi

Key Points

Schwannomas and neurofibromas share common MRN imaging findings.
Differentiating benign from malignant neoplasms of peripheral nerves is problematic; usually, they cannot be distinguished with confidence.
Several non-neoplastic nerve lesions can be specifically diagnosed by MR imaging.

7.1 Introduction

The classification and nomenclature of peripheral nerve tumors have been difficult and confusing; however, advances in MRN imaging have improved the diagnostic work-up, expanding differential diagnostic possibilities and determining whether lesions are intra- or extra-neural. These advances have implications for safe and complete resection of common and uncommon neurogenic and non-neurogenic tumors and for targeted fascicular biopsy.

The clinical appearance of a neurogenic tumor is usually that of a soft tissue mass or nerve enlargement that might be associated with symptoms related to the nerve involved. Peripheral nerve enlargement is a distinctive radiological feature and has multiple differential diagnoses, including peripheral nerve sheath tumors, post-traumatic neuroma, and inflammatory neuropathy, among many other pseudotumoral conditions.

MRN imaging evaluates nerve anatomy, signal intensity, internal pattern, and course, as well as the surrounding tissues and innervated muscles. Normal peripheral nerves appear isointense to the muscle on T1-weighted (T1-w) images and iso- to slightly hyperintense on T2-weighted (T2-w) images—depending on the amount of endoneurial fluid. They also have a fascicular pattern and fail to enhance after gadolinium administration, due to the nerve-blood barrier (Fig. 7.1). On DTI, normal nerves show fractional anisotropy (FA) values of >0.4–0.5 [1].

MRN examination protocols should always include gadolinium administration, since patterns of contrast enhancement can distinguish different types of pathology with similar non-contrast appearances.

D. Binaghi (✉)
Radiology Department, Peripheral Nerve Section, Favaloro University, Favaloro Foundation, Buenos Aires, Argentina

F. Guedes et al. (eds.), *Diagnostic Assessment and Treatment of Peripheral Nerve Tumors*, https://doi.org/10.1007/978-3-030-77633-6_7

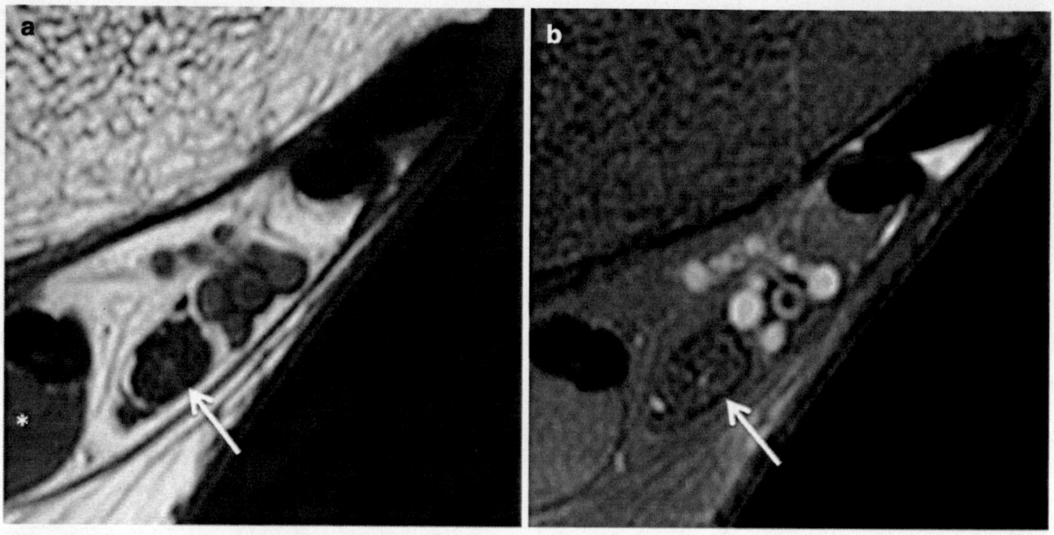

Fig. 7.1 Normal anatomy of the tibial nerve at the level of the ankle. On axial T1-weighted imaging (**a**), it is isointense to the muscle (flexor hallucis longus, asterisk); on STIR (short tau inversion recovery) (**b**), it exhibits mildly high signal intensity (arrows) and a fascicular appearance

7.2 Intraneural Benign Tumors of Neural Sheath Origin

The most common benign peripheral nerve tumors are schwannomas and neurofibromas. It is usually difficult, if not impossible, to reliably differentiate these two lesions on the basis of MRN imaging features, despite their different pathological characteristics. The typical MRN imaging appearance (Fig. 7.2) of a benign peripheral nerve sheath tumor is of a well-defined oval lesion, usually in continuity with the origin nerve, that is less than 5 cm in diameter, and is isointense to the muscle on T1-w, is hyperintense on T2-w, and has prominent enhancement after contrast administration. Often, there is an area of low signal on T2-w imaging, which usually does not show enhancement, representing the classic "target sign" of a benign neurogenic tumor, due to peripheral myxoid material and central fibrous tissue. On diffusion tensor imaging (DTI), these lesions are associated with high apparent diffusion coefficient (ADC) values (>1.1–1.2 10^{-3} mm/s^2) [2, 3]. Also, diffusion tensor tractography (DTT) can be used to visualize the 3D course of nerve fibers and bundles, which are displaced in the presence of a schwannoma and infiltrated in a neurofibroma (Figs. 7.3 and 7.4). DTT is also able to determine a "safe zone," in which dissection can be performed, avoiding damage to normal fascicles. Masses displaying classic imaging features need not be biopsied, unless unusual clinical features appear. Malignancy must be suspected in patients who have tumors that rapidly increase in size, become progressively painful, or produce a new neurologic deficit, especially in those patients who have neurofibromatosis.

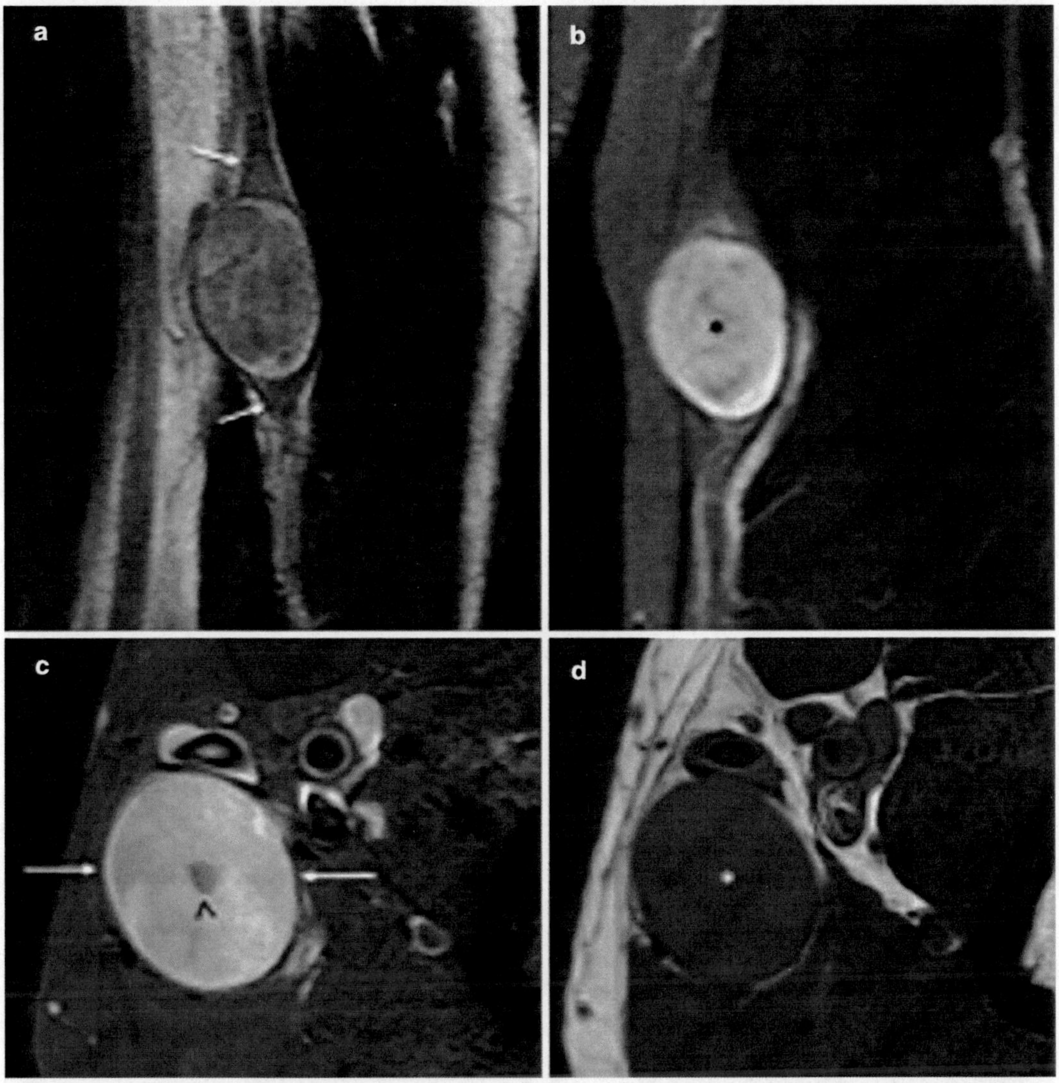

Fig. 7.2 Ulnar nerve benign peripheral nerve sheath tumor. Sagittal T2-weighted imaging (**a**) shows an oval-shaped, well-defined tumor in continuity with the nerve, hyperintense on (**b** – coronal) STIR (**c** – axial) and isointense to the muscle (white asterisk) on T1-w (**d**). Note the typical "target sign" (arrow point) on the axial STIR (**c**)

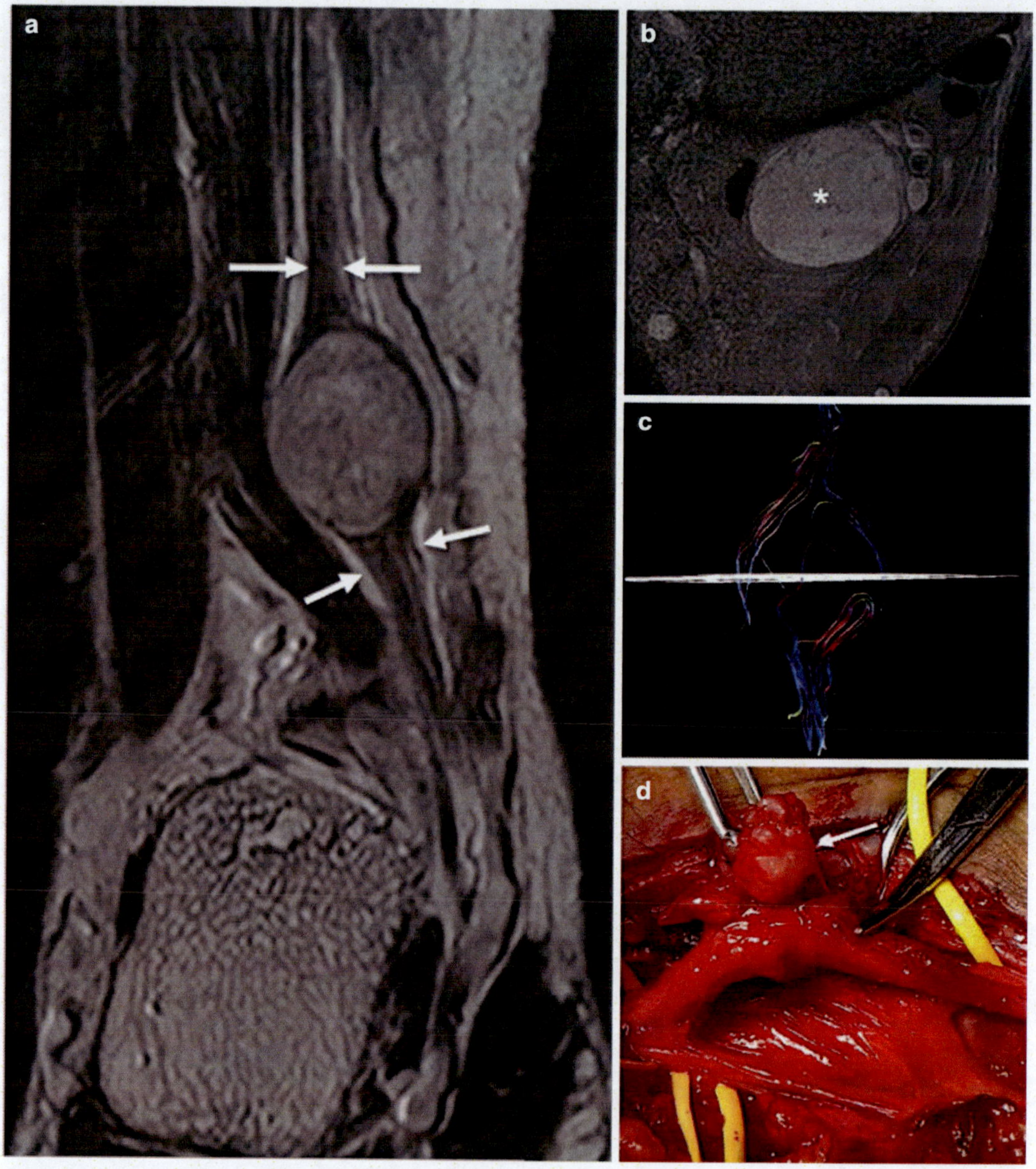

Fig. 7.3 Schwannoma. (**a**) Coronal T2-w imaging shows a well-defined, oval tumor centrally arising from the tibial nerve (arrows), heterogeneously hyperintense (asterisk) on axial PD SPIR (**b**). DTT, overlaid on an MR image (**c**), demonstrates displacement of the normal nerve fascicles. (**d**) Operative appearance

7.3 Intraneural Perineurioma

Intraneural perineurioma is a benign peripheral nerve neoplasm that typically affects teenagers and young adults, with an equal predilection for males and females and upper and lower extremities; it also tends to result in a motor-predominant neuropathy. This tumor is composed of perineurial cells arranged in concentric layers, thereby forming "pseudo-onion bulbs" surrounding axons and their Schwann cells, and is immuno-

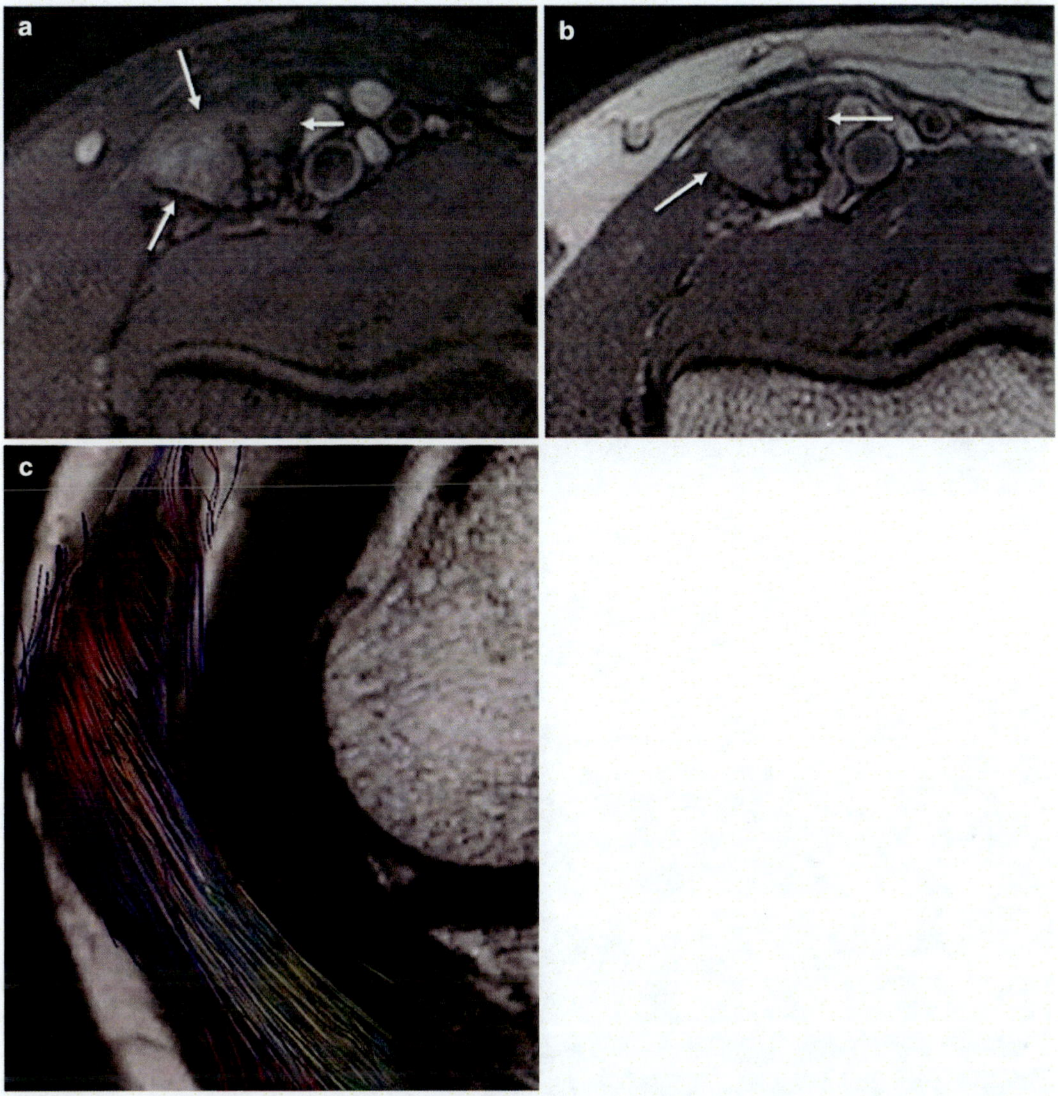

Fig. 7.4 Neurofibroma. Axial PD SPIR (**a**) and PD (**b**) show eccentric enlargement of the median nerve at the elbow, with heterogeneous signal intensity. (**c**) DTT-MR imaging reveals the absence of nerve tract displacement

histochemically EMA (epithelial membrane antigen) positive and S-100 negative (Schwann cell marker). This tumor has likely been underdiagnosed, due to a lack of familiarity among both clinicians and radiologists.

MRN most often shows (Fig. 7.5) nerve enlargement, generally of considerable length—with preservation of the normal fascicular neural structure (honeycomb appearance). These lesions also are isointense on T1-w images, are hyperintense on T2-w images, and exhibit homogeneous, moderate to marked contrast enhancement after intravenous gadolinium injection. Denervation changes in the affected nerve territory are another common finding on MRI. Clinico-radiological diagnosis may be sufficient to obviate a tissue diagnosis [4, 5].

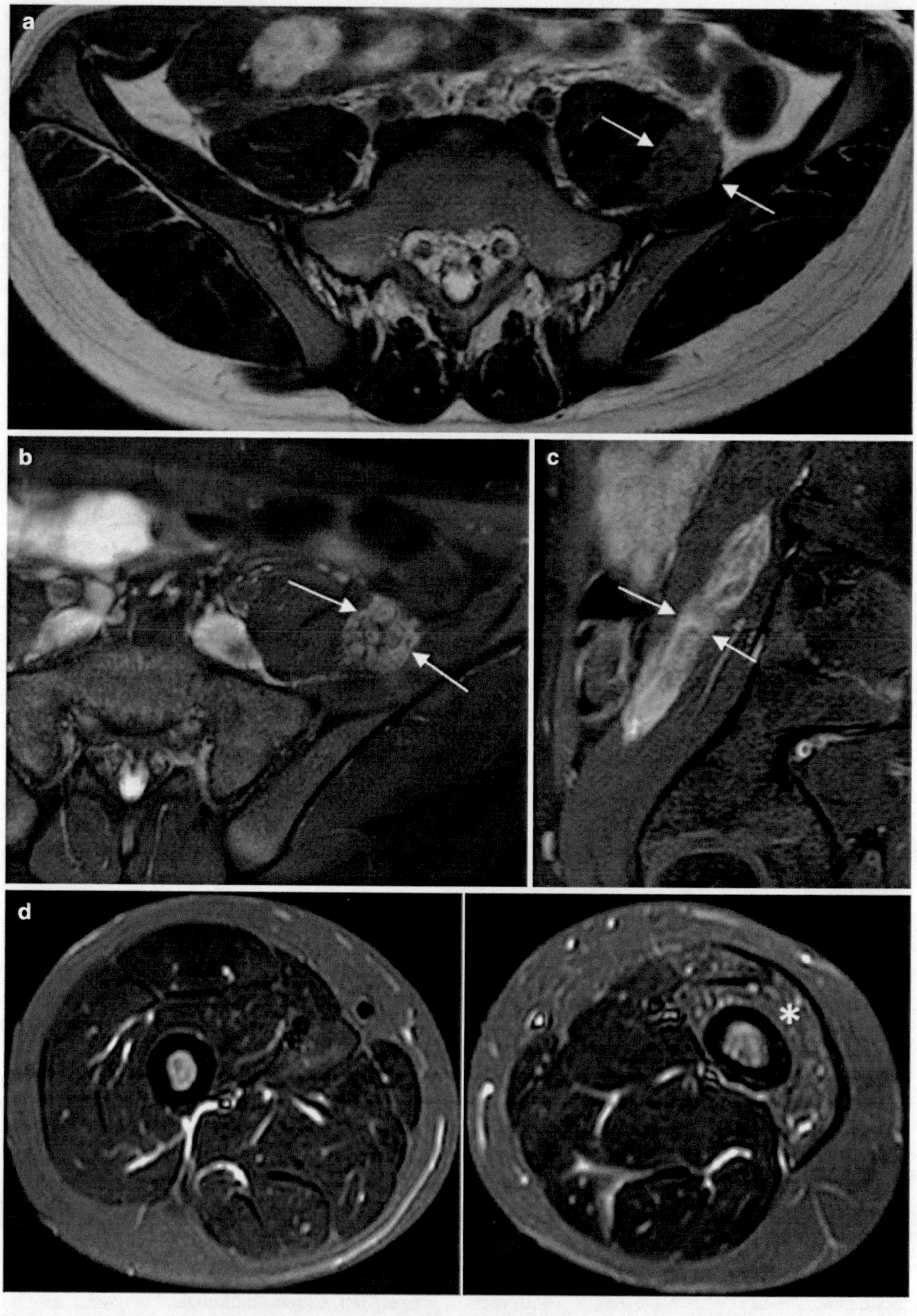

Fig. 7.5 Perineurioma. (**a**) Axial T2-w image shows mark enlargement of the left femoral nerve in the pelvis. (**b**) Axial PD SPAIR demonstrates increased signal intensity (arrows). (**c**) Sagittal T1 SPIR after contrast administration shows prominent enhancement (arrows). (**d**) Axial STIR demonstrates muscle atrophy related to subacute denervation of the anterior compartment of the thigh

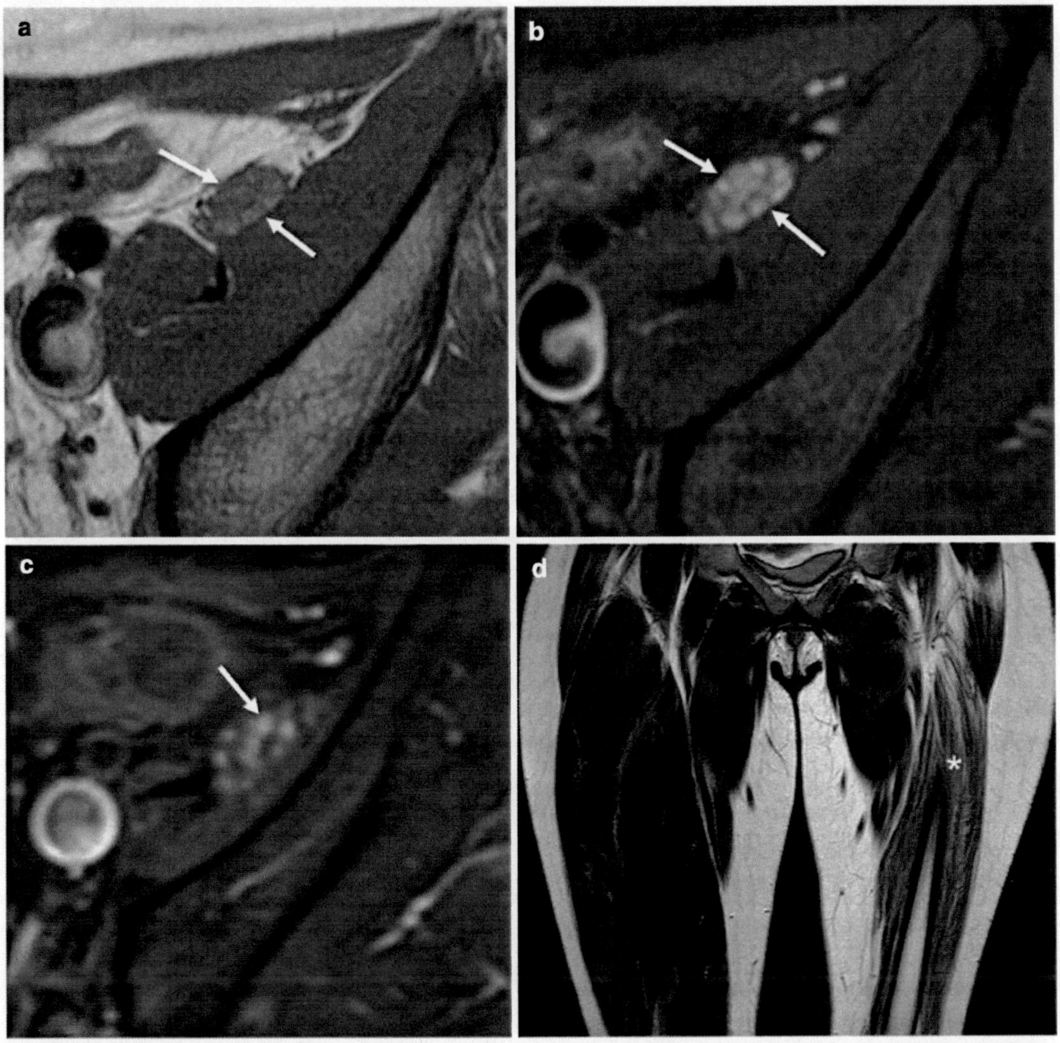

Fig. 7.6 Atypical chronic inflammatory demyelinating polyradiculoneuropathy (CIDP) variant. Axial PD (**a**) and PD SPIR (**b**) show femoral nerve fascicular enlargement and increased signal intensity (arrows), with fascicular enhancement (arrow) after gadolinium injection (axial T1 SPIR, figure **c**). (**d**) Coronal T2-weighted imaging demonstrates muscle denervation changes of the anterior compartment of the left thigh

The differential diagnosis of an intraneural perineurioma is broad and includes other benign nerve tumors, such as neurofibroma, schwannoma, and inherited hypertrophic neuropathy (Charcot-Marie-Tooth and Dejerine-Sottas), as well as acquired processes like focal inflammatory demyelination (Fig. 7.6), traumatic neuroma, sarcoidosis, leukemia, and lymphoma.

7.4 Malignant Peripheral Nerve Sheath Tumors (MPNSTs)

MPNSTs are soft tissue neoplasms that usually arise from peripheral nerves and show variable differentiation toward one of the cellular components of the nerve sheath (Schwann cells, fibroblasts, and perineurial cells). They can occur sporadically

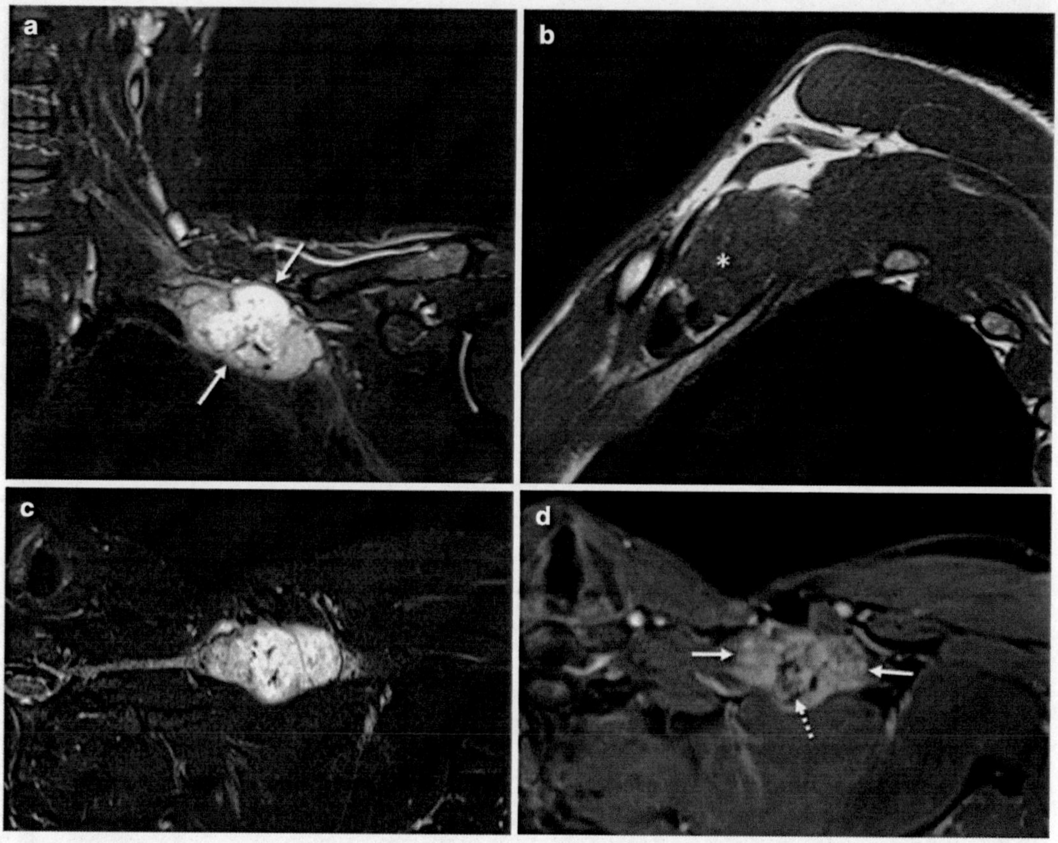

Fig. 7.7 Malignant peripheral nerve sheath tumor (MPNST). Coronal (**a**) and axial (**c**) STIR show a heterogeneous multilobular mass related to the brachial plexus, isointense on T1-w (**b**—sagittal) with heterogeneous gadolinium enhancement (**d**—axial T1 SPIR) due to necrosis (dotted arrow). Courtesy of Sonia Alvarez, MD, Hospital Italiano de Buenos Aires

or in patients with neurofibromatosis type 1 (NF1); and they arise either de novo (Fig. 7.7) or from a preexisting neurofibroma or, rarely, schwannoma. They form a heterogeneous group of neoplasms with a range of morphological characteristics and are often aggressive, with a tendency to recur (recurrence rate up to 40%) and metastasize, not only to distant organs but also with perineural spread along the affected nerve [6].

Unfortunately, MRN differentiation of benign versus malignant peripheral nerve sheath tumors remains challenging. It has been suggested that a combination of two or more MRI features—which include ill-defined or invasive margins, peri-tumoral edema, largest diameter greater than 5 cm, and heterogeneous signal intensity on T1- and T2-weighted images—can serve as indicators of malignancy [7]. Low diffusivity values (ADC < 1.0–1.2 10^{-3}) indicate malignancy on DTI and, on DTT, partial or complete disruption of tracts [2, 3]. Nonetheless, malignancy must be suspected in patients who have tumors that rapidly increase in size, become progressively painful, or produce a new neurologic deficit.

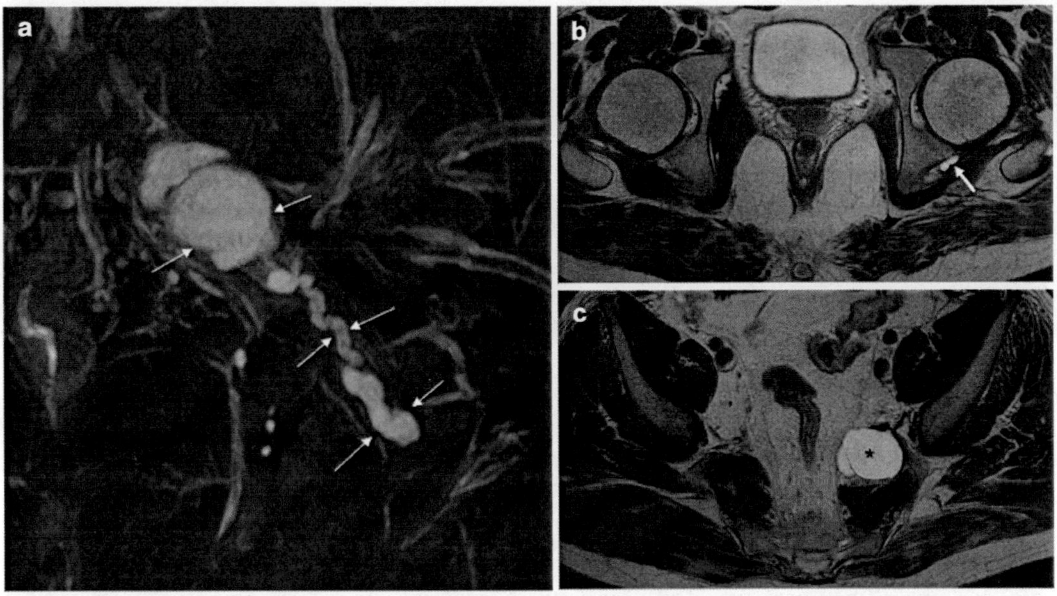

Fig. 7.8 Intraneural ganglion cyst. (**a**) Coronal reformatted STIR image shows the full extent of the cyst from its joint origin extending proximally from the hip joint to the intrapelvic sciatic nerve and lumbosacral plexus (arrows). (**b**) Axial T2-w shows cystic extension into the articular branch. (**c**) Axial T2-w shows intrapelvic extension (asterisk)

7.5 Intraneural Benign Tumors of Non-Neural Sheath Origin

7.5.1 Intraneural Ganglion Cyst

Intraneural ganglion cysts are relatively rare cysts located within the epineurium of peripheral nerves. They most commonly involve the articular branch of the peroneal nerve at the superior tibiofibular joint but can be seen at any joint (Fig. 7.8). Despite a long and controversial history regarding their formation, evidence has substantiated an articular (synovial) origin. On MRN imaging, a nerve sheath ganglion appears as a cyst: hyperintense on T2-w and hypointense on T1-w imaging, unilocular or (most of the time) multilocular, arising from defects in the joint capsule related to the articular branch, and extending via an intraepineurial dissection following the path of least resistance [4]. The fluid dynamics that underlie the formation of the cyst have implications for imaging, since an "isolated" remnant cyst, located away from the articular branch, has been described [8]

.Most of the time, intravenous contrast injection is not required to establish a diagnosis; but when performed, enhancement may be seen about the cyst wall and within thin septation, if present.

7.5.2 Neural Lipomatosis

Adipose lesions involving peripheral nerves represent a constellation of pathologies that, although uncommon, are becoming increasingly recognized as a direct result of the use of high-resolution imaging in patients with neuropathy. Currently, classification and nomenclature for

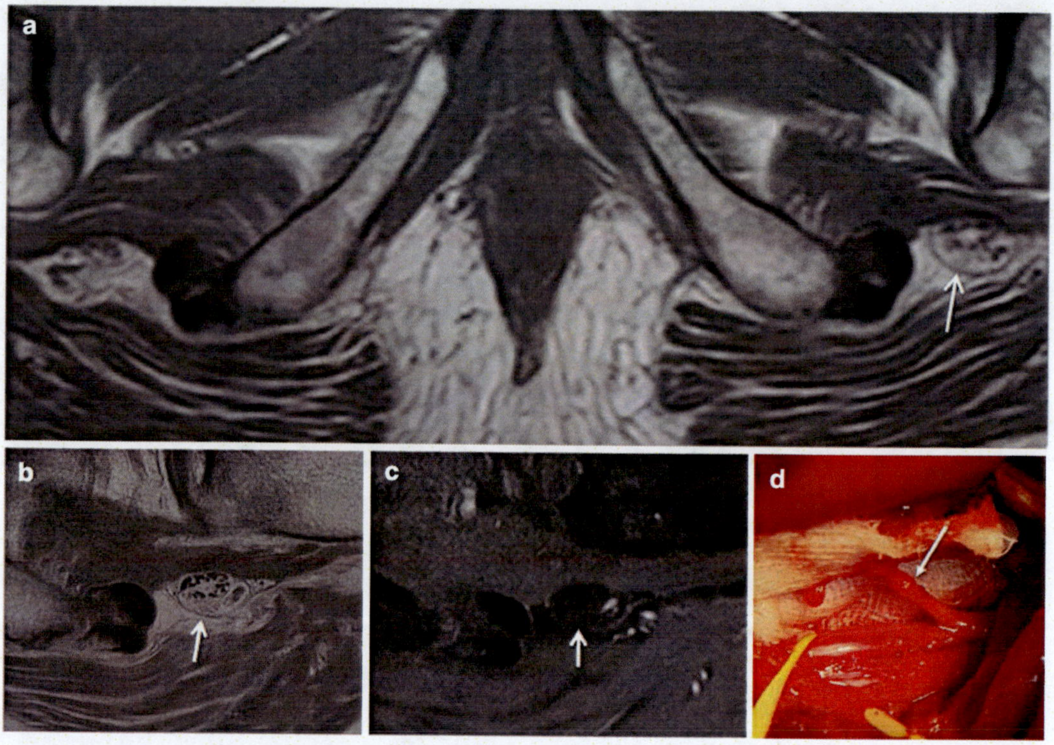

Fig. 7.9 Intraneural lipoma. (**a**) Axial T1-w image shows marked enlargement of the left sciatic nerve at the level of the ischial tuberosity. (**b**) Axial PD demonstrates the presence of fat content tissue within the epineurium. (**c**) Axial PD SPIR shows complete suppression of the tumor (arrow), confirming its adipose nature. (**d**) Operative view (arrow)

these types of lesion are incomplete and confusing. Adipose cells are a normal constituent of peripheral nerves, wherein they reside in the epineurium between fascicles, and could give rise to both lipomatosis and intraneural lipomas.

This discussion will be limited to intraneural lipomas without mesenchymal (soft tissue/osseous) overgrowth.

Intraneural lipomas are adipose lesions within the epineurium that might be encapsulated or may grow and interdigitate between individual fascicles, causing neuropathy secondary to a mass effect. The former can be resected safely and easily using modern microsurgical techniques with good results; the latter are not easily resected and/or separated from the nerve fascicles; as such, the relative pros and cons of surgical treatment should be considered, prior to undertaking surgery. These lesions typically involve the median nerve within the carpal tunnel, although involvement of the ulnar, radial, posterior interosseous, common peroneal, superficial peroneal, brachial plexus, sciatic, and tibial nerves has been reported. [7] MRN imaging is virtually pathognomonic (Fig. 7.9), since an intraneural lipoma shows the same signal intensity as fat, hyperintense on T1- and T2-weighted imaging, with uniform fat suppression on fat-suppressed sequences. Classic findings make routine biopsy of these lesions unnecessary.

7.5.3 Posttraumatic Neuroma

The term *traumatic neuroma* summarizes different forms of non-neoplastic peripheral nerve lesion. Spindle neuromas occur as sequels of a fibroinflammatory response to chronic friction or

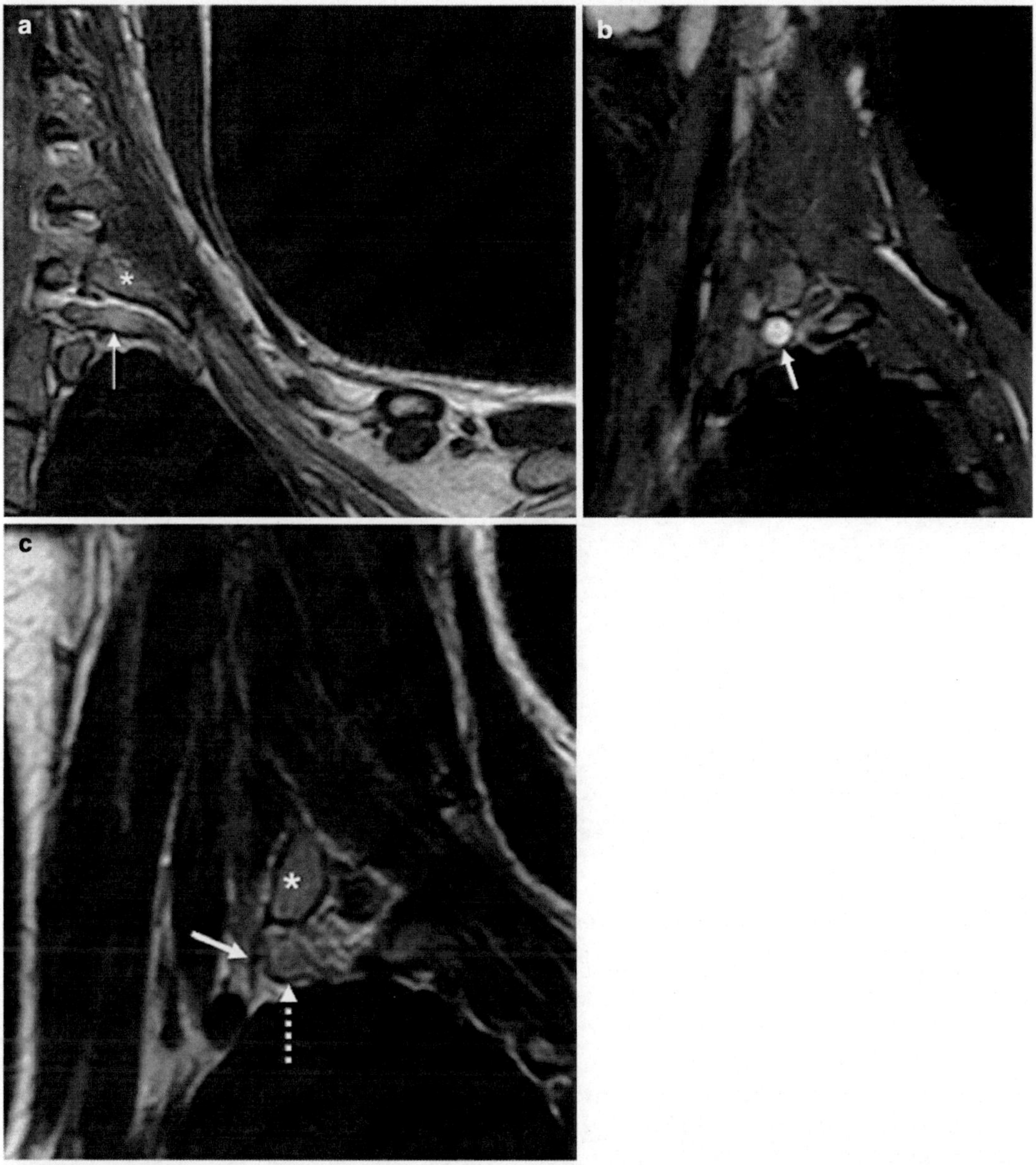

Fig. 7.10 Spindle cell neuroma. (**a**) Coronal T2-w shows an elongated C7 transverse process (asterisk) and C8 nerve root enlargement (arrow). (**b**) Sagittal STIR demonstrates increased signal intensity of the C8 nerve root (arrow). (**c**) Sagittal T2-w demonstrates a thin fibrous band (arrow) causing compression of the C8 nerve root (dotted arrow)

irritation of a non-disrupted nerve trunk (Fig. 7.10), while neuroma-in-continuity and terminal neuromas are the result of severe trauma with either partial disruption (Fig. 7.11) or total transection (Fig. 7.12) of a nerve, in which disorganized proliferation of nerve tissue represents an abortive attempt of the proximal nerve ending to re-establish continuity [9]. The disorganization of the neurogenic tissue seen in posttraumatic neuroma might be the key finding to rule out other pathologies [2]. Traumatic neuromas present loss of normal fascicular architecture; and

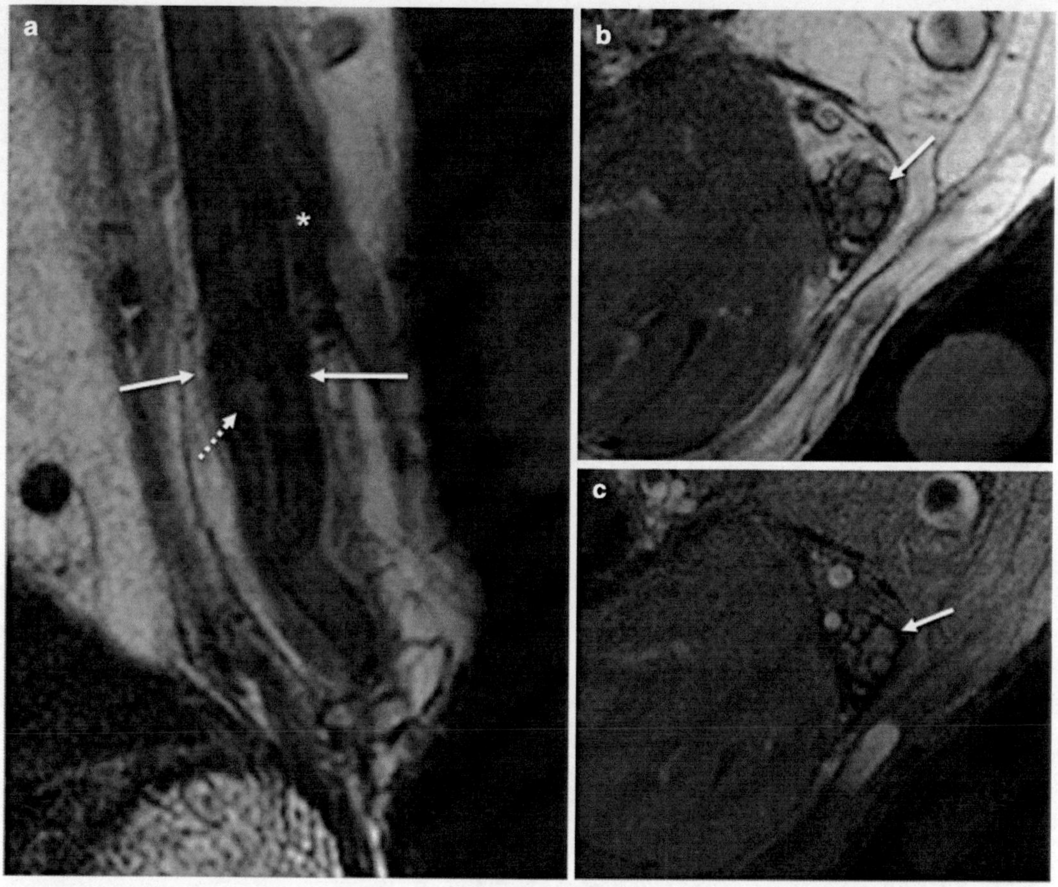

Fig. 7.11 Neuroma-in-continuity. (**a**) Sagittal T2-w shows enlargement of the ulnar nerve (arrows) in the distal arm, due to portal iatrogenic entrance (asterisk). Note the small ulnar nerve neuroma-in-continuity (dotted arrow). (**b**) Axial PD and (**c**) axial PD SPIR show fascicular enlargement consistent with a neuroma-in-continuity (arrows), which shows mild hyperintensity

most are homogenously isointense on T1-w images and heterogeneously hyperintense on fluid-sensitive sequences with variable contrast enhancement.

7.5.4 Morton's Neuroma

Morton's neuromas are the result of perineural fibrosis and degeneration of the plantar digital nerve at the level of the metatarsal head, with the second or third intermetatarsal spaces as the most common locations. Morton's neuromas are centrally located within the interspace, typically extending plantar to the level of the deep transverse intermetatarsal ligament, and show intermediate intensity on T1-w images and intermediate to low signal intensity on T2-w images, due to their high collagen content (Fig. 7.13) [2]. The intravenous administration of gadolinium contrast material has limited use, due to variable enhancement of the lesion. Fluid may be present in the intermetatarsal bursa secondary to associated inflammation [2, 9].

There are imaging mimickers, like intermetatarsal bursitis and fibrotic changes related to metatarsophalangeal plantar plate injury (called a pseudo-Morton's lesion) [10, 11]. The former is a fluid collection centered in the intermetatarsal space—above the level of the deep transverse

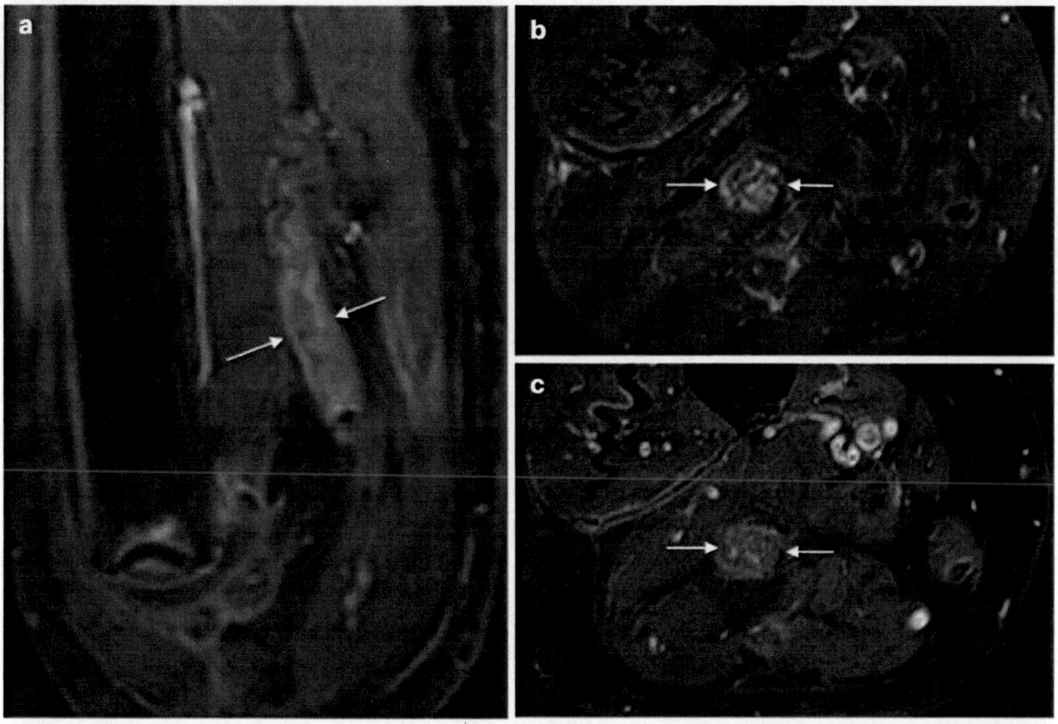

Fig. 7.12 Terminal neuroma. (**a**) Sagittal T1 SPIR contrast-enhanced image shows bulbous enlargement of the distal ending of the sciatic nerve (arrows) in an amputated patient. (**b**) Axial STIR demonstrates loss of fascicular appearance and increased signal intensity (arrows). (**c**) Axial T1 SPIR contrast-enhanced image shows mild heterogeneous enhancement (arrows)

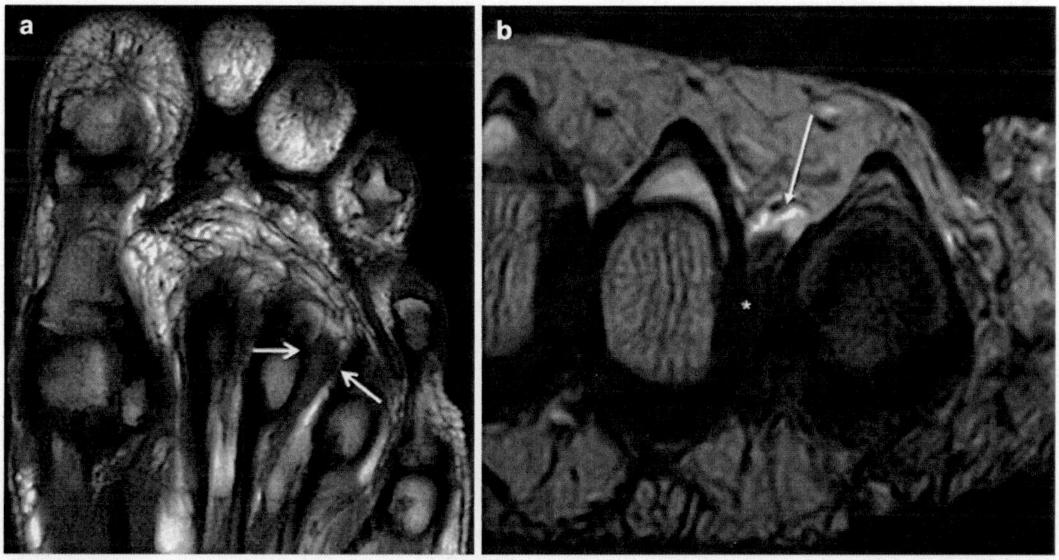

Fig. 7.13 Morton's neuroma. (**a**) Axial T1-w at the level of the metatarsal heads shows isointense fusiform enlargement of the plantar digital nerve (arrows) in the third intermetatarsal space. (**b**) Coronal T2-w demonstrates low signal intensity of the neuroma (asterisk), associated with intermetatarsal bursal fluid (arrow)

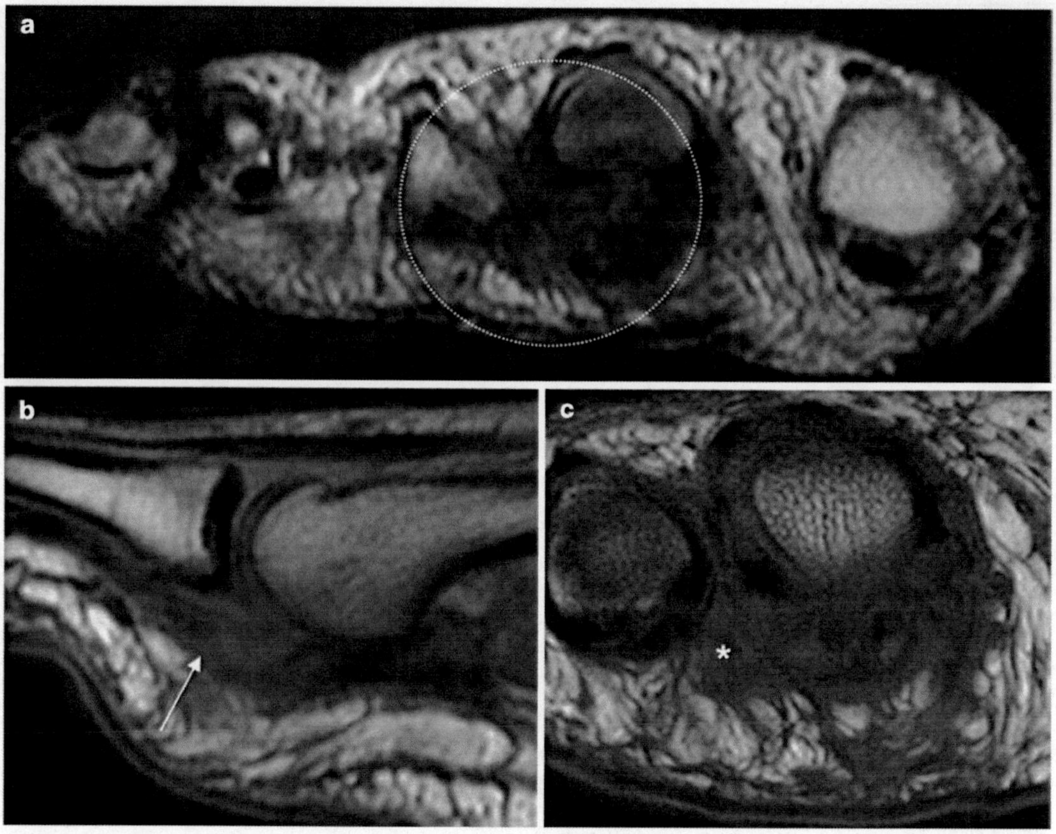

Fig. 7.14 Metatarsophalangeal (MTP) joint plantar plate rupture and pseudo-Morton's lesion. Coronal T2-w (**a**) and T1-w (**c**) show obliteration of the second intermetatarsal space, due to eccentric reactive pericapsular soft tissue thickening (dotted circle and asterisk) related to MTP plantar plate rupture (arrow, **b**—sagittal PD)

ligament—which thus shows high signal intensity on T2-w images; the latter is pericapsular fibrosis eccentrically located within the intermetatarsal space that broadly abuts the plantar lateral and lateral aspects of the metatarsophalangeal joint and exhibits intermediate signal on T1- and T2-weighted images (Fig. 7.14). A correct diagnosis has clinical consequences, as metatarsalgia is commonly treated with a steroid injection that may result in soft tissue atrophy, precipitating a tear in the capsule and/or plantar plate and causing joint instability [10].

7.5.5 Hereditary Neuropathy

Charcot-Marie-Tooth (CMT) syndrome is a rare hereditary motor and sensory neuropathy presented in this chapter, given that its MRN appearance might suggest the presence of a peripheral nerve tumor. This, therefore, renders this lesion a differential diagnosis to consider. The classification remains confusing in many aspects, since it requires constant change due to the identification of new genetic forms. [12] Different genetic forms also have different imaging appearances: the demyelinated/dysmyelinated type (CMT1A) presents with symmetrical and bilateral nerve enlargement (Fig. 7.15) with minimal gadolinium enhancement, whereas the axonal forms (CMT2) show normal size to minimal nerve enlargement, but abnormal hyperintensity on fluid-sensitive sequences [3, 13]. The most "typical" phenotype is characterized by distal weakness, sensory loss, foot deformities (*pes cavus* and hammertoes), and

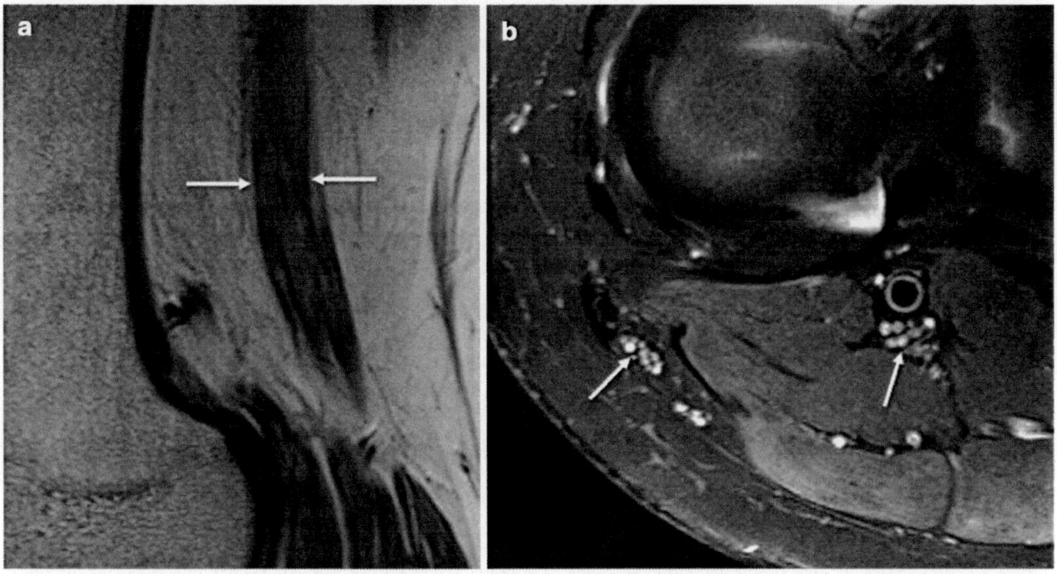

Fig. 7.15 Charcot-Marie-Tooth 1A. (**a**) Sagittal T2-w shows enlargement of the distal sciatic nerve (arrows). (**b**) Axial PD SPIR demonstrates enlargements of individual fascicles in both the tibial and peroneal nerves (arrows)

absent reflexes. The diffuse nature of the clinical and imaging findings is distinctive and should help distinguish CMT from a peripheral nerve tumor.

7.5.6 Inflammatory Neuropathy

The spectrum of immune-mediated polyneuropathies is wide, with various subtypes continuing to be identified. Chronic inflammatory demyelinating polyradiculoneuropathy (CIDP) is relevant as a differential diagnosis of a PN tumor.

CIDP is a rare and heterogeneous but treatable immune-mediated neuropathy; consequently, avoiding diagnostic delay is important to prevent irreversible axonal loss, although misdiagnosis is common. The hallmark of typical CIDP is a chronic progressive, monophasic, or recurrent demyelinating polyradiculoneuropathy with a progressive phase of weakness that exceeds 2 months, often with sensory dysfunction and absent or reduced tendon reflexes [14]. However, there are a variety of clinical phenotypes that can be a diagnostic challenge, for which MRN is particularly useful. The affected nerve is T1 isointense and T2 hyperintense (Fig. 7.6), and variable fascicular damage can be seen and, subsequently, variable degree of enhancement, though the absence of contrast enhancement has been reported more often. CIDP is a differential diagnosis for perineurioma, posttraumatic neuroma, amyloidosis, CMT disease, Dejerine-Sottas disease, etc. Occasionally, targeted fascicular biopsy may be indicated and helpful in those patients who do not respond to first-line treatment.

7.5.7 Infectious Neuropathy

The peripheral nervous system can be affected by infection, but this is rare and does not usually produce mass-like enlargement of the affected nerve. Leprosy is an exception. In most cases, the neural lesion remains a granuloma (Fig. 7.16); however, in tuberculoid leprosy, abscess formation—with the ulnar nerve most commonly affected—can be identified as a nerve tumor with loss of fascicular architecture, along with thickened hypointense epineurium, hypointense on T1- and hyperintense on T2-weighted images,

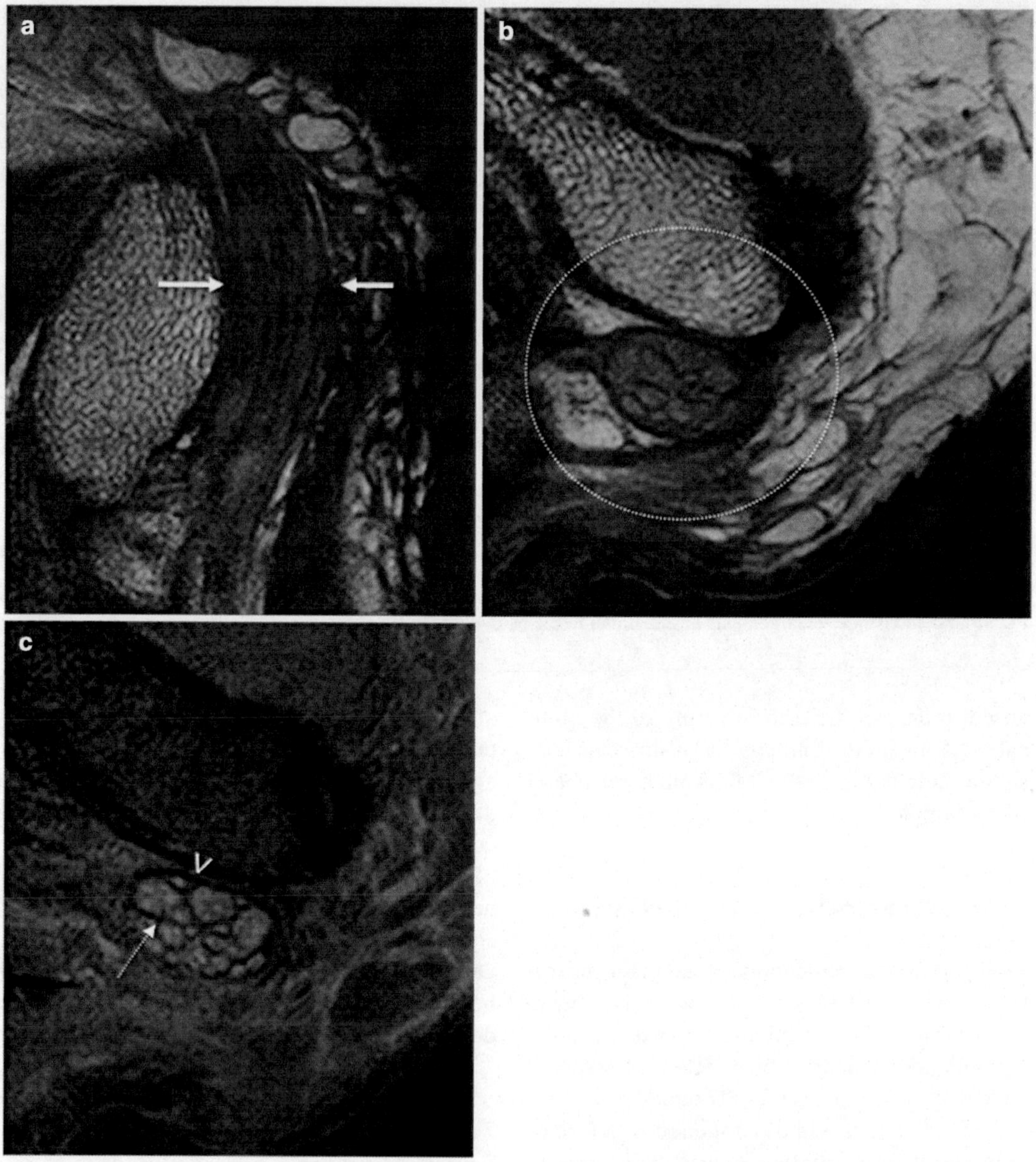

Fig. 7.16 Hansen's disease. (**a**) Sagittal T2-w demonstrates thickening of the ulnar nerve within the cubital tunnel. (**b**) Axial PD and (**c**) axial PD SPIR show swollen fascicules surrounded by the thickened hypointense perineurium (dotted arrow) and epineurium (arrowhead)

with peripheral rim enhancement due to central necrosis [15]. Some of these abscesses may calcify and, therefore, might be seen on X-ray exams. It is important to keep in mind that a nerve abscess as the first manifestation of leprosy is uncommon; therefore, a high index of suspicion is required to make the correct diagnosis.

7.5.8 Endometriosis

Endometriosis is a common gynecological condition, defined as the occurrence of endometriotic tissue (endometrial glands, stroma, or both) outside the uterus in a female of reproductive age. Although an infrequent cause of peripheral neuropathy, it

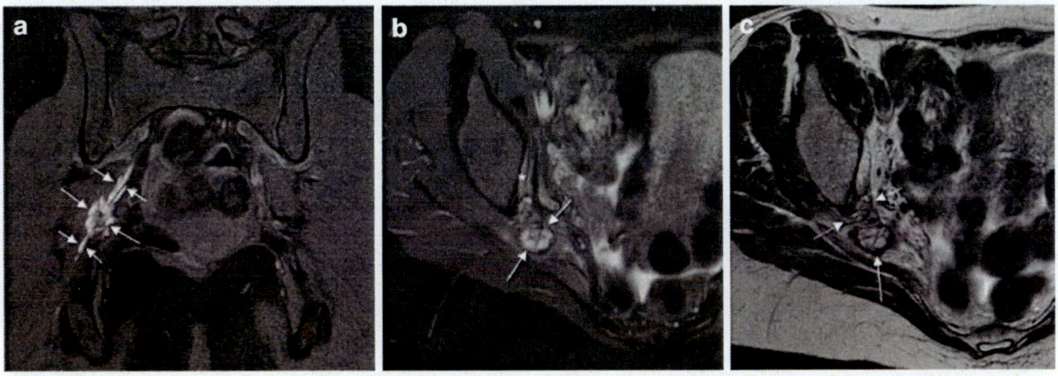

Fig. 7.17 Endometriosis. (**a**) Coronal T1 SPIR identifies a spontaneous hyperintense multilobulated mass at the sciatic notch (arrows). (**b**) Axial PD SPAIR. The sciatic nerve is markedly thickened (arrows) and exhibits fascicular enlargement with increased signal intensity, due to intraneural methemoglobin deposition. Note the denervation changes in the internal obturator muscle (asterisk). (**c**) Axial T2-w shows epineurium thickening and loss of the fat plane around the nerve, due to retractive fibrous tissue (dotted arrows)

should be considered in those patients with cyclic pain linked to their menstrual period [16]. The typical deposits of endometriosis are hyperintense on T1-w images—particularly on T1 fat-suppressed sequences—due to methemoglobin and other blood products, while on T2-w images, the signal can be mixed, based on the age of any associated blood products and the proportions of stromal and endometrial cells and fibrosis (Fig. 7.17). Post-gadolinium enhancement is variable. Denervation signs are also a frequent finding [17, 18].

7.5.9 Malignant Infiltration

Perineural spread is the process of neoplastic invasion of nerves. It also is a marker of poor outcome and, therefore, decreased survival, which can be observed in the absence of lymphatic or vascular invasion [19]. MRN images can be challenging, particularly if the patient has been irradiated. In radiation-induced neuropathy, the area may show (Fig. 7.18) mild nerve enlargement (relative to perineural spread) with T2 hyperintense signal alterations and fascicular and/or homogeneous enhancement after gadolinium administration. Soft tissue edema in the irradiated area is another common finding [20].

With perineural spread, nerves exhibit irregular/infiltrating and nodular contours on T1- and T2-weighted imaging, as well as irregular/heterogeneous perifascicular gadolinium enhancement (Fig. 7.19). Lesions tend to be multiple, and there might also be evidence of other metastases in ganglions, bone, or muscle [20].

7.6 Summary

Advances in MRN imaging have improved the diagnostic work-up of neural and non-neural tumors, expanding differential diagnostic possibilities and facilitating operative interventions—including targeted fascicular biopsies—rendering surgical exploration faster and more straightforward.

The MR imaging characteristics of many peripheral nerve lesions are unique; nevertheless, they should be carefully considered in the context of the neurological examination and laboratory evaluation to enhance outcomes. A multidisciplinary approach to patient care is highly advised.

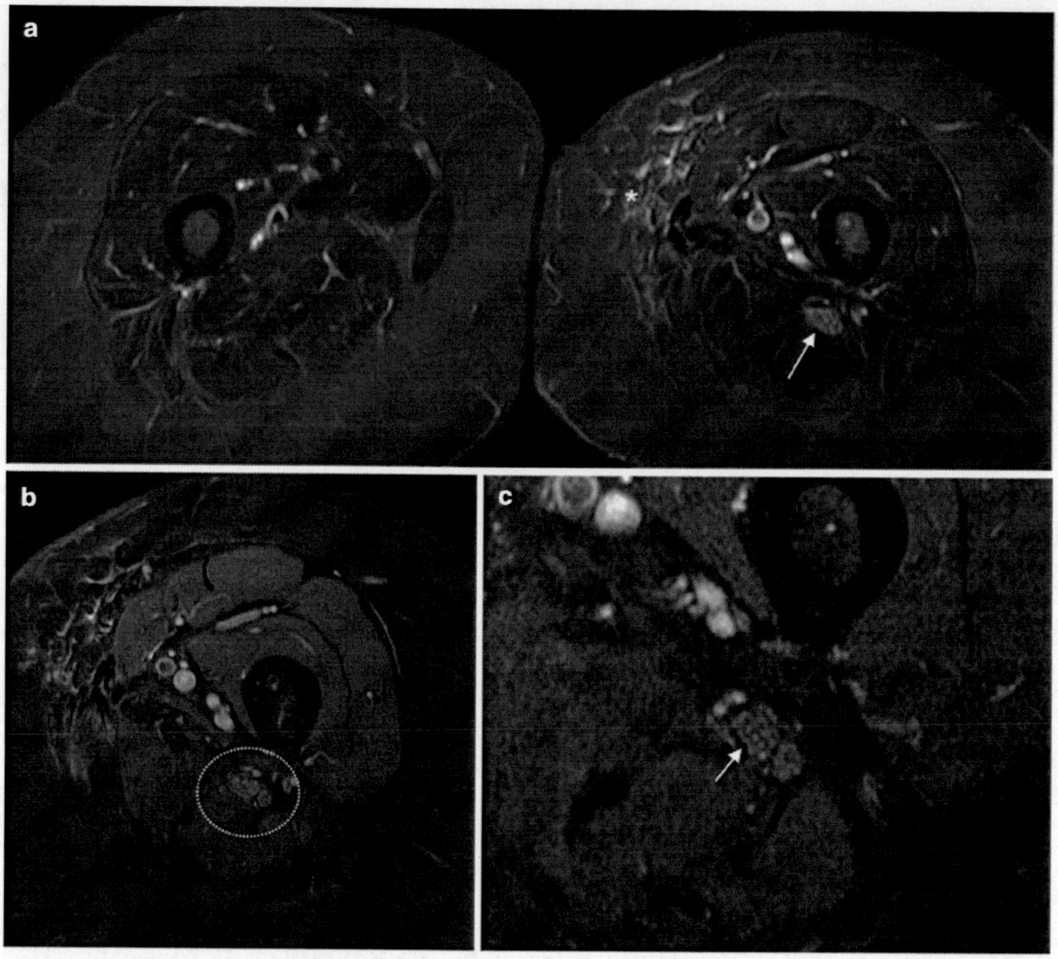

Fig. 7.18 Radiation-induced neuropathy. (**a**) Axial STIR shows marked enlargement of the left sciatic nerve (arrow) and subcutaneous edema (asterisk) related to radiotherapy. (**b**) Axial PD SPAIR. Nerve fascicles show increased signal intensity (dotted circle). (**c**) Axial T1 SPIR exhibits fascicular enhancement after gadolinium injection (arrow)

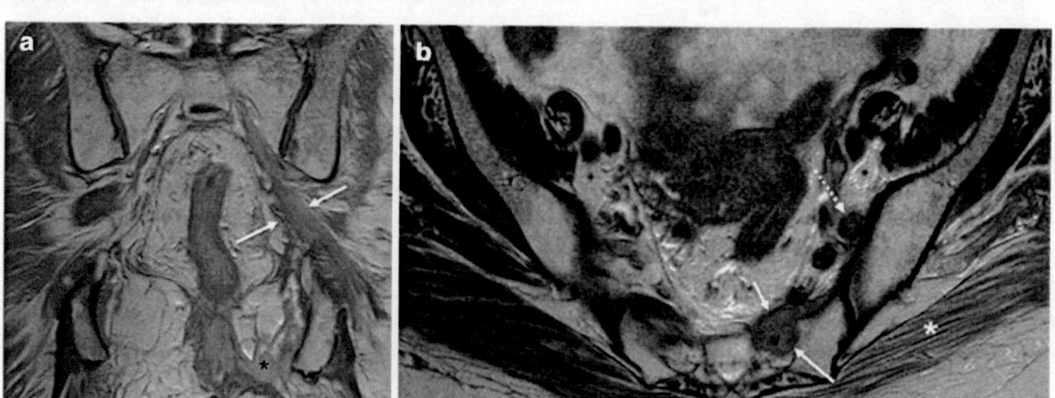

Fig. 7.19 Metastatic endometrial cancer. (**a**) Coronal T1 gadolinium-enhanced image shows the left sciatic nerve enlarged and enhanced. Note inferior hypogastric plexus spread (asterisk). (**b**) Axial T2-w identifies enlargement of S1 (dotted arrow) and S3 (arrows) on the left due to perineural spread. Denervation changes of the gluteus maximus are also seen (asterisk)

References

1. Chhabra A, Peripheral MR. Neurography approach to interpretation. Neuroimaging Clin N Am. 2014;24:79–89.
2. Tagliafico AS, et al. Nerve tumors: what the MSK radiologist should know. Semin Musculoskelet Radiol. 2019;23:76–84.
3. Ahlawat S, Chhabra A, Blakely J. Magnetic resonance neurography of peripheral nerve tumors and tumorlike conditions. Neuroimaging Clin N Am. 2014;24:171–92.
4. Spinner RJ, Amrami KK. What's new in the management of benign peripheral nerve lesions? Neurosurg Clin N Am. 2008;19:517–31.
5. Wilson TJ, et al. Clinico-radiological features of intraneural perineuriomas obviate the need for tissue diagnosis. J Neurosurg. 2018;129(4):1034–40.
6. Puffer RC, et al. Extensive perineural spread of an intrapelvic sciatic malignant peripheral nerve sheath tumor: a case report. Acta Neurochir. 2018;160(9):1833–6.
7. Li C-S, et al. Differentiation of soft tissue benign and malignant peripheral nerve sheath tumors with magnetic resonance imaging. Clin Imaging. 2008;32:121–7.
8. Spinner RJ, et al. Dynamic phases of peroneal and tibial intraneural ganglia formation: a new dimension added to the unifying articular theory. J Neurosurg. 2007;107:296–307.
9. Woertler K. Tumors and tumor-like lesions of peripheral nerves. Semin Musculoskelet Radiol. 2010;14:547–58.
10. Umans H, et al. MRI of lesser metatarsophalangeal joint plantar plate tears and associated adjacent interspace lesions. Skelet Radiol. 2014;43(10):1361–8.
11. Yamada AF, et al. Second and third metatarsophalangeal plantar plate tears: diagnostic performance of direct and indirect MRI features using surgical findings as the reference standard. AJR. 2017;209: W100–8.
12. Pareyson D, Saveri P, Pisciotta C. New developments in Charcot–Marie–tooth neuropathy and related diseases. Curr Opin Neurol. 2017;30(5):471–80.
13. De Smet K, et al. MRI in hypertrophic mono- and polyneuropathies. Clin Radiol. 2013;68(3): 317–22.
14. Bunschoten C, et al. Progress in diagnosis and treatment of chronic inflammatory demyelinating polyradiculoneuropathy. Lancet Neurol. 2019;18: 784–94.
15. Sen D, et al. Ultrasonography and magnetic resonance imaging of ulnar nerve abscess in leprosy. Med J Armed Forces India. 2016;72(1):78–81.
16. Capek S, et al. Sequential imaging of intraneural sciatic nerve endometriosis provides insight into symptoms of cyclical sciatica. Acta Neurochir. 2016;158:507–12.
17. Floyd JR, et al. Cyclic sciatica from extrapelvic endometriosis affecting the sciatic nerve. J Neurosurg Spine. 2011;14:281–9.
18. Siquara de Sousa AC, et al. Magnetic resonance imaging evidence for perineural spread of endometriosis to the lumbosacral plexus: report of 2 cases. Neurosurg Focus. 2015;39(3):E15.
19. Liebig C, et al. Perineural invasion in cancer. Cancer. 2009;115(15):3379–91.
20. Capek S, et al. Perineural spread of pelvic malignancies to the lumbosacral plexus and beyond: clinical and imaging patterns. Neurosurg Focus. 2015;39(3):E14.

8 X-Ray, Computed Tomography (CT), Positron Emission Tomography (PET) Imaging, and Intraoperative Imaging Adjuncts in the Evaluation and Treatment of Peripheral Nerve Tumors

Adela Wu, Thomas J. Wilson, and Michel Kliot

8.1 Introduction

Nerve tumors encompass a broad array of diagnoses, including schwannoma, neurofibroma, malignant peripheral nerve sheath tumor (MPNST), intraneural perineurioma, fibrolipomatous hamartoma, and metastatic disease.

Diagnostic imaging is critical in evaluating and treating peripheral nerve masses. The two mainstays of imaging in the evaluation of peripheral nerve masses are ultrasound and MRI. Prior chapters in this book have demonstrated the clinical utility of ultrasound (Chap. 6) and MRI (Chap. 7) in the identification and treatment of peripheral nerve tumors. In this chapter, we will focus on additional imaging techniques that may, in certain circumstances, be useful in evaluating peripheral nerve tumors, including X-ray, computed tomography (CT), and positron emission tomography (PET) imaging.

A. Wu · T. J. Wilson · M. Kliot (✉)
Department of Neurosurgery, Stanford University, Stanford, CA, USA

8.2 X-Ray

X-rays typically have a limited role in the evaluation of peripheral nerve tumors and are not typically recommended in the standard evaluation of these tumors. However, it is important to recognize direct and indirect signs, when present, on X-rays ordered for other reasons or ordered early in the evaluation of a patient before the presence of a nerve tumor is known.

Nerve tumors can occasionally be visualized on plain X-rays as a hyperdense shadow (Fig. 8.1). These may be recognized on chest or abdominal X-rays ordered for evaluation of chest or abdominal pain, respectively. X-rays do not have the resolution required to appropriately evaluate these tumors. Thus, when identified, X-rays should be followed with a more advanced imaging modality, such as MRI or ultrasound.

When the tumor occurs near the bone, some information can be gleaned. Benign nerve tumors tend to erode the bone in a smooth fashion, and the eroded bone will often have sclerotic margins typical of slow-growing tumors. Malignant nerve tumors often invade nearby bone causing ragged bone erosion, without sclerotic margins. One example is the rib notching that may be associated with intercostal benign nerve sheath tumors [1].

F. Guedes et al. (eds.), *Diagnostic Assessment and Treatment of Peripheral Nerve Tumors*,
https://doi.org/10.1007/978-3-030-77633-6_8

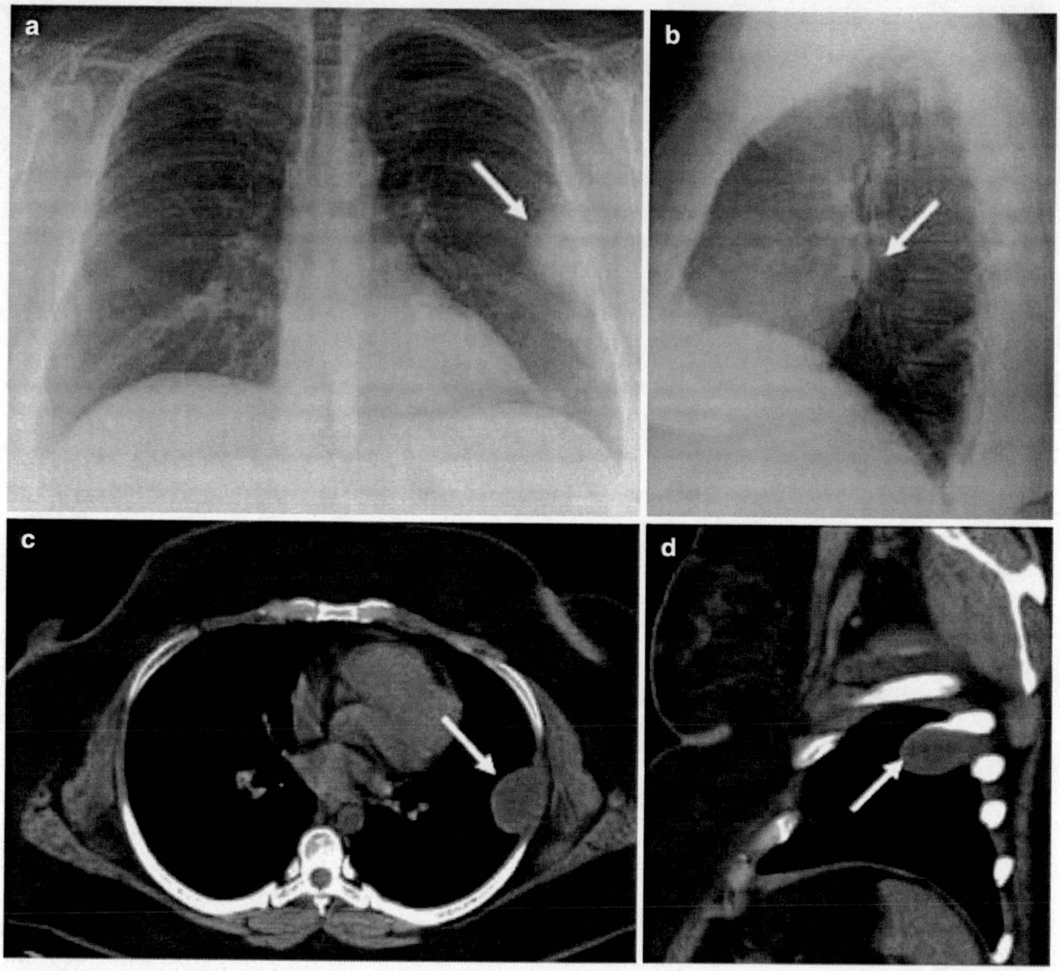

Fig. 8.1 (**a**) AP and (**b**) lateral chest X-ray showing a hyperdense shadow along the rib, ultimately found to be a schwannoma arising from the intercostal nerve. (**c**) Axial and (**d**) sagittal CT of the chest showing the same lesion along the rib, external to the lung parenchyma. The mass is isodense to the nearby muscle, well-circumscribed, and fusiform in shape. This was ultimately diagnosed as a schwannoma arising from the intercostal nerve upon resection

In cases of neurofibromatosis type 1 (NF1), patients will often have neurofibromas at multiple spinal levels. These slow-growing nerve tumors will often erode the bone in the neural foramina, causing enlargement of the foramina and scalloping of the vertebral body (Fig. 8.2). When these changes are visualized at multiple spine levels, this may be indirect evidence for a diagnosis of neurofibromatosis. In these cases, it is often difficult to visualize the tumor directly with plain X-rays.

Fibrolipomatous hamartomas are masses of peripheral nerves that consist of fatty infiltration and proliferation between fascicles of a nerve. This typically results in significant enlargement of the involved nerve [2]. The most common nerve affected is the median nerve, accounting for nearly 60% of the reported cases in the literature [3]. Overgrowth of the soft tissue and bone in the territory of the involved nerve is common, occurring in at least 60% of cases and possibly much higher [3, 4]. As part of this over-

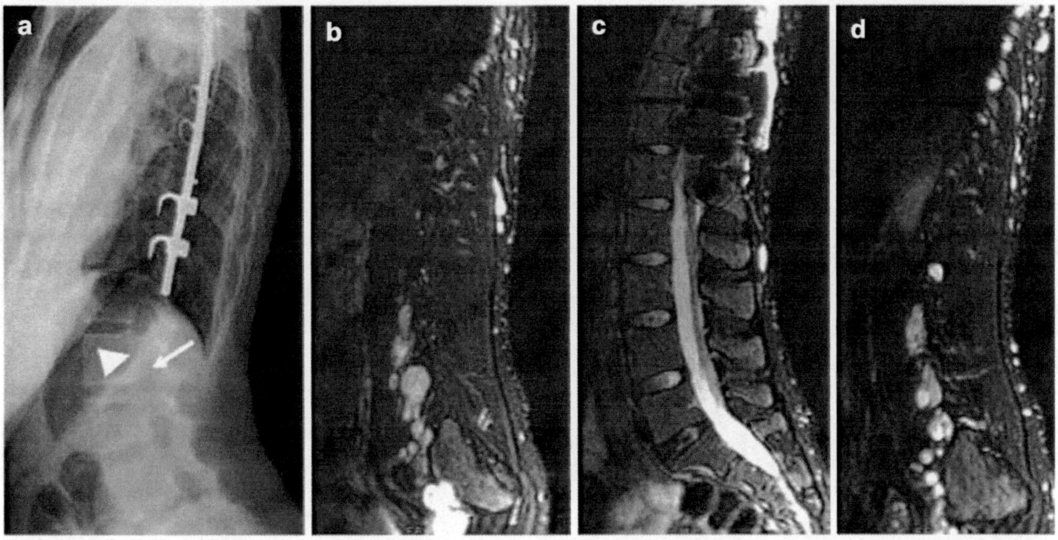

Fig. 8.2 (**a**) Lateral X-ray showing the widening of the neural foramen (arrow) and the scalloping of the vertebral body (arrowhead) that can be seen in association with benign peripheral nerve tumors. (**b**) Left parasagittal, (**c**) mid-sagittal, and (**d**) right parasagittal T2-weighted MRI image showing the associated benign peripheral nerve tumors arising from the neural foramina in this patient with neurofibromatosis type 1

growth, macrodactyly occurs in approximately one-third of cases [5, 6]. There are pathognomonic features of this lesion on MRI. On axial imaging, the involved nerve resembles a coaxial cable, while on coronal imaging, the nerve resembles strands of spaghetti. Nerve fascicles are hypointense on both T1- and T2-weighted images. The fat distribution varies from lesion to lesion but takes on one of two patterns: either distributed between nerve fascicles or distributed peripherally surrounding the nerve fascicles [7–9]. While the tumor cannot be directly visualized on plain X-rays, the soft tissue and bone overgrowth can be imaged and evaluated using plain X-rays (Fig. 8.3).

8.3 CT

While still not as useful as ultrasound and MRI, CT can be useful in the evaluation of peripheral nerve tumors. CT does not provide the same soft tissue resolution as MRI but does provide useful information. Many times, a peripheral nerve tumor may be initially recognized on a CT scan before the presence of a peripheral nerve tumor is known. Furthermore, CT can be useful in evaluating metastatic disease in cases where a malignant nerve tumor is suspected, in showing the relationship of vasculature to the tumor for preoperative planning, in showing bone changes and bone anatomy that may be useful in both diagnosis and preoperative planning, and in cases where there are contraindications to MRI and ultrasound.

On CT, the most common benign peripheral nerve sheath tumors, which are neurofibromas and schwannomas, typically appear as well-circumscribed and solid masses. The shape of the mass is typically either spherical or fusiform and typically occurs in the expected location of a peripheral nerve, though visualization of the entering and exiting peripheral nerves is difficult on CT. The mass is usually hypodense relative to the muscle and classically is described to show moderate to marked contrast enhancement on post-contrast images, though we have also commonly observed faint or no contrast

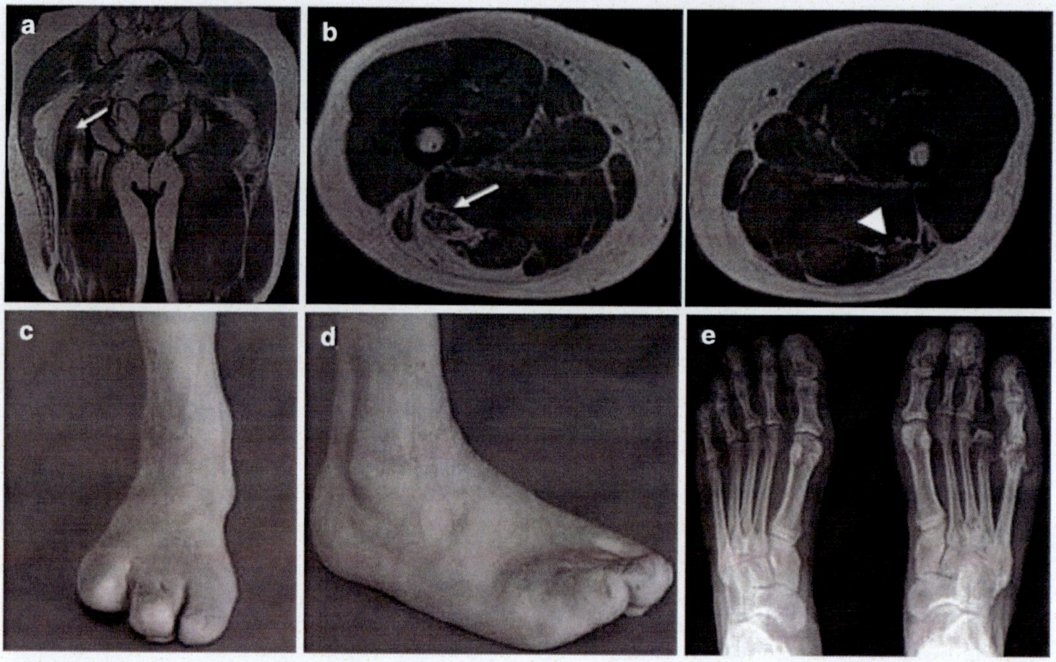

Fig. 8.3 (**a**) Coronal and (**b**) axial T1-weighted MRI showing a fibrolipomatous hamartoma of the right sciatic nerve (arrow). Comparatively, the normal left sciatic nerve is shown on the axial image (arrowhead). On coronal imaging, the nerve resembles strands of spaghetti, while on the axial imaging, the nerve has a coaxial cable-like appearance. (**c, d**) Photographs of the right foot of this patient with a fibrolipomatous hamartoma showing the soft tissue overgrowth and bony abnormalities that can be associated. (**e**) Plain X-rays of the feet of this patient showing the soft tissue overgrowth in the right foot, as well as the bone abnormalities in the phalanges, associated with a fibrolipomatous hamartoma

enhancement (Fig. 8.4). The contrast enhancement may be homogeneous or heterogeneous. Particularly with schwannomas, there can be a cystic component to the tumor, though intratumoral cystic changes should raise the possibility of a malignancy [10].

Comparatively, malignant peripheral nerve sheath tumors (MPNSTs) are usually larger. They also are typically hypodense relative to the muscle but may show areas of central necrosis. Contrast enhancement is variable but often is heterogeneous. The borders of the tumor are typically irregular and may invade surrounding structures. Similar to MRI, CT cannot reliably differentiate between benign nerve tumors and MPNSTs.

Malignant peripheral nerve sheath tumors commonly metastasize to the lung, liver, brain, lymph nodes, and retroperitoneum [11, 12]. Due to the frequency of metastases to the lung and liver, metastatic workup should include a CT scan of the chest, abdomen, and pelvis. In this way, CT is also indirectly valuable in the evaluation of nerve tumors.

8.4 Fluorodeoxyglucose (FDG)-PET

FDG-PET works by the principle that metabolically active cells take up glucose at a higher rate than metabolically quiet cells. By radiolabeling glucose, we are capable of imaging metabolically active cells. Since tumor cells are rapidly dividing and metabolically active, they are well visualized by FDG-PET. FDG-PET can be useful in trying to distinguish between benign and malignant peripheral nerve tumors and can also be useful in evaluating for metastatic disease in cases of

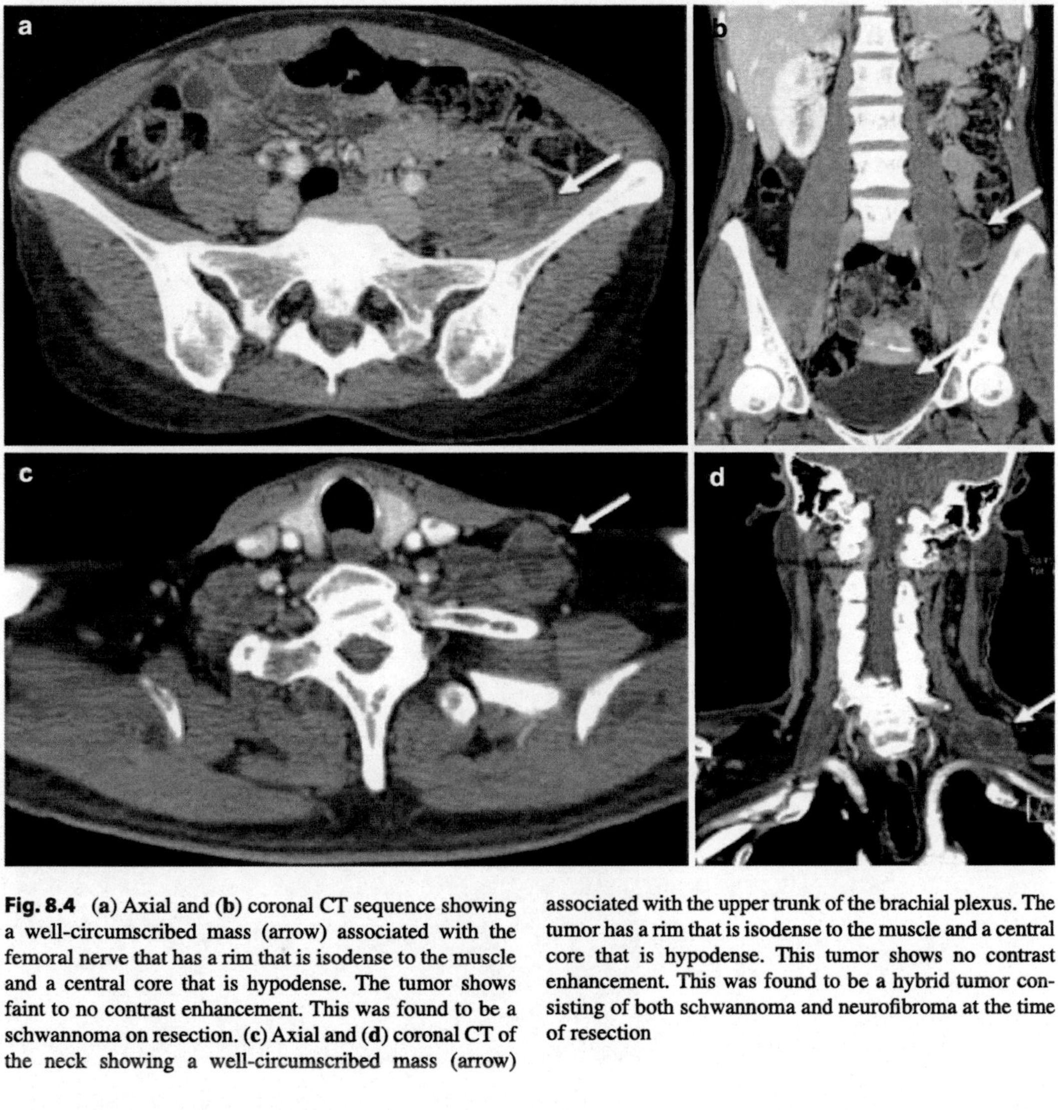

Fig. 8.4 (**a**) Axial and (**b**) coronal CT sequence showing a well-circumscribed mass (arrow) associated with the femoral nerve that has a rim that is isodense to the muscle and a central core that is hypodense. The tumor shows faint to no contrast enhancement. This was found to be a schwannoma on resection. (**c**) Axial and (**d**) coronal CT of the neck showing a well-circumscribed mass (arrow) associated with the upper trunk of the brachial plexus. The tumor has a rim that is isodense to the muscle and a central core that is hypodense. This tumor shows no contrast enhancement. This was found to be a hybrid tumor consisting of both schwannoma and neurofibroma at the time of resection

malignant peripheral nerve tumors. However, while useful in some circumstances, FDG-PET is fraught with problems and cannot reliably distinguish benign from malignant nerve tumors.

Glucose utilization is typically measured using a value known as the standardized uptake value (SUVmax), where a lower SUVmax suggests lower glucose utilization and a benign tumor, whereas a higher SUVmax suggests higher glucose utilization and a potential malignancy (Fig. 8.5). Threshold values have been established. Another value reported on FDG-PET is the tumor-to-liver ratio, which some suggest may be a better predictor of malignancy. In one study, using an SUVmax threshold of 6.1, the sensitivity was 94%, and the specificity was 91% for MPNST [13]. However, the main problem is that there is considerable overlap in SUVmax between MPNSTs and benign neurofibromas, and this problem is magnified by an even greater overlap between schwannomas, which often have a higher SUVmax than neurofibromas, and MPNSTs. A recent study by Ahlawat and colleagues found that the SUVmax for benign tumors included in the study was 3.2, with a standard deviation of 1.8. This means to account for

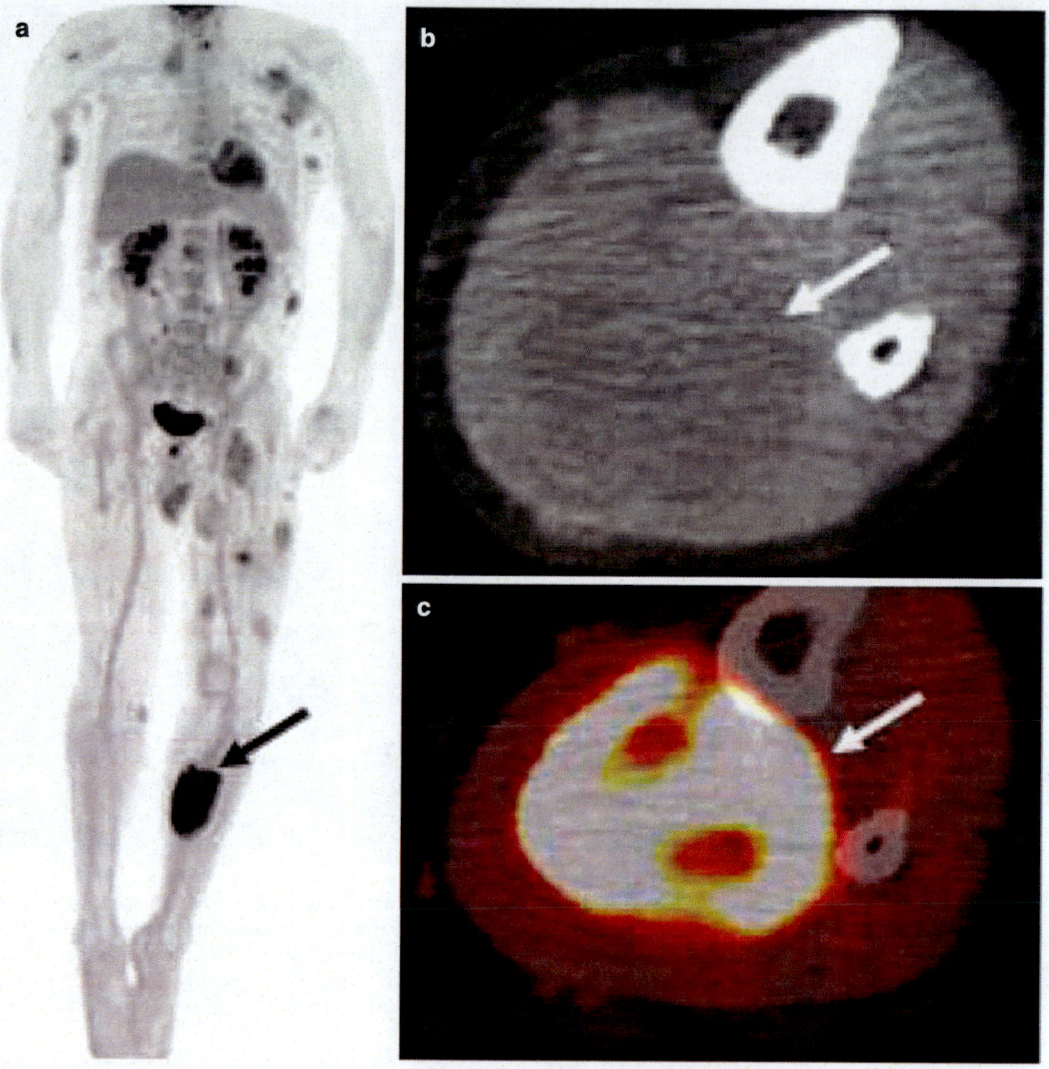

Fig. 8.5 (**a**) Whole-body FDG-PET image showing a hypermetabolic tumor (arrow) in the left calf and numerous other tumors that show varying levels of metabolic activity. (**b**) CT and (**c**) FDG-PET image showing the tumor in the left calf associated with the tibial nerve. The CT shows a mass that is isodense to the surrounding muscle. The FDG-PET image shows that the mass is hypermetabolic, with an SUVmax of 21.3. This suggests a diagnosis of malignant peripheral nerve sheath tumor, which was confirmed at the time of resection

95% of benign tumors (±2 standard deviations) would include a range of 0–6.8. In the same study, the average SUVmax for MPNSTs was 8.0, with a standard deviation of 3.9. This means that 68% of the MPNSTs (±1 standard deviation) fall within the range of 4.1–11.9 [14]. These ranges demonstrate the problem of considerable overlap between benign and malignant. Some authors have suggested that a better and more predictive value is the tumor-to-liver ratio. The consensus threshold seems to be 1.5, with a higher tumor-to-liver threshold being more suggestive of a malignancy [15]. Increased glucose utilization can be patchy within malignant tumors (Fig. 8.6). FDG-PET can also be used to identify potential areas for biopsy.

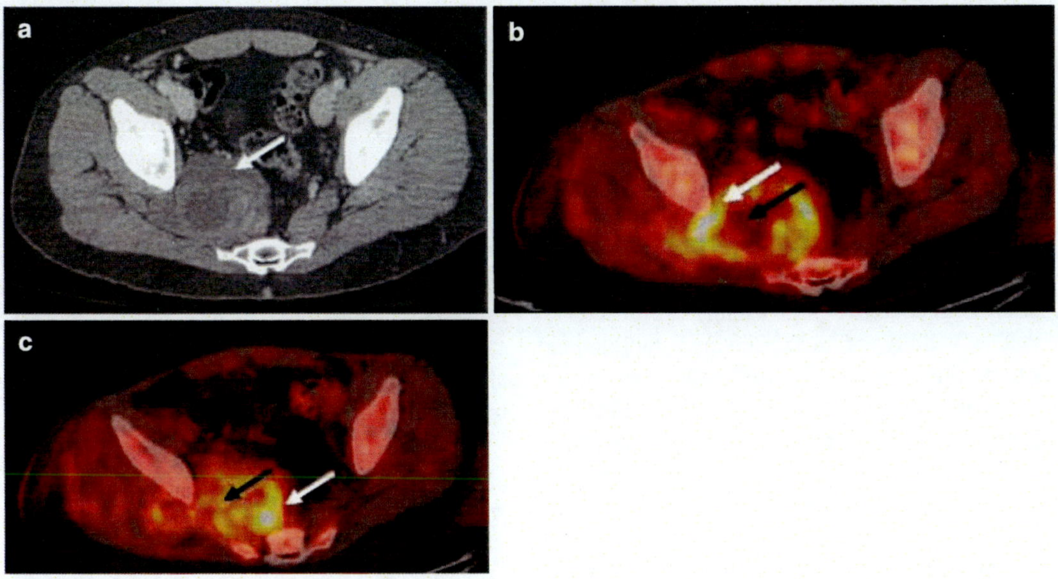

Fig. 8.6 (**a**) CT and (**b**, **c**) FDG-PET images showing a large, irregular mass associated with the right sciatic nerve. The mass shows heterogeneous PET avidity, suggesting some areas of the tumor are more hypermetabolic than others. The SUVmax of this tumor was 12.1. The mass was found to be a malignant peripheral nerve sheath tumor

In fact, some have argued that the SUVmax is a better measure of prognosis and predictor of overall survival than tumor histology itself in malignant peripheral nerve tumors [16]. Brenner et al. found that patients with tumors demonstrating SUV levels less than 3 survived over the entire follow-up course, whereas other patients with the same tumor grade but SUV >3 died within 4–33 months.

Additional information from FDG-PET that may be useful in detecting malignant tumors includes the mean SUV and tracer uptake heterogeneity, which reflects the increased glucose metabolism and cellular activity in malignant tumors [17]. It was found that there was a statistically significant negative correlation between mean SUV and mean ADC on PET imaging, parameters that may provide additional information for defining malignant precursor lesions in the future [18].

FDG-PET also proves useful for asymptomatic patients [19]. In a group of 41 high-risk patients, children and adolescents with plexiform neurofibromas, most did not present with overt symptoms. However, approximately 20% of the patients were diagnosed on PET imaging with malignant peripheral nerve tumors, which were also confirmed histologically [19].

FDG-PET therefore proves to be an extremely useful preoperative imaging modality for patients who are suspected to be at risk for malignant transformation of their peripheral nerve tumors. The novel combination of MRI and PET offers several advantages in diagnosing malignant nerve tumors. MRI provides the detailed resolution and contrast necessary to visualize the tumors' size, appearance, and growth, while ^{18}F-FDG-PET adds a powerful level of monitoring for malignant transformation. Together, this new imaging modality offers patients with peripheral nerve tumors a wealth of information within one setting and without the cumulative risk of radiation over time from CT scans. PET/MRI is as sensitive as PET/CT for depicting peripheral nerve tumors. FDG-avid lesions found on PET/CT were all visible on PET/MRI [20]. Given that patients with

NF1 and other syndromes involving multiple peripheral nerve tumors require serial monitoring, it would be beneficial for them to undergo PET/MRI rather than the cumulative radiation of CT over time. Furthermore, the MRI sequences offer detailed anatomical resolution of the tumors as well [21]. ADC values obtained from MRI have also proven useful, with lower values correlating with increased cellularity and malignancy compared to benign tumors [22].

The validity of metabolic and radiological information provided by PET/MRI was further tested in studies with NF1 patients [23]. One group followed 28 patients with 83 peripheral nerve lesions who were deemed to be at high risk for malignant transformation. This study found a standardized uptake value (SUV) maximum threshold of 2.78 or greater reliably differentiated between benign and malignant tumors [23]. In addition, the tumor growth rate, a factor that could be measured from serial MRI studies, was significantly correlated with the mean SUV, which may allow physicians to critically monitor suspicious lesions over time and allow intervention either before or sooner after malignant transformation.

8.5 Intraoperative Imaging Modalities

Adjunct fluorophores are under investigation as aids during surgical resection of peripheral nerve tumors. Central nervous system tumor resection commonly involves 5-aminolevulinic acid (5-ALA), indocyanine green (ICG), and fluorescein as part of intraoperative imaging. Fluorescein, which acts as a vascular fluorophore, illuminates nerve tumors as yellow green. In one study including 20 patients afflicted with 25 different types of nerve tumors, the addition of fluorescein successfully delineated the boundary between tumor tissue and surrounding nerve in all neurofibromas and 13/14 schwannomas [24]. Other studies have corroborated the safe and effective use of fluorescein in peripheral nerve tumor resection as well [25, 26].

8.6 Conclusion

A great deal of progress has been made in using imaging to distinguish benign from malignant nerve tumors, particularly in the setting of NF1. This distinction is critical in formulating a treatment plan. It is the hope that current and new emerging imaging modalities, combined with longitudinal studies, will provide important information about the natural history of these masses with greater reliability and improve our ability to intervene in a timely manner and to the benefit of the patient.

References

1. Pilavaki M, Chourmouzi D, Kiziridou A, Skordalaki A, Zarampoukas T, Drevelengas A. Imaging of peripheral nerve sheath tumors with pathologic correlation: pictorial review. Eur J Radiol. 2004;52(3):229–39.
2. Razzaghi A, Anastakis DJ. Lipofibromatous hamartoma: review of early diagnosis and treatment. Can J Surg. 2005;48(5):394–9.
3. Marek T, Spinner RJ, Syal A, Mahan MA. Strengthening the association of lipomatosis of nerve and nerve-territory overgrowth: a systematic review. J Neurosurg. 2019:1–9.
4. Marek T, Mahan MA, Carter JM, Amrami KK, Benarroch EE, Spinner RJ. Lipomatosis of nerve and overgrowth: is there a preference for motor (mixed) vs. sensory nerve involvement? Acta Neurochir (Wien) [Internet]. 2019;161(4):679–84. Available from: http://www.ncbi.nlm.nih.gov/pubmed/30798481. [cited 2020 Feb 11].
5. Silverman TA, Enzinger FM. Fibrolipomatous hamartoma of nerve. A clinicopathologic analysis of 26 cases. Am J Surg Pathol. 1985;9(1):7–14.
6. Amadio PC, Reiman HM, Dobyns JH. Lipofibromatous hamartoma of nerve. J Hand Surg Am [Internet]. 1988;13(1):67–75. Available from: http://www.ncbi.nlm.nih.gov/pubmed/3351231. [cited 2020 Feb 11].
7. De Maeseneer M, Jaovisidha S, Lenchik L, et al. Fibrolipomatous hamartoma: MR imaging findings. Skeletal Radiol [Internet]. 1997;26(3):155–60. Available from: http://www.ncbi.nlm.nih.gov/pubmed/9108225. [cited 2020 Feb 11].
8. Marom EM, Helms CA. Fibrolipomatous hamartoma: pathognomonic on MR imaging. Skeletal Radiol [Internet]. 1999;28(5):260–4. Available from: http://www.ncbi.nlm.nih.gov/pubmed/10424331. [cited 2020 Feb 11].
9. Wilson TJ, Joseph JR, Dillman JR, Heider A, Yang LJS. Evaluation and management of fibrofatty tumors

of the extremities: case report. J Neurosurg Pediatr [Internet]. 2016;17(1):66–9. Available from: http://www.ncbi.nlm.nih.gov/pubmed/26451716. [cited 2020 Feb 11]
10. Wasa J, Nishida Y, Tsukushi S, et al. MRI features in the differentiation of malignant peripheral nerve sheath tumors and neurofibromas. Am J Roentgenol [Internet]. 2010;194(6):1568–74. Available from: http://www.ncbi.nlm.nih.gov/pubmed/20489098. [cited 2020 Feb 11]
11. Durbin AD, Ki DH, He S, Look AT. Malignant peripheral nerve sheath tumors. Adv Exp Med Biol. Springer New York LLC. 2016:495–530.
12. Park S-K, Yi H-J, Paik S-S, Kim Y-J, Ko Y, Oh S-J. Metastasizing malignant peripheral nerve sheath tumor initially presenting as intracerebral hemorrhage. Case report and review of the literature. Surg Neurol [Internet]. 2007;68(1):79–84; discussion 84. [cited 2020 Jan 11]. Available from: http://www.ncbi.nlm.nih.gov/pubmed/17586234.
13. Benz MR, Czernin J, Dry SM, et al. Quantitative F18-fluorodeoxyglucose positron emission tomography accurately characterizes peripheral nerve sheath tumors as malignant or benign. Cancer [Internet]. 2010;116(2):451–8. Available from: http://www.ncbi.nlm.nih.gov/pubmed/19924789. [cited 2019 Oct 27].
14. Ahlawat S, Blakeley JO, Rodriguez FJ, Fayad LM. Imaging biomarkers for malignant peripheral nerve sheath tumors in neurofibromatosis type 1. Neurology [Internet]. 2019;93(11):e1076–84. Available from: http://www.ncbi.nlm.nih.gov/pubmed/31395668. [cited 2019 Oct 27].
15. Brahmi M, Thiesse P, Ranchere D, et al. Diagnostic accuracy of PET/CT-guided percutaneous biopsies for malignant peripheral nerve sheath tumors in neurofibromatosis type 1 patients. PLoS One [Internet]. 2015;10(10):e0138386. Available from: http://www.ncbi.nlm.nih.gov/pubmed/26445379. [cited 2020 Feb 11]
16. Brenner W, Friedrich RE, Gawad KA, et al. Prognostic relevance of FDG PET in patients with neurofibromatosis type-1 and malignant peripheral nerve sheath tumours. Eur J Nucl Med Mol Imaging. 2006;33(4):428–32.
17. Derlin T, Tornquist K, Münster S, et al. Comparative effectiveness of 18F-FDG PET/CT versus whole-body MRI for detection of malignant peripheral nerve sheath tumors in neurofibromatosis type 1. Clin Nucl Med. 2013;38(1)
18. Berzaczy D, Mayerhoefer ME, Azizi AA, et al. Does elevated glucose metabolism correlate with higher cell density in neurofibromatosis type 1 associated peripheral nerve sheath tumors? PLoS One [Internet]. 2017;12(12):e0189093. Available from: http://www.ncbi.nlm.nih.gov/pubmed/29206885. [cited 2019 Nov 7].
19. Azizi AA, Slavc I, Theisen BE, et al. Monitoring of plexiform neurofibroma in children and adolescents with neurofibromatosis type 1 by [18F]FDG-PET imaging. Is it of value in asymptomatic patients? Pediatr Blood Cancer. 2018;65(1)
20. Raad R, Lala S, Allen J, et al. Comparison of hybrid 18F-fluorodeoxyglucose positron emission tomography/magnetic resonance imaging and positron emission tomography/computed tomography for evaluation of peripheral nerve sheath tumors in patients with neurofibromatosis type 1. World J Nucl Med. 2018;17(4):241.
21. Fayad LM, Wang X, Blakeley JO, et al. Characterization of peripheral nerve sheath tumors with 3T proton MR spectroscopy. Am J Neuroradiol. 2014;39(5):1035–41.
22. Ahlawat S, Blakeley JO, Rodriguez FJ, Fayad LM. Imaging biomarkers for malignant peripheral nerve sheath tumors in neurofibromatosis type 1. Neurology. 2019;93:e1076.
23. Reinert CP, Schuhmann MU, Bender B, et al. Comprehensive anatomical and functional imaging in patients with type I neurofibromatosis using simultaneous FDG-PET/MRI. Eur J Nucl Med Mol Imaging. 2019;46(3):776–87.
24. Vetrano IG, Acerbi F, Falco J, et al. Fluorescein-guided removal of peripheral nerve sheath tumors: a preliminary analysis of 20 cases. J Neurosurg [Internet]. 2019:1–10. Available from: http://www.ncbi.nlm.nih.gov/pubmed/31812148. [cited 2020 Jan 11].
25. Pedro MT, Eissler A, Schmidberger J, et al. Sodium fluorescein-guided surgery in peripheral nerve sheath tumors: first experience in 10 cases of schwannoma. World Neurosurg [Internet]. 2019; Available from: http://www.ncbi.nlm.nih.gov/pubmed/30660884. [cited 2020 Jan 11].
26. Stone JJ, Graffeo CS, de Ruiter GCW, Rock MG, Spinner RJ. Intraoperative intravenous fluorescein as an adjunct during surgery for peroneal intraneural ganglion cysts. Acta Neurochir (Wien) [Internet]. 2018;160(3):651–4. Available from: http://www.ncbi.nlm.nih.gov/pubmed/29372402. [cited 2020 Jan 11].

9 Indications and Techniques for Preoperative Biopsy in Peripheral Nerve Tumors

Fernando Guedes, Gabriel Elias Sanches, Rodrigo Salvador Vivas Cardoso, and Martijn J. A. Malessy

9.1 Introduction

Soft tissue tumors arising from peripheral nerves may be benign, such as schwannomas, neurofibromas, and perineuriomas, or malignant, such as the malignant peripheral nerve sheath tumors (MPNST). In general, oncological surgeons choose to perform preoperative biopsies in soft tissue tumors for diagnostic and staging purposes, despite the fact that most peripheral nerve tumors (PNT) are benign. These procedures may cause devastating iatrogenic sequelae; therefore, it is crucial to differentiate between benign and malignant lesions. To date, the vast majority of MPNST remain incurable, mainly because of their high rate of recurrence and metastatic potential, although it is important to emphasize that, in recent years, MPNST have been subdivided into two distinct groups with different clinical behavior and prognosis [1].

The so-called low-grade MPNST correspond to around 15%, while the high grade comprehend around 85% of all MPNST [1]. Recent data demonstrate the possibility of clinical control for extended time in low-grade lesions, without the need for wide resections and negative margins [2]. However, to date, it is not possible to establish preoperatively with certainty if a MPNST is low or high grade through clinical examination nor through imaging exams. Therefore, only histopathological analysis is adequate for establishing if a MPNST is low or high grade. It is also important to bring attention to other entities, such as atypical neurofibromas, hybrid tumors, or the cellular neurofibromas and cellular schwannomas, which may resemble MPNST [3–5].

The World Health Organization (WHO) classifies MPNST as a soft tissue sarcoma in its latest editions of the series "WHO Classification of Tumours." Thus, the general approach is still guided by oncological surgery protocols, which, as stated, propose preoperative biopsies [1]. In practice, it is possible to observe situations in which biopsies were performed in benign tumors, which in turn produced iatrogenic lesions to fascicles or worsening of pain or in many circumstances resulted in an inconclusive diagnosis. The same is true for malignant tumors, because given their geographical heterogeneity, biopsies performed in atypical or low-grade regions of the tumor may not reach other areas with clearly high-grade characteristics [6]. For that reason, depending on the area targeted by the biopsy, the given diagnosis may be inaccurate. In advanced referral centers, it is possible to perform image-guided biopsies, using CT, MRI, or PET-CT. However, such techniques are not universally available.

F. Guedes (✉) · G. E. Sanches · R. S. V. Cardoso
Division of Neurosurgery, Department of Surgery, Gaffrée e Guinle University Hospital (HUGG), School of Medicine, Federal University of Rio de Janeiro State (UNIRIO), Rio de Janeiro, RJ, Brazil

M. J. A. Malessy
Department of Neurosurgery, Leiden University Medical Center, Leiden, The Netherlands

F. Guedes et al. (eds.), *Diagnostic Assessment and Treatment of Peripheral Nerve Tumors*,
https://doi.org/10.1007/978-3-030-77633-6_9

This chapter discusses indications and limitations of peripheral nerve tumor biopsies, bringing attention to the critical need for clinical correlation and imaging exams, so that unnecessary biopsies are not performed in benign tumors, which in turn are more prevalent in the general population [7]. There are different techniques in which to perform biopsy of a tumoral lesion in a peripheral nerve, and their benefits and complications will be discussed below.

9.2 Why Perform Biopsy in Presumed Peripheral Nerve Sheath Tumors?

The possibility of a tumor intrinsic to a nerve must be considered whenever a mass is situated in the anatomic site of a major peripheral nerve or plexus. A positive Tinel sign, thus, may indicate that the nerve is affected, although it does not provide certainty about the tumor's origin, requiring the use of MR imaging to answer this question. If the mass, then, is likely to be a PNST, special considerations must be made when deciding to biopsy it or not, as these masses are usually studied in the context of soft tissue tumors, although they possess some peculiarities.

Given the lack of a consensus for an approach concerning such tumors, we thus suggest that biopsy should only be performed when clinical and imaging evidence supports the hypothesis of malignancy. This is because clinical and imaging parameters, when considered together, are able to quite effectively predict malignancy, therefore ruling out the need for biopsies in evidently benign lesions. These procedures are also not innocuous and may produce worsening of symptoms [8, 9] and increased risk of neurological deficits, in case surgery is later required [10]. Such understanding that only presumed malignant PNT should be biopsied is shared by recent guidelines for the management of soft tissue sarcomas [11]. Nonetheless, clinical and imaging parameters must be followed, especially in the setting of NF1, for previously benign lesions may undergo malignant transformation.

When a presumed PNST, after a thorough clinical and imaging examination, is likely to be a BPNST, the risks of a biopsy may outweigh its benefits, due to the several complications it harbors, such as new-onset or worsening of pain, neurological deficit, fibrosis, and hemorrhage along the biopsy needle track, which can later hinder the tumor's resection. Moreover, in cases of BPNST in which surgery is already indicated, as when there is associated neurological deficit, biopsies provide little to no benefit. However, when clinical and imaging parameters indicate malignancy, preoperative biopsy can be performed so as to guide surgical decision-making and the operative approach. For example, when a lesion is proved to be a MPNST on biopsy, tumor spill should be avoided, and in toto resection should then be performed with sacrifice of the neural element of origin. Sometimes, however, such goal is impossible to be achieved due to the location of the lesion (e.g., brachial or lumbosacral plexus). In addition, the requirement of neoadjuvant therapy may also be guided by the biopsy's result [12]. Some authors, however, prefer to perform upfront resection of presumed MPNST, given the fact that biopsies may be less accurate in large and heterogenous tumors [13].

Another role of performing a biopsy in a presumed MPNST is to identify its grade, because surgical approach may be guided by this information [14–16]. One important aspect concerns the differentiation among high- and low-grade MPNST and pre-malignant lesions termed "atypical neurofibromatous neoplasm with unknown biologic potential" (ANNUBP). ANNUBP may be defined as a Schwann cell neoplasm with at least two of the following features: loss of neurofibroma architecture, cytological atypia, hypercellularity, and a mitotic index between 1/50 and 3/10 high-power fields (HPFs) [17]. Low-grade MPNST in turn display the same features as ANNUBP, but with a higher mitotic index between 3/10 and 9/10 HPF [17]. MPNST presenting with necrosis or with a mitotic index over 10/10 HPF are considered high-grade MPNST [17].

Bernthal et al. demonstrated no prognostic value for surgical margin status in the context of low-grade MPNST [2]. This group reported a disease-specific survival (DSS) of 100% in low-grade MPNST, with a median follow-up of 47 months after surgery, independently of margin status. In addition, Watson et al. reported a DSS of 100% in 12 patients with low-grade MPNST, after a follow-up of 5 years, and 4 of these patients presented R1 (microscopically positive) and/or R2 (macroscopically positive) surgical margins [18]. It is not possible, however, to determine whether these lesions were low-grade MPNST or ANNUBP according to more recent classifications. Nelson et al. also presented a series of 16 surgically treated atypical neurofibromas, ANNUBP, and low-grade MPNST in which a safe marginal resection technique was conducted with overall little morbidity and no recurrence after a median follow-up of 2.45 years [19]. These results indicate that perhaps it is not imperative to obtain negative margins in less agressive lesions, allowing for preservation of adjacent structures and functionality of the inflicted peripheral nerve.

9.3 Biopsy Techniques and Their Complications

There is a range of techniques used to perform biopsies in masses thought to be PNST, such as fine-needle aspiration cytology (FNAC), core-needle biopsy (CNB), incisional biopsy, and excisional biopsy (Table 9.1).

Both fine-needle aspiration cytology (FNAC) and core-needle biopsy (CNB) have been shown to be of useful predictive value for detection of malignancies and correct diagnosis of soft tissue tumors and more specifically of PNST. CNB has been shown to be consistently superior and should be the method of choice for presumed MPNST, if there is the possibility to perform it in an image-guided fashion [20–30]. FNAC, in fact, has been shown not to be reliable in the specific context of head and neck schwannomas, concerning its diagnostic yield and diagnostic accuracy [31–33]. Therefore, some authors suggest that CNB, and not FNAC, should be performed prior to open biopsy in soft tissue tumors [34–36], which is in line with the fact that percutaneous biopsy tends to result in fewer complications than open biopsy in soft tissue masses [35, 37–39]. Nonetheless, when considering PNST (especially those located in deeper planes), it is not clear whether the benefits of percutaneous biopsy outweigh its risks, as these tumors can often present as a diagnostic challenge [40] and are located inside peripheral nerves, which may result in direct damage to fascicles or compression by hematoma caused by the needle (Fig. 9.1). This may in turn result in impaired function, persistent pain, and a higher risk of neurological deficits if surgery is later performed [8–10, 41, 42]. Other complications may follow, such as seroma and infection [27, 35, 37–39]. Moreover, Ogose et al. describe that the track of the needle is often contaminated by tumor cells; therefore, the needle track ought to be excised along with the lesion during definitive resection [25].

Open biopsies, in turn, are also useful in the context of presumed MPNST. The risk of damaging functional nerve fibers is reduced, as the surgeon is usually able to more accurately identify the tumor's location and to aim the biopsy at its nonfunctional electrically silent regions, as assessed through electrical stimulation. This technique, however, also harbors risks such as spillage of tumor cells in the surrounding tissue, which may make total resection difficult or impossible in the future. Therefore, tumor manip-

Table 9.1 Different techniques for biopsy of PNT [57]

Excisional biopsy	Incisional biopsy	Core-needle biopsy	Fine-needle aspiration cytology
The lesion is removed as a whole, for both diagnostic and therapeutic purposes. It is usually reserved for small (<5 cm in diameter) and superficial lesions, and it is important to include a margin of normal tissue to the excision	Consists in surgically removing a wedge of the lesion, after surgical opening of the skin and subcutaneous tissues	Several specimens of the lesion are obtained by a needle inserted through a small incision of the skin. The larger the needle, the more optimal the specimens are, although this technique tends to underestimate the tumor's grade, better assessed by the excised specimen	It is performed by insertion of a fine needle directly to the lesion, in order to obtain cells through aspiration. Although considered a minor and very safe surgical procedure, it is unable to inform about the tumor's architecture and mitotic index, limiting its use in determining histologic subtype and grade

ulation should be thoroughly avoided in order to minimize the risk of seeding of neoplastic cells.

Concerning the proper diagnosis of the tumor's grade, there have been reports of excisional biopsies that identified different regions with different grades in each of them [6, 43]. A biopsy by needle, in such instances of progression into malignancy, might then fail to correctly assess the tumor's grade, as it might be confined to a region in which the tumor is benign or low grade. In addition, biopsying the tumor in different quadrants further improves the accuracy of the technique, as a more representative sample of the tumor is obtained.

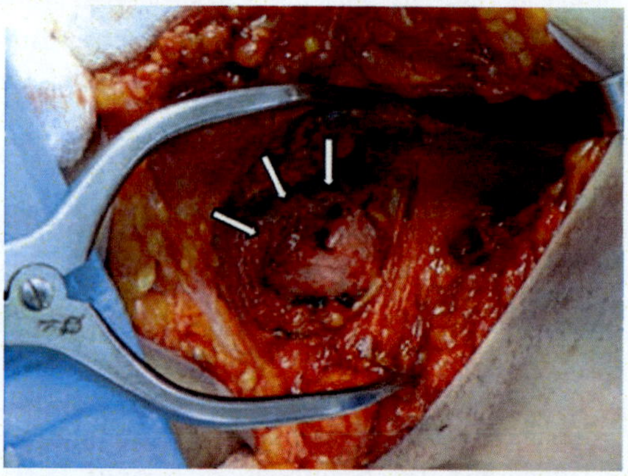

Fig. 9.1 Surgical photograph during exposition of a tumor of the ulnar nerve in the right arm during its definitive surgical resection. White arrows indicate the different aspect of the previously biopsied area. This patient was submitted to a core-needle biopsy under local anesthesia elsewhere, which was not conclusive. During the preoperative biopsy, the patient complained of acute electric pain irradiating to the hand, which did not decrease for the following weeks, when definitive surgical resection of the tumor was conducted at our institution. The final histopathological diagnosis was of a schwannoma

Novel techniques, introducing the use of CT, MRI, ultrasonography (USG), and PET-CT, to assist percutaneous biopsies have been reported. For instance, Rimondi et al. reported the use of percutaneous CT-guided biopsy in a series of 2027 cases of musculoskeletal lesions, with an accuracy rate of 77.3% in first attempts and of 94% when another biopsy was performed in previously undiagnosed lesions. This study reported only 22 complications, 18 of which were transient paresis, although the proportion of PNT among all lesions is not specified [44]. The efficacy of this technique was further demonstrated in PNST by Pianta et al. [45]. Also, two separate studies, consisting of 45 and 24 MRI-guided needle biopsies of musculoskeletal lesions, found good results, with only 1 complication in the former: exacerbation of neuropathic pain in a PNST [9, 46]. USG is also useful to guide biopsy for superficial lesions [47] (Fig. 9.2). Moreover, Brahmi et al. described a technique utilizing PET/CT to guide core-needle biopsy in 26 NF1 patients with clinical suspicion of MPNST, with no complications observed [43]. There are also other techniques with high accuracy which rely on the usage of high-resolution MRI to guide the biopsy of fascicles and branches of main peripheral nerves [48–51]. The accuracy and complications of percutaneous biopsies in different settings are summarized in Table 9.2. Image-guided biopsies are,

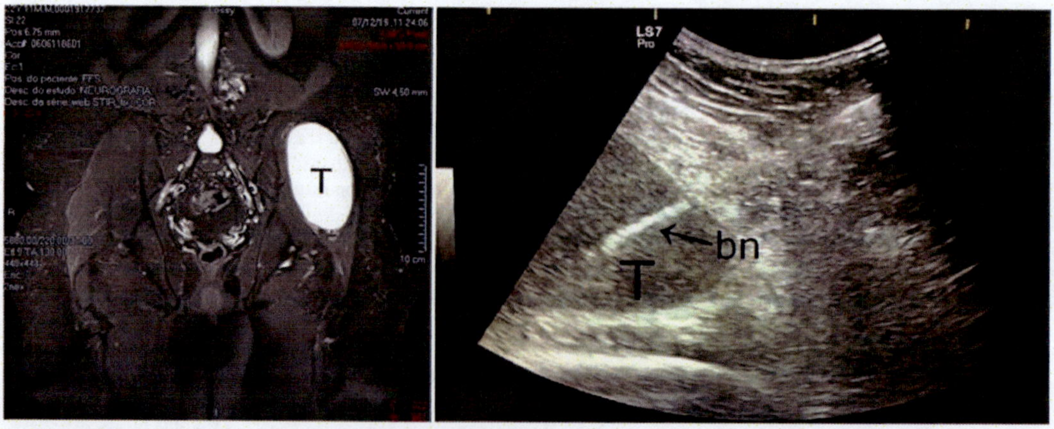

Fig. 9.2 Left: STIR-weighted MRI of a patient with a tumor over the course of the left sciatic nerve at the level of the gluteal region. Right: USG-guided biopsy of the lesion. *T* Tumor, *bn* Biopsy needle

Table 9.2 Accuracy and complications of percutaneous biopsy

Study	Number of lesions	Types of lesion studied	Technique	Accuracy in identification of malignancies	Accuracy in the identification of the lesion's histologic type	Rate of complications (%)	Complications
Ball AB et al. [38]	52	Soft tissue tumors	CNB	98%	94%	1.9%	Severe bleeding
Resnick et al. [22]	39	PNST	FNAC (19)	45%	13.8%	Not informed	N/A
			CNB (20)	60%	50%	Not informed	N/A
Welker et al. [35]	173	Musculoskeletal lesions	CNB (90)	92.4%	72.7%	1.1%	Bleeding and persistent drainage
			CT-guided CNB (55)				
			Fluoro-guided CNB (28)				
Yang and Damron [50]	50	Musculoskeletal lesions	FNAC (50)	88%	74%	Not informed	N/A
			CNB (50)	93%	90%		
Carrino et al. [9]	45	Musculoskeletal lesions	MR-guided FNAC (4)	N/A	75.5%	2.2%	Exacerbation of neuropathic pain in a PNST
			MR-guided CNB (10)				
			Both (31)				
Strauss et al. [26]	426	Soft tissue tumors	CNB	97.6%	88.7%	0.4%	Bleeding
Adams et al. [27]	252	Bone and soft tissue tumors	CNB	91%	80.7%	0%	N/A
Rimondi et al. [42]	2027	Musculoskeletal lesions	CT-guided CNB	N/A	77.3%	0.09%	Transient paresis and hematomas
Liu et al. [31]	20	Head and neck schwannomas	FNAC	50%	20%	Not informed	N/A
Wakely et al. [28]	56	MPNST	FNAC	N/A	30–70–93%[a]	Not informed	N/A
Yasumatsu et al. [32]	12	Head and neck schwannomas	FNAC	N/A	25%	Not informed	N/A
Layfield et al. [29]	257	Musculoskeletal lesions	FNAC (62)	N/A	81.5%	Not informed	N/A
			CNB (130)		78.3%		
			Open (111)		89.2%		
Pianta et al. [43]	41	PNST	CT-guided CNB	N/A	100%	12%	Increased pain (later resolved)
Brahmi et al. [41]	26	MPNST	PET/CT-guided CNB	N/A	96%	0%	N/A
Zheng et al. [51]	56	Schwannomas	FNAC	N/A	33.9%	Not informed	N/A
Ahn et al. [33]	81	Head and neck schwannomas	FNAC	N/A	19.2%	25%	Neurological events associated with the nerve of origin
			CNB	N/A	96.6%	34.6%	

CNB Core-needle biopsy
FNAC Fine-needle aspiration cytology
N/A Not applicable
[a]Respectively, from primary, metastatic, and locally recurrent lesions

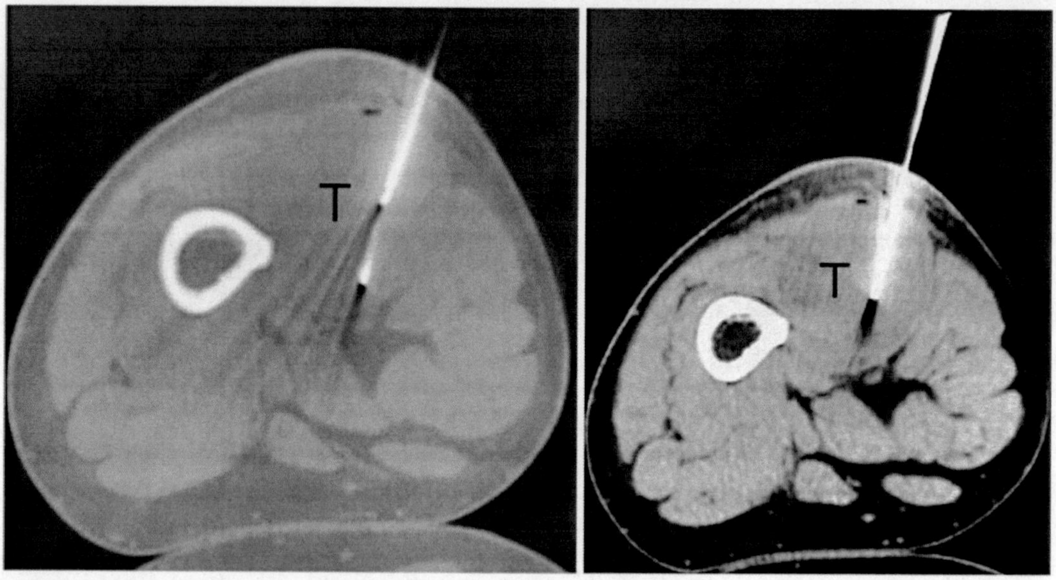

Fig. 9.3 CT-guided core-needle biopsy performed for a lesion later diagnosed as a sarcoma of the thigh compressing the sciatic nerve. *T* Tumor

perhaps, the most efficient techniques reported to date to perform preoperative biopsies in presumed MPNST (Fig. 9.3), considering their ability to assess the tumor's malignancy status and histopathological type and the small risks they pose to patients. Nonetheless, the possibility of using such expensive equipment in this preoperative biopsy setting is not feasible for many services in the world. We therefore recommend these techniques in case they are available; if not, open biopsy should be conducted with wide exposure of the tumor, and tissue should be obtained from different quadrants in order to guarantee a more representative sample of the lesion.

9.4 Final Considerations

When a MPNST is suspected upon clinical and imaging criteria (on MRI, USG, and PET-CT, if available), the patient should be transferred to a multidisciplinary referral center for soft tissue sarcomas with an additional unit for peripheral nerve surgery. A screening of these patients is critical and should include thorax and abdomen CT to evaluate systemic disease. After the decision for biopsy has been made, MRI and PET-CT are helpful in order to guide it at specific areas of the tumor which present characteristics associated with malignancy (necrotic, hemorrhagic, and hypermetabolic regions). In general, for lesions suspected to be malignant, the approach should be based on the acquisition of a pathological specimen for diagnosis and staging.

It is important to stress that PNST are rare and heterogeneous and, therefore, the great majority of pathologists do not possess enough experience to evaluate these lesions, sometimes with small fragments of tissue. Nonetheless, nowadays, a series of immunohistochemical markers, such as SOX10, TLE1, HMGA2, and others, have been useful to distinguish these different tumors and to confirm the diagnosis [52]. Loss of H3K27 methylation has also been shown to be very specific for MPNST [53–55], although this feature may not be suitable to distinguish them from melanomas [56].

According to our experience, FNAC should not be used in the context of PNT, as it is often inconclusive and may result in neurological deficit and neuropathic pain; on the other hand, image-guided (MRI, USG, or PET-CT) CNB is considered a safe and accurate procedure. Yet, from our experience, the amount of obtained material is not always sufficient for the correct diagnosis, and many patients do develop intense neuropathic pain after the procedure.

In our institution, when confronted with a presumed MPNST, the case is discussed along with the surgical oncology group. If, on MRI, the lesion appears not to be neurogenic, the case will be conducted by surgical oncology, and a CNB will probably be performed. However, if the lesion appears to arise from a peripheral nerve, the case will be conducted by the neurosurgery team. In these instances, if the lesion is likely malignant by clinical and imaging criteria, our policy is to perform incisional biopsies in quadrants, thoroughly avoiding tumor manipulation and thereby minimizing the risk of seeding of neoplastic cells to its surroundings. If intraoperative frozen section anatomopathological examination of the material shows a MPNST, we then stop the procedure, close the wound, and wait for the definitive histopathological diagnosis. Such incisional biopsies must be performed in areas of tumor found to be electrically silent, as evaluated by electrical stimulation during the surgical procedure.

An algorithm summarizing our policy when confronting patients harboring potential PNT is presented in Fig. 9.4.

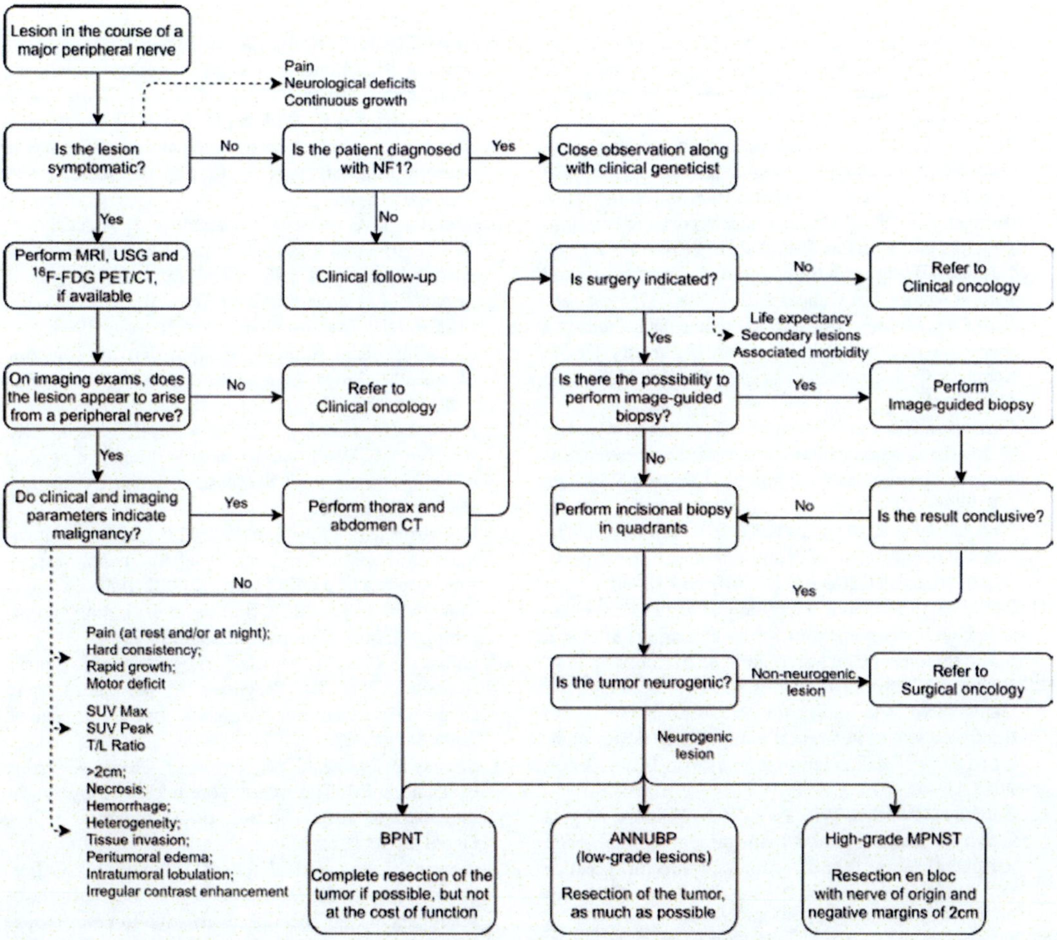

Fig. 9.4 An algorithm to help in the decision-making process concerning possible PNT

References

1. Louis DN, Ohgaki H, Wiestler OD, Cavenee WK, editors. Weltgesundheitsorganisation. WHO classification of tumours of the central nervous system. Revised 4th edition. Lyon: International Agency for Research on Cancer; 2016.
2. Bernthal NM, Putnam A, Jones KB, Viskochil D, Randall RL. The effect of surgical margins on outcomes for low grade MPNSTs and atypical neurofibroma: outcomes of intermediate nerve sheath tumors. J Surg Oncol. 2014;110:813–6.
3. Woodruff JM, Godwin TA, Erlandson RA, Susin M, Martini N. Cellular schwannoma: A variety of schwannoma sometimes mistaken for a malignant tumor. Am J Surg Pathol [Internet]. 1981;5. Available from: https://journals.lww.com/ajsp/Fulltext/1981/12000/Cellular_schwannoma__A_variety_of_schwannoma.1.aspx
4. Chimelli LMC, Guedes-Correa JF, Siquara-de-Sousa AC. Hybrid peripheral nerve sheath tumor—case report. Brain Pathol (ICN 2014 Suppl).
5. Lang SS, Zager EL, Coyne TM, Nangunoori R, Kneeland B, Nathanson KL. Hybrid peripheral nerve sheath tumor: case report and review of the literature. J Neurosurg. 2012;117(5):890–6.
6. Tajima S, Koda K. A neurogenic tumor containing a low-grade malignant peripheral nerve sheath tumor (MPNST) component with loss of p16 expression and homozygous deletion of CDKN2A/p16: a case report showing progression. Int J Clin Exp Pathol. 2015;8(5):5113–20.
7. Hajdu SI. Benign soft tissue tumors: classification and natural history. CA Cancer J Clin. 1987;37(2):66–76.
8. Kim DH, Murovic JA, Tiel RL, Kline DG. Operative outcomes of 546 Louisiana State University Health Sciences Center peripheral nerve tumors. Neurosurg Clin North Am. 2004;15:177–92.
9. Carrino J, Khurana B, Ready J, Silverman S, Winalski C. Magnetic resonance imaging-guided percutaneous biopsy of musculoskeletal lesions. J Bone Jt Surg Am. 2007;89:2179–87.
10. Levi AD, Ross AL, Cuartas E, Qadir R, Temple HT. The surgical management of symptomatic peripheral nerve sheath tumors. Neurosurgery. 2010;66:833–40.
11. Dangoor A, Seddon B, Gerrand C, Grimer R, Whelan J, Judson I. UK guidelines for the management of soft tissue sarcomas. Clin Sarcoma Res. 2016;6:20.
12. Bishop AJ, Zagars GK, Torres KE, Bird JE, Feig BW, Guadagnolo BA. Malignant peripheral nerve sheath tumors: a single institution's experience using combined surgery and radiation therapy. Am J Clin Oncol. 2018;41:465–70.
13. Bethany C Prudner, Tyler Ball, Richa Rathore, Angela C Hirbe. Diagnosis and management of malignant peripheral nerve sheath tumors: Current practice and future perspectives. Neuro-Oncology Advances 2020;2:(Supplement_1):i40–i49.
14. Ducatman BS, Scheithauer BW, Piepgras DG, Reiman HM, Ilstrup DM. Malignant peripheral nerve sheath tumors. A clinicopathologic study of 120 cases. Cancer. 1986;57:2006–21.
15. Wong WW, Hirose T, Scheithauer BW, Schild SE, Gunderson LL. Malignant peripheral nerve sheath tumor: analysis of treatment outcome. Int J Radiat Oncol Biol Phys. 1998;42:351–60.
16. Anghileri M, Miceli R, Fiore M, Mariani L, Ferrari A, Mussi C, et al. Malignant peripheral nerve sheath tumors: Prognostic factors and survival in a series of patients treated at a single institution. Cancer. 2006;107:1065–74.
17. Miettinen MM, Antonescu CR, Fletcher CDM, Kim A, Lazar AJ, Quezado MM, et al. Histopathologic evaluation of atypical neurofibromatous tumors and their transformation into malignant peripheral nerve sheath tumor in patients with neurofibromatosis 1—a consensus overview. Hum Pathol. 2017;67:1–10.
18. Watson KL, Al Sannaa GA, Kivlin CM, Ingram DR, Landers SM, Roland CL, et al. Patterns of recurrence and survival in sporadic, neurofibromatosis Type 1-associated, and radiation-associated malignant peripheral nerve sheath tumors. J Neurosurg. 2017;126:319–29.
19. Charlie N. Nelson, Eva Dombi, Jared S. Rosenblum, Markku M. Miettinen, Tanya J. Lehky, Patricia O. Whitcomb, Christina Hayes, Gretchen Scott, Sarah Benzo, Brigitte C. Widemann, Prashant Chittiboina, Safe marginal resection of atypical neurofibromas in neurofibromatosis type 1. Journal of Neurosurgery 133(5):1516–26.
20. Miralles T, Gosalbez F, Menéndez P, Astudillo A, Torre C, Buesa J. Fine needle aspiration of soft-tissue lesions. Acta Cytol. 1986;30:671–8.
21. Logan PM, Connell DG, O'Connell JX, Munk PL, Janzen DL. Image-guided percutaneous biopsy of musculoskeletal tumors: an algorithm for selection of specific biopsy techniques. Am J Roentgenol. 1996;166:137–41.
22. Resnick JM, Fanning CV, Caraway NP, Varma DGK, Johnson M. Percutaneous needle biopsy diagnosis of benign neurogenic neoplasms. Diagn Cytopathol. 1997;16(1):17–25.
23. Kilpatrick SE, Geisinger KR. Soft tissue sarcomas: the usefulness and limitations of fine-needle aspiration biopsy. Am J Clin Pathol. 1998;110:50–68.
24. Wakely PE Jr, Kneisl JS. Soft tissue aspiration cytopathology. Cancer Cytopathol. 2000;90:292–8.
25. Ogose A, Hotta T, Morita T, Higuchi T, Umezu H, Imaizumi S, et al. Diagnosis of peripheral nerve sheath tumors around the pelvis. Jpn J Clin Oncol. 2004;34:405–13.
26. Strauss DC, Qureshi YA, Hayes AJ, Thway K, Fisher C, Thomas JM. The role of core needle biopsy in the diagnosis of suspected soft tissue tumours. J Surg Oncol. 2010;102:523–9.
27. Adams SC, Potter BK, Pitcher DJ, Temple HT. Office-based core needle biopsy of bone and soft tissue malignancies: an accurate alternative to open biopsy with infrequent complications. Clin Orthop Relat Res. 2010;468:2774–80.

28. Wakely PE, Ali SZ, Bishop JA. The cytopathology of malignant peripheral nerve sheath tumor: a report of 55 fine-needle aspiration cases. Cancer Cytopathol. 2012;120:334–41.
29. Layfield LJ, Schmidt RL, Sangle N, Crim JR. Diagnostic accuracy and clinical utility of biopsy in musculoskeletal lesions: a comparison of fine-needle aspiration, core, and open biopsy techniques: diagnostic accuracy and clinical utility of biopsy. Diagn Cytopathol. 2014;42:476–86.
30. Kaur I, Handa U, Kundu R, Garg S, Mohan H. Role of fine-needle aspiration cytology and core needle biopsy in diagnosing musculoskeletal neoplasms. J Cytol. 2016;33:7.
31. Liu H-L, Yu S-Y, Li GK-H, Wei WI. Extracranial head and neck schwannomas: a study of the nerve of origin. Eur Arch Otorhinolaryngol. 2011;268:1343–7.
32. Yasumatsu R, Nakashima T, Miyazaki R, Segawa Y, Komune S. Diagnosis and management of extracranial head and neck schwannomas: a review of 27 cases. Int J Otolaryngol. 2013;2013:1–5.
33. Ahn D, Lee GJ, Sohn JH, Jeong JY. Fine-needle aspiration cytology versus core-needle biopsy for the diagnosis of extracranial head and neck schwannoma. Head Neck. 2018;40:2695–700.
34. Yao L, Nelson SD, Seeger LL, Eckardt JJ, Eilber FR. Primary musculoskeletal neoplasms: effectiveness of core-needle biopsy. Radiology. 1999;212:682–6.
35. Welker JA, Henshaw RM, Jelinek J, Shmookler BM, Malawer MM. The percutaneous needle biopsy is safe and recommended in the diagnosis of musculoskeletal masses. Cancer. 2000;89(12):2677–86.
36. Torriani M, Etchebehere M, Amstalden EMI. Sonographically guided core needle biopsy of bone and soft tissue tumors. J Ultrasound Med. 2002;21:275–81.
37. Moore TM, Meyers MH, Patzakis MJ, Terry R, Harvey JPJ. Closed biopsy of musculoskeletal lesions. JBJS [Internet]. 1979;61:375–80. Available from: https://journals.lww.com/jbjsjournal/Fulltext/1979/61030/Closed_biopsy_of_musculoskeletal_lesions_.10.aspx
38. Ball ABS, Fisher C, Pittam M, Watkins RM, Westbury G. Diagnosis of soft tissue tumours by Tru-Cut® biopsy. Br J Surg. 1990;77:756–8.
39. For the members of the Musculoskeletal Tumor Society. The hazards of the biopsy, revisited. J Pediatr Orthop [Internet]. 1996;16. Available from: https://journals.lww.com/pedorthopaedics/Fulltext/1996/11000/THE_HAZARDS_OF_THE_BIOPSY,_REVISITED__FOR_THE.60.aspx
40. Rodriguez FJ, Folpe AL, Giannini C, Perry A. Pathology of peripheral nerve sheath tumors: diagnostic overview and update on selected diagnostic problems. Acta Neuropathol. 2012;123:295–319.
41. de Sousa ACS, Guedes-Correa JF, Costa JP, Amorim RMP, Santos LL, Pereira MRC. Preoperative biopsies in peripheral nerve tumor: clinical consequences. Brain Pathol. 2014;24(Suppl. 1):39–103.
42. Guedes-Corrêa JF, Amorim RP, Pereira MR da C, Cardoso RSV, Costa FD, Bianchi B de S, et al. Multimodal treatment of an extremely rare desmoplastic small round cell tumor primary to the brachial plexus—a case report and review of literature. Surg Neurol Int. 2019;10:140.
43. Brahmi M, Thiesse P, Ranchere D, Mognetti T, Pinson S, Renard C, et al. Diagnostic accuracy of PET/CT-guided percutaneous biopsies for malignant peripheral nerve sheath tumors in neurofibromatosis type 1 patients. PLoS One. 2015;10:e0138386.
44. Rimondi E, Rossi G, Bartalena T, Ciminari R, Alberghini M, Ruggieri P, et al. Percutaneous CT-guided biopsy of the musculoskeletal system: results of 2027 cases. Eur J Radiol. 2011;77:34–42.
45. Pianta M, Chock E, Schlicht S, McCombe D. Accuracy and complications of CT-guided core needle biopsy of peripheral nerve sheath tumours. Skeletal Radiol. 2015;44:1341–9.
46. Wu H-TH, Chang C-Y, Chang H, Yen C-C, Cheng H, Chen PC-S, et al. Magnetic resonance imaging guided biopsy of musculoskeletal lesions. J Chin Med Assoc. 2012;75:160–6.
47. Tøttrup M, Eriksen JD, Hellfritzsch MB, Sørensen FB, Baad-Hansen T. Diagnostic accuracy of ultrasound-guided core biopsy of peripheral nerve sheath tumors. J Clin Ultrasound. 2020;48:134–8.
48. Capek S, Amrami KK, James P, Dyck B, Spinner RJ. Targeted fascicular biopsy of the sciatic nerve and its major branches: rationale and operative technique. Neurosurg Focus FOC. 2015;39:E12.
49. Laumonerie P, Capek S, Amrami KK, James P, Dyck B, Spinner RJ. Targeted fascicular biopsy of the brachial plexus: rationale and operative technique. Neurosurg Focus FOC. 2017;42:E9.
50. Marek T, Howe BM, Amrami KK, Spinner RJ. From targeted fascicular biopsy of major nerve to targeted cutaneous nerve biopsy: implementing clinical anatomy can catalyze a paradigm shift. Clin Anat. 2018;31:616–21.
51. Marek T, Stone JJ, Amrami KK, Spinner RJ. Targeted nerve biopsy: a technique in evolution. Clin Anat. 2018;31:1200–4.
52. Guedes-Corrêa J, Cardoso R. Immunohistochemical markers for schwannomas, neurofibromas and malignant peripheral nerve sheath tumors—what can the recent literature tell us? Arq Bras Neurocir. 2018;37:105–12.
53. Makise N, Sekimizu M, Kubo T, Wakai S, Hiraoka N, Komiyama M, et al. Clarifying the distinction between malignant peripheral nerve sheath tumor and dedifferentiated liposarcoma: a critical reappraisal of the diagnostic utility of MDM2 and H3K27me3 status. Am J Surg Pathol. 2018;42:656.
54. Mito JK, Qian X, Doyle LA, Hornick JL, Jo VY. Role of histone H3K27 trimethylation loss as a marker for malignant peripheral nerve sheath tumor in fine-needle aspiration and small biopsy specimens. Am J Clin Pathol. 2017;148:179–89.
55. Schaefer I-M, Fletcher CD, Hornick JL. Loss of H3K27 trimethylation distinguishes malignant

peripheral nerve sheath tumors from histologic mimics. Mod Pathol. 2016;29:4–13.
56. Le Guellec S, Macagno N, Velasco V, Lamant L, Lae M, Filleron T, et al. Loss of H3K27 trimethylation is not suitable for distinguishing malignant peripheral nerve sheath tumor from melanoma: a study of 387 cases including mimicking lesions. Mod Pathol. 2017;30:1677–87.
57. Fisher C, Montgomery EA, Thway K. Biopsy interpretation of soft tissue tumors. In: Wolters Kluwer (UK) Ltd. Philadelphia, PA; 2012.

10 Fundamental Aspects of the Surgical Techniques for the Resection of Peripheral Nerve Tumors

Harley Brito da Silva,
Francisco Flávio Leitão de Carvalho Filho,
and Rajiv Midha

10.1 Introduction

Most of the difficulties in any type of surgical procedure arise with the unfamiliarity of the surgeons on how to manage a specific problem. Because of their relative rarity, that is one of the problems most surgeons face with the management of peripheral nerve tumors. Peripheral nerve tumors account for 8–12% of the benign soft tissue neoplasms [1, 2], and malignant peripheral nerve tumors account for less than 5% of the malignant soft tissue neoplasms [3]. Thus, these types of neoplasms are infrequently surgically managed, unless a strong referral center for neurofibromatosis patients is present at the hospital [4]. Thus, this chapter will address some of the key points that surgeons must be aware when facing peripheral nerve tumors.

Furthermore, one possible challenging difficulty for most surgeons is the unfamiliarity with the detailed anatomy required to operate on these neoplasms. Knowledge of peripheral nerve, surrounding vessel, and muscle anatomy is required for a successful resection of both superficial and deep-seated tumors. This is of utmost importance in particular for the benign tumors, since the goal is not only the resection of the neoplasm but also the preservation of the neurological function [5]. Therefore, before approaching these tumors, the surgeon involved in the management should thoroughly review all the anatomy of the involved peripheral nerve or nerves and of the surrounding structures, and ideally cadaveric dissection prior to the surgery should be performed by the less experienced.

The first step should be, as always, history taking and a complete neurological examination. Most peripheral nerve tumors will be slow-growing masses that can be palpated by the surgeon, and these masses are usually soft and mobile. Pain is the most common complaint along with radiating dysesthesia or paresthesia. Sensory deficits or mild motor deficits may be documented. However, an adherent and fast-growing mass, associated with evolving motor deficit, is a warning sign of the possibility of a

H. Brito da Silva
Department of Neurological Surgery, Harborview Medical Center, University of Washington, Seattle, USA

Neurosurgical Service Hospital Instituto José Frota, Fortaleza, Brazil

F. F. Leitão de Carvalho Filho
Neurosurgical Service Hospital Instituto José Frota, Fortaleza, Brazil

Neurosurgical Service Hospital Geral de Fortaleza, Fortaleza, Brazil

R. Midha (✉)
Department of Clinical Neurosciences, Division of Neurosurgery, Hotchkiss Brain Institute, University of Calgary, Calgary, AB, Canada
e-mail: rajmidha@ucalgary.ca

F. Guedes et al. (eds.), *Diagnostic Assessment and Treatment of Peripheral Nerve Tumors*,
https://doi.org/10.1007/978-3-030-77633-6_10

malignant lesion. This concern is heightened with a previous history of radiation therapy and in the setting of NF1, where there may be a malignant transformation of a benign tumor into a malignant one [6, 7].

The advancements in imaging and neurophysiology offer the possibility of a safe resection of peripheral nerve system (PNS) tumors and preservation of function [5]. MRI can give the surgeon the necessary information regarding precise location, size, and relation to adjacent anatomical and bypassing fascicular structures [8]. Furthermore, MRI scans along with PET scans can occasionally be useful to differentiate schwannomas from neurofibromas and benign from malignant tumors. Ultrasound [9] is also another very useful diagnostic tool, as it can identify tumor and vessels, and can be useful as an adjunct in the operating room. Electrodiagnostic methods such as electromyography and nerve conduction studies may both help to objectively assess the degree of neurological deficit preoperatively but are not indicated if the neurological exam is normal. More important, however, is the use of intraoperative monitoring of the specific muscle groups that could be affected during the PNS tumor resection [10]. More detailed information regarding pathology, imaging, and electrophysiology is presented in other chapters of this book.

It is worth noting that most frequently the surgeon will encounter a benign subtype of schwannomas (Figs. 10.1 and 10.2) or neurofibromas (Figs. 10.3 and 10.4) at surgery. However, a surgeon can encounter other intrinsic peripheral nerve sheath tumors such as perineuromas [11], dermal nerve sheath myxomas, and hybrid nerve sheath tumors. Additionally, peripheral non-nerve sheath tumors can be found, for example, meningiomas, lipomas, ganglioneuromas, epidermoid cysts, angiomas, solitary fibrous tumors/hemangiopericytomas, glomus tumors, and other rarer entities [12]. Finally, some inflammatory and infective pathologies such as sarcoid granulomas and leprosy can present itself along the PNS mimicking nerve neoplasia.

Particular aspects related to the clinical indication and to the surgical technique required for the resection of benign PN tumors will be discussed below. However, a detailed explanation of the surgery of specific tumor types will be discussed elsewhere in this book.

10.2 Clinical Indications for Surgery

The key to a successful surgical intervention starts with the appropriate clinical indication. Considering that as mentioned above benign schwannomas and neurofibromas are the most frequently encountered types of peripheral nerve tumors, then it is of paramount importance that the surgeons know when and how to operate on these cases. The surgeon must be able to remove these benign lesions in the vast majority of cases without incurring a permanent neurological deficit. Therefore, caution is warranted when deciding for a surgical procedure, with an appropriate informed decision between the surgeon and the patient.

Thus, one should start with the case for the conservative treatment. A patient with a single small non-growing or slow-growing tumor with no neurological symptoms or signs should not be operated on, and this patient should be followed up serially. If the patient has a family history of NF1 or NF2, then one can proceed with a thorough physical examination to find syndromic signs and to exclude other tumors. A referral to a genetic specialized clinic to establish if that patient carries gene mutations may be warranted. In the case that the patient arrives at the surgical clinic already with a pre-established diagnosis of NF1/NF2 and still has one or a couple of small tumors and again with no neurological symptoms or signs, then conservative management still is the best option. One important distinction should be made here. In the presence of multiple tumors [13], the physician should order a cranial MRI, because of the higher probability of intracranial tumors; if otherwise, a yearly follow-up is recommended. For these patients, a chart identifying the exact location of the tumor(s) and the size of it is extremely helpful for future follow-ups [2].

The next group are those patients with larger tumors and/or minimal neurological deficit. These are the patients that present themselves with paresthesia and dysesthesias, but with no pain complaint and no muscle weaknesses caused by the tumor. These patients can be also treated conservatively, in particular if the tumor is relatively small. In cases of larger lesions and ones that are demonstrating progressive growth, elective surgical resection is appropriate. Normally, these patients will already have some degree of pain, and it is important to remind the patient of all the surgical risks involved in the resection of the tumor, including augmentation of paresthesia and dysesthesia, as well the small risk of new postoperative neurological deficits. For these larger masses where it is elected not to do surgery *and* where the imaging is concerning, the option of doing an image-guided core needle biopsy to establish the diagnosis should be discussed with the patient. Otherwise, as in the above group, half-yearly or yearly follow-up is recommended.

A third group of patients consist of patients that have one or multiple tumors of any size with uncontrolled pain but no muscle weakness. These patients constitute a group that requires appropriate surgical treatment. The goal of surgery is to remove the tumor causing the painful syndrome and yet preserve function. Sometimes this entails removing the dominant symptom provoking tumor in a multinodular schwannoma or multifascicular neurofibroma, but leaving behind smaller non-symptomatic lesions (Fig. 10.3). Patients with peripheral nerve tumors that present with pain and minor sensory and/or motor should be operated. That is the classical indication for surgery of peripheral nerve tumors. Moreover, if multiple symptomatic tumors are present and if the anatomical location permits, then it is possible to approach it in the same day, as we do for cases of schwannomatosis [1] in one limb or regional area. Otherwise, staged procedures can be scheduled.

There is a special group of patients that need to be considered, and these are patients with deep-seated tumors. While peripheral nerve tumors along the limbs are easy to diagnose and detect, deep-seated tumors in the thoracic and abdominal regions and also in the brachial plexus and lumbosacral plexus regions are usually diagnosed when presenting as large masses. Clinically one of the following or all of them are associated with these cases: pain, paresthesia, dysesthesia, and muscle weakness. These tumors often compress vascular structures and can be difficult to approach. Although these are challenging tumors for the surgeon, there is no doubt about the surgical indication, when they are large, growing, and/or symptomatic [14]. Conversely, small and non-growing (even large) asymptomatic lesions should simply be followed. A biopsy prior to surgical resection could be performed to differentiate between a benign and a malignant lesion. Surgical resection in both cases should be performed, and in particular, for malignant tumors, the goal is to perform a radical resection (with margins) [6].

The advantages and disadvantages of the surgical procedure should be always presented to the patient. Among the listed advantages are the establishment of a pathological diagnosis, pain reduced or abolished, possible improvement of paresthesia and dysesthesia, avoidance of progression of a benign tumor to a malignant tumor [7], resection before tumor growth size that causes muscle weakness, and, in case of muscle weakness already present, improvement of muscle weakness or even complete restoration of the motor function. The other side of this is the risk of furthering sensory and motor deficits and, worse, even creating new deficits after the tumor resection.

10.3 Fundamental Aspects of the Surgical Technique

For the safe resection of peripheral nerve tumors, there are some very important points to be observed. First, the surgical exposure should allow the surgeon to identify tumor-free margins of the nerve, with sufficient proximal and distal length exposed (Fig. 10.1). That is relatively easy and straightforward for tumors localized along the limbs. The incision should be large enough then to allow this exposure. Magnification can be used already at the moment of the skin incision either through loupes or the surgical microscope; however, once the nerve is found and tumor dissection initiated, the surgeons should immediately start using the surgical microscope. Also, colored vessel loops are used once vascular and nerve structures are found in order to facilitate the proper identification of the structures.

The approach to deep-seated peripheral nerve tumors could pose a problem, and it is not in the scope of this chapter to describe surgical approaches to such lesions, but it is important to notice that often the best choice of approach for deep-seated tumors in the thoracic or abdominal region requires a multidisciplinary team including thoracic surgeons or general surgeons [15]. However, once the involved nerve and tumor are localized, from that moment on, the procedure should be performed by the surgeon experienced with microsurgery. A useful advice is to have easy access to vascular clamps for those cases which there is a tumor adjacent to a major vessel. An emergency arterial wall repair is not something to be underestimated, and the use of clamping will be necessary for it.

Previously the senior author (RM) has called the attention to the importance of distinguishing between the two main types of tumors, eccentric tumors, exemplified by schwannomas (Figs. 10.1 and 10.2), and mostly centrally located tumors, exemplified by neurofibromas (Figs. 10.3 and 10.4), in regard to surgical technique [16].

Traditionally, under the microscope, the surgeon initially identifies both distally and proximally a nerve region which presents no tumor involvement of the fascicles that is followed by the longitudinal opening of the *epineurium* overlying the tumor. This is done using magnification with an operating microscope to evaluate for a fascicle-free zone which is aided with mapping of the surface using direct electrical stimulation and looking for an absence of motor evoked response. Recently Stone et al. published [17] a paper regarding the technique for the interfascicular dissection of benign peripheral nerve sheath tumors, similar to which the senior author has used for the past two decades. The step-by-step technique consists of the following:

1. Fascicle-free window is identified on the tumor through visual and intraoperative monitoring.
2. The pseudocapsule layers are divided with sharp instrument until a smooth and shiny true capsule layer is found.

3. Then, this plane which has minimal resistance is dissected circumferentially until the tumor is completely enucleated.
4. At the poles, the surgeon looks for a single non-functioning nerve fascicle; if there is more than one fascicle, then the surgeon proceeds once more to repeat step 2.
5. The non-functioning entering or exiting fascicle or fascicles are cut.
6. The sides of the pseudocapsule are spread in opposite directions to evaluate for residual tumor, and then if there is any, it is safely removed.

Thc most frequently encountered benign tumors bypassing fascicles are white in comparison to the yellowish coloration of the tumors [17, 18] (Fig. 10.2). It is important that the dissection is performed with frequent testing of the function of these fascicles and continuing intraoperative monitoring. During this stage of the surgery, often, the neurophysiologist will mention to the surgeon some neurophysiological changes when manipulating the fascicles. When that happens, the surgeon should proceed with the fascicle/tumor capsule dissection at another area of the nerve. Most of the time, these are transitory chances, and the careful resection can be continued for that particular fascicle. The technique to dissect the fascicle from capsule can vary; most of the time, blunt microtechnique using either a micro-forceps or a micro-dissector is the safest, but certainly there could be occasions that the use of a micro-scissor or a knife is warranted when trying to obtain a complete resection. For really large tumors, tumor debulking is the best way to proceed in order to avoid extreme and potentially hazardous mobilization of the involved nerve. Once most of the tumor is debulked, then the surgeon can use the steps described above. The final dissection of the tumor from a fascicle can be performed through sharp cut, aided by judicious coagulation.

Special problems arise for the cases in which fascicles enter directly into the tumor; this situation requires the help of the neurophysiologist. If there are many fascicles involved, and these are functioning (motor) fascicles responding to neurophysiological stimuli, then it is advisable to carefully remove in a piecemeal fashion as much tumor as it is possible to do safely and leave the tumor part involving the functioning fascicles (as in Fig. 10.3 example). If only, from a neurophysiological perspective, *non-functioning* fascicles are involved and cannot be separated from tumor capsule, then if the goal is to achieve a complete removal, these fascicles could be sacrificed, and again either cutting or coagulation is possible (Fig. 10.1).

There are several surgical and pathological contraindications for the use of the above technique including multiple prior surgeries, which makes the identification of pseudocapsule and capsule very difficult, and an atypical lesion, i.e., malignant tumors. When prior surgery makes morphological identification of the capsule difficult, careful interfascicular dissection starting at either end of normal nerve and then arriving at the nerve-tumor interface may be warranted to find the correct dissection plan. Of course, in cases of malignant lesions, an en bloc or wide excision is warranted, and entering the tumor capsule is to be avoided.

Summarizing, the fundamental technique for tumor resection always requires careful tumor resection away from bypassing fascicles using microsurgery with the help of intraoperative monitoring in order to properly identify functioning from non-functioning fascicles.

10.4 Illustrative Cases

10.4.1 Case 1 Radial Nerve Schwannoma

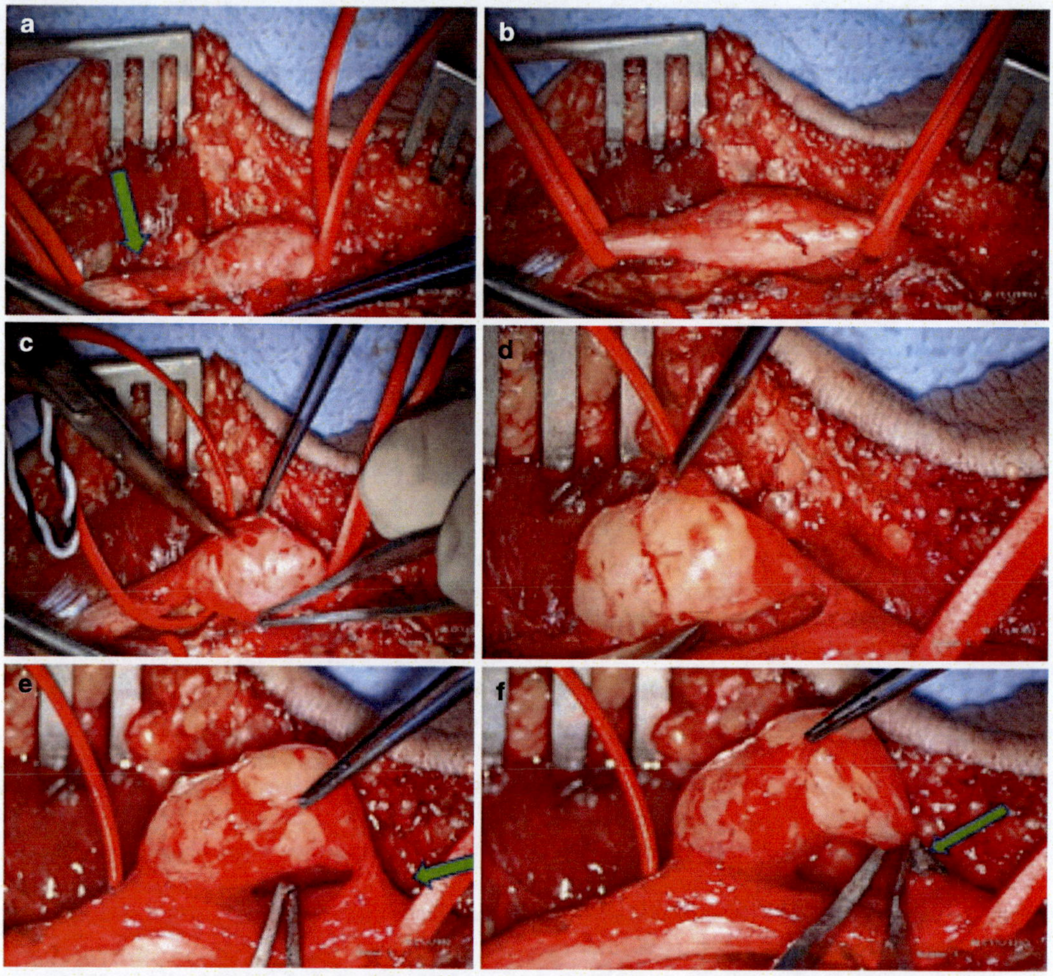

Fig. 10.1 Isolation of the nerve (green arrow) and the tumor after the soft tissue dissection (**a**). Schwannoma is inspected circumferentially after the mobilization of nerve and tumor, searching for fascicle-free zones (**b**). Schwannoma capsule is dissected initially (**c**), with further capsular dissection circumferentially (**d**). Schwannoma is lifted from the nerve trunk, and entering and exiting fascicles (green arrows) can be visualized (**e**). Coagulation of the exiting fascicle (**f**), prior to its division

10.4.2 Case 2 Peroneal Nerve Schwannoma

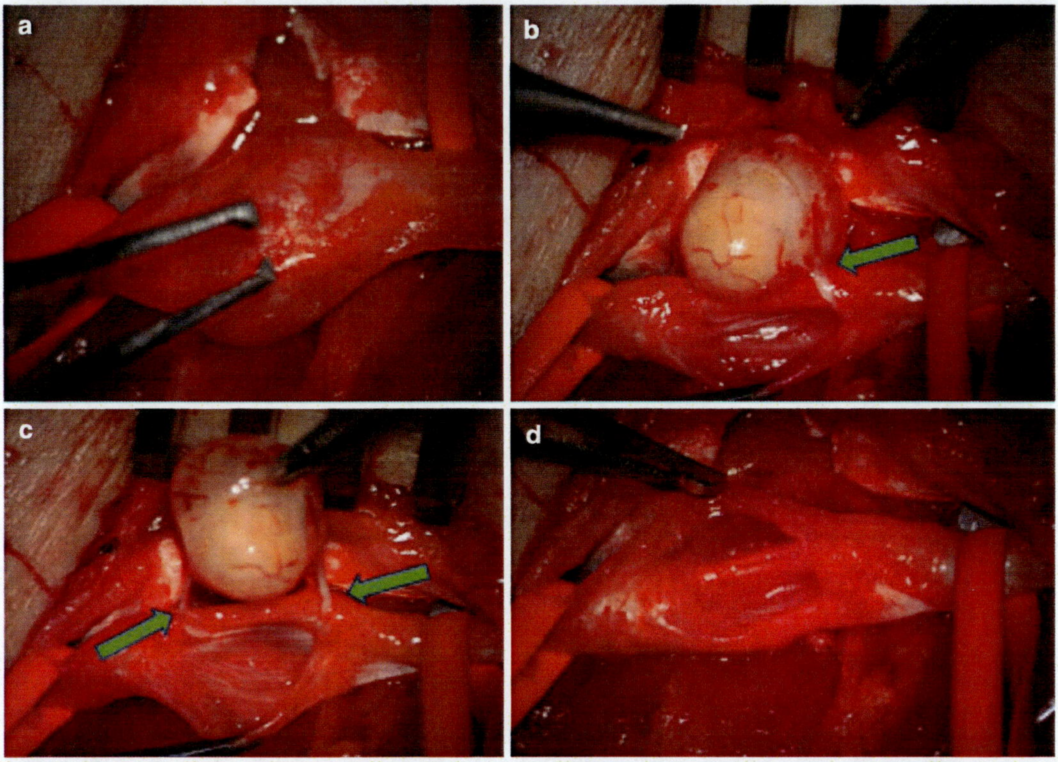

Fig. 10.2 Photograph of the peroneal nerve schwannoma and surface fascicles prior to resection (**a**). Peroneal nerve schwannoma dissection off of the fascicles, yellowish color for the tumor and white-colored fascicles (green arrows) (**b**, **c**), with entering and exiting fascicles seen clearly in panel (**c**). Preserved nerve along with bypassing fascicles after schwannoma removal (**d**)

10.4.3 Case 3 Ulnar Nerve Neurofibroma

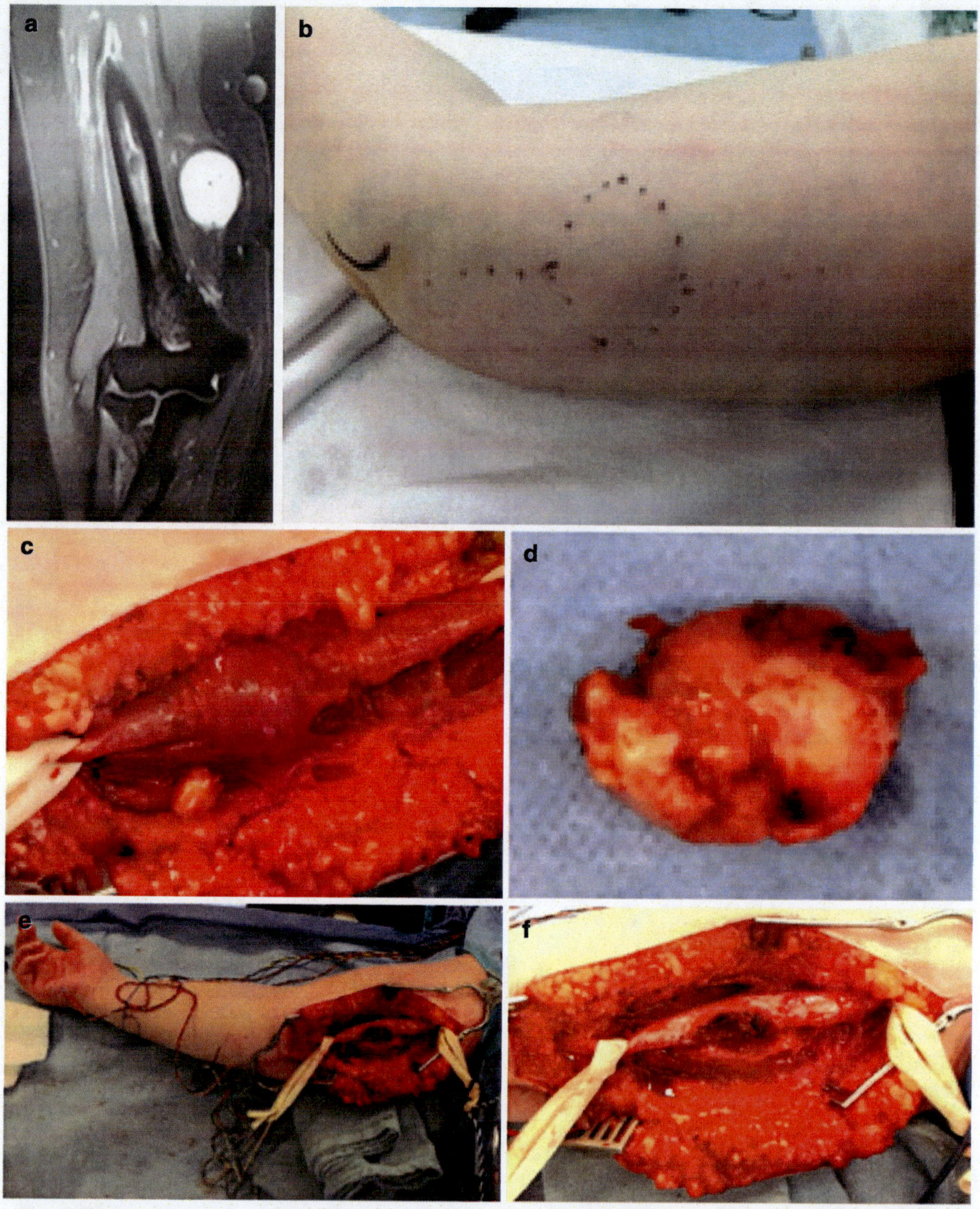

Fig. 10.3 MRI of the ulnar nerve neurofibroma (**a**). Marking of the skin incision and the approximate location of the tumor (**b**). After soft tissue dissection, the ulnar nerve and neurofibroma are exposed (**c**). Photograph of the resected neurofibroma (**d**). After the microsurgical resection, one can see in the arm the needle electrodes on the hand muscles for EMG recording of the ulnar muscle groups. This allowed successful removal of the dominant neurofibroma from the ulnar nerve and selective non-resection of small neurofibromas in conducting fascicles which were causing EMG activation. Postoperatively the patient had a motor deficit which is now resolved, and the pain which was there prior to surgery is no longer there (**e**). The ulnar nerve post tumor resection (**f**)

10.4.4 Case 4 Solitary Radial Nerve Neurofibroma

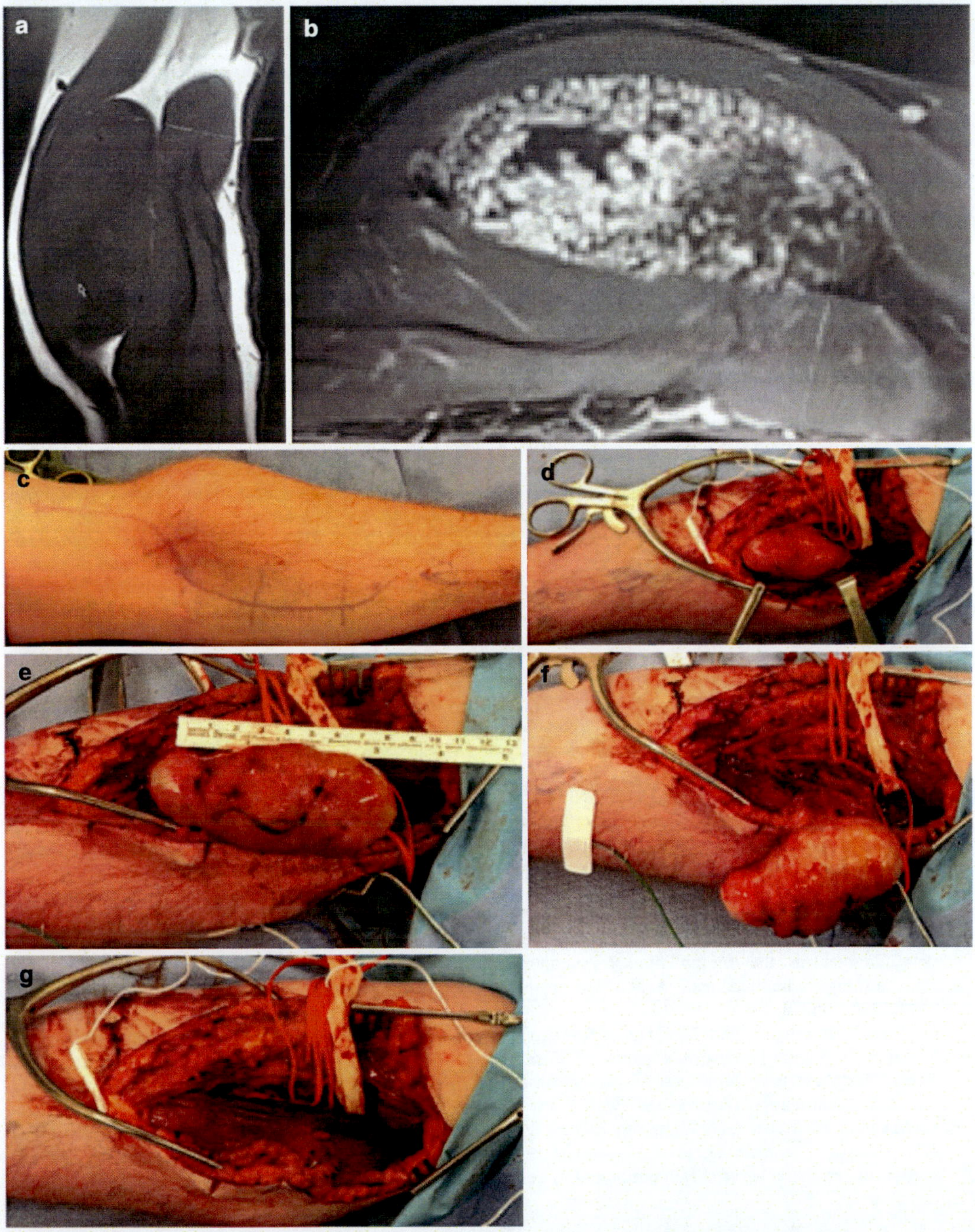

Fig. 10.4 MR image of the solitary neurofibroma (**a**, **b**). Skin marked for incision showing the use of an extensile skin incision for this case (**c**). Surgical site showing the isolated tumor. It was a SOLITARY neurofibroma from forearm branches of the radial nerve, and the senior author achieved complete resection sparing all branches by using intraoperative stimulation of bypassing nerve branches and recording evoked EMGs (**d**). Neurofibroma and radial nerve; the neurofibroma was approximately 8.5 cm long (**e**), and it was removed as one large sample (**f**). Radial nerve and branches after the complete removal of the neurofibroma (**g**)

10.5 Conclusion

The fundamental aspect of proper resection of peripheral nerve tumors is the use of a good microsurgical technique that allows the safe resection of the tumor and preservation of the nerve functions. In order for that to happen, several steps are necessary. Through clinical history and physical examination, detailed MRI and ultrasound imaging are the preoperative steps, along with carefully selecting patients for surgery. Microsurgery techniques for interfascicular dissection are to be mastered, while intraoperative monitoring of the nerve function is an important tool during surgery in order to achieve the best possible outcome of complete nerve tumor resection and absence of a new neurological deficit and further improvement of the existing deficits. The following chapters in this book present detailed information about the management of different types of peripheral nerve tumors.

References

1. MacCollin M, Woodfin W, Kronn D, Short MP. Schwannomatosis: a clinical and pathologic study. Neurology. 1996;46(4):1072–9.
2. MacCollin M, Chiocca EA, Evans DG, Friedman JM, Horvitz R, Jaramillo D, et al. Diagnostic criteria for schwannomatosis. Neurology. 2005;64(11):1838–45.
3. Lewis JJ, Brennan MF. Soft tissue sarcomas. Curr Probl Surg. 1996;33(10):817–72.
4. Rodriguez FJ, Scheithauer BW, George D, Midha R, MacCollin M, Stemmer-Rachamimov AO. Superficial neurofibromas in the setting of schwannomatosis: nosologic implications. Acta Neuropathol. 2011;121(5):663–8.
5. Martinez F, Dominguez-Paez M, Cuadros-Romero M, Moragues R, Segura-Fernandez Nogueras M, Casales N, et al. Peripheral nerve tumours: a 66-case retrospective study. Neurocirugia (Astur). 2020;31:105–11.
6. McLaughlin EJ, Heuer GG, Whitmore RG, Birknes JK, Belasco J, Sterman D, et al. Treatment of a malignant peripheral nerve sheath tumor and its complications through a multidisciplinary approach. J Neurosurg Pediatr. 2011;7(5):543–8.
7. Simmermacher S, Vordermark D, Kegel T, Strauss C. Malignization of a vestibular schwannoma 13 years after radiation therapy. HNO. 2017;65(Suppl 2):153–7.
8. Humhej I, Ibrahim I, Lodin J, Sames M, Cizmar I. Image possibilities of the peripheral nerve tumor using magnetic resonance imaging—case report. Acta Chir Plast. 2019;60(1):9–13.
9. Battaglia PJ, Carbone-Hobbs V, Guebert GM, Mackinnon SE, Kettner NW. High-resolution ultrasonography and shear-wave sonoelastography of a cystic radial nerve schwannoma. J Ultrasound. 2017;20(3):261–6.
10. Kwok K, Davis B, Kliot M. Resection of a benign brachial plexus nerve sheath tumor using intraoperative electrophysiological monitoring. Neurosurgery. 2007;60(4 Suppl 2):316–20; discussion 20-1
11. Vajtai I, Hewer E, Andres R, Neuenschwander M, Kappeler A, Gugger M. Meningial perineurioma: a benign peripheral nerve sheath tumor in a previously unrecognized central nervous system location, mimicking meningioma. Pathol Res Pract. 2011;207(9):592–6.
12. Friedrich RE, Diekmeier C. Peripheral nerve sheath tumors of the upper extremity and hand in patients with neurofibromatosis type 1: topography of tumors and evaluation of surgical treatment in 62 patients. GMS Interdiscip Plast Reconstr Surg DGPW. 2017;6:Doc15.
13. Nunes F, MacCollin M. Neurofibromatosis 2 in the pediatric population. J Child Neurol. 2003;18(10):718–24.
14. Vucemilo L, Lajtman Z, Mihalj J, Plascak J, Mahovic Lakusic D, Muzinic D. Brachial plexus schwannoma—case report and literature review. Acta Clin Croat. 2018;57(2):366–71.
15. Freitas B, Figueiredo R, Carrerette F, Acioly MA. Retroperitoneoscopic resection of a lumbosacral plexus schwannoma: case report and literature review. J Neurol Surg A Cent Eur Neurosurg. 2018;79(3):262–7.
16. Midha R. Entrapment neuropathies and peripheral nerve tumors. In: Ellenbogen R, editor. Principles of neurological surgery. 4th ed. London: Elsevier; 2018.
17. Stone JJ, Puffer RC, Spinner RJ. Interfascicular resection of benign peripheral nerve sheath tumors. JBJS Essent Surg Tech. 2019;9(2):e18.
18. Stone JJ, Spinner RJ. Go for the gold: a "plane" and simple technique for resecting benign peripheral nerve sheath tumors. Oper Neurosurg (Hagerstown). 2020;18:60–8.

11 Neurophysiological Monitoring during Surgery

Carlos Alberto Rodríguez Aceves
and Armando Tello Valdés

11.1 Introduction

The goal of surgical resection of nerve tumors is to achieve complete removal of the tumor while preserving nerve function. In the past, the surgical treatment of nerve tumors was a difficult task, because of a lack of complete understanding of the tumor biology and its microscopic anatomy and the absence of adequate surgical tools for a safest resection [1, 2].

Different neurophysiological preoperative tests exist, as mentioned in Chap. 5. After they were first described for the surgical management of peripheral nerve injuries in 1960 by Kline et al. [3, 4], they have been integrated routinely as multimodal intraoperative monitoring (MIOM) during peripheral nerve surgery in selected cases. These techniques can be adapted to different surgical procedures allowing a continuous identification and quantification of distinct parameters to clearly reveal functional status of nerve structures during nerve surgery [5].

MIOM is particularly useful for some peripheral nerve lesions that constitute a surgical challenge. It is essential to establish the baseline neurological status, the regional anatomy, and the type of anesthesia used. At present, its use is widespread for the surgical management of peripheral nerve tumors to minimize damage to functional neural elements [5–7].

MIOM consists of two elements: mapping for the timely identification of nerve structures that must be preserved and continuous monitoring of the functional integrity of a specific nerve pathway for early detection of variations that call for modification of surgical maneuvers [5].

11.2 Intraoperative Monitoring Techniques

Neurophysiological techniques follow the same principles as preoperative evaluation; however, stimulation and recording electrodes in the surgical field must be sterile [5] (Fig. 11.1).

Communication between the surgical and monitoring teams is imperative, since the correct positioning of electrodes in the muscles or nerve of interest, the application of stimuli, how to perform manipulation of the studied nerve, the use of total intravenous anesthesia (TIVA) during surgery without muscle relaxant medication, and avoiding the use of tourniquets are fundamental factors for an optimal registry [5, 8] (Fig. 11.2).

C. A. Rodríguez Aceves (✉)
Neurosurgery Department, Neurological Center, The American British Cowdray Medical Center, Mexico City, Mexico

Peripheral Nerve Committee, World Federation of Neurosurgical Societies, Mexico City, Mexico

A. Tello Valdés
Head of Clinical Neurophysiology Department, Hospital Español de México, Mexico City, Mexico

F. Guedes et al. (eds.), *Diagnostic Assessment and Treatment of Peripheral Nerve Tumors*,
https://doi.org/10.1007/978-3-030-77633-6_11

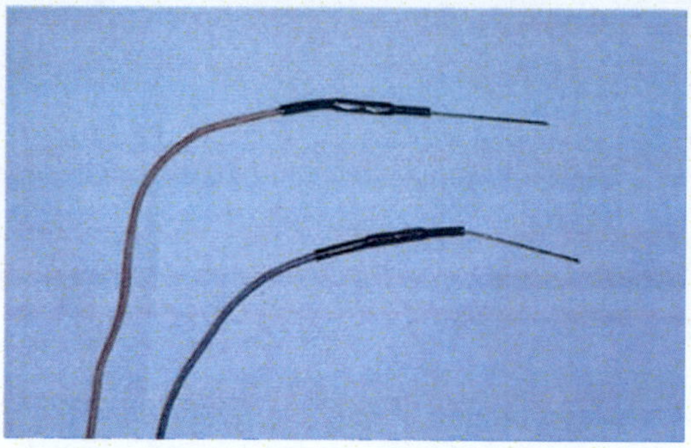

Fig. 11.1 Monopolar intramuscular needle for EMG recording

Recording techniques are divided according to bioelectrical signals: (1) spontaneous EMG activity and (2) evoked responses—somatosensory evoked potentials (SSEPs), motor evoked potentials (MEPs), evoked EMG potentials, and nerve action potential (NAP). Thus, evoked responses can be recorded at the cerebral cortex, spinal cord, muscle, or peripheral nerve. The selection of the specific monitoring technique will depend on the structure we need to evaluate [5, 9, 10]. The following section of this chapter will refer to the most useful techniques for peripheral nerve tumor surgery.

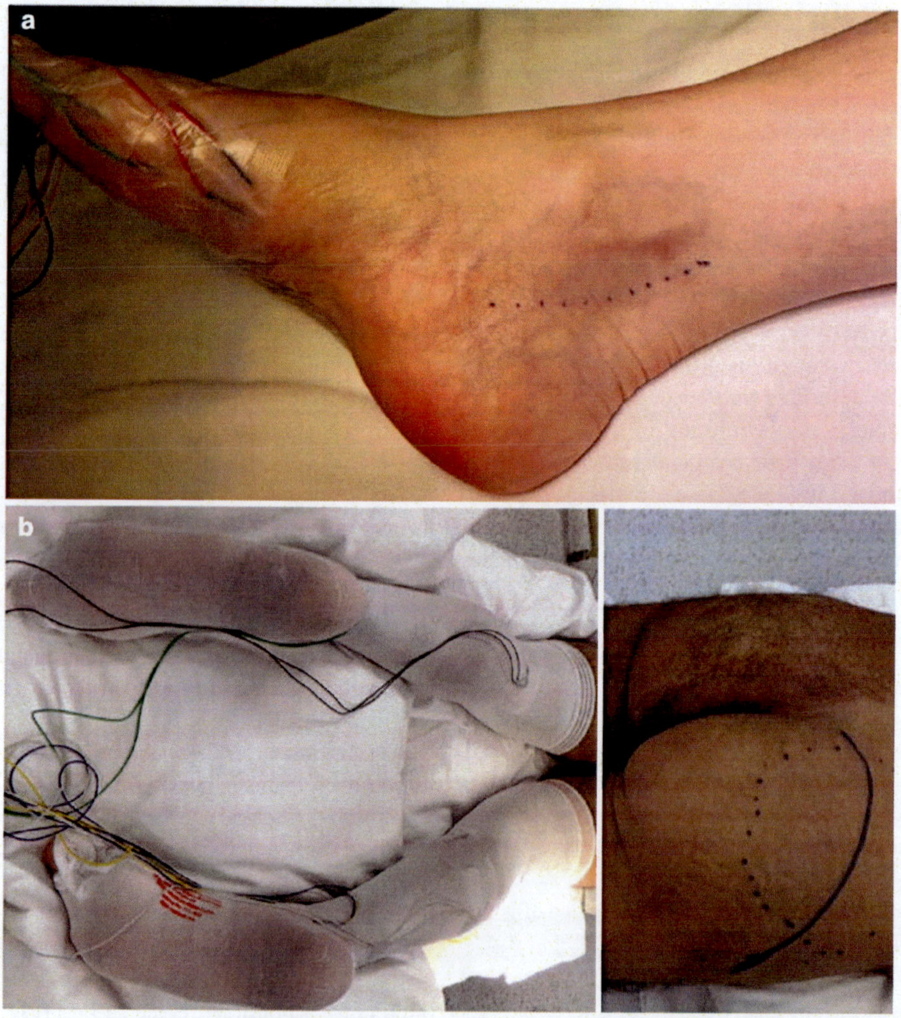

Fig. 11.2 Electrode placement in selected muscles away from surgical field after positioning and anesthesia induction. (**a**) For resection of distal tibial nerve tumor and (**b**) For resection of proximal sciatic nerve tumor

11.2.1 Continuous Intraoperative Electromyography (EMG)

Continuous EMG is the uninterrupted recording of the electrical activity of the muscle or muscles of interest. It provides dynamic real-time information to surgeons if during intraneural tumor resection, retraction injury, nerve compression, or vascular insult occurs. It may also indicate nerve proximity in the case of extraneural tumor resection. It is used to avoid nerve trunk or fascicular damage during surgical manipulation. When nerve irritation occurs, by mechanical, thermal, or metabolic trauma, muscle activity increases and can be displayed on a digital screen and as an audible signal, so that the surgeon becomes aware of any harmful manipulation of the nerve in real time. Surgical manipulation must be interrupted if sustained tonic activity (neurotonic discharges) is present. These discharges appear as rapid, irregular bursts, lasting several milliseconds, or prolonged trains [5, 8, 11, 12] (Fig. 11.3).

11.2.2 Stimulus-Triggered Intraoperative Electromyography (tEMG)

tEMG is useful for mapping nerve or fascicle identification. A brief, low-intensity electrical stimulation is applied to a nerve, with subsequent recording of a compound muscle action potential (CMAP) using the same electrodes as for continuous EMG. tEMG helps to identify nerve structures in a more precise way than visual muscle contraction. The stimulator may be a monopolar or bipolar sterile device and is used by the surgeon; bipolar electrodes deliver a more focal stimulation, with less current spread to nearby neural structures [5, 11] (Fig. 11.4).

Despite the fact that CMAP recording is easier than NAP recording, it is recommended that the surgeon palpate and observe the target muscles, because EMG cannot sample all motor units during stimulation [6].

11.2.3 Nerve Action Potential

Like CMAP, registry of NAP is obtained by direct stimulation of the nerve trunk proximal to the site of injury, and recording takes place along the course of the stimulated nerve, distal to the site of injury. Using the same principle, NAP can be recorded in a single fascicle or group of fascicles in tumor resection. With this technique, some surgeons have demonstrated the absence of electrical response across the fascicle(s) involved in certain types of tumors. However, its application is not as useful as for traumatic injuries, since sometimes these are technically challenging for several reasons, including problems related to access to an appropriate length of the fascicle segment, distortion of anatomy, presence of a stimulus artifact, and flawed recording parameters [5, 13, 14]. These problems can sometimes be resolved by using stimulating electrodes with three poles (tripolar) with anode-cathode-anode array, which reduces the stimulus artifact when the recording electrode is near the stimulus.

11.2.4 Somatosensory and Motor Evoked Potentials

In SSEPs, the responses are produced by applying an electrical stimulus to a peripheral nerve and subsequently recording the response at cortical level of the sensory pathway or upper relay stations. Intraoperatively, those responses are compared with baseline reference values obtained before the beginning of the surgical procedure. A decrease of more than 50% in amplitude or an increase of more than 10% in latency of responses is associated with an adverse neural function. One limitation of SSEPs is that the value is based on the calculated averages of stimuli which may take several minutes to change following an acute insult [15, 16].

When SSEPs are used to evaluate the somatosensory pathways at risk during peripheral nerve tumor resection, a decrease in the responses may be indicative of stretching or compression of the

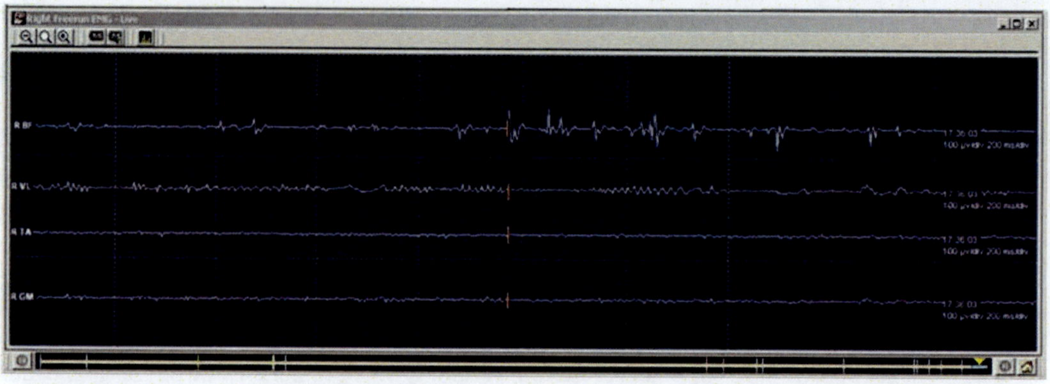

Fig. 11.3 Continuous EMG during resection of an extraneural tumor mass compressing proximal sciatic nerve showing neurotonic discharges due to mechanical irritation by manipulation. Source: Neurophysiology archives, The American British Cowdray Medical Center

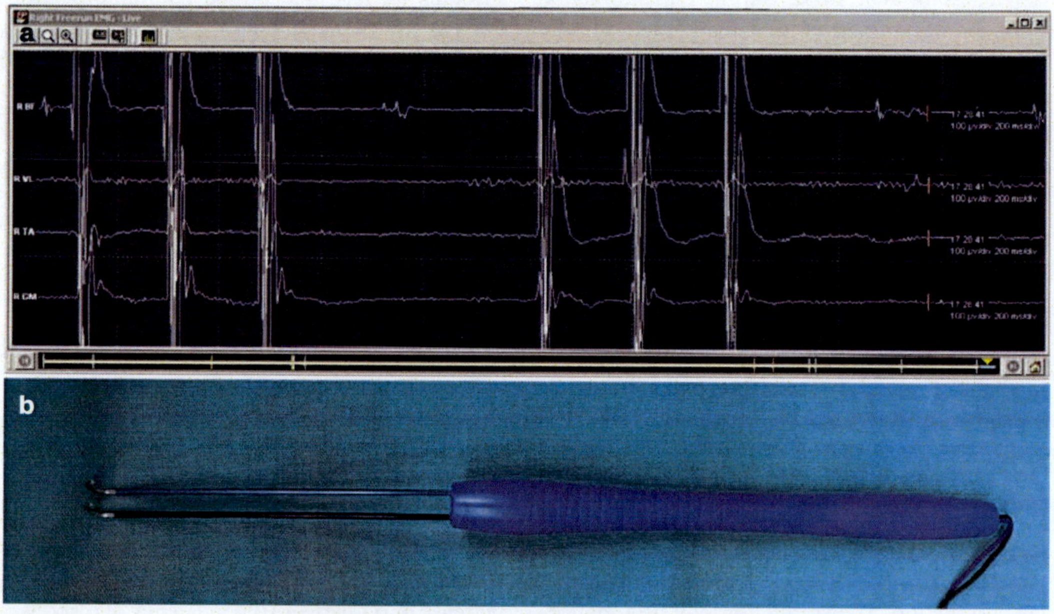

Fig. 11.4 (**a**) Evoked EMG during resection of a proximal sciatic nerve tumor. Source: Neurophysiology archives, The American British Cowdray Medical Center. (**b**) Bipolar hook electrodes

nerve trunk. Therefore, its most useful application is during resection of neighboring extraneural lesions, in which the nerve trunk may not be visible to the surgeon (Fig. 11.5).

MEPs are obtained using high-voltage, short-duration repetitive stimulation, over the motor cortex, with electrodes placed on the scalp (transcranial MEPs) to evaluate motor responses within the monitored muscles. Since individual muscles are often innervated by motor fibers from more than one nerve root, its use for peripheral nerve tumor resection usually is limited to the assessment of the proximal segments of the nerve trunks or plexuses. Nevertheless, some sur-

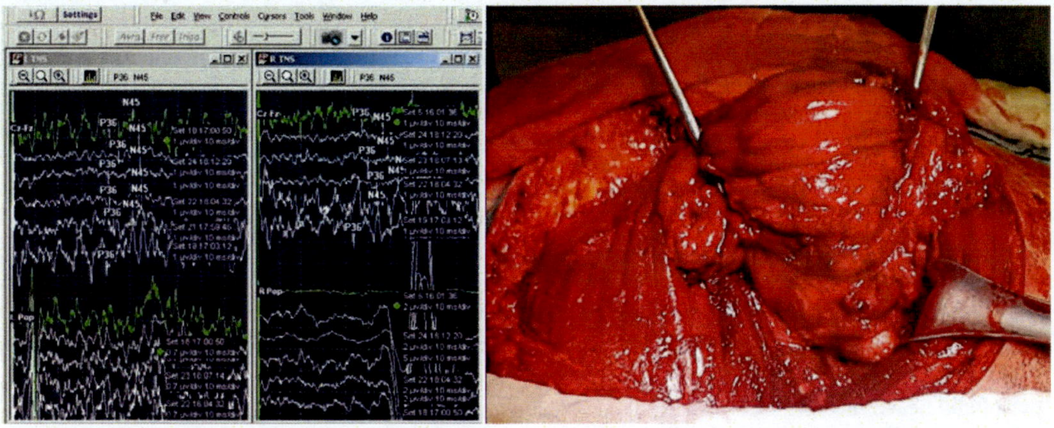

Fig. 11.5 SSEPs during resection of a right sided gluteal liposarcoma with intrapelvic extension through sciatic foramen compressing proximal sciatic nerve. White lines represent baseline responses and green ones represent final responses for left and right tibial nerves respectively. Source: Neurophysiology archives, The American British Cowdray Medical Center

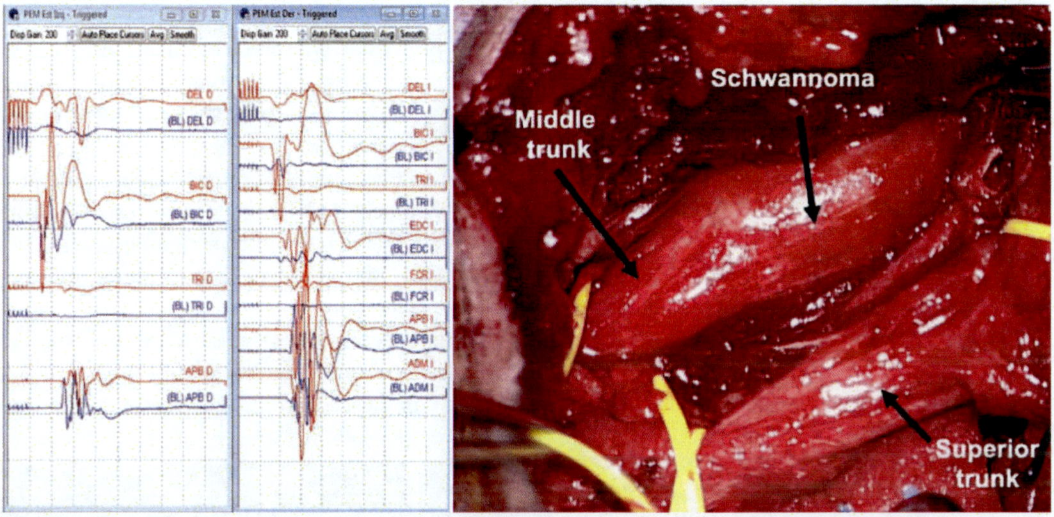

Fig. 11.6 MEPs during resection of a left sided C7-Middle trunk extraforaminal schwannoma. Blue lines represent baseline responses and red ones represent final responses for left and right muscles innervated by C5 to T1 roots respectively. Source: Neurophysiology archives, The American British Cowdray Medical Center

geons advocate the utility of intraoperative MEPs in predicting neurological deficits following the surgical enucleation of peripheral nerve schwannoma and also demonstrate that even if a nerve is not transected or injured, traction or compression may induce ischemia with the resultant decrease in MEP response [15, 17, 18] (Fig. 11.6).

11.3 Surgical Applications in Tumor Resection

MIOM can assist the surgeon to preserve critical nerve function during intraneural or extraneural tumor resection and to select nonfunctional fascicles when a nerve biopsy is needed [19, 20].

Before surgery, it is necessary to select the muscles that will be monitored. The anesthesiologist must be instructed to use only short-acting muscle relaxants for anesthetic induction, and once the patient is intubated, no muscle relaxants must be used during the rest of the surgery; anesthetic blocks also must be avoided. For hemostasis and bleeding control, it is preferred to use proper careful bipolar coagulation and direct compression during surgery, since the use of tourniquets interferes with normal nerve conduction [8, 21–23].

As mentioned in previous chapters, benign peripheral nerve sheath tumors (BPNSTs) are the most frequent type of tumors within peripheral nerves, and these are represented by schwannomas and neurofibromas, the first being the most common BPNST [24].

Schwannomas and neurofibromas arise from a single or multiple fascicles, respectively, allowing for microsurgical removal with no or a low risk of permanent postoperative deficit [25].

After exposure of the nerve trunk and tumor as needed, direct electrical stimulation at low setting (0.5–2 mA) on the tumor surface is performed prior to dissection. In this mapping stage, continuous EMG and CMAP registry are critical to avoid damage to functional fascicles (Fig. 11.7). To identify a safe zone of entry before opening the nerve trunk, the surgeon should look for any electrical response or muscle contraction, either visible or palpable after electrical stimulation. After exposing the tumor within the nerve, the dissection stage is carried out also guided by continuous EMG. Compression and traction of functional fascicles will elicit EMG discharges. If EMG discharges occur, the surgical maneuver should be stopped and modified to avoid damage to these fascicles, until proximal entering and distal exiting fascicles of the tumor are reached. Stimulation with triggered EMG and recording of NAP of these fascicles allows the surgeon to confirm their lack of functionality or the existence of any motor response in the case of multiple fascicles seen in neurofibromas; if they exist, an attempt to reconstruct the fascicle should be done [6, 13, 26–31] (Fig. 11.8).

At the end of the procedure, any of the evoked responses described previously can aid in confirming the integrity of the neural function.

When a more diffuse tumor (such as plexiform neurofibroma or perineurioma) or malignant peripheral nerve sheath tumor is present, the same principles are employed using direct electrical stimulation and continuous and triggered EMG with recording of CMAPs to identify and preserve functional fascicles. Nevertheless, the nature of these types of tumors reduces the possibility of accomplishing surgical resection with complete preservation of function despite the use of MIOM, but they may help to predict postoperative outcome.

The resection of extraneural tumors (such as desmoid tumors) in the vicinity of a nerve trunk can be monitored by using continuous

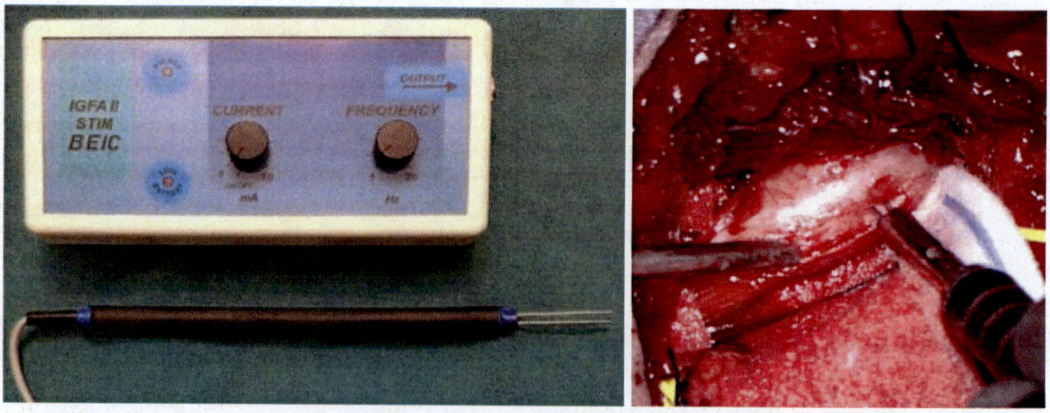

Fig. 11.7 Mapping of schwannoma surface to identify a safe zone of entry by direct electrical stimulation with the IGFA II Stim™ nerve stimulator device by BEIC

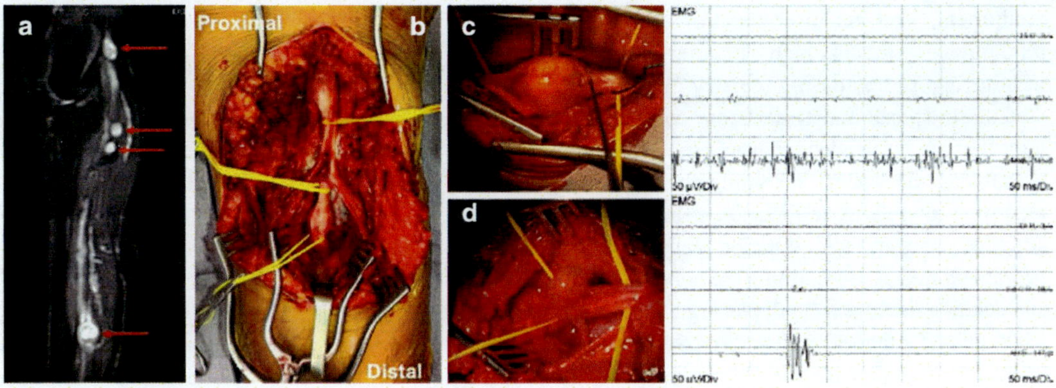

Fig. 11.8 Dissection stage of one of multiple schwannomas (red arrows) arising from right tibial nerve in a patient with schwannomatosis. (**a**) Sagittal STIR sequence MRI with multiple tumors arising from tibial nerve. (**b**) Surgical exposure of proximal tibial nerve showing multiple schwannomas, two at the popliteal fossa, and one more distally. (**c**) Continuous EMG neurotonic discharges of the right abductor hallucis during dissection of proximal pole of one of the tumors. (**d**) Continuous EMG with brief neurotonic discharge of the right abductor hallucis during final steps of enucleation of tumor. Source: Neurophysiology archives, Hospital Español de México

EMG and evoked responses such as MEPs and SSEPs. In these cases, mobilization or manipulation of the tumor can cause inadvertent damage to adjacent nerves. MIOM allows the detection and protection of nerves that may be difficult to identify, at a stage when a neurological deficit is reversible [19].

Nerve tumor biopsy was discussed in Chap. 9. When necessary, MIOM is also helpful to avoid damage by identifying functional fascicles at risk [14].

11.4 Potential Pitfalls

MIOM may yield preventable false-positive or false-negative responses. As mentioned in the previous section of this chapter, communication among the surgical team is the first step to avoid registry errors. The clinical neurophysiologist needs to be capable of interpreting electrical changes during surgery, discriminating and reducing artifacts, identifying peak waves, and integrating the diverse monitoring modalities [9, 22].

A clear knowledge of the regional anatomy and innervation territories is mandatory for the selection of the correct muscles to be monitored, as well as the proper application of recording electrodes outside the surgical field. These two initial steps avoid the possibility of incorrect registry in muscles not related to the affected nerve and also obstruction of the surgical field for the surgeon or detachment of electrodes during surgery.

TIVA with a combination of propofol and opioids is the preferred general anesthetic technique for any procedure that requires the use of neurophysiological monitoring, since with balanced dosage, the neuromuscular junction and cortex remain functional. Inhalation anesthesia, anesthetic blocks, and muscle relaxants interfere with neural pathway responses and muscle contraction causing delayed or reduced neural responses [31–33].

Some peripheral nerve surgeons use tourniquets for bleeding control; nevertheless, when MIOM is employed, their use may interfere with normal neurophysiological responses due to nerve ischemia. Thus, if a tourniquet is employed, deflation of the cuff is necessary at least 20 min before the registry of nerve evoked responses [34]. Low temperature can also affect the registry by slowing conduction; thus, cold irrigation is not recommended.

Equipment failure can never be eliminated completely and should always be considered by the neurophysiology team. Therefore, qualified, experienced personnel are needed to identify and correct any errors made in setting up the recording equipment, such as disconnections, as well as recognizing artifacts (such as cautery, anesthetic monitoring, lights) during registry [35].

Current spread and artifacts are common problems that can be avoided by using bipolar or tripolar stimulating electrodes, increasing the stimulating-recording interelectrode distance, using the lowest stimulus intensity and duration necessary for a supramaximal response, lifting the nerve away from surrounding tissue and fluid, placing a ground electrode, and orienting electrodes correctly; these are all technical considerations that neurophysiologists must bear in mind [36].

11.5 Summary

Communication among the surgical team (surgeon, neurophysiologist, and anesthesiologist) is imperative for the selection of the most useful neurophysiological techniques to accomplish optimal MIOM during peripheral nerve or neighboring tumor resection surgery. This strategy must be based on the biological nature (probable origin) of the tumor, its anatomical localization, and its topographical relation with the nerve trunks (neural or extraneural). This information can be obtained with an adequate preoperative diagnostic approach [8]. In spite of its cost and time-consuming labor, MIOM provides information that cannot be obtained by other intraoperative tools [13, 19].

Since peripheral nerve tumor surgery can be a difficult task, even for experienced surgeons, to optimize the results, in addition to the correct application of the microsurgical technique, the surgeon must rely on the different intraoperative neurophysiological modalities to perform a safe resection and avoid complications, reducing the risk of inadvertent lesions in the nerve trunks or functional fascicles inside the nerve.

References

1. Powers CJ, Friedman AH. A brief history of surgery for peripheral nerve sheath tumors. Neurosurg Focus. 2007;22(6):E1.
2. Little KM, Zomorodi AR, Selznick LA, Friedman AH. An eclectic history of peripheral nerve surgery. Neurosurg Clin N Am. 2004;15(2):109–23.
3. Zouridakis G, Papanicolau A. A concise guide to intraoperative monitoring. Boca Raton: CRC Press LLC; 2012.
4. Galloway GM, Nuwer MR, López JR. Intraoperative neurophysiologic monitoring. New York: Cambridge University Press; 2010.
5. Rodríguez-Aceves CA, Domínguez-Páez M, Fernández-Sánchez VE. Electrodiagnostic pre-, intra-, and postoperative evaluations. In: Socolovsky M, Rasulic L, Midha R, Garozzo D, editors. Manual of peripheral nerve surgery: from the basics to complex procedures. New York: Thieme Medical Publishers; 2017. p. 48–57.
6. Russel SM. Preserve the nerve: microsurgical resection of peripheral nerve sheath tumors. Neurosurgery. 2007;61:ONS 113-ONS 118.
7. Crum BA, Strommen JA. Intraoperative peripheral nerve stimulation and recording. In: Nuwer MR, editor. Intraoperative monitoring of neural function handbook of clinical neurophysiology. Boston: Elsevier; 2008. p. 364–70.
8. Maniker AH. Diagnostic steps, imaging, and electrophysiology. Neurosurg Clin N Am. 2004;15(2):133–44.
9. Kim SM, Kim SH, Seo DW, Lee KW. Intraoperative neurophysiologic monitoring: basic principles and recent update. J Korean Med Sci. 2013;28(9):1261–9.
10. Brown MS, Brown DS. Intraoperative monitoring technician: a new member of the surgical team. AORN J. 2011;93(2):242–8.
11. Holland NR. Intraoperative electromyography. J Clin Neurophysiol. 2002;19(5):444–53.
12. Strommen JA, Crum BA. Intraoperative monitoring with free-running EMG. In: Nuwer MR, editor. Intraoperative monitoring of neural function handbook of clinical neurophysiology. Boston: Elsevier; 2008. p. 396–403.
13. Wang H, Spinner RJ. Intraoperative testing and monitoring during peripheral nerve surgery. In: Nuwer MR, editor. Intraoperative monitoring of neural function handbook of clinical neurophysiology. Boston: Elsevier; 2008. p. 764–73.
14. Crum BA, Strommen JA. Peripheral nerve stimulation and monitoring during operative procedures. Muscle Nerve. 2007;35(2):159–70.
15. Koht A, Sloan TB. Evoked response monitoring. In: Prabhakar H, editor. Neuromonitoring techniques: quick guide for clinicians and residents. London: Academic Press; 2018. p. 147–77.
16. Rodríguez-Aceves CA, Collado-Ortiz MA, Correa Márquez LI. Monitoreo intreoperatorio multimodal y su aplicación en cirugía de nrevios periféricos:¿Cuándo es de utilidad? An Med(Mex). 2016;6(2):123–31.
17. Sasaki H, Nagano S, Yokouchi M, Setoguchi T, et al. Utility of intraoperative monitoring with

motor-evoked potential during the surgical enucleation of peripheral nerve schwannoma. Oncol Lett. 2018;15(6):9327–2.
18. Burkholder LM, Houlden DA, Midha R, Weiss E, et al. Neurogenic motor evoked potentials: role in brachial plexus surgery. Case report. J Neurosurg. 2003;98(3):607–10.
19. Wang H, Bishop AT, Shin AY, Spinner RJ. Intraoperative testing and monitoring during brachial plexus surgery. In: Nuwer MR, editor. Intraoperative monitoring of neural function handbook of clinical neurophysiology. Boston: Elsevier; 2008. p. 720–30.
20. Spinner RJ. Complication avoidance. Neurosurg Clin N Am. 2004;15(2):193–202.
21. Sharma JP, Salhotra R. Tourniquets in orthopedic surgery. Indian J Orthop. 2012;46(4):377–83.
22. Ali Z. Intraoperative neurophysiologic monitoring and anesthetic implications. Indian J Anaesth. 2019;63(2):81–3.
23. Van Der Walt JJN, Thomas JM, Figaji AA. Intraoperative neurophysiological monitoring for the anaesthetist. South Afr J Anaesth Analg. 2013;19(4):197–202.
24. Skovronsky DM, Oberholtzer JC. Pathologic classification of peripheral nerve tumors. Neurosurg Clin N Am. 2004;15(2):157–66.
25. Guha D, Davidson B, Nadi M, Alotaibi M, et al. Management of peripheral nerve sheath tumors: 17 years of experience at Toronto Western hospital. J Neurosurg. 2018;128(4):1226–34.
26. Ijichi K, Kawakita D, Maseki S, Beppu S, et al. Functional nerve preservation in extracranial head and neck schwannoma surgery. JAMA Otolaryngol Head Neck Surg. 2016;142(5):479–83.
27. Kim D-H, Choi J-G, Son B-C. Identification of safe zone with intraoperative neurophysiological monitoring during surgical removal of peripheral nerve tumor. The Nerve. 2016;2(2):78–80.
28. Tiel R, Kline D. Peripheral nerve tumors: surgical principles, approaches, and techniques. Neurosurg Clin N Am. 2004;15(2):167–75.
29. Ball JR, Biggs MT. Operative steps in management of benign nerve sheath tumors. Neurosurg Focus. 2007;22(6):E7.
30. Kwok K, Davis B, Kliot M. Resection of a benign brachial plexus nerve sheath tumor using intraoperative electrophysiological monitoring. Neurosurgery. 2007;60(4 Suppl 2):316–20.
31. Scheufler KM, Zentner J. Total intravenous anesthesia for intraoperative monitoring of the motor pathways: an integral view combining clinical and experimental data. J Neurosurg. 2002;96(3):571–9.
32. Eroglu A, Apan A, Ertuk E, Ben-Shlomo I. Comparison of the anesthetic techniques. ScientificWorldJournal. 2015;2015:650684.
33. Husain AM. A practical approach to neurophysiologic intraoperative monitoring, 2nd ed. Demos Medical Publishing; 2014.
34. Jahangiri FR. Multimodality neurophysiological monitoring during tibial/fibular osteotomies for preventing peripheral nerve injuries. Neurodiagn J. 2013;53(2):153–68.
35. Schramm J, Møller AR. Intraoperative neurophysiologic monitoring in neurosurgery. Berlin Heidelberg: Springer-Verlag; 1991.
36. Galloway G, Nuwer MR, López JR, Zamel KM. Intraoperative neurophysiologic monitoring. New York: Cambridge University Press; 2010.

12 Complications after Tumor Resection

Javier Robla Costales, Mariano Socolovsky, and Fernando Martínez Benia

Peripheral nerve tumors constitute an important field in peripheral nerve surgery. It is important to know how to resect them and the complications that can occur secondary to the procedure.

Many complications can be avoided if the surgeon acquires broad knowledge about peripheral nerve tumors, including decision-making and operative skills. Major nerve complications typically relate to resecting a benign nerve sheath tumor unnecessarily or resecting a nerve unnecessarily as part of an extraneural lesion. These serious complications frequently stem from a lack of understanding of basic principles of tumor surgery [1].

Approximately 90% of all peripheral nerve tumors are benign, and most of the remaining can be classified within the malignant peripheral nerve sheath tumor (MPNST) group (2). Within the benign category, neurofibromas and schwannomas represent the vast majority of all tumors, most being sporadic and unassociated with either neurofibromatosis type 1 (NF1) or type 2 (NF2) [3].

Schwannomas and neurofibromas can be completely resected with acceptable morbidity (Table 12.1). Surgery is successful at preserving function in 90% of schwannomas, 80% of neurofibromas, and 66% of neurofibromas in those with NF1 [4].

Schwannomas typically are eccentrically located, and there is frequently a single entering and exiting fascicle into the tumor. Reconstruction of this fascicle is not necessary, because it has been demonstrated to be electrophysiologically nonfunctional [3, 4]. Schwannoma excision through intracapsular enucleation may produce temporary sensory and/or motor dysfunction, but few have long-term neurological deficits [3–5]. Siqueira et al. have demonstrated a higher risk of complications after schwannoma resection in patients under 50 years old and when the tumor is greater than 3 cm in greatest diameter [6]. Occasionally, several or multiple fascicles are involved, which may occur sporadically or in patients with NF2 or schwannomatosis [3, 7].

Patients who had previously undergone a biopsy have a significantly higher risk of sensory loss or a motor deficit and poorer outcomes after subsequent tumor resection [8, 9].

Contrary to schwannomas, in neurofibromas, there are typically several fascicles involved in the tumor that remain functional, making resection generally riskier than with schwannomas [3].

J. Robla Costales (✉)
Department of Neurosurgery, Hospital HM Regla/HM San Francisco, León, Spain

M. Socolovsky
WFNS Peripheral Nerve Surgery Committee, Peripheral Nerve & Brachial Plexus Surgery Program, Department of Neurosurgery, University of Buenos Aires School of Medicine, Buenos Aires, Argentina

F. Martínez Benia
Department of Neurosurgery, Hospital de Clínicas "Dr. Manuel Quintela", Montevideo, Uruguay

F. Guedes et al. (eds.), *Diagnostic Assessment and Treatment of Peripheral Nerve Tumors*,
https://doi.org/10.1007/978-3-030-77633-6_12

Table 12.1 Incidence of complications after resection of different nerve tumors in published series

Author	Year	Tumor	Cases	Complications (%)	Type of complications
Siqueira et al. [6]	2013	Sch	72	15.2	Sensory disturbances
Martínez et al. [22]	2019	Various	66	15	Dysesthesia, motor deficit
Hirai et al. [23]	2019	Sch	141	34.8	Sensory disturbances, motor weakness
Nelson et al. [24]	2019	At NF	21	12	Sensory disturbances
Yuce et al. [25]	2019	SchPB	11	0	
Kim et al. [26]	2012	Sch	30	76.7[a]/36.7[b]	Pain, motor weakness, hypesthesia

Comp Complications, *Sch* Schwannoma, *At NF* Atypical Neurofibromas, *SchPB* Brachial plexus Schwannomas (<3 cm).
[a]Immediately
[b]At 58 months of follow-up

Interfascicular dissection can typically preserve most functioning fascicles. The tumor may be removed as a solitary mass once the correct plane has been defined and the entering and exiting fascicles are identified. In a situation in which functioning fascicles are lost, but proximal and distal portions of the nerve can be identified, reconstruction can be performed using inter-positional grafts [4]. As with schwannomas, recurrence after neurofibroma excision is uncommon.

Plexiform lesions involve more fascicles and appear beaded. Cellular subtypes may have high mitotic rates and, although benign, may have a higher recurrence rate than other histologic types [3]. These lesions, which affect multiple fascicles, generally are not completely resectable without major neurological deficit, unless they are located within expendable branches [4]. Plexiform lesions should be managed nonoperatively or debulked selectively in cases of refractory neuropathic pain. Rapidly growing masses which produce pain and progressive neurological deficits should be considered for biopsy and/or resection [3, 4]. Trying to resect an "unresectable" tumor like a plexiform neurofibroma in other circumstances will lead to a functional deficit for sure [1].

Excellent results may be obtained without complications in patients with extraneural tumors like lipomas, hemangiomas, or ganglion cysts, which extrinsically compress a peripheral nerve [1]. These conditions can all be treated surgically with microscopic neurolysis and excision of the mass, without resultant nerve function loss.

Hemangiomas and arteriovenous malformations are vascular anomalies that result in a benign space-occupying mass. Due to the common proximity of nerves and vessels, a tumor arising from a vessel may be mistaken as a nerve tumor [10]. Despite originating from neighboring vessels, reports have documented that the malformation may also encompass and infiltrate a nerve [11]. In addition, a vascular malformation may directly involve the nerve through its vasa nervorum. The primary treatment goal is excision of the hemangioma free from the nerve, in order to relieve symptoms and maintain nerve function. However, if an appropriate plane of dissection is not present, sole decompression of the nerve may help to relieve symptoms while preserving the nerve's integrity. Extreme care should be taken when dissecting the malformation to identify any accessory nerves, as reports have indicated an association between vascular malformations and bifurcated nerves [12, 13].

Peripheral nerve lipomas can exist in any nerve distribution but are most commonly described involving the median nerve. This fibrofatty tumor is present circumferentially around the nerve. Microsurgical neurolysis, surgical debulking, and precise removal of tissue are possible, preserving nerve function, as mentioned previously [4].

A different clinical entity is the fibrolipomatous hamartoma (FLH). These lesions are characterized by fibrofatty proliferation causing epineural and perineural fibrosis. Magnetic resonance imaging (MRI) characteristics of fibrolipomatous hamartomas are pathognomonic, obviating the need for biopsy for diagnosis. Resection should be indicated as a first option only in rare occasions, when the FLH occurs in an expendable nerve. It is important to keep in mind that significant neurological deficit is inevitable after excision of this benign lesion. Typical management is several surgeries over years, progressing from decompression to neurolysis and finally resection and reconstruction only in cases of severe pain and dysfunction [4].

Intraneural ganglion cysts are benign lesions filled with mucinous content and located inside the epineurium of peripheral nerves. The peroneal nerve at the fibular head is the most commonly affected nerve [14]. Spinner et al. published their articular theory, implicated in the formation and frequent recurrence of these lesions after surgical treatment [15]. Since then, the operative approach includes dissection of the cyst and its articular branch to the joint of origin, limited decompression of the cyst through a longitudinal epineurotomy away from the fascicles, and disconnection of the articular branch near the joint [16]. Resection of the cyst and its cyst wall, as was suggested in the past, should be avoided because of the risks of a postoperative nerve function deficit [14, 16]. Cyst decompression by itself, also widely performed in the past, is destined to fail, with cyst recurrence inevitable (1).

Perineuriomas are rare benign peripheral nerve tumors. They typically present in adolescents or young adults and cause a gradually progressive but painless neuropathy, affecting motor fibers more than sensory fibers [3, 4, 17]. Fascicular biopsy based on MRI abnormalities may be indicated to establish a diagnosis; but when classic clinical and MRI findings are present, biopsy may not be indicated, and patients can merely be followed up, avoiding the risk associated with a nerve biopsy. Some have advocated resecting and grafting focal lesions; but tendon transfers can be considered in the majority of cases to compensate for any neurological deficit [3].

Neural loss is often unavoidable when dealing with locally infiltrating tumors (e.g., desmoids) or malignant tumors, despite optimal surgical conditions, as nerve fascicles are involved and it is very difficult to separate them from the mass [1].

Malignant peripheral nerve sheath tumors (MPNSTs) arise from major or minor peripheral nerve branches or sheaths of peripheral nerve fibers and are derived from Schwann cells or pluripotent cells of neural crest origin [4]. The need for adequate resection of the tumor to obtain negative microscopic margins leads to sacrifice of neural tissue and ensuing functional deficits.

Importantly, surgeons should not perform radical resection of a nerve (or amputation of a limb) based on the histologic interpretation of a frozen section. Sometimes it is not easy for pathologists to differentiate certain benign tumors from malignancy on frozen section. Instead, tissue should be held over for permanent section and reviewed again in detail [1].

Additionally, one frequent complication after peripheral nerve tumor resection is neuropathic pain, whether the tumor is benign or malignant [8, 18, 19]. The incidence of this complication has been reported to range from 5.7% to 17.6% in different series, and there have been reported discrepancies concerning whether or not this incidence is higher after excision of neurofibromas, when compared to schwannomas [8, 19]. Patients suffering from this condition should be ideally referred to a specialized pain management service, and several drugs may be used for its control. Pregabalin and gabapentin, among others, are usually first-line options, whereas tramadol stands as second line and strong opioids as third line [20, 21].

References

1. Spinner RJ. Complication avoidance. Neurosurg Clin N Am. 2004;15:193–202. vii
2. Kim DH, Murovic JA, Tiel RL, et al. A series of 397 peripheral neural sheath tumors: 30-year experience at Louisiana State University health sciences center. J Neurosurg. 2005;102:246–55.
3. Spinner RJ, Hébert-Blouin M, Zager EL. Peripheral nerve tumors. In: Siqueira M, Socolovsky M, Malessy M, Devy I, editors. Treatment of peripheral nerve lesions. Prism Publications; 2011.
4. Barbour JR, Boyd KU. Tumors of the peripheral nervous system. In: Mackinnon SE, editor. Nerve surgery. 1st ed. New York: Thieme Medical Publishers, Inc.; 2017. p. 530–71.
5. Ozdemir O, Ozsoy MH, Kurt C, et al. Schwannomas of the hand and wrist: long-term results and review of the literature. J Orthop Surg (Hong Kong). 2005;13:267–72.

6. Siqueira MG, Socolovsky M, Martins RS, et al. Surgical treatment of typical peripheral schwannomas: the risk of new postoperative deficits. Acta Neurochir. 2013;155:1745–9.
7. Tang CYK, Fung B, Fok M, Zhu J. Schwannoma in the upper limbs. Biomed Res Int. 2013;2013:167196.
8. Levi AD, Ross AL, Cuartas E, et al. The surgical management of symptomatic peripheral nerve sheath tumors. Neurosurgery. 2010;66:833–40.
9. Guedes-Corrêa JF, Lourenço Torrao FJ, Barbosa D. Benign peripheral nerve tumors. In: Socolovsky M, Rasulic L, Midha R, editors. Manual of peripheral nerve surgery: from the basics to complex procedures. Stuttgart: Thieme Medical Publishers; 2017.
10. Nuthakki S, Fessell D, Lal N, et al. Epithelioid hemangioendothelioma mimicking a nerve sheath tumor clinically and on MR imaging. Skeletal Radiol. 2007;36(Suppl 1):S58–62.
11. Hariri A, Cohen G, Masmejean EH. Venous malformation involving median nerve causing acute carpal tunnel syndrome. J Hand Surg Eur Vol. 2011;36:431–2.
12. Ranalli NJ, Huang JH, Lee EB, Zhang PJ, Siegelman ES, Zager EL. Hemangiomas of the brachial plexus: a case series. Neurosurgery. 2009;65(4 Suppl):A181–8. https://doi.org/10.1227/01.NEU.0000335643.41581.1D.
13. Gutowski KA, Olivier WA, Mehrara BJ, Friedman DW. Arteriovenous malformation of a persistent median artery with a bifurcated median nerve. Plast Reconstr Surg. 2000;106:1336–9.
14. Robla-Costales J, Socolovsky M, Dubrovsky A, et al. Intraneural cysts of the peroneal nerve in childhood: report of 2 cases and literature review. Neurocirugia (Astur). 2011;22:324–31.
15. Spinner RJ, et al. Peroneal intraneural ganglia: the importance of the articular branch. Clinical series. J Neurosurg. 2003;99(2):319–29.
16. Spinner RJ, Amrami KK. What's new in the management of benign peripheral nerve lesions? Neurosurg Clin N Am. 2008;19:517–31; v
17. Mauermann ML, Amrami KK, Kuntz NL, et al. Longitudinal study of intraneural perineurioma—a benign, focal hypertrophic neuropathy of youth. Brain. 2009;132:2265–76.
18. Desai KI. The surgical management of symptomatic benign peripheral nerve sheath tumors of the neck and extremities: an experience of 442 cases. Clin Neurosurg. 2017;81:568–80.
19. Guha D, Davidson B, Nadi M, et al. Management of peripheral nerve sheath tumors: 17 years of experience at Toronto Western Hospital. J Neurosurg. 2018;128:1226–34.
20. Cruccu G, Truini A. A review of neuropathic pain: from guidelines to clinical practice. Pain Ther. 2017;6:35–42.
21. Murnion BP. Neuropathic pain: current definition and review of drug treatment. Aust Prescr. 2018;41:60–3.
22. Martínez F, Domínguez-Páez M, Cuadros-Romero M, et al. Peripheral nerve tumours: a 66-case retrospective study. Neurocirugia. 2020;31:105–11.
23. Hirai T, Kobayashi H, Akiyama T, et al. Predictive factors for complications after surgical treatment for schwannomas of the extremities. BMC Musculoskelet Disord. 2019;20:166.
24. Nelson CN, Dombi E, Rosenblum JS, et al. Safe marginal resection of atypical neurofibromas in neurofibromatosis type 1. J Neurosurg. 2019:1–11.
25. Yuce I, Kahyaoglu O, Mertan P, et al. Ultrasound-guided microsurgical excision for brachial plexus schwannomas: short-term clinical study. Turk Neurosurg. 2019;29:594–7.
26. Kim S-M, Seo S-W, Lee J-Y, Sung K-S. Surgical outcome of schwannomas arising from major peripheral nerves in the lower limb. Int Orthop. 2012;36:1721–5.

13 Management of Painful Conditions Associated with Nerve Tumors

Anna C. Filley and Christopher J. Winfree

13.1 Introduction

Pain is a common complication of peripheral nerve tumors and may be secondary to ongoing physical compression or aberrant electrical activity causing heightened transmission of pain signals. Focal compressive neuropathies are often associated with a palpable mass and a positive Tinel sign, characterized by radiating pain in the distribution of the nerve that can be reproduced with percussion of the mass. When charged with the management of painful conditions occurring in the setting of nerve tumors, it is important to consider the etiology and type of pain, the relationship of symptoms to the location of lesion(s), and the underlying risk of malignancy or other diagnoses that may influence management and degree of aggressiveness of treatment.

Peripheral nerve sheath tumors (PNSTs), including the benign neurofibroma and schwannoma, and the more aggressive malignant peripheral nerve sheath tumor (MPNST) are primary neural tumors that inherently arise and grow in close proximity to peripheral nerves. As a result of primary neural involvement and mass effect by the growing tumor, patients commonly develop pain or paresthesias in the distribution of the affected nerve, which may become debilitating [1, 2]. Pain is, in fact, the most common presenting complaint in patients with peripheral nerve tumors and far more frequent than motor deficits [3, 4]. The time course and severity of symptoms are heavily influenced by the growth rate, size, and location of the tumor. Tumors arising in focally stenotic locations or more superficially in the head, neck, or extremities tend to become apparent earlier; in contrast, those arising from deeper structures within the chest, abdomen, and pelvis may remain asymptomatic until becoming quite large. Benign lesions tend to have a more gradual progression of symptoms when compared to the acute onset and rapid deterioration seen with malignant lesions. This is further evidenced by the nodular growth pattern of most benign tumors that tends to displace adjacent structures, thus remaining asymptomatic for a longer period of time than those with more invasive phenotypes. Another important clinical scenario to keep in mind is the potential for malignant transformation of a known benign lesion, which commonly presents with rapid enlargement and severe, unrelenting pain.

PNSTs most commonly arise as isolated, spontaneous lesions; the presence of multiple tumors in a single patient should raise suspicion of an underlying neurocutaneous syndrome, including neurofibromatosis (NF) types 1 and 2 and schwannomatosis. Management of painful aspects of disease in the setting of a genetic tumor predisposition syndrome is challenging, as these

A. C. Filley · C. J. Winfree (✉)
Department of Neurological Surgery, Columbia University, New York, NY, USA
e-mail: cjw12@cumc.columbia.edu

F. Guedes et al. (eds.), *Diagnostic Assessment and Treatment of Peripheral Nerve Tumors*,
https://doi.org/10.1007/978-3-030-77633-6_13

patients have a greater tumor burden and may experience a more aggressive disease course. In addition to predisposing to the development of PNSTs, these genetic disorders may also be associated with unique pain syndromes that the clinician should be aware of. Patients may experience diffuse, multifocal pain that is poorly localized; more recent molecular and genetic studies are beginning to identify altered expression of inflammatory, cytokine, and other neuromodulating factors that may underlie the exaggerated pain levels experienced by some patients; however, there is still much to be done in the way of developing therapeutic interventions. However, even with maximal medical management including surgery, radiation, and medications, many patients still experience debilitating chronic pain that significantly impacts quality of life.

Chronic nerve pain may also be a postoperative complication following tumor biopsy or attempted resection. Severe surgical pain has been observed in up to 20% of patients undergoing resection of PNSTs [3]. Most cases are related to iatrogenic injury and intraoperative manipulation of the nerve and spontaneously resolve. In rare cases, however, pain is a lasting complication of operative nerve damage; this is more frequently observed with invasive or malignant tumors in which some intentional sacrifice of neural tissue is performed.

Fundamentally underlying the peripheral nerve surgeon's role in management of painful conditions associated with PNSTs is the distinction between operative and non-operative scenarios. Tumor-related pain is classically managed with surgery, which can be less ideal in settings of multiple or invasive tumors. Broadly speaking, the management of compressive neuropathies that can be attributed to mass lesion is primarily operative and directed toward alleviating ongoing pressure on the nerve. Particularly in the setting of isolated, spontaneous lesions, complete surgical resection is curative and leads to resolution of symptoms. Overall, the fundamental principle of surgery for PNSTs is optimizing the trade-off between symptom relief and risk of iatrogenic nerve injury. The potential for iatrogenic damage becomes of greater consideration for patients with multiple lesions and for tumors arising from deeper structures in the abdomen and pelvis that are poorly accessible to the surgeon as well as large, invasive tumors or those that encase critical structures that could not be sacrificed. In these cases, subtotal resections or nerve decompressions may provide a degree of relief. Chronic pain related to unresectable disease, widespread neuropathy of a neurocutaneous syndrome, or nerve injury may be managed with neuropathic pain medications, topical anesthetics, or nerve blocks. In certain medically refractory cases, the peripheral nerve surgeon may consider neuromodulation with a peripheral nerve stimulator (PNS), spinal cord stimulator (SCS), or dorsal root ganglion (DRG) stimulator.

13.2 Pain Secondary to Local Tumor Mass Effect

Benign nerve tumors most commonly occur as isolated, sporadic lesions within cranial, autonomic, or peripheral nerves essentially anywhere in the body. Their progressive growth can eventually lead to neural compression and the subsequent development of pain. The vast majority of nerve tumors are benign lesions that exhibit slow growth rates. Typically, the patient will become aware of an area of the body that, when bumped, produces a sudden, radiating pain. This radiating pain is often easily reproduced on physical examination, referred to as a Tinel sign (Fig. 13.1). The pain may radiate locally or distally down an extremity, depending on the sensory distribution of the affected nerve. One interesting exam finding is that multiple Tinel signs can occur when multiple nerves run together, as in the upper arm. It is not unusual for a nerve tumor involving the median nerve in the medial upper arm to yield a Tinel that radiates into the median nerve territory of the hand as well as one that radiates into the medial forearm. This occurs because a median nerve tumor in this location can also compress and irritate the adjacent medial antebrachial cutaneous nerve. In many cases, the patient realizes that there is an associated mass that is the source

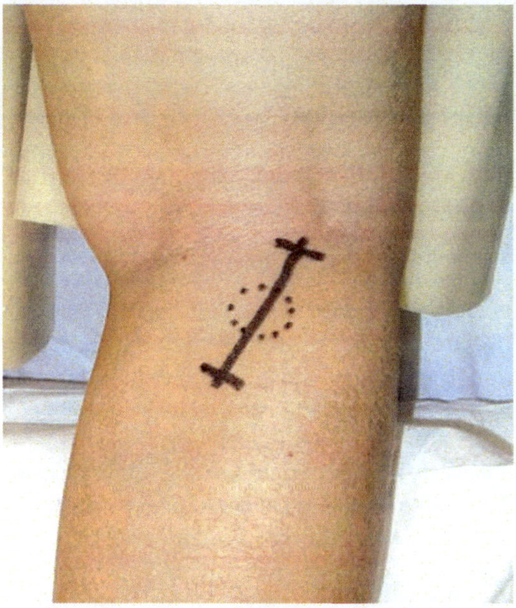

Fig. 13.1 Intraoperative photograph demonstrating a patient with a lateral sural cutaneous nerve schwannoma, indicated by the dotted circle. The planned skin incision is indicated by the straight line. On examination, the patient reported a painful Tinel sign radiating onto the lateral foot and ankle when the lesion was tapped

of the pain; however, if the lesion is sufficiently deep, then the mass may remain occult.

For example, schwannomas are the most frequently diagnosed nerve tumors. They classically appear as small, well-circumscribed nodules growing eccentric to a parent nerve in the skin or underlying soft tissues. With progressive growth, they may cause pain, paresthesia, and eventually sensorimotor deficits. Symptoms usually appear gradually with mild, relatively nonspecific findings, and lesions are often misdiagnosed in early stages. As a result, schwannomas may be the underlying cause of nonspecific chronic nerve pain [5]. Symptomatic lesions, particularly of the extremities, classically present after a relatively prolonged time course with pain, most often in the setting of a palpable mass [3, 6]. Particularly characteristic of peripheral nerve schwannomas is a positive Tinel sign [2, 7–9]. This physical exam finding may be seen with other tumor types but is most commonly associated with schwannomas [6].

Given the benign, slow-growing nature of most peripheral nerve tumors, the decision to remove the lesion is often based on the presence of a significant pain syndrome. For example, a patient with an axillary schwannoma may find the lesion uncomfortable when they keep their arm in an adducted position. Similarly, a patient with a benign tumor in the back of the thigh might find sitting in a chair painful. It is appropriate to offer surgical excision to the nerve tumor patient with pain that is provoked during normal life activities. The prognosis for isolated, symptomatic tumors tends to be quite good, and most patients experience resolution of symptoms [4]. Recurrence is rare following complete resection of benign lesions.

13.3 Pain Secondary to Schwannomatosis

Schwannomatosis is a genetic neurocutaneous disorder characterized by the presence of multiple non-intradermal schwannomas in patients who do not meet diagnostic criteria for NF2 [10]. Features characteristic of NF2 that are notably absent in schwannomatosis are intracranial meningiomas and schwannomas of the vestibular nerve, which are present in nearly all patients with NF2, commonly bilateral, and pathognomonic of the disease [11]. Schwannomatosis is also genetically distinct from NF2 and most commonly arises as a spontaneous rather than familial disease. Germline mutations in two genes, SMARCB1 and LZTR1, have been linked with the development of schwannomatosis [12]. Relatively uncommon in the general population, only 2–5% of patients undergoing resection of a peripheral nerve schwannoma meet criteria for a diagnosis of schwannomatosis [13, 14]. However, it is imperative to identify these patients given a significantly higher propensity to develop chronic, treatment-refractory pain syndromes, which in many cases become functionally debilitating [10, 12, 15, 16].

The pathophysiology underlying this propensity for treatment-refractory pain syndromes in schwannomatosis is poorly understood. Recent cohort analysis of germline mutations demonstrated that over similar overall tumor burdens, a significant association exists between a painful phenotype and LZTR1-mutated disease [17]. Other studies have associated painful lesions with differential levels of cytokines and other factors postulated to modulate nociceptive neuron responsiveness [18]. Among these is vascular endothelial growth factor (VEGF), which is known to contribute to angiogenesis and inflammatory responses [18]. More recently, VEGF has been shown to be upregulated in peripheral nerve injury and is thought to underlie a component of neuropathic pain [19]. Current investigational studies of VEGF antagonists have shown reduced tumor burden and improved pain in a small number of treated patients [20, 21].

Chronic pain is reported by most patients with schwannomatosis [17] and commonly involves both localized and multifocal or diffuse symptoms. Of note, this pain is often not associated with a discrete mass [10]. In other cases, the pain is clearly associated with nerve tumors. On history, patients may indicate resection of one or more prior lesions. On physical exam, multiple palpable nodules may be noted, prompting further workup and diagnosis. Imaging studies may reveal the presence of additional asymptomatic lesions [22]. On MRI, schwannomas appear as small, well-circumscribed nodules distributed along the course of one or more peripheral nerves (Fig. 13.2) [11].

Management of pain in the setting of schwannomatosis is complicated by the presence of numerous lesions as well as a component of nonfocal pain for which a causative mass lesion cannot be identified. As for the non-syndromic patient, operative intervention is typically offered for symptomatic lesions, with asymptomatic lesions managed conservatively [10, 11, 14, 22–24]. There can be exceptions to this based on clinical need, however. For example, a patient with a steadily growing nerve tumor that is exerting mass effect on surrounding structures may elect to undergo surgery to avoid subsequent problems should the tumor continue to enlarge. To illustrate, one would not need to wait for a retroperitoneal tumor that is observed progressively, but asymptomatically, compressing the renal pelvis to actually cause symptomatic hydronephrosis before surgical removal. But these circumstances should be fairly rare. Nevertheless, most schwannomatosis patients ultimately undergo multiple procedures, with the most common indication for resection being intractable pain [10, 11, 25].

Interestingly, the nerve tumors may be exquisitely painful even when quite small. This can lead to the awkward scenario where the surgeon finds themself operating on tiny lesions that in a non-syndromic patient would almost certainly be asymptomatic. The surgeon may even wonder if such a small lesion could be causing such a painful condition in their patient. If pain can be localized to specific lesions, surgery often improves symptoms to some degree [11, 25]. However, complete relief is achieved in less than half of patients, and up to 75% experience recurrence of symptoms, either at the resection site or with development of additional tumors [10]. In our experience, surgical excision of the painful schwannomas, no matter how small, can be an effective treatment for the pain syndrome associated with the individual lesions but may have little impact on the more diffuse pain syndromes not attributable to individual lesions.

Schwannomatosis patients that have a pain syndrome not clearly caused by a specific tumor may benefit from a nonsurgical pain management strategy. Pharmacotherapy with neuropathic pain medications, often as part of a multimodal strategy, is often needed. Most patients with schwannomatosis have trialed multiple pain medications (mean of 3), although 20% of patients have tried six to ten medications and 7% have trialed more than ten different medications for chronic pain [10]. Opiates, anti-inflammatories, anticonvulsants, and antidepressant agents are most cited; not uncommon are muscle relaxants and topical lidocaine patches. Some patients underwent more invasive pain procedures such as spinal blocks or radiofrequency lesioning [10]. However, even with early surgical resection of symptomatic lesions and exhaustive pharmacologic strategies, many patients are left with chronic, debilitating pain [10, 12, 15, 16].

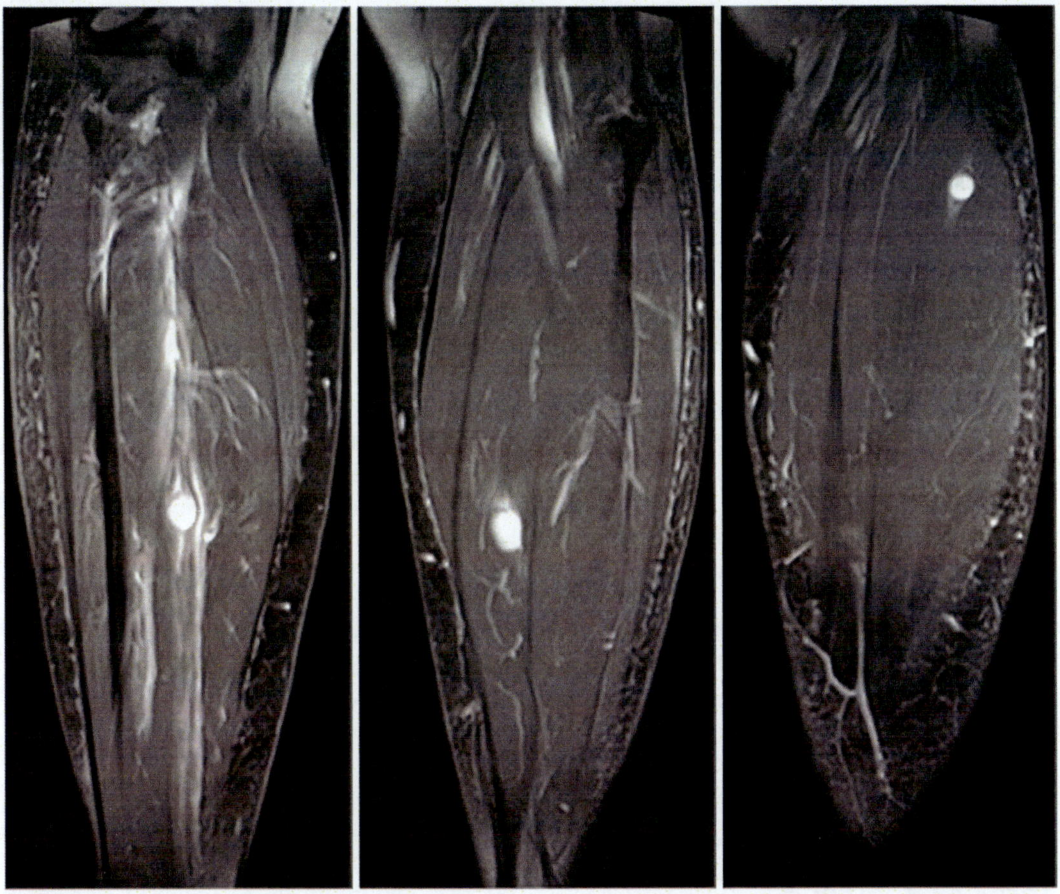

Fig. 13.2 T1 coronal, fat-suppressed, contrast-enhanced MRI of the legs in a patient with multiple painful schwannomas in the setting of schwannomatosis

13.4 Pain Secondary to Neurofibromatosis Type 1

Most patients with NF1 report a relatively longstanding history of chronic pain that is in most cases multifocal [26–29]. Symptoms are most frequently localized to the upper extremities (70%) and least likely to be reported in the pelvic region (35%) [26]. Patients with NF1 are predisposed to developing multiple cutaneous, subcutaneous, and plexiform neurofibromas [30]. The course of these lesions differs from isolated PNSTs in that these lesions are numerous and larger in size and tend to recur; as a result, patients with NF1 tend to undergo numerous surgical procedures and experience chronic pain that often begins at a relatively young age. Pain is a prominent feature of plexiform neurofibromas, which can be the source of significant morbidity even for children [31]. Chronic pain may begin in the pediatric and adolescent years; in a survey of young adults with NF1 and their caregivers, ~1/3 of participating NF1 patients regularly took pain medications; of these patients, 90% required prescription medication as a component of therapy. However, most patients (59%) and their caregivers (73%) reported persistent pain-limited daily function [27]. By adulthood, a history of opiate use for NF1-associated pain becomes fairly common; unfortunately, of the 17% of respondents who endorsed an active prescription, 85% described these agents as having "little to no" effect [26].

Even relatively benign lesions, like neurofibroma, may end up causing significant discomfort. Present in nearly all patients with NF1, cutaneous neurofibromas arise during puberty [32] and increase in size and number with age [33]. They may be associated with itching and mild pain and are often numerous in NF1 patients [34]. Discomfort and cosmetic concerns prompt most patients to seek definitive treatment with surgical resection (65%) or laser ablation (38%) [32]. However, recurrence rates are extremely high, and patients often undergo numerous procedures to address lesions, reporting frequent complications. In one large survey of 255 adults with NF1, 55% reported at least 1 surgery in the prior year. Of all patients, 43% noted complications occurring in all prior procedures including some degree of permanent weakness in the majority [26].

Diffuse symptoms in the absence of focal lesions are rarely observed in NF1; in one large study, 2.3% of patients had characteristics of a diffuse peripheral neuropathy, which was associated with proximal, large neurofibromas and a higher propensity to develop MPNST [28].

13.5 Pain Secondary to Entrapment Neuropathy

Nerve tumors that occur arising at the typical sites of peripheral nerve entrapment may produce an entrapment neuropathy. Nerve tumors can precipitate nerve entrapments anywhere entrapments normally occur. Entrapment neuropathy can occur with sporadic lesions as well as with those in the setting of neurofibromatosis [35] or schwannomatosis. Symptoms arise from direct mechanical compression by the lesion or intracompartmental pressure elevation within an enclosed space, eventually leading to nerve compression or ischemia. Patients may present with episodic pain that worsens in settings of increased edema or positions that may further narrow the entrapment site.

Careful physical examination usually reveals the presence of a mass within the area of entrapment. Sometimes, especially in patients of generous body habitus, the lesion is not palpable. In these cases, imaging studies, including ultrasonography and MR neurography, may reveal the presence of a nerve tumor in a patient who otherwise presents as a nerve entrapment [36]. This can be quite helpful for surgical planning, and there are typically notable differences in the surgical techniques used for simple nerve decompressions vs. nerve tumor excisions. For example, we utilize general anesthesia for most nerve tumor cases, as the procedures often require direct electrical stimulation of the nerve and significant nerve manipulation, both of which can be painful in the sedated patient. These techniques are rarely needed for simple nerve decompressions. Similarly, the operating microscope can be helpful for many tumor cases, whereas it is rarely needed for routine nerve entrapment release. It is certainly suboptimal for the surgeon to perform a routine nerve decompression procedure, only to unexpectedly encounter a nerve tumor in the surgical field, ill-equipped to resect it with maximal safety and efficacy.

Classical symptoms of carpal tunnel syndrome including nocturnal pain and paresthesia may occur with lesions arising near the carpal tunnel [35]. Lesion resection and sparing of nerve fascicles may result in resolution of symptoms [37]. Performing carpal tunnel release as well may facilitate recovery [38–40]. A peroneal nerve tumor arising behind the fibular head can mimic a standard peroneal neuropathy at that location (Fig. 13.3). Patients may experience pain or paresthesia in the distribution of the peroneal nerve that may be worse with prolonged, exaggerated bending of the knee, crouching, or physical activity. Symptoms may arise in relation to an enlarging palpable mass in that location, often with a positive Tinel sign given superficial location [41, 42]. Surgical resection and decompression of the associated lesion tend to resolve symptoms [37]. In most cases, we recommend performing a formal nerve decompression across the site of entrapment when performing nerve tumor excision in these locations. This helps ensure that any nerve swelling that might occur after lesionectomy won't result in nerve compression at the site of entrapment.

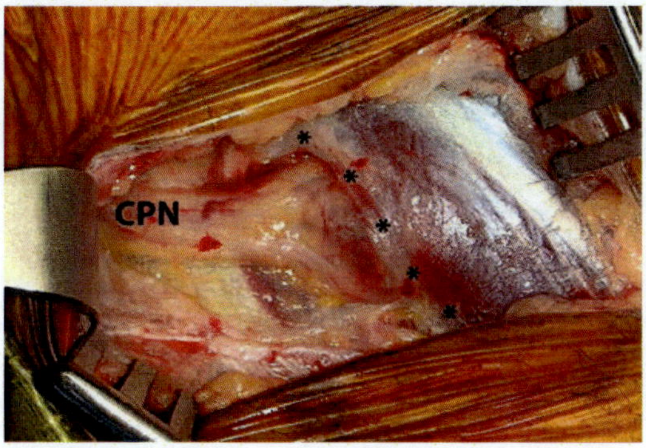

Fig. 13.3 Intraoperative photograph demonstrating a schwannoma located within the common peroneal nerve (CPN). The lesion is located at the exact spot where the nerve dives under the posterior border of the peroneus longus fascia, indicated by the asterisks (*). This site represents the usual site of entrapment for the common peroneal nerve. This patient was treated with peroneal nerve decompression and tumor resection

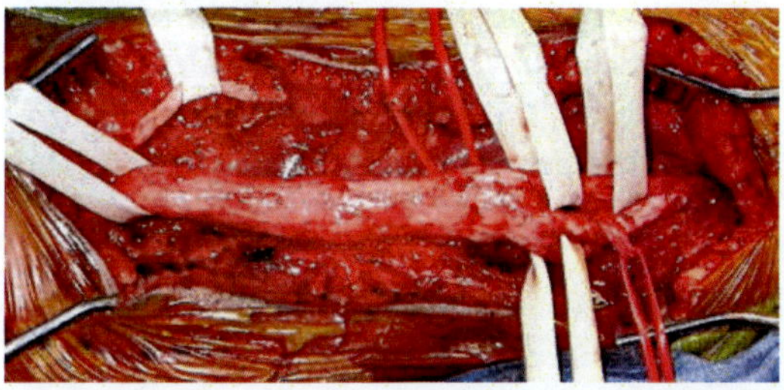

Fig. 13.4 Intraoperative photograph demonstrating a plexiform neurofibroma located within the common peroneal nerve. The lesion involves the segment of nerve across the fibular head at its usual site of entrapment. This patient was treated with peroneal nerve decompression without tumor resection

It is important to note that plexiform neurofibromas have an extensively infiltrative growth pattern, often involving multiple fibers over longer lengths to the degree that surgical removal is not possible without sustaining significant loss of function. Nevertheless, these lesions can cause nerve compression if they occur at a typical site of nerve entrapment (Fig. 13.4). In these cases, simple decompression of the nerve and tumor mass may be sufficient to relieve the patient's symptoms [8]. Tumor debulking may be performed if there are resectable nodules, but aggressive reduction of tumor burden in these cases risks neurological injury. Surgical intervention is associated with increased morbidity and risk of permanent deficits, particularly for more extensive vs. partial resections [43]. Resection has been shown to benefit from intraoperative monitoring [6].

13.6 Pain Secondary to Malignancy

Malignant peripheral nerve sheath tumors (MPNSTs) are highly aggressive soft tissue sarcomas that present with rapid onset and progression of focal deficits and most notably severe and unrelenting pain. Severe pain or rapid enlargement of previously quiescent tumor, particularly a plexiform neurofibroma in the setting of neurofibromatosis, should prompt concern for malignancy [29, 44–47]. Plexiform neurofibromas (PNF) are large, complex masses that form as extensive networks of nodular growths extending along the course of a nerve and its branches. They carry a lifetime risk of malignant transformation of about 15% [48]. In these cases, patients classically present with an enlarging mass and new severe, refractory pain [49, 50].

As we have described above, pain can be present in the context of benign nerve tumors. The key is to distinguish a pain pattern that suggests a malignant lesion. Pain that is only present when the lesion is tapped is suggestive of a benign lesion. Pain that mimics a nerve entrapment in the setting of a nerve tumor at the site of entrapment, especially when tapped or with change in limb position, also suggests a benign process. Radiating or localized pain that is unremitting, even at rest or worse at night, suggests a malignant process. It is important to note that the combination of clinical presentation, physical examination, and imaging characteristics of the lesion may be necessary to distinguish benign from malignant lesions. Ultimately, pathological analysis of the tumor specimen is the most reliable method.

The prognosis for these lesions is extremely poor and as such is managed aggressively; surgical resection with wide margins is performed when possible [6]. The ability to achieve a complete resection is heavily influenced by the location of the tumor and degree of involvement of surrounding structures; tumors of the extremities are more amenable to resection than those arising from abdominopelvic or paraspinal structures [51]. However, MPNSTs have a highly infiltrative pattern of growth that often makes a complete resection impossible, even if some degree of sacrifice of neural elements is accepted. Often, debulking with subtotal resection and decompression of neural elements become the primary goals of surgery, which can provide patients with meaningful relief of symptoms [8, 52, 53]. In addition to tumor debulking, which is usually subtotal, palliative radiation and chemotherapy have been attempted without clear benefit [53, 54]. Local recurrences occur in 40–65% of cases, and metastatic disease develops in 40–68% [48]. Recurrent tumors are characterized by increased rates of subcutaneous tissue (80%) and muscle (65%) edema [55] which can contribute to symptomatic presentations. Continued progression tends to lead to subsequent involvement of additional adjacent structures and worsening deficits including intractable chronic pain [29].

13.7 Pain Secondary to Cranial Nerve Tumors

Nerve tumors, such as schwannomas and neurofibromas, may rarely involve the trigeminal nerve (CN V). The resultant pain condition may mimic classic trigeminal neuralgia and consist of lancinating facial pain. In other cases, the resultant pain condition may mimic atypical trigeminal neuralgia and consist of more constant facial pain [56]. Trigeminal neurofibromas may initially be asymptomatic and painless, though with growth may cause bony destruction and pain or swelling [57]. Plexiform lesions may cause "massive expansion of these tissues," and patients may have significant associated pain in the distribution of the branches affected [49].

Treatment of trigeminal nerve tumors can consist of some combination of pharmacological pain management, surgical resection, or stereotactic radiosurgery. Radiosurgical options may include tumor dose regimens (14–15 Gy) applied to the tumor to achieve growth arrest of the lesion or nerve dose regimens (75–80 Gy) applied to the nerve to control the pain.

13.8 Pain After Nerve Tumor Surgery

Postoperative neuropathic pain syndromes are rare but potentially debilitating complications of nerve tumor surgery [6, 29]. Immediate postoperative pain or mild deficits have been reported in 5.7–17.6% of procedures across multiple large series. In the vast majority of cases, symptoms are transient and thought to be secondary to minor iatrogenic injury and edema sustained during intraoperative nerve manipulation [3, 4, 6, 58].

Rarely, more significant damage is incurred, and patients experience prolonged courses of neurogenic pain [3]. This is more frequently seen in lesions with greater degrees of neural involvement, as evidenced by postoperative pain syndromes occurring at rates of 3.5%, 8.6%, and 10.5% in a study contrasting complications in schwannoma, neurofibroma, and MPNST, respectively [6]. Other features that have been associated with higher rates of neurologic deficits include larger tumors [9, 24, 59, 60], degree of preoperative symptoms, proximal locations (brachial plexus) [61], and a history of prior biopsy or surgery in that area [3, 6, 8]. This risk can be reduced with the use of intraoperative monitoring [6].

Initial management of postoperative pain involves a conservative strategy that utilizes physical therapy and pain medications. First-line pharmacotherapy includes traditional neuropathic pain medications like anticonvulsants (e.g., gabapentin, pregabalin), tricyclic antidepressants (e.g., nortriptyline, amitriptyline), and serotonin/norepinephrine reuptake inhibitors (e.g., duloxetine). With persistent symptoms, other agents may be added in combination, including GABA-b receptor agonists (e.g., baclofen), NMDA antagonists (e.g., ketamine), and low-dose opioid medications (e.g., tramadol, hydrocodone)[11, 25, 62, 63]. Medication doses may be titrated and trialed in combination prior to attempting more invasive pain management strategies. Local delivery methods may be particularly helpful as adjunct therapies, avoiding side effects associated with systemic treatment. Transdermal application of lidocaine patches and topical capsaicin have demonstrated efficacy in relief of neuropathic pain in a portion of patients [63–65].

If conservative management and pharmacotherapy do not provide adequate relief, more invasive procedures may be performed to deliver targeted analgesia via nerve block or intrathecal injection. Limited by duration of action, multiple sessions may be necessary to achieve the desired effect, as was seen in a case report of progressively improving pain relief with recurrent nerve block in a patient with medication-refractory pain following S1 nerve root schwannoma resection [66]. Nerve blocks are also used to treat cancer-related pain in unresectable tumors [67]. For more severe or persistent symptoms, alternative options are chemical or thermal ablative or surgically destructive procedures, also for refractory cancer-related pain [29, 64].

Neurostimulation is a well-established method of treating medically refractory chronic neuropathic pain using application of an electric current to modulate transmission and perception of pain signals. Options include peripheral nerve stimulation (PNS), dorsal root ganglion (DRG) stimulation, or spinal cord stimulation (SCS) [68]. Patients being considered for neurostimulator implant first undergo placement of the electrode stimulator as a trial; if successful, the battery or generator can be permanently implanted to provide chronic access. Major risks of these systems include infection and a tendency to lose effectiveness over time [39].

Of the three modalities, peripheral nerve stimulation has the most distal target. The electrode is inserted directly over the target nerve, proximal to the site of injury, which can be achieved with a minimally invasive percutaneous procedure, using fluoroscopic or ultrasound guidance to improve accuracy [69]. PNS is particularly useful for cranial (trigeminal) and proximal upper extremity (brachial plexus), and success ranges from 50 to 80% [39].

Slightly more invasive, the electrodes of a SCS are inserted into the posterior epidural space in order to deliver electrical impulses to the dorsal columns in order to obscure the transmission and perception of pain; of note, this does introduce the sensation of paresthesia, which may be uncomfortable to some patients. The success of this method relies on the function overlap between the stimulated territory and the region of pain, which introduces a complication with certain pain distributions [68]. Classic indications for SCS are failed back surgery syndrome, complex regional pain syndrome (CRPS) type 1 (no nerve injury), CRPS type 2 (nerve injury), intractable angina, limb ischemia, and arachnoiditis [70].

Dorsal root ganglion (DRG) stimulation has further improved the ability to localize coverage to a particular area, yielding better results in patients with post-surgical pain and peripheral nerve damage [71–73]. Stimulation of the DRG was shown to be superior to dorsal column SCS in patients with CRPS, demonstrating less postural variation in signaling and less sensory discomfort [74]. Advances in technology continue to improve the precision and personalization of pain relief of neuromodulators. Closed-loop spinal cord stimulator systems utilize real-time evoked responses in the dorsal column as continuous feedback that modulates the magnitude of stimulus output applied in order to optimize therapeutic intervention [75].

Ultimately, if neurostimulation is ineffective at relieving chronic pain, then intrathecal pharmacotherapy may be indicated. These systems consist of a refillable, programmable pump connected to an intrathecal spinal catheter. Continuous administration of intrathecal opioid (e.g., morphine, hydromorphone) and/or non-opioid medications (e.g., ziconotide, bupivacaine) may provide sufficient pain relief when other strategies are unsuccessful [76].

13.9 Conclusion

Pain is common in the setting of peripheral nerve tumors and may be associated with focal compression or entrapment, malignancy, neurocutaneous syndrome, or nerve injury. The presence of a tumor syndrome may predispose patients to developing a higher tumor burden and more treatment-refractory symptoms. Ultimately, the management of painful conditions in the setting of peripheral nerve tumors relies on addressing the underlying pathology. Operative intervention is the foundation for tumor-related pain and is directed toward relieving compression on affected nerve(s). Approaches may range from complete resection to minimally invasive decompression of entrapment sites. Severe, chronic pain may also be managed with a combination of medications, local delivery of analgesics, or neuromodulation procedures. Unfortunately, even with maximal medical management, many patients still experience persistent pain. Ongoing studies have shown some promise in novel therapies to treat medically refractory pain in these patients.

References

1. Omezzine SJ, et al. A rare cause of non discal sciatica: schwannoma of the sciatic nerve. Orthop Traumatol Surg Res. 2009;95(7):543–6.
2. Nawabi DH, Sinisi M. Schwannoma of the posterior tibial nerve: the problem of delay in diagnosis. J Bone Joint Surg Br. 2007;89(6):814–6.
3. Desai KI. The surgical management of symptomatic benign peripheral nerve sheath tumors of the neck and extremities: an experience of 442 cases. Neurosurgery. 2017;81(4):568–80.
4. Gosk J, et al. Peripheral nerve tumours: 30-year experience in the surgical treatment. Neurosurg Rev. 2015;38(3):511–20; discussion 521.
5. Rhanim A, et al. A rare cause of chronic sciatic pain: Schwannoma of the sciatic nerve. J Clin Orthop Trauma. 2013;4(2):89–92.
6. Levi AD, et al. The surgical management of symptomatic peripheral nerve sheath tumors. Neurosurgery. 2010;66(4):833–40.
7. Eroglu U, et al. Sciatic nerve schwannoma: case report. Turk Neurosurg. 2014;24(1):120–2.
8. Donner TR, Voorhies RM, Kline DG. Neural sheath tumors of major nerves. J Neurosurg. 1994;81(3):362–73.
9. Park MJ, Seo KN, Kang HJ. Neurological deficit after surgical enucleation of schwannomas of the upper limb. J Bone Joint Surg Br. 2009;91(11):1482–6.
10. Merker VL, et al. Clinical features of schwannomatosis: a retrospective analysis of 87 patients. Oncologist. 2012;17(10):1317–22.
11. MacCollin M, et al. Diagnostic criteria for schwannomatosis. Neurology. 2005;64(11):1838–45.
12. Alaidarous A, et al. Segmental schwannomatosis: characteristics in 12 patients. Orphanet J Rare Dis. 2019;14(1):207.
13. Antinheimo J, et al. Population-based analysis of sporadic and type 2 neurofibromatosis-associated meningiomas and schwannomas. Neurology. 2000;54(1):71–6.
14. Huang JH, et al. Management of patients with schwannomatosis: report of six cases and review of the literature. Surg Neurol. 2004;62(4):353–61; discussion 361.
15. Merker VL, et al. Relationship between whole-body tumor burden, clinical phenotype, and quality of life in patients with neurofibromatosis. Am J Med Genet A. 2014;164A(6):1431–7.
16. MacCollin M, et al. Schwannomatosis: a clinical and pathologic study. Neurology. 1996;46(4):1072–9.
17. Jordan JT, et al. Pain correlates with germline mutation in schwannomatosis. Medicine (Baltimore). 2018;97(5):e9717.
18. Ostrow KL, et al. The secretomes of painful versus nonpainful human schwannomatosis tumor cells differentially influence sensory neuron gene expression and sensitivity. Sci Rep. 2019;9(1):13,098.
19. Kiguchi N, et al. Vascular endothelial growth factor signaling in injured nerves underlies peripheral sensitization in neuropathic pain. J Neurochem. 2014;129(1):169–78.
20. Tamura R, et al. A VEGF receptor vaccine demonstrates preliminary efficacy in neurofibromatosis type 2. Nat Commun. 2019;10(1):5758.
21. Blakeley J, et al. Clinical response to bevacizumab in schwannomatosis. Neurology. 2014;83(21):1986–7.
22. Yamamoto T, Maruyama S, Mizuno K. Schwannomatosis of the sciatic nerve. Skeletal Radiol. 2001;30(2):109–13.
23. Molina AR, et al. Multiple schwannomas of the upper limb related exclusively to the ulnar nerve in a patient with segmental schwannomatosis. J Plast Reconstr Aesthet Surg. 2013;66(12):e376–9.
24. Siqueira MG, et al. Surgical treatment of typical peripheral schwannomas: the risk of new postoperative deficits. Acta Neurochir (Wien). 2013;155(9):1745–9.
25. Li P, et al. Clinical features of spinal schwannomas in 65 patients with schwannomatosis compared with 831 with solitary schwannomas and 102 with neurofibromatosis Type 2: a retrospective study at a single institution. J Neurosurg Spine. 2016;24(1):145–54.
26. Buono FD, et al. Pain symptomology, functional impact, and treatment of people with Neurofibromatosis type 1. J Pain Res. 2019;12:2555–61.
27. Wolters PL, et al. Pain interference in youth with neurofibromatosis type 1 and plexiform neurofibromas and relation to disease severity, social-emotional functioning, and quality of life. Am J Med Genet A. 2015;167A(9):2103–13.
28. Drouet A, et al. Neurofibromatosis 1-associated neuropathies: a reappraisal. Brain. 2004;127(Pt 9):1993–2009.

29. Creange A, et al. Neurological complications of neurofibromatosis type 1 in adulthood. Brain. 1999;122(Pt 3):473–81.
30. Sabatini C, et al. Treatment of neurofibromatosis type 1. Curr Treat Options Neurol. 2015;17(6):355.
31. Kongkriangkai AM, et al. Substantial pain burden in frequency, intensity, interference and chronicity among children and adults with neurofibromatosis Type 1. Am J Med Genet A. 2019;179(4):602–7.
32. Guiraud M, et al. Cutaneous neurofibromas: patients' medical burden, current management and therapeutic expectations: results from an online European patient community survey. Orphanet J Rare Dis. 2019;14(1):286.
33. Cannon A, et al. Cutaneous neurofibromas in neurofibromatosis type I: a quantitative natural history study. Orphanet J Rare Dis. 2018;13(1):31.
34. Varni JW, Nutakki K, Swigonski NL. Pain, skin sensations symptoms, and cognitive functioning predictors of health-related quality of life in pediatric patients with neurofibromatosis type 1. Qual Life Res. 2019;28(4):1047–52.
35. Freitas D, et al. Carpal tunnel syndrome due to a plexiform neurofibroma of the median nerve in a neurofibromatosis type 1 patient: clinical approach. BMJ Case Rep. 2013:2013.
36. Shapeero LG, et al. Post-treatment complications of soft tissue tumours. Eur J Radiol. 2009;69(2):209–21.
37. Nkaoui M, Sasbou Y. Entrapment neuropathy in the foot revealing schwannoma of the superficial peroneal nerve: outcome of conservative surgical treatment. Pan Afr Med J. 2017;28:161.
38. Kutahya H, et al. Schwannoma of the median nerve at the wrist and palmar regions of the hand: a rare case report. Case Rep Orthop. 2013;2013:950106.
39. Hubert J, Landes G, Tardif M. Schwannoma of the median nerve. J Plast Surg Hand Surg. 2013;47(1):75–7.
40. Ochsner F, Baumann RP, Kuntzer T. Carpal tunnel syndrome with an unusual cause: a malignant nerve sheath tumor of the median nerve. Rev Neurol (Paris). 2001;157(12):1547–9.
41. Nascimento G, et al. Ancient Schwannoma of superficial peroneal nerve presenting as intermittent leg pain: a case report. Int J Surg Case Rep. 2015;6C:19–22.
42. van Zantvoort AP, Cuppen P, Scheltinga MR. Management and patients perspective regarding a common peroneal nerve schwannoma: a rare cause of lower leg pain in a young individual. BMJ Case Rep. 2017:2017.
43. Prada CE, et al. Pediatric plexiform neurofibromas: impact on morbidity and mortality in neurofibromatosis type 1. J Pediatr. 2012;160(3):461–7.
44. Valeyrie-Allanore L, et al. Symptoms associated with malignancy of peripheral nerve sheath tumours: a retrospective study of 69 patients with neurofibromatosis 1. Br J Dermatol. 2005;153(1):79–82.
45. Topsakal C, et al. Malignant schwannoma of the sciatic nerve originating in a spinal plexiform neurofibroma associated with neurofibromatosis type 1--case report. Neurol Med Chir (Tokyo). 2001;41(11):551–5.
46. Evans DG, et al. Malignant peripheral nerve sheath tumours in neurofibromatosis 1. J Med Genet. 2002;39(5):311–4.
47. Ganju A, et al. Outcomes in a consecutive series of 111 surgically treated plexal tumors: a review of the experience at the Louisiana State University Health Sciences Center. J Neurosurg. 2001;95(1):51–60.
48. Pacelli J, Whitaker CH. Brachial plexopathy due to malignant peripheral nerve sheath tumor in neurofibromatosis type 1: case report and subject review. Muscle Nerve. 2006;33(5):697–700.
49. Korf BR. Plexiform neurofibromas. Am J Med Genet. 1999;89(1):31–7.
50. Tonsgard JH, et al. CT imaging in adults with neurofibromatosis-1: frequent asymptomatic plexiform lesions. Neurology. 1998;50(6):1755–60.
51. Baehring JM, Betensky RA, Batchelor TT. Malignant peripheral nerve sheath tumor: the clinical spectrum and outcome of treatment. Neurology. 2003;61(5):696–8.
52. Kitano D, et al. Two cases of debulking surgery for lower limb diffuse plexiform neurofibroma with transcatheter arterial embolisation. Int J Surg Case Rep. 2019;55:132–5.
53. Zou C, et al. Clinical, pathological, and molecular variables predictive of malignant peripheral nerve sheath tumor outcome. Ann Surg. 2009;249(6):1014–22.
54. Pourtsidis A, et al. Malignant peripheral nerve sheath tumors in children with neurofibromatosis type 1. Case Rep Oncol Med. 2014;2014:843749.
55. Sedaghat S, et al. Malignant peripheral nerve sheath tumours in magnetic resonance imaging: primary and recurrent tumour appearance, post-treatment changes, and metastases. Pol J Radiol. 2020;85:e196–201.
56. MacNally SP, et al. Trigeminal schwannomas. Br J Neurosurg. 2008;22(6):729–38.
57. Sleiman Z, et al. Mandibular neurofibroma: case report of a rare tumor. Clin Pract. 2019;9(4):1143.
58. Kim DH, et al. A series of 397 peripheral neural sheath tumors: 30-year experience at Louisiana State University Health Sciences Center. J Neurosurg. 2005;102(2):246–55.
59. Kim SM, et al. Surgical outcome of schwannomas arising from major peripheral nerves in the lower limb. Int Orthop. 2012;36(8):1721–5.
60. Oberle J, Kahamba J, Richter HP. Peripheral nerve schwannomas–an analysis of 16 patients. Acta Neurochir (Wien). 1997;139(10):949–53.
61. Sawada T, et al. The relationship between preoperative symptoms, operative findings and postoperative complications in schwannomas. J Hand Surg Br. 2006;31(6):629–34.
62. Hua C, et al. Sirolimus improves pain in NF1 patients with severe plexiform neurofibromas. Pediatrics. 2014;133(6):e1792–7.
63. Baron R, Binder A, Wasner G. Neuropathic pain: diagnosis, pathophysiological mechanisms, and treatment. Lancet Neurol. 2010;9(8):807–19.

64. Bates D, et al. A comprehensive algorithm for management of neuropathic pain. Pain Med. 2019;20(Suppl 1):S2–S12.
65. Bardo-Brouard P, et al. High-concentration topical capsaicin in the management of refractory neuropathic pain in patients with neurofibromatosis type 1: a case series. Curr Med Res Opin. 2018;34(5):887–91.
66. Naja Z, et al. Repetitive nerve block for neuropathic pain management: a case report. Scand J Pain. 2018;18(1):125–7.
67. Sirohiya P, et al. Early intervention for the management of chronic pain in a patient with recurrent schwannoma foot. Indian J Palliat Care. 2020;26(1):145–6.
68. Cruccu G, et al. EFNS guidelines on neurostimulation therapy for neuropathic pain. Eur J Neurol. 2007;14(9):952–70.
69. Deer TR, et al. A review of the bioelectronic implications of stimulation of the peripheral nervous system for chronic pain conditions. Bioelectron Med. 2020;6:9.
70. Epstein LJ, Palmieri M. Managing chronic pain with spinal cord stimulation. Mt Sinai J Med. 2012;79(1):123–32.
71. Morgalla MH, et al. Dorsal root ganglion stimulation (DRGS) for the treatment of chronic neuropathic pain: a single-center study with long-term prospective results in 62 cases. Pain Physician. 2018;21(4):E377–87.
72. Liem L, et al. A multicenter, prospective trial to assess the safety and performance of the spinal modulation dorsal root ganglion neurostimulator system in the treatment of chronic pain. Neuromodulation. 2013;16(5):471–82; discussion 482.
73. Morgalla MH, et al. Dorsal root ganglion stimulation used for the treatment of chronic neuropathic pain in the groin: a single-center study with long-term prospective results in 34 cases. Neuromodulation. 2017;20(8):753–60.
74. Deer TR, et al. Dorsal root ganglion stimulation yielded higher treatment success rate for complex regional pain syndrome and causalgia at 3 and 12 months: a randomized comparative trial. Pain. 2017;158(4):669–81.
75. Maheshwari A, et al. Advanced methods of spinal stimulation in the treatment of chronic pain: pulse trains, waveforms, frequencies, targets, and feedback loops. Expert Rev Med Devices. 2019;16(2):95–106.
76. Deer TR, et al. The polyanalgesic consensus conference (PACC): recommendations on intrathecal drug infusion systems best practices and guidelines. Neuromodulation. 2017;20(2):96–132.

14 Indications for Radiotherapy and Chemotherapy in Malignant Tumors

James Feghali, Daniel Lubelski, and Allan J. Belzberg

14.1 Introduction

Malignant peripheral nerve sheath tumors (MPNSTs) constitute a subcategory of soft tissue sarcomas with complex genomics and are known to have elevated recurrence rates and poor prognosis [1, 2]. Approximately 5% of the 15,000 incident cases of soft tissue sarcomas yearly in the United States are MPNSTs [3]. Approximately half of the cases occur in patients with neurofibromatosis type 1 (NF1) with a lifetime risk of about 16%, while the rest arise sporadically or as a result of radiotherapy [1, 4]. Even with multimodal therapy, the prognosis of MPNST is poor with a 5-year survival rate of 35%–50% [5–7]. Most studies have demonstrated poorer disease-specific survival in NF1-associated MPNST when compared to sporadic disease [5, 8, 9]. Currently, the only proven curative approach to treatment is complete surgical resection with wide negative margins [2, 10, 11], but the viability of this treatment option can be compromised by factors such as lesion size, location, and metastasis. Although the efficacy and role of radiotherapy and chemotherapy in the management of MPNST largely remain unclear, we offer in this chapter a general overview of their indications and potential use.

J. Feghali · D. Lubelski · A. J. Belzberg (✉)
Department of Neurosurgery, Johns Hopkins University School of Medicine, Baltimore, MD, USA
e-mail: abelzbe1@jhmi.edu

14.2 Radiotherapy

Radiotherapy is often recommended as adjuvant treatment in intermediate- or high-grade tumors that are more than 5 cm in size or after marginal excision of low-grade lesions (e.g., R1 resection) with the aim of improving local control [12]. The majority of retrospective studies evaluating the effect of adjuvant or neoadjuvant radiotherapy have shown no significant association with improved local disease control or survival (Table 14.1) [5, 7, 13–37]. The most common form of radiotherapy used is adjuvant external beam radiotherapy (EBRT) with cumulative doses ranging between 12.5 and 90 Gy, but other modalities such as brachytherapy have also been employed [38]. A retrospective study by Wong et al. on 134 patients found that radiation dose and the use of intraoperative high-energy electron irradiation or brachytherapy were associated with improved local control of disease but not with overall survival on multivariable analysis [26]. Namely, patients with a cumulative dose that surpassed 60 Gy had a local control rate of 73% after 5 years compared to 50% for lesser doses [26]. Only three retrospective analyses have demonstrated evidence of a survival benefit with the use of radiotherapy in MPNST with a hazard ratio (HR) of 0.22–0.63 [6, 39, 40]. In another study by Arshi et al. of 374 patients with head and neck MPNSTs extracted from the Surveillance, Epidemiology, and End Results (SEER) cancer

F. Guedes et al. (eds.), *Diagnostic Assessment and Treatment of Peripheral Nerve Tumors*,
https://doi.org/10.1007/978-3-030-77633-6_14

Table 14.1 Retrospective studies analyzing the effect of radiotherapy on outcome in malignant peripheral nerve sheath tumors

Authors	Year	No. of patients (% with NF1)	Radiation (% of patients)	Radiation effect on prognosis[a]
Storm et al.	1980	20 (70)	50	NS
Sordillo et al.	1981	165 (40)	39	–
Ducatman et al.	1986	120 (52)	49	NS
Hruban et al.	1990	43 (53)	35	NS
Wanebo et al.	1993	28 (54)	18	NS
Doorn et al.	1995	22 (50)	45	–
deCou et al.	1995	28 (39)	46	NS
Wong et al.	1998	134 (24)	54	S
Kourea et al.	1998	25 (60)	44	–
Casanova et al.	1999	24 (29)	50	NS
Ramanathan et al.	1999	29 (100)	83	NS
Baehring et al.	2003	54 (22)	69	S
Carli et al.	2005	167 (17)	38	NS
Anghileri et al.	2006	205 (22)	44	S
Okada et al.	2007	53 (45)	30	NS
Hagel et al.	2007	52 (73)	-	NS
Zou et al.	2009	140 (55)	49	NS
Porter	2009	123 (27)	61	NS
Longhi et al.	2010	62 (35)	48	NS
Stucky et al.	2012	175 (32)	63	NS
LaFemina et al.	2013	105 (40)	61	NS
Dunn et al.	2013	23 (100)	91	–
Ren et al.	2013	26 (4)	77	NS
Kahn et al.	2014	33 (55)	61	NS
Fan et al.	2014	146 (12)	29	NS
Wang et al.[b]	2015	43 (14)	35	NS
Arshi et al.[c]	2015	374 (-)	43	S[d]
Valentin et al.	2016	294 (36)	57	NS
Watson et al.	2017	274 (52)	51	NS
Chou et al.[b]	2017	29 (–)	66	NS
Yuan et al.	2017	159 (44)	57	NS
Mowery et al.	2019	2858 (–)	-	NS
Martin et al.	2019	3267 (–)	37	NS
Martin et al.	2019	784 (27)	44	NS
Miao et al.	2019	280 (28)	68	S

NS Nonsignificant, *S* Significantly improved prognosis
[a]Local control or survival in multivariable analysis
[b]All evaluated tumors located in the spine
[c]All evaluated tumors located in the head and neck
[d]Only significant on subgroup analysis

database, radiotherapy failed to show a significant benefit in survival when analyzed in the complete cohort but demonstrated improved overall survival (OS) and disease-specific survival (DSS) in the subgroup of patients with a lesion greater than 5 cm (HR for OS = 0.4; HR for DSS = 0.05) and the subgroup of patients with stage III/IV cancer (HR for OS = 0.32; HR for DSS = 0.13) [41]. However, the temporal relationship between radiotherapy and surgery could not be determined because of the data availability in this administrative database. The major bias inherent in the retrospective nature of these studies is that tumors treated with radiotherapy are more extensive, of relatively higher grade, and more likely to have been resistant to other therapies, so the true effect of radiotherapy on the general population of MPNST patients may not be captured.

There have been no prospective studies dedicated exclusively for MPNST, but there have been some evaluating the effect of radiotherapy on soft tissue sarcomas in general. A prospective study that randomized 91 patients with high-grade soft tissue sarcomas of the extremity (malignant schwannoma, $n = 9$) to either receive or not receive EBRT following surgical resection and chemotherapy reported significantly lower local recurrence rates in the radiotherapy group but no difference in overall survival in the entire sample [42]. Given the small number of included MPNSTs, no subgroup analysis was carried out. Yang et al. prospectively randomized a total of 141 patients with non-MPNST soft tissue sarcomas of the extremity to either receive or not receive adjuvant radiotherapy following limb-sparing surgical resection and chemotherapy [42]. In both the high-grade and low-grade tumor subgroups, there was a significantly lower incidence of local recurrence in the radiotherapy group but no significant difference in overall survival [42]. From review of the current literature, it is clear that the role of radiotherapy in the management of MPNSTs remains to be defined. Given the lack of head-to-head comparisons and standardization of radiotherapy protocols, evidence-based guidelines for optimal indications, cumulative dosages, fraction numbers, and timing remain unknown.

14.3 Chemotherapy

The main use of chemotherapy in MPNST is in metastatic disease and in cases where preoperative chemotherapy may downstage tumors to improve surgical outcome [12]. Several agents with different mechanisms of action have been used in MPNST, and these include doxorubicin, cyclophosphamide, ifosfamide, dactinomycin, vincristine, and etoposide [7]. Monotherapy with doxorubicin and doxorubicin combined with ifosfamide have demonstrated superior response rates in MPNST compared to other regimens, and they are often used as first-line therapy in high-grade MPNST and high-grade soft tissue sarcomas in general [43, 44]. A recent international randomized controlled trial failed to demonstrate any improvement in disease-free or overall survival when using MPNST-tailored high-dose ifosfamide chemotherapy compared to standard chemotherapy of epirubicin plus ifosfamide used in most soft tissue sarcomas [45]. While MPNSTs are generally chemoresistant with response rates near 20% [44], studies suggest that NF1-associated tumors are more resistant to chemotherapy when compared to sporadic disease [7, 46]. As in radiotherapy, most studies in the literature have failed to demonstrate a survival benefit with the use of chemotherapy [6, 8, 18, 19, 26, 39, 47]. One randomized trial evaluating the use of adjuvant chemotherapy in soft tissue sarcomas in general showed that a regimen consisting of five cycles of epirubicin and ifosfamide following local therapy (combinations of radiation and surgery/amputation) led to improved median overall survival (75 months versus 46 months) [48]. Given the proximity to vital organs and anatomical structures, retroperitoneal soft tissue sarcomas represent a subset of tumors where chemotherapy may improve treatment outcomes [49], and that is currently being investigated in several trials [50]. Other future studies will continue to characterize the indications for chemotherapy as well as the optimal agents and treatment protocols.

14.4 Targeted Therapy

With the expanding knowledge acquired on the genetics and pathophysiology of soft tissue sarcomas in general and MPNSTs in particular, targeted agents are being investigated for their potential benefit in treating these aggressive diseases. Clinical trials with erlotinib [51], sorafenib [52], imatinib [53], and dasatinib [54] did not demonstrate a significant survival benefit. However, ongoing trials evaluating other agents such as bevacizumab and ganetespib may identify novel therapies that ameliorate outcome [55].

The RAS/RAF/MEK/ERK pathway that translates extracellular inputs into increased cellular growth and proliferation has been a recent therapeutic target of interest for MPNST. The protein product of the *NF1* gene, which is commonly mutated in both NF1-associated and sporadic diseases, is neurofibromin, which negatively regulates the previously mentioned pathway by accelerating GTP hydrolysis on Ras proteins [56]. MEK inhibitors in particular have demonstrated antitumor properties in MPNST cells in vitro and in MPNST mouse models [57]. Moreover, selumetinib, an oral selective inhibitor of MEK 1 and 2, led to a decrease in the burden of inoperable plexiform neurofibromas in a clinical trial involving children with NF1 [58]. Given these promising results, MEK inhibitors are being used as adjuvant therapy in some centers. Currently, an ongoing phase II trial (SARC031, NCT03433183) involving patients with metastatic or inoperable sporadic or NF1-associated MPNST is evaluating the efficacy of selumetinib in combination with an mTOR kinase inhibitor [59]. Immune checkpoint blockade, an approach commonly used in glioma therapy, is also being investigated in MPNST, and pembrolizumab, a PD-1 inhibitor, is being evaluated in an ongoing phase II trial on locally advanced and unresectable MPNST (NCT02691026) [59]. Over the last 20 years, treatment outcomes for MPNST have failed to improve significantly. Moving forward, a clearer understanding of MPNST genetics and the identification of novel druggable targets can help establish novel combination therapies that prolong survival.

14.5 Conclusion

Although guidelines for the use of radiotherapy and chemotherapy in MPNST are lacking, we have provided a general overview of the relevant literature along with the most common indications for using these adjunct therapies. Understanding that there are several therapeutic avenues to manage MPNST including surgery, radiotherapy, chemotherapy, and targeted therapy is crucial. Optimal outcomes are achieved in a multidisciplinary setting that combines expertise of surgeons, oncologists, radiologists, radiation oncologists, and pathologists with extensive knowledge in sarcoma treatment.

References

1. Widemann BC, Italiano A. Biology and management of undifferentiated pleomorphic sarcoma, myxofibrosarcoma, and malignant peripheral nerve sheath tumors: state of the art and perspectives. J Clin Oncol. 2018;36:160–7. https://doi.org/10.1200/JCO.2017.75.3467.
2. Farid M, Demicco EG, Garcia R, et al. Malignant peripheral nerve sheath tumors. Oncologist. 2014;19:193–201. https://doi.org/10.1634/theoncologist.2013-0328.
3. Prudner BC, Ball T, Rathore R, Hirbe AC. Diagnosis and management of malignant peripheral nerve sheath tumors: current practice and future perspectives. Neuro-Oncology Adv. 2019; https://doi.org/10.1093/noajnl/vdz047.
4. Uusitalo E, Rantanen M, Kallionpaa RA, et al. Distinctive cancer associations in patients with neurofibromatosis type 1. J Clin Oncol. 2016;34:1978–86. https://doi.org/10.1200/JCO.2015.65.3576.
5. Ducatman BS, Scheithauer BW, Piepgras DG, et al. Malignant peripheral nerve sheath tumors. A clinicopathologic study of 120 cases. Cancer. 1986;57:2006–21. https://doi.org/10.1002/1097-0142(19860515)57:10<2006::aid-cncr2820571022>3.0.co;2-6.
6. Anghileri M, Miceli R, Fiore M, et al. Malignant peripheral nerve sheath tumors: prognostic factors and survival in a series of patients treated at a single institution. Cancer. 2006;107:1065–74. https://doi.org/10.1002/cncr.22098.
7. Carli M, Ferrari A, Mattke A, et al. Pediatric malignant peripheral nerve sheath tumor: the Italian and German soft tissue sarcoma cooperative group. J Clin Oncol. 2005;23:8422–30. https://doi.org/10.1200/JCO.2005.01.4886.

8. Sordillo PP, Helson L, Hajdu SI, et al. Malignant schwannoma—clinical characteristics, survival, and response to therapy. Cancer. 1981;47:2503–9. https://doi.org/10.1002/1097-0142(19810515)47:10<2503::aid-cncr2820471033>3.0.co;2-3.
9. Evans DGR, Baser ME, McGaughran J, et al. Malignant peripheral nerve sheath tumours in neurofibromatosis 1. J Med Genet. 2002;39:311–4. https://doi.org/10.1136/jmg.39.5.311.
10. Scaife CL, Pisters PW. Combined-modality treatment of localized soft tissue sarcomas of the extremities. Surg Oncol Clin N Am. 2003;12:355–68. https://doi.org/10.1016/s1055-3207(03)00003-6.
11. Gupta G, Mammis A, Maniker A. Malignant peripheral nerve sheath tumors. Neurosurg Clin N Am. 2008;19:533–43. https://doi.org/10.1016/j.nec.2008.07.004.
12. Ferner RE, Gutmann DH. International consensus statement on malignant peripheral nerve sheath tumors in neurofibromatosis. Cancer Res. 2002;62:1573–7.
13. Kahn J, Gillespie A, Tsokos M, et al. Radiation therapy in management of sporadic and neurofibromatosis type 1-associated malignant peripheral nerve sheath tumors. Front Oncol. 2014;4:324. https://doi.org/10.3389/fonc.2014.00324.
14. Fan Q, Yang J, Wang G. Clinical and molecular prognostic predictors of malignant peripheral nerve sheath tumor. Clin Transl Oncol. 2014;16:191–9. https://doi.org/10.1007/s12094-013-1061-x.
15. Ren X, Wang J, Hu M, et al. Clinical, radiological, and pathological features of 26 intracranial and intraspinal malignant peripheral nerve sheath tumors. J Neurosurg. 2013;119:695–708. https://doi.org/10.3171/2013.5.JNS122119.
16. LaFemina J, Qin L-X, Moraco NH, et al. Oncologic outcomes of sporadic, neurofibromatosis-associated, and radiation-induced malignant peripheral nerve sheath tumors. Ann Surg Oncol. 2013;20:66–72. https://doi.org/10.1245/s10434-012-2573-2.
17. Stucky C-CH, Johnson KN, Gray RJ, et al. Malignant peripheral nerve sheath tumors (MPNST): the Mayo Clinic experience. Ann Surg Oncol. 2012;19:878–85. https://doi.org/10.1245/s10434-011-1978-7.
18. Longhi A, Errani C, Magagnoli G, et al. High grade malignant peripheral nerve sheath tumors: outcome of 62 patients with localized disease and review of the literature. J Chemother. 2010;22:413–8. https://doi.org/10.1179/joc.2010.22.6.413.
19. Zou C, Smith KD, Liu J, et al. Clinical, pathological, and molecular variables predictive of malignant peripheral nerve sheath tumor outcome. Ann Surg. 2009;249:1014–22. https://doi.org/10.1097/SLA.0b013e3181a77e9a.
20. Porter DE, Prasad V, Foster L, et al. Survival in malignant peripheral nerve sheath tumours: a comparison between sporadic and neurofibromatosis type 1-associated tumours. Sarcoma. 2009;756395:2009. https://doi.org/10.1155/2009/756395.
21. Okada K, Hasegawa T, Tajino T, et al. Clinical relevance of pathological grades of malignant peripheral nerve sheath tumor: a multi-institution TMTS study of 56 cases in Northern Japan. Ann Surg Oncol. 2007;14:597–604. https://doi.org/10.1245/s10434-006-9053-5.
22. Hagel C, Zils U, Peiper M, et al. Histopathology and clinical outcome of NF1-associated vs. sporadic malignant peripheral nerve sheath tumors. J Neurooncol. 2007;82:187–92. https://doi.org/10.1007/s11060-006-9266-2.
23. Mowery A, Clayburgh D. Malignant peripheral nerve sheath tumors: analysis of the national cancer database. Oral Oncol. 2019;98:13–9. https://doi.org/10.1016/j.oraloncology.2019.09.010.
24. Ramanathan RC, Thomas JM. Malignant peripheral nerve sheath tumours associated with von Recklinghausen's neurofibromatosis. Eur J Surg Oncol. 1999;25:190–3. https://doi.org/10.1053/ejso.1998.0625.
25. Casanova M, Ferrari A, Spreafico F, et al. Malignant peripheral nerve sheath tumors in children: a single-institution twenty-year experience. J Pediatr Hematol Oncol. 1999;21:509–13.
26. Wong WW, Hirose T, Scheithauer BW, et al. Malignant peripheral nerve sheath tumor: analysis of treatment outcome. Int J Radiat Oncol Biol Phys. 1998;42:351–60. https://doi.org/10.1016/s0360-3016(98)00223-5.
27. deCou JM, Rao BN, Parham DM, et al. Malignant peripheral nerve sheath tumors: the St. Jude Children's Research Hospital experience. Ann Surg Oncol. 1995;2:524–9. https://doi.org/10.1007/bf02307086.
28. Wanebo JE, Malik JM, SR VB, et al. Malignant peripheral nerve sheath tumors. A clinicopathologic study of 28 cases. Cancer. 1993;71:1247–53. https://doi.org/10.1002/1097-0142(19930215)71:4<1247::aid-cncr2820710413>3.0.co;2-s.
29. Hruban RH, Shiu MH, Senie RT, Woodruff JM. Malignant peripheral nerve sheath tumors of the buttock and lower extremity. A study of 43 cases. Cancer. 1990;66:1253–65. https://doi.org/10.1002/1097-0142(19900915)66:6<1253::aid-cncr2820660627>3.0.co;2-r.
30. Storm FK, Eilber FR, Mirra J, Morton DL. Neurofibrosarcoma. Cancer. 1980;45:126–9. https://doi.org/10.1002/1097-0142(19800101)45:1<126::aid-cncr2820450122>3.0.co;2-u.
31. Martin E, Muskens IS, Coert JH, et al. Treatment and survival differences across tumor sites in malignant peripheral nerve sheath tumors: a SEER database analysis and review of the literature. Neuro-oncology Pract. 2019;6:134–43. https://doi.org/10.1093/nop/npy025.
32. Martin E, Coert JH, Flucke UE, et al. A nationwide cohort study on treatment and survival in patients with malignant peripheral nerve sheath tumours. Eur J Cancer. 2019;124:77–87. https://doi.org/10.1016/j.ejca.2019.10.014.

33. Yuan Z, Xu L, Zhao Z, et al. Clinicopathological features and prognosis of malignant peripheral nerve sheath tumor: a retrospective study of 159 cases from 1999 to 2016. Oncotarget. 2017;8:104,785–95. https://doi.org/10.18632/oncotarget.18975.
34. Watson KL, Al Sannaa GA, Kivlin CM, et al. Patterns of recurrence and survival in sporadic, neurofibromatosis type 1-associated, and radiation-associated malignant peripheral nerve sheath tumors. J Neurosurg. 2017;126:319–29. https://doi.org/10.3171/2015.12.JNS152443.
35. Chou D, Bilsky MH, Luzzati A, et al. Malignant peripheral nerve sheath tumors of the spine: results of surgical management from a multicenter study. J Neurosurg Spine. 2017;26:291–8. https://doi.org/10.3171/2016.8.SPINE151548.
36. Valentin T, Le Cesne A, Ray-Coquard I, et al. Management and prognosis of malignant peripheral nerve sheath tumors: the experience of the French Sarcoma Group (GSF-GETO). Eur J Cancer. 2016;56:77–84. https://doi.org/10.1016/j.ejca.2015.12.015.
37. Wang T, Yin H, Han S, et al. Malignant peripheral nerve sheath tumor (MPNST) in the spine: a retrospective analysis of clinical and molecular prognostic factors. J Neurooncol. 2015;122:349–55. https://doi.org/10.1007/s11060-015-1721-5.
38. Hong J, Pisapia J, Niziolek PJ, et al. Malignant peripheral nerve sheath tumors. In: Socolovsky M, Lukas R, Rajiv M, Debora G, editors. Manual of peripheral nerve surgery: from the basics to complex procedures. New York: Thieme Medical Publishers; 2017. p. 196–209.
39. Baehring JM, Betensky RA, Batchelor TT. Malignant peripheral nerve sheath tumor: the clinical spectrum and outcome of treatment. Neurology. 2003;61:696–8. https://doi.org/10.1212/01.wnl.0000078813.05925.2c.
40. Miao R, Wang H, Jacobson A, et al. Radiation-induced and neurofibromatosis-associated malignant peripheral nerve sheath tumors (MPNST) have worse outcomes than sporadic MPNST. Radiother Oncol. 2019;137:61–70. https://doi.org/10.1016/j.radonc.2019.03.015.
41. Arshi A, Tajudeen BA, St John M. Malignant peripheral nerve sheath tumors of the head and neck: demographics, clinicopathologic features, management, and treatment outcomes. Oral Oncol. 2015;51:1088–94. https://doi.org/10.1016/j.oraloncology.2015.08.012.
42. Yang JC, Chang AE, Baker AR, et al. Randomized prospective study of the benefit of adjuvant radiation therapy in the treatment of soft tissue sarcomas of the extremity. J Clin Oncol. 1998;16:197–203. https://doi.org/10.1200/JCO.1998.16.1.197.
43. In GK, Hu JS, Tseng WW. Treatment of advanced, metastatic soft tissue sarcoma: latest evidence and clinical considerations. Ther Adv Med Oncol. 2017;9:533–50. https://doi.org/10.1177/1758834017712963.
44. Kroep JR, Ouali M, Gelderblom H, et al. First-line chemotherapy for malignant peripheral nerve sheath tumor (MPNST) versus other histological soft tissue sarcoma subtypes and as a prognostic factor for MPNST: an EORTC soft tissue and bone sarcoma group study. Ann Oncol Off J Eur Soc Med Oncol. 2011;22:207–14. https://doi.org/10.1093/annonc/mdq338.
45. Gronchi A, Ferrari S, Quagliuolo V, et al. Histotype-tailored neoadjuvant chemotherapy versus standard chemotherapy in patients with high-risk soft-tissue sarcomas (ISG-STS 1001): an international, open-label, randomised, controlled, phase 3, multicentre trial. Lancet Oncol. 2017;18:812–22. https://doi.org/10.1016/S1470-2045(17)30334-0.
46. Ferrari A, Miceli R, Rey A, et al. Non-metastatic unresected paediatric non-rhabdomyosarcoma soft tissue sarcomas: results of a pooled analysis from United States and European groups. Eur J Cancer. 2011;47:724–31. https://doi.org/10.1016/j.ejca.2010.11.013.
47. Moretti VM, Crawford EA, Staddon AP, et al. Early outcomes for malignant peripheral nerve sheath tumor treated with chemotherapy. Am J Clin Oncol. 2011;34:417–21. https://doi.org/10.1097/COC.0b013e3181e9c08a.
48. Frustaci S, Gherlinzoni F, De Paoli A, et al. Adjuvant chemotherapy for adult soft tissue sarcomas of the extremities and girdles: results of the Italian randomized cooperative trial. J Clin Oncol. 2001;19:1238–47. https://doi.org/10.1200/JCO.2001.19.5.1238.
49. Group T-ARW. Management of primary retroperitoneal sarcoma (RPS) in the adult: a consensus approach from the Trans-Atlantic RPS Working Group. Ann Surg Oncol. 2015;22:256–63. https://doi.org/10.1245/s10434-014-3965-2.
50. van Houdt WJ, Raut CP, Bonvalot S, et al. New research strategies in retroperitoneal sarcoma. The case of TARPSWG, STRASS and RESAR: making progress through collaboration. Curr Opin Oncol. 2019;31:310–6. https://doi.org/10.1097/CCO.0000000000000535.
51. Albritton KH, Rankin C, Coffin CM, et al. Phase II study of erlotinib in metastatic or unresectable malignant peripheral nerve sheath tumors (MPNST). J Clin Oncol. 2006;24:9518. https://doi.org/10.1200/jco.2006.24.18_suppl.9518.
52. Maki RG, D'Adamo DR, Keohan ML, et al. Phase II study of sorafenib in patients with metastatic or recurrent sarcomas. J Clin Oncol. 2009;27:3133–40. https://doi.org/10.1200/JCO.2008.20.4495.
53. Chugh R, Wathen JK, Maki RG, et al. Phase II multicenter trial of imatinib in 10 histologic subtypes of sarcoma using a bayesian hierarchical statistical model. J Clin Oncol. 2009;27:3148–53. https://doi.org/10.1200/JCO.2008.20.5054.
54. Schuetze SM, Wathen JK, Lucas DR, et al. SARC009: Phase 2 study of dasatinib in patients with previously treated, high-grade, advanced sarcoma. Cancer. 2016;122:868–74. https://doi.org/10.1002/cncr.29858.
55. Bradford D, Kim A. Current treatment options for malignant peripheral nerve sheath tumors. Curr Treat

Options Oncol. 2015;16:328. https://doi.org/10.1007/s11864-015-0328-6.

56. Carroll SL. Molecular mechanisms promoting the pathogenesis of Schwann cell neoplasms. Acta Neuropathol. 2012;123:321–48. https://doi.org/10.1007/s00401-011-0928-6.
57. Jessen WJ, Miller SJ, Jousma E, et al. MEK inhibition exhibits efficacy in human and mouse neurofibromatosis tumors. J Clin Invest. 2013;123:340–7. https://doi.org/10.1172/JCI60578.
58. Dombi E, Baldwin A, Marcus LJ, et al. Activity of selumetinib in neurofibromatosis type 1-related plexiform neurofibromas. N Engl J Med. 2016;375:2550–60. https://doi.org/10.1056/NEJMoa1605943.
59. Natalie Wu LM, Lu QR. Therapeutic targets for malignant peripheral nerve sheath tumors. Future Neurol. 2019;14:FNL7. https://doi.org/10.2217/fnl-2018-0026.

Part II

Peripheral Nerve Tumors in the General Population

15 Schwannomas of the Extremities

Mario Siqueira, Roberto Martins, and Luciano Foroni

15.1 Introduction

Schwann cells provide insulation for both the motor and the sensory peripheral nerve conductions. These cells constitute the myelin sheath, which is biochemically composed of distinct proteins that protect and insulate peripheral axon as the action potential (neural sign) travels down the nodes of Ranvier [1]. Schwannomas are benign tumors of peripheral nerve sheaths that arise from Schwann cells anywhere in the peripheral nervous system (cranial nerves, spinal nerve roots and plexuses, and peripheral nerves). These tumors are also known as neurilemmomas, neurilemomas, neurolemmoma, neurinomas, Schwann cell tumor, peripheral glioma, and peripheral fibroblastoma.

Schwannomas occur sporadically as well as in conjunction with genetic neurocutaneous syndromes [2, 3]. Most lesions are solitary, asymptomatic, and characterized by a slow and non-infiltrating pattern of growth [4–7]. They are usually smaller than 5 cm in diameter, but deep-seated tumors can grow to impressive sizes [8]. Malignant transformation is known to be exceptionally rare [5, 9–11].

This chapter will be related exclusively with peripheral nerve schwannomas of the extremities.

15.2 Historic Data

In 1811, Louis Odier first used the term “neuroma” [12] to describe deep-seated, circumscribed nerve tumors, but many other authors applied this term indiscriminately to both primary and metastatic tumors involving nerves, as well as to traumatic neuromas [13]. It was Rudolph Virchow in 1863 [14] that clarified the misnomer by proposing that a true neuroma contains nerve cells and a false neuroma (tumor) arises from nerve sheaths.

In 1839, Theodor Schwann, a young German physiologist, aged 29, published his momentous book *Mikroskopische Untersuchungen über die Übereinstimmung in der Struktur und dem Wachstum der Thiere und Pflanzen* (Microscopical Researches into the Accordance in the Structure and Growth of Animals and Plants) [15], where he described the discovery of a new type of cell surrounding the axons of nerve fibers.

In 1910, based on his observations of the appearance of the cells under light microscopy of the tumorous type of “neuroma,” Jose Juan Verocay, a Uruguayan physician, postulated that they arise from Schwann cells and that they should be histologically distinguished from

M. Siqueira (✉) · R. Martins · L. Foroni
Peripheral Nerve Surgery Unit, Department of Neurosurgery, University of São Paulo Medical School, São Paulo, SP, Brazil
e-mail: mgsiqueira@uol.com.br

F. Guedes et al. (eds.), *Diagnostic Assessment and Treatment of Peripheral Nerve Tumors*,
https://doi.org/10.1007/978-3-030-77633-6_15

neurofibromas and described the eponymous Verocay bodies [16].

The French pathologist Pierre Masson was the first to use the term "schwannoma" to designate these tumorous "neuromas" in 1923 [17].

The first description of the surgical management of a schwannoma can probably be credited to the British surgeon William Cheselden [18]. In 1741, in his book *The Anatomy of the Human Body*, Cheselden described a tumor that occupied the center of a "cubital" nerve, displacing the nerve fibers to the periphery. This seems to be a description of a schwannoma, but there is not enough clinical or histological information to draw this conclusion definitively. Despite recognizing the distinction between the nerve fibers and the tumor tissue itself, Cheselden seems to have excised the tumor "en bloc" with the nerve.

15.3 Incidence and Location

Schwannomas are relatively rare. They can be seen at any age but are more commonly diagnosed during early and middle adulthood, with no apparent racial and gender predilection [19, 20]. It represents approximately 5% of all benign soft tissue tumors in adults and occurs sporadically in 95% of cases [7, 21, 22]. The remainder of schwannomas are related to genetic neurocutaneous syndromes, including neurofibromatosis type 1, neurofibromatosis type 2, and schwannomatosis [23]. These tumors are usually solitary but can be multiple, with several lesions located along the nerve (Fig. 15.1a and b) or arising in different nerves. Multiple tumors should always raise suspicion of familial conditions. Owing to its low incidence and its clinical signs and symptoms, schwannomas are often misunderstood and associated with other soft tissue tumors [24].

Schwannomas are considered the most common tumor arising from peripheral nerves [3–5, 7, 23, 25–27], but in a few series, the neurofibromas predominate [28–32]. Schwannomas can be found in the cranial, spinal, and peripheral nerves and sympathetic nerve roots. The most common sites of occurrence, in order of frequency, include the spinal roots and peripheral nerves in the neck and on the flexor area of the upper limbs and the posterior aspect of the lower limbs [33, 34]. While more frequent in the upper limb (70%) [9, 27, 35] and mostly affecting large nerve trunks [9, 21, 27], ultimately any nerve can be affected. Eventually, schwannomas may arise from very small and unidentifiable nerve branches.

The analysis of 10 large series from the literature (1261 tumors) demonstrated that in upper extremity, the most common locations in order of frequency are brachial plexus and ulnar, median, and radial nerves. In the lower limbs, the sequence was sciatic, peroneal, tibial, and femoral [4, 8, 9, 26, 27, 36–40].

15.4 Diagnosis

Most peripheral schwannomas are solitary, slow-growing small lesions (<3 cm) that are incidentally discovered or present with mild to moderate sensorimotor symptoms. When symptomatic, the diagnosis is usually straightforward, based upon physical examination and imaging studies.

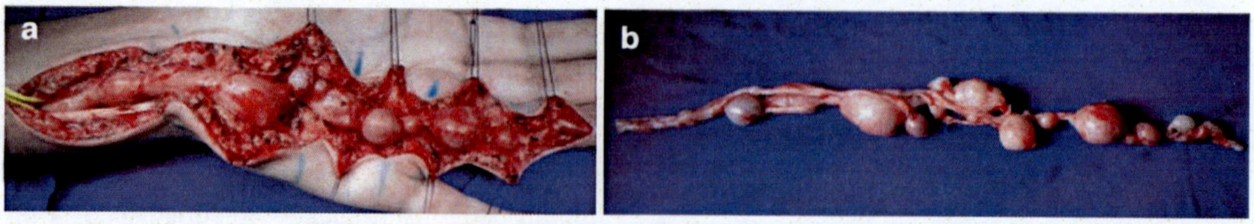

Fig. 15.1 Multiple tumors arising from the sensory part of the ulnar nerve. (**a**) Surgical picture. (**b**) Tumors after removal

15.4.1 Symptoms and Clinical Signs

Clinical presentation is mostly nonspecific. The majority of patients complain at admission of a slow-growing mass that causes symptoms of compression in surrounding tissues and tingling sensations in the distribution of the involved nerve [5]. The symptoms usually depend on the site and size of the lesion. The small size and the slow growth pattern of most schwannomas allow for adaptation of nerve function to the pressure effects, explaining the usual absence of neurological deficits. But at a certain point of their growth (usually when surpassing 25–30 mm in diameter), most tumors start to induce neurological symptoms due to compression of neighboring nerve fibers [41, 42]. In some occasions, smaller tumors may also be symptomatic, especially when they occur in a confined space. The most frequent presentation of schwannoma is a mass located over the course of a nerve (Fig. 15.2), painful to pressure. The tumor is mobile from side to side but not in the axis of the nerve. Percussion induces painful paresthesia in the territory of the nerve of origin, similar to the Tinel sign [30]. As the tumor grows larger and exerts local pressure on the nerve of origin, dysesthesia, neuropathic pain, sensory loss, and weakness can occur [20]. Eventually, the tumor may cause severe neuropathic pain, particularly when it arises in areas exposed to frequent pressure (i.e., the sole of the foot or in the buttock).

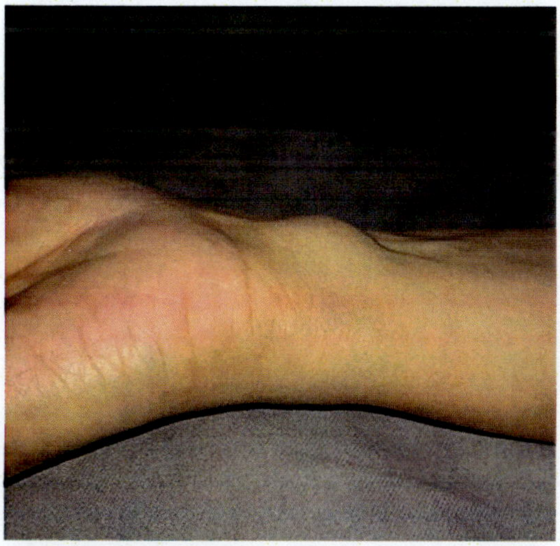

Fig. 15.2 Mass painful to pressure located over the course of the median nerve, proximal to the wrist, on the flexor area of the forearm

15.4.2 Electroneuromyography

The role of preoperative electroneuromyography in patients with schwannomas is very limited. The exam may provide evidence of a nerve lesion in advanced cases where it can demonstrate localized slowing or a block of conduction on stimulation of the nerve along its course, in conjunction with profuse denervation activity when a needle electrode is inserted into the muscle. However, more commonly, only a few fibers are affected by the disease process, such that electroneuromyographic studies usually are normal [43, 44]. Even so, the exam should be made because it provides a baseline for comparison in cases of new neurological deficits after tumor resection [26, 45].

15.4.3 Imaging Studies

Although meticulous physical examination and a history of long symptom duration are often sufficient to point to the diagnosis, an appropriate diagnostic imaging study is usually needed for confirmation. Several imaging modalities can provide useful information for preoperative assessment, such as computerized tomography scan (CT scan), magnetic resonance imaging (MRI), and sonography [23, 46]. However, no image is specific of schwannoma [35, 46–48]; the non-centered nature of the tumor relative to the nerve, which is usually assessed on axial images, appears to be the most defining feature of a schwannomatous nerve tumor [34].

We usually start the image evaluation with ultrasonography. Recent advances in ultrasound technology provided higher spatial resolution identifying the localization of the nerve tumor, its origin from a nerve fascicle, and its relationship with non-involved nerve fascicles [42, 49, 50]. Ultrasonography can eliminate the vast majority of false tumor lesions and allows for differentiation between lymphadenopathy, neuroma, and liquid tumor (hematoma, abscess, or thrombosed aneurysm); however, it is more operator-dependent than MRI. As a general rule, peripheral nerves are more visible when surrounded by tissues of a different echostructure. Peripheral nerves appear as tubular structures made of hypoechoic nerve fascicles embedded in a hyperechoic connective tissue corresponding to the epineurium. Longitudinally, ultrasonography images present a fascicular pattern, and transversely, fascicles appear rounded or oval in shape, giving the nerve the typical honeycomb appearance [51, 52]. Characteristic sonographic findings of schwannomas include a globoid mass with clearly defined margins, off-centered along the nerve, with a homogeneous or a more or less heterogeneous hypoechoic structure, depending on their cystic or solid internal appearance, in direct contact with the echogenic nerve structure [51, 53–55] (Fig. 15.3a). The uniform cellular pattern is responsible for the typical homogeneous and decreased echogenicity and the moderate to marked sound through-transmission [54]. The use of color Doppler ultrasound also provides the surgeon with valuable information regarding the presence of intralesional flow and helps in differentiating solid and cystic lesions [50, 55] (Fig. 15.3b). Additionally, ultrasound is cheaper, does not expose the patient to radiation, and is widely available compared to computed tomography and MRI [38, 50]. Although useful, the ultrasonography examination can provoke local pain and peripheral paresthesia through the pressure of the transducer on the mass and cannot replace MRI for determining the topography, the exact extent of tumor formation, or the presence of invasion [55]. The neural origin of a mass from a small nerve (single hypoechoic fascicle) is also very difficult to determine, particularly in superficial lesions [56]. Ultrasound does not allow definitive differentiation from a neurofibroma [55].

Owing to its high spatial resolution and multiplanar imaging options, the MRI is capable of imaging the tumor, its capsule, the nerve from which the tumor arises, and its relations with surrounding tissues. Many authors consider MRI the most helpful method in confirming the diagnosis of schwannoma preoperatively [5, 57–61]. However, when they arise from cutaneous or other small nerves, the nerve may be obliterated by the mass on MR imaging [62]. The appearance of schwannomas in MRI is an eccentric globular mass located in relation to a nerve. They usually have smooth margins and show iso- or hypo-signal intensity to the muscle on T1-weighted images (Fig. 15.4a) and high intensity in T2-weighted image, homogeneous or heterogeneous, depending on intrinsic changes in

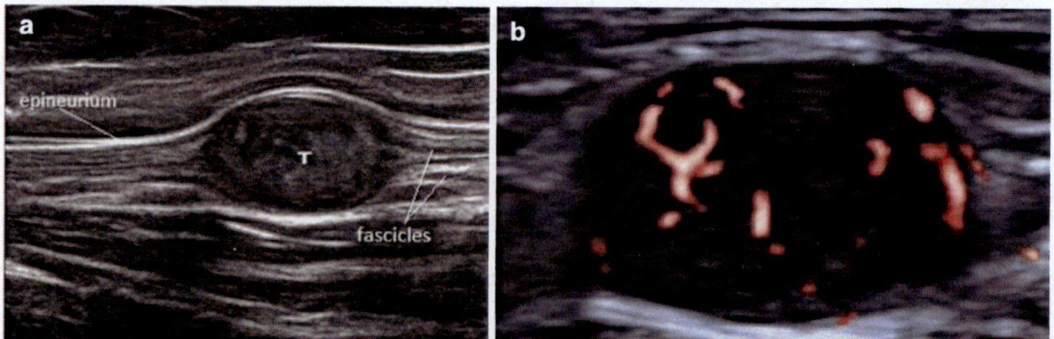

Fig. 15.3 Ultrasonographic image of a median nerve schwannoma in the arm. (**a**) Longitudinal image showing a slightly heterogeneous hypoechoic globoid mass with clearly defined margins, connected to a nerve. The nerve appears as a tubular structure made of hypoechoic nerve fascicles embedded in a hyperechoic connective tissue corresponding to the epineurium. (**b**) Color Doppler ultrasound demonstrating deep and peripheral intralesional flow. T, tumor (Courtesy of Dr. Renato Sernik)

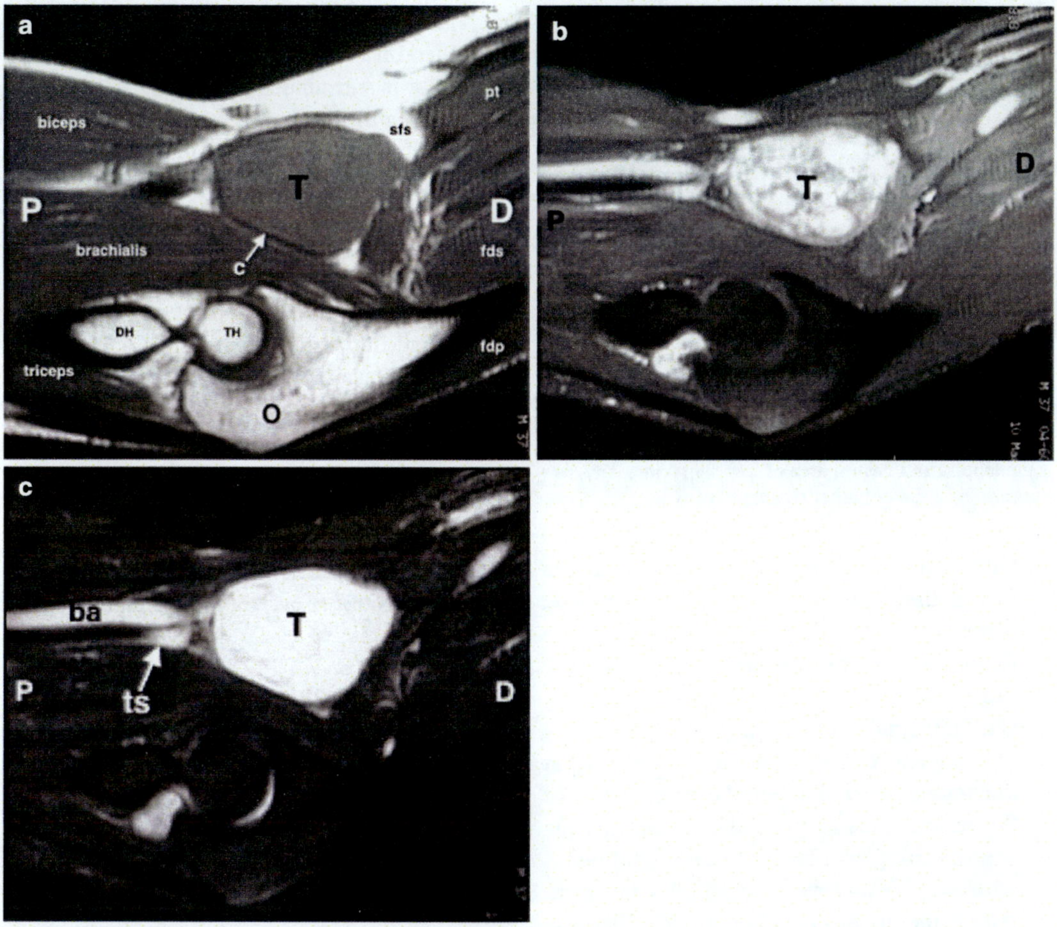

Fig. 15.4 Magnetic resonance image of a schwannoma of the median nerve at the cubital fossa. (**a**) T1-weighted image of a homogeneous globular mass with smooth margins and a slightly hypointense signal in relation to adjacent muscles. (**b**) T2-weighted image showing a high intensity heterogeneous sign inside the tumor. (**c**) T1-weighted image after the infusion of contrast (gadolinium) demonstrating an intense and homogeneous enhancement of the lesion. *Ba* Brachial artery, *C* Capsule, *D* Distal, *DH* Distal humerus, *fdp* Flexor digitorum profundus, *fds* Flexor digitorum superficialis, *O* Olecranon, *P* Proximal, *pt.* Pronator teres, *sfs* "Split fat sign," *T* Tumor, *TH* Trochlea of humerus, *ts* "Tail sign"

the tumor (Fig. 15.4b) [59, 63–66]. Most of the time, a well-defined hypointense capsule at the margin of the tumor is visible (Fig. 15.4a) [36, 67]. After infusion of contrast (gadolinium), the tumor usually shows an intense and homogeneous enhancement (Fig. 15.4c). In tumors with necrotic or cystic areas, the enhancement will be heterogeneous.

Some signs on MRI can help in the diagnosis of schwannomas: the target sign, the tail sign, and the split fat signal.

- Although more common in neurofibromas [10, 43], a "target sign" is also present in schwannomas. The sign is portrayed on T2-weighted images as a central area of low or intermediate signal intensity, surrounded by a rim of higher signal intensity (Fig. 15.5) [68, 69]. Postcontrast, there is central enhancement with persistent peripheral hypointensity [47]. The pathological basis of the target sign in schwannomas is a central distribution of the more cellular Antoni type A tissue pattern,

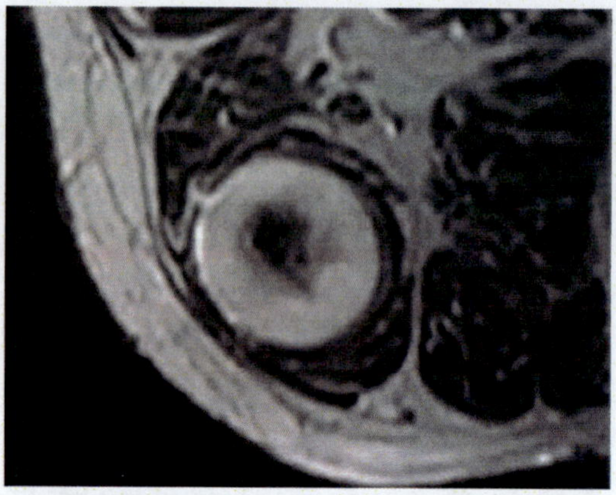

Fig. 15.5 The "target sign." In a T2-weighted image, the sign appears as a central area of low signal intensity, surrounded by a rim of higher signal intensity

with a surrounding rim of hypocellular Antoni type B tissue pattern [36, 42, 70]. The target pattern is usually absent in large masses and in tumors with cystic, hemorrhagic, or necrotic degeneration [66].

- The "tail sign" on MR images oriented along the long axis of the tumor consists of a linear thickening formed from the extremities of the lesion, consisting of the nerve entering and/or exiting neoplasm, which is contiguous with the parent nerve, resembling a tail coming off the tumor [71] (Fig. 15.4c). Virtually pathognomonic for peripheral nerve sheath tumors (both benign and malignant), this feature is usually easy to detect in lesions affecting large deep nerves but is often difficult or impossible to assess in superficial or in small lesions [64].
- Because neurovascular bundles are normally surrounded by fat, benign masses arising in relation to these structures usually maintain a thin rim of fat about them as they slowly enlarge and remodel the surrounding fat plane. Usually seen on T1-weighted images, the rim separates the tumor from the surrounding muscle tissue and appears more prominent at the tapering margins (poles) of the neoplasm. Known as the "split fat sign," this configuration is frequent in neurofibromas, but less common in schwannomas [71] (Fig. 15.4a).

A thin hypointense capsule is occasionally identified on T2-weighted images, particularly if the tumor is surrounded by fat (Fig. 15.4a). This sign is highly suggestive of peripheral nerve sheath tumor and slightly more common in schwannomas than in neurofibromas [62].

While US is the primary imaging modality, due to its ease of use, low price, and accessibility, MRI remains the gold standard as it is able—in the vast majority of cases—to identify the type of tumor and, importantly, determine its resectability [64]. However, despite many advances in MRI, many authors agree that it is difficult to definitively differentiate between malignant and benign neoplasms as well as between different types of benign tumors solely on the basis of MRI findings [21, 72, 73].

On CT scan, a schwannoma seems like a well-demarcated round or oval mass that frequently demonstrates prominent cystic degeneration [59, 74]. On contrast-enhanced CT, the tumor demonstrates homogeneous hypodensity with thin-smooth contrast enhancement at the margin and irregular enhancement at the centrum. We seldom use the CT scan for the diagnosis of a schwannoma.

Eventually radiographs can be performed to rule out any bony involvement or abnormalities [75].

15.4.4 Biopsy

Although the diagnosis of a soft tissue tumor is usually confirmed by a percutaneous biopsy, this diagnostic technique is not recommended when a peripheral nerve sheath tumor is presumed. Besides the moderate sensitivity of these biopsies, whether by fine-needle aspiration or by needle core [76], or even by open biopsy, this procedure carries a risk of hemorrhage within the tumor, damage to viable fascicles, the seeding of cells along the needle track in cases of malignant tumors, and possible scarring that distorts the pathological anatomy of the tumor-nerve interface and thereby increases the challenge of definitive surgical removal [40, 77, 78]. Additionally, the patient can have worsening of the neurogenic pain and development of new neurological deficits, either secondary to hemorrhage or from direct trauma to the susceptible fascicles stretched by the tumor [8].

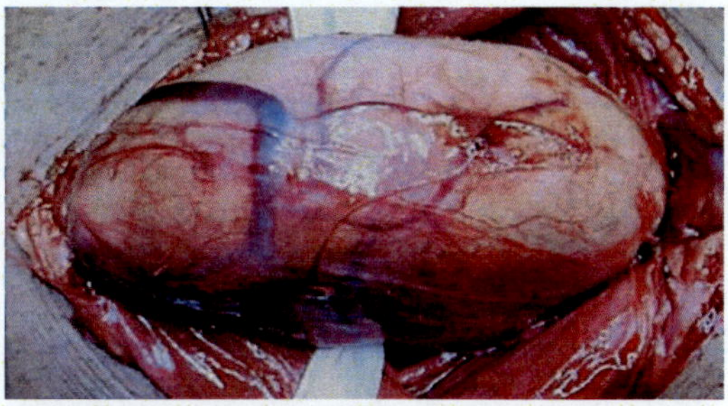

Fig. 15.7 Surgical picture of a schwannoma demonstrating the frequent engorged and tortuous blood vessels coursing over the capsule of the tumor

15.5 Pathology

Schwannomas are derived from the sheath of peripheral nerves and are composed almost entirely of Schwann cells. Macroscopically they are fusiform or round masses, usually less than 5 cm in diameter, that are eccentrically located in relation to the nerve [40, 49, 79] (Fig. 15.6). The tumor is well enveloped by a true capsule which consists of fibrous perineurium of the nerve bundle of origin. The frequent epineurial blood vessels coursing over the capsule of the tumor are usually engorged and tortuous (Fig. 15.7). The capsule is surrounded by a condensation of the deepest layers of the epineurium. Eventually the remaining intact nerve fascicles are generally spread over the capsule of the tumor, instead of concentrating in a specific area [29, 80, 81] (Fig. 15.8).

The cut surface of a schwannoma is similar to that of many mesenchymal neoplasms, with a yellowish, "fish flesh" soft appearance (Fig. 15.9). In larger tumors, the surface may be cystic. Besides the cystic formation, other degenerative changes may occur in larger tumors, like hemorrhage, calcification, and hyalinization.

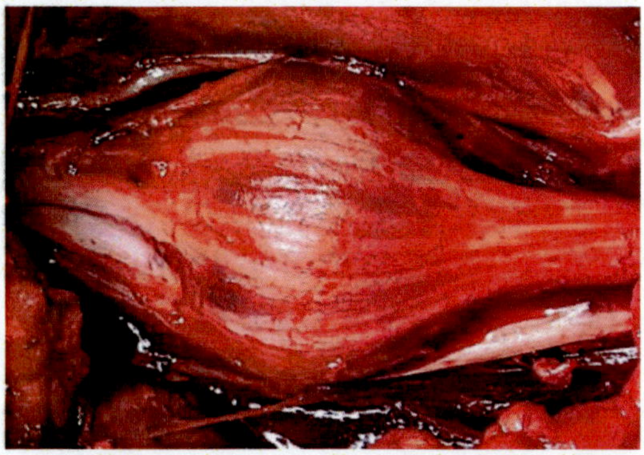

Fig. 15.8 Surgical picture showing a less common distribution of the intact fascicles spread over the entire capsule of the tumor

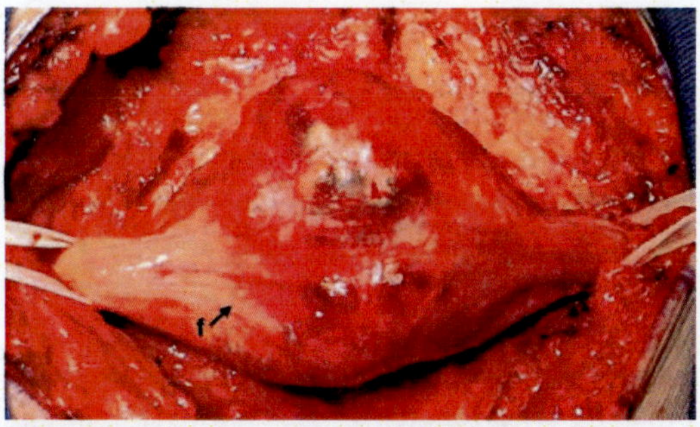

Fig. 15.6 Surgical picture of a typical schwannoma: rounded mass eccentrically located in relation to the nerve, dislocating the fascicles. *f* Fascicle

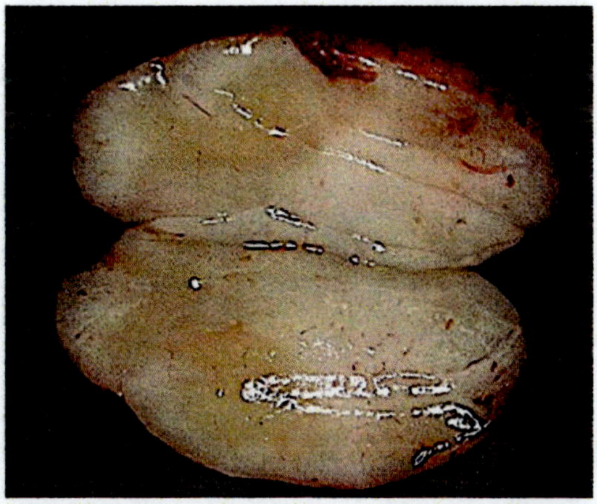

Fig. 15.9 Cut surface of a schwannoma with the typical yellowish, "fish flesh," soft appearance

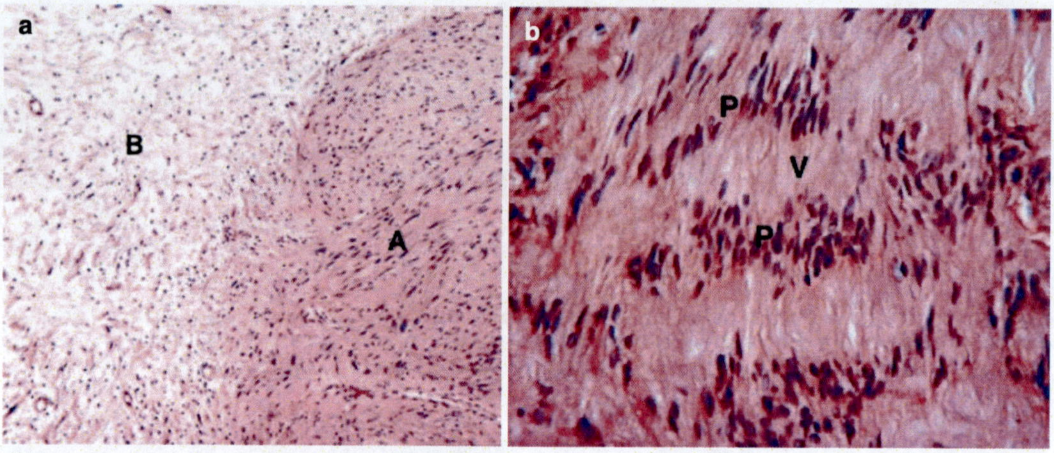

Fig. 15.10 Microscopic aspects of schwannomas: (**a**) usual low-power microscopic aspect of schwannomas showing two distinct patterns of cellular architecture—(i) dense cellular area of closely packed spindle cells (Antoni A) and (ii) area with fewer cells loosely arranged in a mucinous-like matrix (Antoni B). (**b**) High-power microscopy depicting parallel compact rows of elongated nuclei called palisades (P) with a clear area without nuclei between the two zones of palisades called Verocay bodies (V)

Schwannomas contain varying proportions of two distinct patterns of cellular architecture in the tumors, the so-called Antoni A and Antoni B (Fig. 15.10a), described by Nils Antoni, a Swedish physician, in 1920, based on analysis of 30 cases of schwannomas [82]. The Antoni A component is a densely cellular area of closely packed spindle cells which form rows of elongated nuclei (palisades) and compact parallel rows of elongated nuclei alternated with clear anuclear zones containing cell processes, the Verocay bodies (Fig. 15.10b). The Antoni B area has fewer cells loosely arranged in a mucinous-like matrix [10, 73, 83–85]. One area is usually predominant in every tumor [57].

Apart from the classical type, some rarer histological variants of schwannoma have been described including the cellular, ancient, epithelioid, melanotic, and plexiform types [84].

Ancient schwannoma is an uncommon variant with a course typical of a slow-growing neoplasm [57]. This subtype is characterized by extensive cystic degeneration, hemorrhage, fibrosis, and diffuse hypocellular areas, these changes being probably related to the long time of development of these tumors [86, 87]. They are usually large and, owing to its nuclear atypia (large and hypochromatic nucleus), might be confused with malignant tumors [36]. This mistake can be made also in cases of schwannomas formed exclusively from Antoni A tissue type (the "cellular" variety). Immunohistochemical analysis is useful in the differential diagnosis of peripheral nerve tumors. It is performed using monoclonal antibodies against proteins: S-100, CD31, CD34, and GFAP. The cellular areas of schwannomas strongly express the S-100 protein, which is useful especially in the differentiation of the large tumors from soft tissue sarcomas [88].

15.6 Differential Diagnosis

Solitary neurofibromas should always be considered in the differential diagnosis. Peripheral schwannomas and neurofibromas cause virtually identical symptoms and signs, and no single imaging finding or combination allows definite diagnosis to distinguish these tumors [62].

Unlike neurofibromas, the schwannomas are typically encapsulated and do not have multiple cell types inherent to the tumor [62]. Detection of a capsule in the MRI, which causes a low intensity rim at the margin of the tumor, and the presence of the nerve along one side of the mass could help to differentiate schwannomas from neurofibromas [28, 57].

Besides solitary neurofibroma, the differential possibilities for schwannomas should include any soft tissue mass that can cause a compressive effect, like sarcomas, ganglion cyst, fibroma, myxoma, and lipoma [9, 20, 24]. Tumors producing important motor deficit and pain should always raise a high suspicion of malignancy [42].

15.7 Treatment

In the last decades, the majority of papers in the literature about schwannomas consisted in case reports or small series, and only a few large series have been reported [3, 9, 26, 29, 40]. The current treatment of these lesions is based on papers describing in detail the possibilities of treatment and its results.

The treatment of peripheral schwannomas can be conservative or surgical. The decision to operate or observe a patient with schwannoma should be based on balancing the risks of surgery against those associated with more conservative management, always taking into account patient wishes. Risks related to the common practice of continuous conservative management of schwannomas include the possibility of progressive neurological dysfunction, malignant change (albeit rare), and increasing complexity of the surgery as the tumor grows. On the other hand, patients undergoing surgery for a schwannoma are exposed to the risks of anesthesia, wound complications, and neurological injury. Experienced nerve surgeons have demonstrated that schwannomas can be resected completely and safely from major peripheral nerves in most cases. However, as nerve tumors are relatively rare, the number of surgeons with extensive experience in this field is small, which explains some of the complications related to its treatment that can result in lost function. Patients with small, incidental, and asymptomatic tumors should be treated conservatively with periodic outpatient evaluation and imaging studies (at least once a year). However, when the lesion is symptomatic, progressing in size, cosmetically displeasing, or causing pain, the surgical treatment is indicated [9]. Usually the tumor size alone is not an indication for surgery in asymptomatic patients [26].

The surgical excision of schwannomas ranges from subtotal or partial resection (50% or more) to gross total excision (>90% of the tumor) leaving behind the tumor capsule adherent to the neural fascicles to total excision of the tumor along with the tumor capsule. The principal goal for surgical treatment of a schwannoma is to excise the tumor without inflicting any neurological deficit [44].

Surgical Technique—The rationale for surgical resection of nerve sheath tumors includes the preservation, or improvement, of neurological function, the treatment of neuropathic pain, and a pathological diagnosis [38]. The operation should be performed under general anesthesia, avoiding pharmacological muscle relaxation. Magnification (surgical loupes and microscope) and the use of microsurgical techniques are of paramount importance. A lengthy linear skin incision is centered over the tumor and extended along the anatomic course of the involved nerve, to properly expose the tumor and the proximal and distal extent of the affected nerve and local vessels. Proximity to a flexion crease demands an alternative incision. For tumors not readily palpable, transdermal ultrasound can help localize the incision directly over the tumor [60]. A complete exposure of a schwannoma (360°) should be achieved before intraneural dissection (Fig. 15.11a). During the exposition of a schwannoma, important sensory nerves are often encountered in or near the operative field. Damage to these nerves from transection, retraction, cautery, or suture misplacement is a significant source of avoidable morbidity [80]. By virtue of having completely dissected the tumor free of surrounding soft tissues and other nerve elements, the nerve can be gently rotated, allowing for the search of a fascicle-free area [89]. This rotation should not exceed 180 degrees, to avoid possible nerve injury, and the nerve should be returned to its original orientation before closure [60].

At this point, the location of fascicles splaying over the tumor surface is carefully noted. Using a nerve stimulator on a low setting (e.g., 0.5 mA),

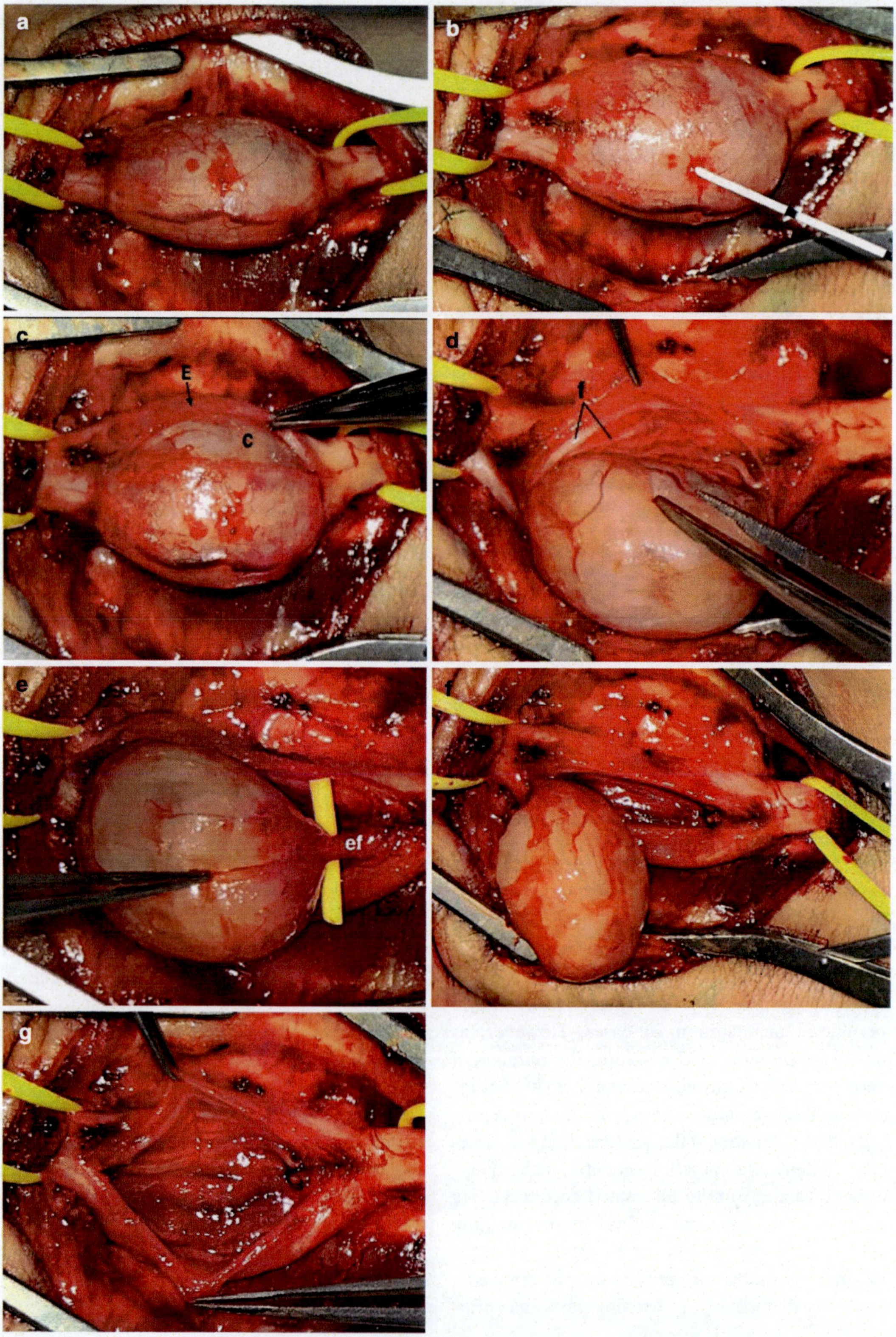
a
b
c
E
c
d
f
e
ef
f
g

it is possible to identify functioning and non-functioning fascicles (Fig. 15.11b). An area with both the least number of visible fascicles and no electrical response to the stimulation is selected for the nerve incision. This area is usually the most prominent part of the tumor. A longitudinal incision parallel to the nerve is made in the epineurium with a number 15 scalpel, until the shiny surface of the tumor is exposed (Fig. 15.11c). The incision is lengthened with microscissors at either end where the tumor tapers into normal nerve with care not to damage any fascicles as they coalesce here [60]. It should extend along the length of the tumor and involved nerve [89, 90]. Bleeding is controlled with a fine-tipped bipolar.

From this point, two main approaches have been reported: extracapsular and intracapsular enucleation.

(a) Extracapsular enucleation: The perineural connective tissue generates a well-formed capsule around the tumor, and usually the tumor is not adherent. Gentle dissection along the plane of cleavage between the tumor capsule and the epineurium should be performed, dissecting bluntly and retracting extracapsularly the uninvolved nerve fibers splayed around the tumor (Fig. 15.11d). In this way, the tumor can be shelled out as a whole without disturbing the nerve fascicles. Filmy adhesions are bluntly dissected with the aid of a small dissector or sharply cut as needed with microscissors. The plane of dissection is maintained by small cottonoid strips or pledgettes [89]. In this manner, the tumor is completely dissected (360 degrees) out from the nerve, leaving the surrounding fascicles intact. The violation of the tumor capsule is usually heralded by herniation of tumor through its capsule followed by tumor hemorrhage.

Next, the surgeon should direct the dissection to the poles of the tumor, where usually one (but sometimes two) small fascicle can be seen entering and leaving the tumor. An interfascicular dissection with magnification is performed at the proximal and distal poles of the tumor to isolate at least 3 or 4 mm of the fascicles (Fig. 15.11e). The entering fascicle is then electrically stimulated and should elicit no muscular contraction [89]. The entering fascicle and leaving fascicle are then coagulated and transected, and the tumor is removed (Fig. 15.11e) [44]. In the rare occasion of a contraction observed during the electrical stimulation, an attempt to separate the entering fascicle from the tumor should be done. If it is not possible, this motor fascicle has to be reconstructed with a graft after the removal of the tumor [91]. In a few cases, despite meticulous dissection, one or more small fascicles can be found to pass through the body of the tumor and have to be sacrificed to allow a total resection, usually without causing additional neurological deficits [38]. At the end of tumor resection, there is no need for reapproximation of the epineurial edges (Fig. 15.11f) [89]. Extracapsular enucleation is generally believed to be routinely possible, producing little or no damage to the underlying nerve fascicles [3, 5, 77].

(b) Intracapsular enucleation: When fascicles seem unusually adherent to the capsule or the bulk of large tumors (Fig. 15.12a) is an obstacle for seeing the cleavage planes of dissection, the risk of transient or permanent neurological damage increases [44, 61, 78].

Fig. 15.11 Surgical pictures of a schwannoma extracapsular resection. (**a**) Complete exposure of the tumor and the proximal and distal extent of the affected nerve. (**b**) Electrical stimulation of the surface of the tumor to find an area without functioning fascicles. (**c**) Longitudinal incision of the epineurium, exposing the tumor capsule. (**d**) Blunt dissection along the cleavage plane between the tumor capsule and the epineurium. Note the uninvolved fascicles splayed around the tumor have been gently retracted extracapsularly. (**e**) After complete dissection of the tumor, leaving the surrounding fascicles intact, an interfascicular dissection is made to isolate the fascicle entering the tumor. (**f**) The entering fascicle is electrically stimulated, coagulated, and transected, allowing the dislocation of the tumor and dissection of the leaving fascicle. (**g**) After coagulation of the leaving fascicle and "en bloc" resection of the tumor, there is no need for reapproximation of the epineurial edges. *C* Tumor capsule, *E* Epineurium, *ef* Entering fascicle, *f* Fascicle

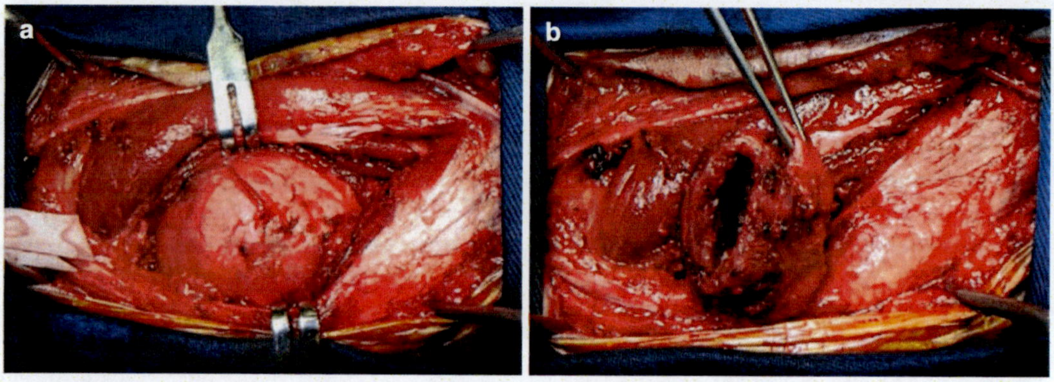

Fig. 15.12 Surgical pictures of a schwannoma intracapsular resection. (**a**) The bulk of this large tumor is an obstacle to achieve the cleavage planes of dissection. (**b**) The center of the tumor was removed piece by piece to allow its dissection

In these cases, "en bloc" resection should be discarded, and an intracapsular enucleation is the best option. The capsule is opened longitudinally, and the tumor contents are enucleated by using suction, forceps and scissors, or an ultrasonic surgical aspirator (Fig. 15.12b). The center of the tumor is removed piece by piece as much as possible. The downside of this internal dissection ("debulking") is the associated bleeding that usually accompanies this technique. The capsule can then be dissected away from the spared fascicles and epineurium and finally total or partially removed.

When for some reason, in both techniques, the capsule of the tumor (or part of it) remains, it can either be left alone as part of the tumor bed or an attempt can be made to remove it. Conceptually, its presence might contribute to an increased rate of recurrence, but this has never been proved [89].

The techniques of extracapsular or intracapsular enucleation of schwannomas have been described by several authors to date, and good results have been reported with each technique [5, 29, 44, 57, 77, 78, 90]. However, few authors [90] found that neurological deficit after enucleation was significantly lower using the intracapsular compared with the extracapsular technique. To minimize the risk of nerve injury, "en bloc" resection should not be used because according to these authors, the main purpose of schwannoma surgery is the relief of symptoms, not tumor resection. We prefer the extracapsular enucleation in most case, performing the intracapsular enucleation only when the previous technique is not possible. Independent of the type of excision applied, after tumor removal, the tumor bed is gently irrigated with saline, and brief applications of low-power bipolar coagulation with a fine-tipped forceps are used to stop any persistent bleeding [60]. A perfect hemostasis is very important to prevent hematoma formation and scarring around the nerves. In general, the extremity fascia is not sutured so as not to cause secondary nerve compression.

A simple, occlusive dressing is applied and maintained for 3 days. There is no need for postoperative immobilization by casts, splints, or compressive dressings, and patients are encouraged to gently use the affected limb immediately after surgery, to reduce subsequent tethering of the nerve by scar tissue [92]. Whenever possible, the involved extremity should be elevated above the heart during the initial postoperative period, to minimize edema. During the first two postoperative weeks, only range-of-motion exercises should be performed. After this initial period, a physical therapy regimen aiming progressive strengthening exercises for both the affected and supportive musculature is started.

15.8 Postoperative Course

Often, the patient complains of slight paresthesias in the distribution of the nerve related to the tumor that usually disappear in the first or second postoperative week.

Patients with subtotal or gross total excision of a schwannoma should be regularly assessed for the detection of complications or recurrence of the tumor. Three months after surgery, a clinical examination and MRI should be done to confirm the extent of tumor excision. If the tumor was totally resected, the patient should be evaluated clinically and with a new MRI every 12 months, for some years. In cases of partial resection, this follow-up evaluation should be done every 6 months, for many years.

15.9 Outcome and Complications

There is a common belief that meticulous dissection of a schwannoma leads to complete removal of the tumor without increasing the neurological loss, if present [5]. Careful resection of schwannomas usually resolves the patient's symptoms, and regardless of the nerve from which the tumor arose, baseline function after resection can be preserved the majority of the time. Although true in most cases, even when the tumor is carefully dissected from the involved nerve, incomplete nerve palsies sometimes occur [3, 5, 41], especially in patients with large tumors [40, 42, 61, 78, 79]. The incidence of complications in the surgical treatment of peripheral schwannomas reported in the literature is extremely variable, ranging from 1.5% to 80%, with an average of 32.4% [3, 5, 9, 26, 30, 38, 40, 44, 61, 78, 79, 90]. Although a number of preoperative symptoms and signs are mentioned as predictable factors for the occurrence of complications, tumor size is the most important. The transection of fascicles entering the tumor substance is believed to be the major cause of postoperative neurological deficit [6, 38, 79, 93], but there are other possible reasons for its occurrence: the longitudinal incision, employed during dissection of the tumor, can damage small fascicles [61], and intact fascicles, preserved from the tumor growth, may be compressed during its surgical enucleation resulting in a neuropraxic injury [27, 61, 93]. Although in a few cases these deficits may be troublesome, most of the complications are transient and related to sensation. Sensibility should recover after a period of a few months to 1 year in most of the cases, as largely reported in the literature [5, 27, 44, 61, 77–79]. Even the persistent residual symptoms or signs at final follow-up usually are tolerable (i.e., mild hypoesthesia or paresthesia) and do not seem to interfere with activities of daily living. The uncommon preoperative motor weakness usually improves with the surgical treatment [26, 44].

The reported incidence of postoperative neurogenic pain following nerve tumor excision ranges from 5.7% to 13% [3, 20, 37–39, 89]. The severity of the pain is variable and in some cases can be quite annoying. It is attributed to edema and damage to the peripheral nerve during handling of the nerve for tumor excision.

The incidence of complications in our series was acceptable (15.2%) [40], but higher numbers of adverse outcomes should be minimized with appropriate selection of patients and meticulous operative technique. Although transient in the majority of cases, permanent neurological deficits can develop in some patients following surgery, and for this reason, all candidates for surgical excision of a schwannoma must be informed about the potential risk of complications. Recurrences after schwannoma resection are very rare [11, 83], even when it is partially enucleated [90].

15.10 Conclusions

. Schwannomas located in extremities arise predominantly from major peripheral nerves and occur mostly in the upper limb, with higher incidence in the brachial plexus and ulnar, median, and radial nerves. In the lower limb, the most affected nerves are the sciatic, peroneal, and tibial. The risk of exacerbation of compression neuropathy caused by gradual tumor growth justifies surgical intervention in symptomatic schwannomas. A schwannoma arising from a major peripheral nerve usually can be excised with an acceptable risk of nerve injury. Improvement of nerve function after the excision of a schwannoma is usually achieved. Meticulous attention to detail is required for large-sized schwannomas, because these tumors seem to have a higher risk of fascicular injury during dissection. As schwannomas are relatively rare, these tumors should be treated at specialized centers by an experienced peripheral nerve surgeon to achieve the best results with less morbidity.

With attention to basic principles, knowledge of surgical approaches, and skillful mastery of the gentle techniques of nerve tumor resection, the surgical treatment of patients harboring intraneural tumors can be quite satisfying to the patient and the surgeon [89].

References

1. Balice-Gordon RJ, Bone LJ, Scherer SS. Functional gap junctions in the Schwann cell myelin sheath. J Cell Biol. 1998;142:1095–104.
2. Halliday AL, Sobel RA, Martuza RL. Benign spinal nerve sheath tumors: their occurrence sporadically and in neurofibromatosis types 1 and 2. J Neurosurg. 1991;74:248–53.
3. Artico M, Cervoni L, Wierzbicki V, D'Andrea V, Nucci F. Benign neural sheath tumours of major nerves: characteristics in 119 surgical cases. Acta Neurochir. 1997;139:1108–16.
4. Das Gupta TK, Brasfield RD, Strong EW, Hadju SI. Benign solitary schwannomas (neurilemmomas). Cancer. 1969;24:355–66.
5. Kang HJ, Shin SJ, Kang ES. Schwannomas of the upper extremity. J Hand Surg Br. 2000;25:604–7.
6. Takase K, Yamamoto K, Imakiire A. Clinical pathology and therapeutic results of neurilemmoma in the upper extremity. J Orthop Surg (Hong Kong). 2004;12:222–5.
7. Weiss SW, Goldblum JR, Enzinger FM. Benign tumors of the peripheral nerves. In: Weiss SW, Goldblum JR, editors. Enzinger and Weiss's soft tissue tumors. 4th ed. St Louis: Mosby; 2001. p. 1111–208.
8. Birch R. Surgical disorders of the peripheral nerves. 2nd ed. London: Springer; 2011.
9. Knight DM, Birch R, Pringle J. Benign solitary schwannomas: a review of 234 cases. J Bone Joint Surg Br. 2007;89:382–7.
10. Viola E, Solà M, Stroppa S, Mosconi M, Benazzo F. Malignant schwannoma in the posterior tibial nerve. Foot (Edinb). 2006;16:216–7.
11. Woodruff JM, Selig AM, Crowley K, Allen PW. Schwannoma (neurilemoma) with malignant transformation: a rare distinctive peripheral nerve tumor. Am J Surg Pathol. 1994;18:882–95.
12. Odier L. Manuel de Medecine Pratique, ed 2. Paris: J. Paschoud; 1811.
13. Walker AE. A history of neurological surgery. Baltimore: Williams & Wilkins; 1951.
14. Virchow R. Die krankhaften Geschwulste, vol. 1–3. Berlin: A Hirschwald; 1863–1867.
15. Schwann T. Mikroskopische Untersuchungen über die Übereinstimmung in der Struktur und dem Wachsthum der Thiere und Pflanzen. Berlin: Sander; 1839.
16. Verocay J. Zur Kenntnis der Neurofibroma. Beitr Pathol Anat. 1910;48:1–69.
17. Masson P. Traité de Pathologie Medicale et de′ Therapeutique Applique′ e/XXVII, Diagnostics de′ Laboratoire. II. Tumeurs—Diagnostics Histologiques. Paris: A. Maloine; 1923.
18. Cheselden W. The anatomy of the human body, ed 6. London: William Bowyer; 1741.
19. Campbell R. Tumors of peripheral and sympathetic nerves. In: Youmans JR, editor. Neurological surgery, vol. 1990. 3rd ed. Philadelphia: WB Saunders; 1990. p. 3667–75.
20. Lai CS, Chen IC, Lan HC, Lu CT, Yen JH, Song DY, Tang. Management of extremity neurilemmomas: clinical series and literature review. Ann Plast Surg. 2013;71:S37–42.
21. Forthman CL, Blazar PE. Nerve tumors of the hand and upper extremity. Hand Clin. 2004;20:233–42.
22. Kransdorf MJ. Benign soft-tissue tumors in a large referral population: distribution of specific diagnoses by age, sex, and location. AJR Am J Radiol. 1995;164:395–402.
23. Giannini C. Tumors and tumor-like conditions of peripheral nerves. In: Dyck PJ, Thomas PK, editors. Peripheral neuropathy. 4th ed. Philadelphia: Elsevier Saunders; 2005. p. 2585–606.
24. Rockwell GM, Thomas A, Salama S. Schwannoma of the hand and wrist. Plast Reconstr Surg. 2003;3:1227–32.
25. Chick G, Alnot JY, Silbermann-Hoffman O. Benign solitary tumors of the peripheral nerves. Rev Chir Orthop Reparatrice Appar Mot. 2000;86:825–34.
26. Desai KI. The surgical management of symptomatic benign peripheral nerve sheath tumors of the neck and extremities: an experience of 442 cases. Neurosurgery. 2017;81:568–80.
27. Sandberg K, Nilsson J, Søe Nielsen N, Dahlin LB. Tumours of peripheral nerves in the upper extremity: a 22- year epidemiological study. Scand J Plast Reconstr Surg Hand Surg. 2009;43:43–9.
28. Beaman FD, Kransdorf MJ, Menke DM. Schwannoma: radiologic-pathologic correlation. Radiographics. 2004;24:1477–81.

29. Kim DH, Murovic JA, Tiel RL, Moes G, Kline DG. A series of 397 peripheral neural sheath tumors: 30-year experience at Louisiana State University health sciences center. J Neurosurg. 2005;102:246–55.
30. Levi AD, Ross AL, Cuartas E, Qadir R, Temple HT. The surgical management of symptomatic peripheral nerve sheath tumors. Neurosurgery. 2010;66:833–40.
31. Lin J, Martel W. Cross-sectional imaging of peripheral nerve sheath tumors: characteristic signs on CT, MR imaging, and sonography. AJR Am J Roentgenol. 2001;176:75.
32. Murphey MD, Smith WS, Smith SE, Kransdorf MJ, Temple HT. Imaging of musculoskeletal neurogenic tumors: radiologic-pathologic correlation. Radiographics. 1999;19:1253–128.
33. Birch R, Booney G, Wynn Parry CB. Surgical disorders of the peripheral nerves. Edinburg: Churchill Livingstone; 1998.
34. Tchernin D, Aubert S, Lesage E, Spas-Defasque E, Degrugillier-Chopinet C, Cohen M, et al. Tumeurs des tissus mous. In: Cotton A, editor. Imagerie Musculosquelettique—Pathologies Générales. Paris: Elsevier Masson; 2013. p. 529–96.
35. Nilsson J, Sandberg K, Soe Nielsen N, Dahlin LB. Magnetic resonance imaging of peripheral nerve tumours in the upper extremity. Scand J Plast Surg Hand Surg. 2009;43:153–9.
36. Adani R, Tarallo R, Mugnai R, Colopi S. Schwannomas of the upper extremity: analysis of 34 cases. Acta Neurochir. 2014;156:2325–30.
37. Gosk J, Gutkowska O, Mazurek P, Koszewicz M, Ziolkowski P. Peripheral nerve tumors: 30-year experience in the surgical treatment. Neurosurg Rev. 2015;38:511–20.
38. Kim SM, Seo SW, Lee JY, Sung KS. Surgical outcome of schwannomas arising from major peripheral nerves in the lower limb. Int Orthop (SICOT). 2012;36:1721–5.
39. Montano N, D'Alessandris QG, D'Ercole M, et al. Tumors of the peripheral nervous system: analysis of prognostic factors in a series with long-term follow-up and review and review of the literature. J Neurosurg. 2016;125:363–71.
40. Siqueira MG, Socolovsky M, Martins RS, Robla-Costales J, Di Masi G, Heise CO, Cosamalón JG. Surgical treatment of typical peripheral schwannomas: the risk of new postoperative deficits. Acta Neurochir. 2013;155:1745–9.
41. Kehoe NJ, Reid RP, Semple JC. Solitary benign peripheral-nerve tumours. Review of 32 years' experience. J Bone Joint Surg Br. 1995;77:497–500.
42. Ogose A, Hotta T, Morita T, Yamamura S, Hosaka N, Kobayashi H, Hirata Y. Tumors of peripheral nerves: correlation of symptoms, clinical signs, imaging features, and histologic diagnosis. Skelet Radiol. 1999;28:183–8.
43. Brooks D. Clinical presentation and treatment of peripheral nerve tumors. In: Dyck P, Lambert E, Thomas P, editors. Peripheral neuropathy. Philadelphia: WB Saunders Philadelphia; 1984. p. 2236–51.
44. Donner TR, Voorhies RM, Kline DG. Neural sheath tumors of major nerves. J Neurosurg. 1994;81:362–73.
45. Maniker AH. Diagnostic steps, imaging, and electrophysiology. Neurosurg Clin N Am. 2004;15:133–44.
46. Amrami KK, Felmlee JP, Spinner RJ. MRI of peripheral nerves. Neurosurg Clin N Am. 2008;19:559–72.
47. Jee WH, Oh SN, McCauley T, Ryu KN, Suh JS, Lee JH, Park JM, Chun KA, Sung MS, Kim K, Lee YS, Kang YK, Ok IY, Kim JM. Extraaxial neurofibromas versus neurilemmomas: discrimination with MRI. AJR Am J Roentgenol. 2004;183:629–33.
48. Singh T, Kliot M. Imaging of peripheral nerve tumors. Neurosurg Focus. 2007;22:E6.
49. Kuo YL, Chiu HY, Yao WJ, Shieh SJ. Ultrasound for schwannoma in the upper extremity. J Hand Surg Eur. 2009;34:697–8.
50. Kuo YL, Yao WJ, Chiu HY. Role of sonography in the preoperative assessment of neurilemmoma. J Clin Ultrasound. 2005;33:87–9.
51. Bianchi S. Ultrasound of the peripheral nerves. Joint Bone Spine. 2008;75:643–9.
52. Martinoli C, Bianchi S, Cohen M, Graif M. Ultrasound of peripheral nerves. J Radiol. 2005;86:1869–78.
53. Fornage BD. Peripheral nerves of the extremities: imaging with US. Radiology. 1988;167:179–82.
54. Simonovsly V. Peripheral nerve schwannoma preoperatively diagnosed by sonography: report of three cases and discussion. Eur J Radiol. 1997;25:47.
55. Garcia J, Bianchi S. Diagnostic imaging of tumors of the hand and wrist. Eur Radiol. 2001;11:1470–82.
56. Valle M, Zamorani MP. Nerve and blood vessels. In: Bianchi S, Martinelli C, editors. Ultrasound of the musculoskeletal system. Berlin: Springer-Verlag; 2007. p. 97–134.
57. Adani R, Baccarani A, Guidi E, Tarallo L. Schwannomas of the upper extremity: diagnosis and treatment. Chir Organi Mov. 2008;92:85–8.
58. Hems TEJ, Burge PD, Wilson DJ. The role of magnetic resonance imaging in the management of peripheral nerve tumors. J Hand Surg Br. 1997;22:57–60.
59. Pilavaki M, Chourmouzi D, Kiziridou A, et al. Imaging of peripheral nerve sheath tumors with pathologic correlation: pictorial review. Eur J Radiol. 2004;52:229–39.
60. Russell SM. Preserve the nerve: microsurgical resection of peripheral nerve sheath tumors. Neurosurgery. 2007;61:ONS-113–8.
61. Sawada T, Sano M, Ogihara H, Omura T, Miura K, Nagano A. The relationship between pre-operative symptoms, operative findings and post-operative complications in schwannomas. J Hand Surg Br. 2006;31:629–34.
62. Ahlawat S, Chhabra A, Blakely J. Magnetic resonance neurography of peripheral nerve tumors and tumor like conditions. Neuroimaging Clin N Am. 2014;24:171–92.

63. Cerofolini E, Landi A, De Santis G. MR of benign peripheral nerve sheath tumors. J Comput Assist Tomogr. 1991;15:593–7.
64. Chhabra A, Soldatos T, Durand DJ, Carrino JA, McCarthy EF, Belzberg AJ. The role of magnetic resonance imaging in the diagnostic evaluation of malignant peripheral nerve sheath tumors. Indian J Cancer. 2011;48:328–34.
65. Soderlund V, Göranson H, Bauer HC. Imaging of benign peripheral nerve sheath tumors. Acta Radiol. 1994;35:282–6.
66. Varma DG, Moulopoulos A, Sara AS, Leeds N, Kumar R, Kim EE, Wallace S. MR imaging of extracranial nerve sheath tumors. J Comput Assist Tomogr. 1992;16:448–53.
67. Woertler K. Tumors and tumor-like lesions of peripheral nerves. Semin Musculosket Radiol. 2010;14:547–58.
68. Stull MA, Moser RP, Kransdorf MJ, Bogumill GP, Nelson MC. Magnetic resonance appearance of peripheral nerve sheath tumours. Skelet Radiol. 1991;20:9.
69. Koga H, Matsumoto S, Manabe J, Tanizawa T, Kawaguchi N. Definition of the target sign and its use for the diagnosis of schwannomas. Clin Orthop Relat Res. 2007;464:224–2.
70. Kakkar C, Shetty CM, Koteshwara P, Bajpai S. Telltale signs of peripheral neurogenic tumors on magnetic resonance imaging. Indian J Radiol Imaging. 2015;25:453–8.
71. Soldatos T, Fisher S, Karri S, Ramzi A, Sharma R, Chhabra A. Advanced MR imaging of peripheral nerve sheath tumors including diffusion imaging. Semin Musculoskelet Radiol. 2015;19:179–90.
72. Kubiena H, Entner T, Schmidt M, Frey M. Peripheral neural sheath tumors (PNST)—what a radiologist should know. Euro J Radiol. 2013;82:51–5.
73. Villanova JC, Woertler K, Narvaez JA, Barceló S, Martinez SJ, Villalón M, Miró J. Soft-tissue tumors update: MR imaging features according to the WHO classification. Euro Radiol. 2007;17:125–38.
74. Agrawal A, Singh GK, Rauniyar RK, Singh I. CT characteristics of dumbbell schwannoma arising from the fifth cervical nerve root. Eur J Gen Med. 2009;6:123–6.
75. Albert P, Patel J, Badawy K, Weissinger W, Brenner M, Bourhill I, Parnell J. Peripheral nerve schwannoma: a review of varying clinical presentations and imaging findings. J Foot Ankle Surg. 2017;56:632–7.
76. Resnick JM, Fanning CV, Caraway NP, Varma DG, Johnson M. Percutaneous needle biopsy diagnosis of benign neurogenic neoplasms. Diagn Cytopathol. 1997;16:17–25.
77. Ozdemir O, Ozsoy MH, Kurt C, Coskunol E, Calli I. Schwannomas of the hand and wrist: long-term results and review of the literature. J Orthop Surg (Hong Kong). 2005;13:267–72.
78. Oberle J, Kahamba J, Richter HP. Peripheral nerve schwannomas—an analysis of 16 patients. Acta Neurochir. 1997;139:949–53.
79. Park MJ, Seo KN, Kang HJ. Neurological deficit after surgical enucleation of schwannomas of the upper limb. J Bone Joint Surg Br. 2009;91:1482–6.
80. Spinner RJ. Complication avoidance. Neurosurg Clin N Am. 2004;15:193–202.
81. Spinner RJ, Amrami KK. What's new in the management of benign peripheral nerve lesions? Neurosurg Clin N Am. 2008;19:517–31.
82. Antoni NRE. Über Rückenmarksteumoren und Neurofibrome. JF Bergmann: Munich; 1920.
83. Enzinger FM, Weiss SW. Soft tissue tumors. CV Mosby: St Louis; 1988.
84. Rodriguez FJ, Folpe AL, Giannini C, Perry A. Pathology of peripheral nerve sheath tumors: diagnostic overview and update on selected diagnostic problems. Acta Neuropathol. 2012;123:295–319.
85. Wippold FJ 2nd, Lubner M, Perrin RJ, Lämmle M, Perry A. Neuropathology for the neuroradiologist: Antoni a and Antoni B tissue patterns. AJNR Am J Neuroradiol. 2007;28:1633–8.
86. Isobe K, Shimizu T, Akahane T, Kato H. Imaging of ancient schwannoma. AJR Am J Roentgeol. 2004;183:331–6.
87. Vlychou MI, Dailiana ZH. Ancient schwannoma of the hand. J Hand Surg Am. 2011;36:2030–3.
88. Folpe AL, Gowan K. Immunohistochemistry for analysis of soft tissue tumors. In: Weiss SW, Goldblum JR, editors. Enzinger and Weiss' soft tumors. 4th ed. St Louis: Mosby; 2001. p. 119–246.
89. Tiel R, Kline D. Peripheral nerve tumors: surgical principles, approaches, and techniques. Neurosurg Clin N Am. 2004;15(2):167–75.
90. Date R, Muramatsu K, Ihara K, Taguchi T. Advantages of intra-capsular micro-enucleation of schwannoma arising from extremities. Acta Neurochir. 2012;154:173–8.
91. Lusk MD, Kline DG, Garcia CA. Tumors of the brachial plexus. Neurosurgery. 1987;21:439–53.
92. Millesi H, Zoch G, Rath T. The gliding apparatus of peripheral nerve and its clinical significance. Ann Chir Main Memb Super. 1990;9:87–97.
93. Mizushima H. Neurological deficits before and after surgical resection of schwannomas in the upper extremities. J Reconstr Microsurg. 2016;32:371–7.

Neurofibromas

16

Lukas Rasulic, Milan Lepić, Andrija Savić,
and Miroslav Samardžić

16.1 Introduction

Neurofibroma is the second most common and most prevalent peripheral nerve tumor. As is the case with all tumors of peripheral nerve origin, it arises from the Schwann cells of the peripheral nerve sheath, but, unlike schwannoma, neurofibroma also comprises fibroblasts, perineurial cells, and mast cells in a variably myxoid background [1]. It is typically sporadic, but in 10% of cases, it occurs syndromically in the course of neurofibromatosis. The deletion in the NF1 gene is responsible for the tumor development in both sporadic and syndromic cases [2]. The lesions are usually in the form of a palpable mass and cause no specific symptoms. Surgery is considered curative, and malignant alteration is rare in sporadic cases [3].

L. Rasulic (✉) · A. Savić · M. Samardžić
Faculty of Medicine, University of Belgrade, Belgrade, Serbia

Department of Peripheral Nerve Surgery, Functional Neurosurgery and Pain Management Surgery, Clinic for Neurosurgery, University Clinical Center of Serbia, Belgrade, Serbia

M. Lepić
Medical Faculty of the Military Medical Academy, University of Defence, Belgrade, Serbia

Clinic for Neurosurgery, Military Medical Academy, Belgrade, Serbia

16.2 Classification

According to the WHO classification of tumors of the nervous system, neurofibroma belongs to the group of tumors of peripheral nerves, along with the subgroup of plexiform neurofibroma. Morphology codes of the International Classification of Diseases for Oncology (ICD-O) and the Systematized Nomenclature of Medicine (SNOMED) are 9540 and 9550 for the neurofibroma and plexiform neurofibroma, respectively. Behavior is coded as 0 (benign tumor) [4].

There is no strict clinical classification of neurofibromas, but the localization-based classification is usually taken into consideration as a starting point (Fig. 16.1).

Localized neurofibroma occurs, as a rule, as a sporadic lesion in the absence of neurofibromatosis. There are two forms that include cutaneous and intraneural neurofibroma. Localized forms usually do not interfere with the remaining axons. When indicated, surgery is curative and malignant alteration is rare [5].

Cutaneous neurofibroma is the most common type of all neurofibromas. It arises from the small cutaneous nerves. The tumor grows quickly and is well circumscribed, but not encapsulated, and therefore diffusely infiltrates the surrounding soft tissues. Probably due to the specific tissue characteristics, the cutaneous neurofibroma is often positioned in the dermis and subcutis skin layers [6]. The lesion will usually remain asymptomatic,

F. Guedes et al. (eds.), *Diagnostic Assessment and Treatment of Peripheral Nerve Tumors*,
https://doi.org/10.1007/978-3-030-77633-6_16

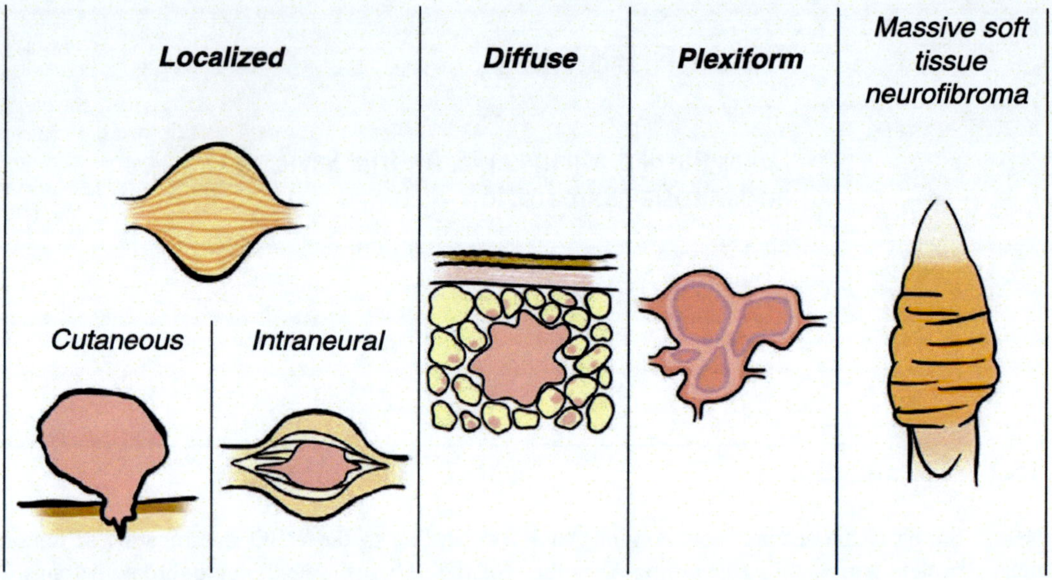

Fig. 16.1 Classification of neurofibromas

the axons may be identified traversing within it, and it will not grow larger than 2 cm [6].

Intraneural neurofibroma is the second most common type. It is characterized by segmental or fusiform nerve enlargement. Due to the developed true capsule, adjacent tissues are usually not involved, and the residual axons remain within the lesion [1].

Diffuse neurofibroma is an ill-defined form, which usually occurs in the head and neck regions [7]. The main characteristic is a diffuse growth pattern with infiltration of the adjacent subcutaneous tissues [8]. Only a minority of patients bear the NF1 disease. Malignant alteration is rare [9].

Plexiform neurofibroma is a third classical form. It appears almost exclusively in patients with NF1 and is characterized by irregular cylindrical or fusiform enlargement of a subcutaneous or deep nerve with the macroscopic appearance of a "bag of worms" [10]. The tumor is constrained to the nervous tissue, but its diffuse component is usually present through the extension into the subcutaneous tissues. Epineural fibroblasts are the main cells of origin of plexiform neurofibromas and are more primitive than Schwann cells; therefore, these tumors exhibit more aggressive growth patterns. Their sources are several motor and/or sensory fascicles or fascicular groups involving the nerve elements. Contrary to previous opinions, these lesions do contain a capsule [6]. The lifetime risk of malignant transformation is considered to be 5–10%. It is important to emphasize that the plexiform neurofibroma is appropriately diagnosed through the histopathological exam only in the presence of macroscopic appearance; therefore, the microscopic finding of plexiform characteristics should not be interpreted alone in order to confirm NF1 [11].

Massive soft tissue neurofibromas are considered a separate form by some authors, but these are more likely to represent a variation and combination of the classical forms. The massive tumor infiltrates the subcutaneous soft tissues and may cause *elephantiasis neuromatosa* with the underlying plexiform and diffuse neurofibroma components [12].

In addition to the classical forms, there are also numerous variations described in the literature, as summarized in Table 16.1. These usually occur in the localized form but may sometimes

Table 16.1 The most common variations associated with neurofibromas

Variation	Characteristics
Cellular	Increased cellularity, but without increase in mitotic activity; atypia may be present
Pigmented	Melanin production
Atypical/bizarre	Hyperchromatic, pleomorphic, atypical nuclei with degenerative changes. Lamellar distribution
Epithelioid	Cohesive epithelioid tumor cell nests
Granular cell	Eosinophilic and similar granular cells to those comprising granular cell tumors
Lipomatous	Present intrinsic adipocytes
Dendritic cell	Dendritic cell morphology with pseudorosettes
Hybrid neurofibroma/schwannoma	Schwannoma nodules

be present in diffuse neurofibromas. Their significance is usually limited to microscopic appearance, rather than an alteration in the course of the disease [13]. A hybrid form has also been described with small schwannoma nodules found within a neurofibroma [14]. These too do not increase the risk of malignant transformation, but their microscopic appearance might arise in the differential diagnosis of malignant peripheral nerve sheath tumor (MPNST) [13].

16.3 Epidemiology

The reported prevalence of neurofibromas is 10–24% of all isolated nerve tumors and 5% of all soft tissue tumors [15]. Neurofibromas affect men and women equally, and there is neither racial nor ethnic predilection. The age of onset is variable; however, young adult age 20–30 years is considered the most commonly associated. Localized lesions usually occur in adults aged 20–40 years, while the diffuse and plexiform types occur in small children [12].

16.4 Etiology/Genetics/Pathophysiology

Neurofibroma arises from the peripheral nerve sheath Schwann cells, probably those of non-myelinated nerve fibers. The genetic origin is due to the homozygotic loss of the NF1 gene on chromosome 17. This mutation leads to hyperplasia of the Schwann cells, which involves other cell types, developing ultimately into the neurofibroma [3, 16].

16.5 Neurofibromatosis

There are two forms of neurofibromatosis (NF): NF1 and NF2. NF1, or Von Recklinghausen disease, is a syndrome (with clear diagnostic criteria) that includes specific "café au lait" macules and additional nerve and musculoskeletal changes. The germline mutation of the NF1 (tumor suppressor gene) on chromosome 17 presents the genetic basis. Individual mutation is considered to cause neurofibroma, while the disease is caused by the more profound germline mutation. Fifty percent of NF1 cases are autosomal dominant, and the rest are a result of a new mutation. The importance of the identification of patients with NF1 concerns the risk for malignant transformation and the development of an MPNST [17]. Neurofibromatosis 2 is almost never associated with the presence of neurofibromas [3].

Neurofibromin is homologous to the GAP protein that influences cell cycling by downregulating the p21 RAS gene. It is encoded by the NF1 gene and is typically present in neurofibromas of patients with NF1, while it is absent in neurofibromas that undergo malignant transformation [17].

Solitary neurofibromas are almost never associated with NF1, whereas presentation with multiple neurofibromas should prompt consideration of possible NF1. Plexiform neurofibromas are almost pathognomonic for NF1 [18].

16.6 Histopathology

Neurofibromas are essentially benign nerve sheath tumors. Unlike schwannomas, neurofibromas are composed of differentiated neoplastic Schwann cells and an additional mixture of non-neoplastic components. The most common—localized—form is characterized by nodular and well-demarcated lesions, growing along the nerve, confined within the epineurium. Diffuse form neurofibromas infiltrate the surrounding soft tissues [19]. Plexiform neurofibromas are characterized by multiple fascicles involved within the tumor (filled with collagen and tumor cells) and contain centrally located residual nerve fibers [19].

Neoplastic Schwann cells are small, with curved or elongated nuclei, while the remaining tissue of neurofibroma is composed of fibroblasts within myxoid or collagen matrix in variable proportions. The Schwann cell component shows expression of S100 and Sox10 proteins [20].

Variations of both localized and diffuse forms with increased cellularity, pigmentation, nuclear atypia, and occasional mitotic figures may resemble low-grade MPNST and present a significant diagnostic dilemma [13].

16.7 Immunohistochemical Evaluation

The Schwann cells of neurofibroma are typically S100 protein positive. Some admixed perineurial cells may be positive for epithelial membrane antigen. Generally residual nerve twigs can be demonstrated with neurofilament stains. Neurofibromas usually contain a significant subpopulation of spindle cells, which are immunopositive for CD34 presenting with the specific "fingerprint" [21].

The resemblance of a human fingerprint is due to positive staining between whorled collagen bundles. If present in more than 60% of the lesion, it is useful in diagnosing neurofibroma and distinguishing neurofibroma from early desmoplastic melanoma [22].

Overview of histopathological and immunohistochemical characteristics is given in Fig. 16.2.

General	*Localized*		*Diffuse*	*Plexiform*	*Immunophenotype*
	Cutaneous	*Intraneural*			
Loose and haphazard spindled cells with poorly defined cell borders Myxoid to pale pink collagenous matrix Coarse collagen bundles "shredded carrots" Low to moderate cellularity Mast cells within the lesion Small, hyperchromatic, wavy nuclei "diving dolphins", "buckled" or "comma-shaped" sometimes with nuclear enlargement and smudgy chromatin Multinucleated giant cells (rare Absent to minimal mitoses	Arise from small cutaneous nerves Typically, unencapsulated with a "grenz zone" of uninvolved dermis between lesion and epidermis Overrun axons may be identified within May contain fat 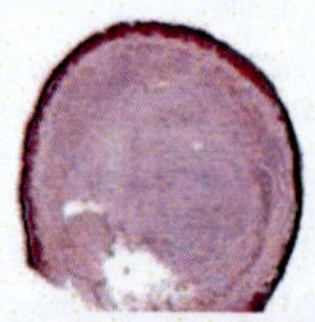	Subcutaneous lesions often have a true capsule Residual axons traverse through lesion Neurofilament immunohistochemistry and Bielschowsky stain show axons within center of lesion Often contains coarse, refractile collagen 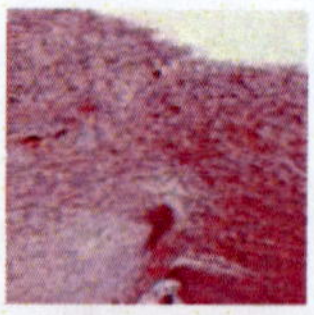	Poorly defined, expansile proliferation around adnexal structures, extending into the subcutaneous tissue and infiltrating adipose May entrap nerves or remain within Uniform matrix of fine, fibrillary collagen Shorter, rounder Schwann cells Pseudomeissnerian corpuscles, comprised of fibrillary and whorled Schwann cells	Multiple intertwined hypertrophic nerve fascicles Serpentine pattern with multiple nodules Predominantly myxoid or edematous background with thick collagen fibers Ma have atypia (nuclear enlargement, hyperchromasia)	S100 (+) in Schwann cells (approximately 50% of tumor cells) CD34 (+) in spindled fibroblasts with distinct "fingerprint" immunopositivity. EMA (+) in occasional perineurial cells Myelin basic protein (+) Neurofilament protein (+) in intratumoral axons Acid mucopolysaccharides (+) in mucinous stroma
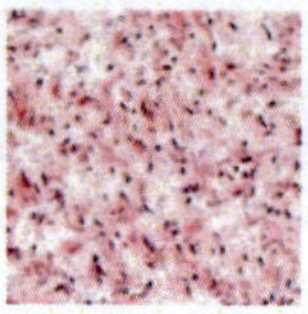	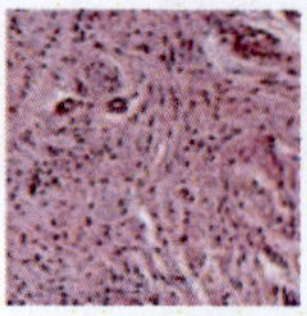	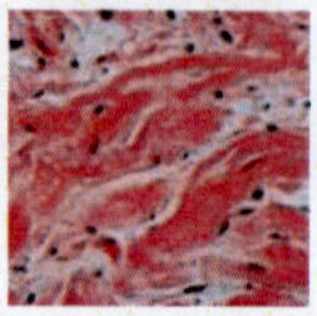	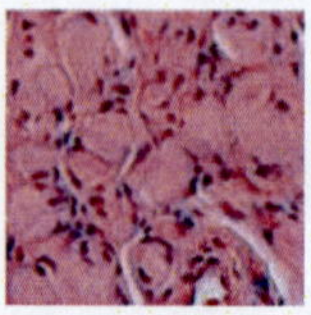	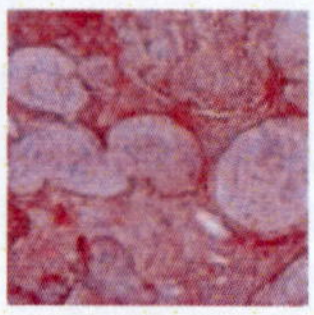	

Fig. 16.2 Histopathologic appearances of various forms of neurofibromas with their characteristics

16.8 Clinical Presentation

Neurofibroma usually presents as a solitary flesh-colored papule. Apart from the palpable mass, neurofibromas will in most cases remain silent. However, pain, disfigurement, and neurological deficits are much more common with neurofibroma than schwannoma, presumably due to infiltrating nature [21]. Discrete neurofibromas may sometimes cause discomfort and/or itching as they grow. In rare cases, due to the compression of a motor nerve, distal weakness may develop [23].

Multiple and plexiform neurofibromas are characteristic of neurofibromatosis in the pediatric age group. Plexiform neurofibromas present as superficial masses, with a tendency to occur in the head and neck.

The massive soft tissue neurofibroma variant is associated with redundant folds of skin and diffuse thickening of adjacent tissue (elephantiasis neuromatosa), while the MPNSTs and malignant transformed neurofibromas are commonly associated with pain [12, 23].

16.9 Imaging

16.9.1 Computerized Tomography (CT)

Neurofibromas appear as hypodense circumscribed masses with minimal or no contrast enhancement on CT, due to the presence of lipids in both nervous and fat tissues included in the tumor. Reliable differentiation between benign and malignant forms is not possible, and the CT is usually used for clarification only in cases related to bones or blood vessels [25].

16.9.2 Magnetic Resonance Imaging (MRI)

On MRI, the characteristic image is hypointense in T1 sequence and hyperintense in T2 with heterogeneous contrast enhancement, resulting in a target sign (central hypointense area in an overall homogeneous hyperintense space-occupying lesion in T2). The sign is a characteristic presentation of peripheral nerve tumors, especially subcutaneous neurofibroma, and is attributed to the accumulation of dense collagen-rich stroma in the center of the lesion [26]. In addition, when neurofibroma involves a larger nerve, two more characteristic signs may be detected: "fascicular sign," as a hyperintense mass with hypointense central foci presenting involved fascicles, and "split fat sign" presenting the peripheral rim of fat tissue [24] (Fig. 16.3).

Irregular contrast medium enhancement is considered characteristic of MPNST, but it may also be seen in plexiform neurofibromas due to the heterogeneous tumor structure [25].

16.9.3 Ultrasound

Peripheral nerve sheath tumors may be visualized with ultrasound as a mass arising from the nerve. Usually, a target sign may be present within the central fibrotic, relatively hyperechoic, area, surrounded by a hypoechoic rim of myxoid tissue. Doppler sonography may be used to distinguish between neurofibromas and schwannomas, since the former appears as a better vascularized lesion, although this technique is not very reliable [27].

Localized forms present no challenge to visualize, although in cutaneous neurofibromas, the nerve of origin may sometimes be hard to differentiate due to its small size. Multiple neurofibromas are usually found within the skin and subcutaneous tissue. Diffuse forms appear as ill-defined areas of subcutaneous infiltration and thickening, in typical localizations.

Pathognomonic appearance with multiple mass lesions arising from the fascicles of a large nerve trunk (bag of worms) is seen in plexiform neurofibromas. The finding of multiple convoluted masses may be followed over a long distance, extending to the terminal nerve branches [28] (Fig. 16.4).

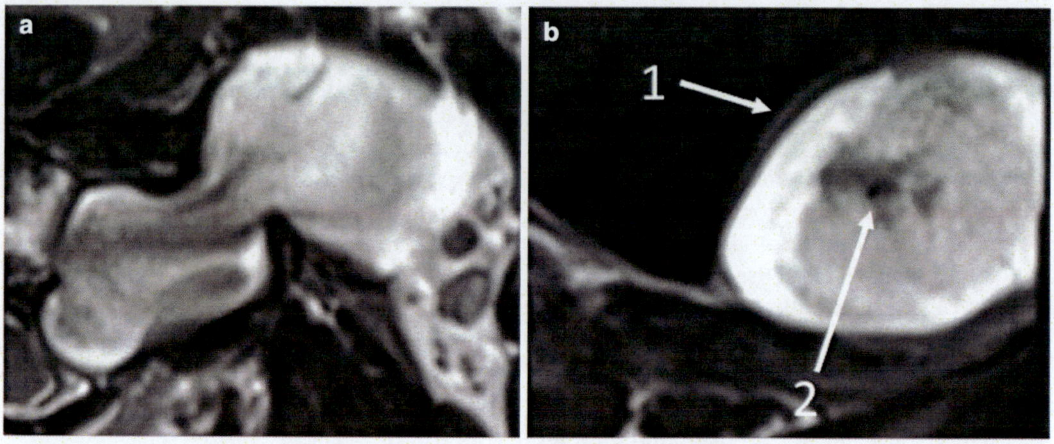

Fig. 16.3 The characteristic appearance of neurofibromas as seen with MRI. (**a**) Plexiform neurofibroma arising from the spinal nerve root (T2W). (**b**) Solitary neurofibroma arising from the intercostal nerve (T2W). The arrows indicate (1) the split fat sign and (2) the hypointense central focus inside a hyperintense mass

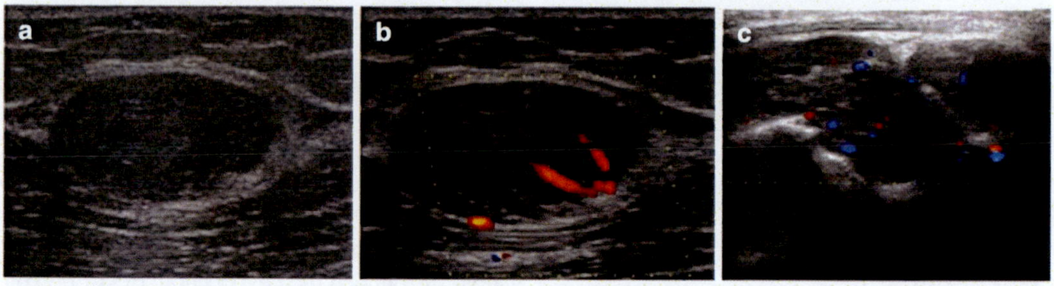

Fig. 16.4 The appearance of neurofibromas of various types visualized with the ultrasound. (**a**) Solitary neurofibroma. (**b**) Additional Doppler sonographic evaluation with only limited vascularization. (**c**) Plexiform neurofibroma

16.9.4 Management

A conservative approach is advocated for small tumors with no or minimal clinical manifestations. However, the fact that a surgical procedure is generally easier in small tumors should be kept in mind [29]. Neurofibromas should be considered for surgical treatment with the aim of complete or partial resection only if they are symptomatic. Significant discomfort or the localization in exposed or stigmatizing areas is also an indication for resection. In most cases, a clinical follow-up would be sufficient.

Resection of plexiform neurofibromas is indicated if they cause cosmetic disfigurement, pain, or compromise of function. Achieving complete resection is difficult due to the frequently present diffuse component. The involvement of large nerves or nerve roots may sometimes be considered as a contraindication for surgical treatment due to the foreseen deficit [23].

Biopsy should not be considered, except in cases highly suggestive of malignancy. To date, no successful chemotherapy has been identified, although ongoing clinical trials have shown promising results, especially with the use of selumetinib in the treatment of NF1-related lesions [30]. Rather than causing any beneficial effect, irradiation may even sometimes stimulate the growth of neurofibromas and should therefore be avoided. The role of adjuvant therapy in MPNSTs is discussed in Chap. 14.

16.10 Surgical Technique and Complications

The surgical procedure is planned individually in accordance with the physical and neurological findings and additional diagnostic procedures. Interventional embolization of feeding arteries may sometimes be considered, when significant bleeding is expected, most often in plexiform neurofibromas.

The aim of surgical treatment is the removal or the reduction of the tumor and functional preservation or recovery, depending on the initial status. When the tumors are located in exposed areas, the aesthetic outcome is most significant, with the temptation of complete tumor removal. Sometimes, skin expanders or reconstructive procedures may be used to avoid or minimize visible skin defects [12].

16.11 Principles of Surgical Treatment

There are some basic principles when planning the surgical procedure for the neurofibroma, including the following and presented in Fig. 16.5:

- Lengthy longitudinal incision over the mass should expose both proximal and distal healthy nerve parts.
- Incision should extend to the tumor capsule with partial excision of the epineurium.
- Microsurgical dissection is started at one of the tumor poles.
- Interfascicular neurolysis.
- Displaced and thinned fascicles are dissected away from the tumor capsule.
- Entering and exiting fascicles are sacrificed after evaluation using intraoperative

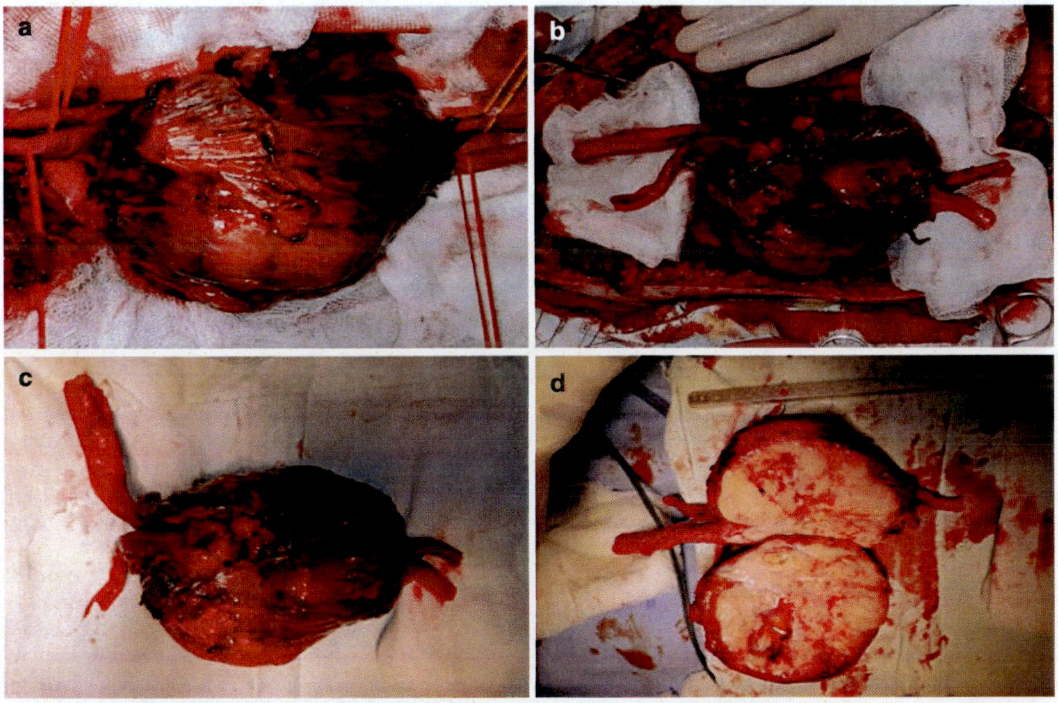

Fig. 16.5 Surgical procedure for the complete removal of the solitary intraneural neurofibroma. (**a**) Dissected tumor. (**b**) Resected tumor with sacrificed fascicles (in situ). (**c**) Resected and removed tumor with sacrificed fascicles. (**d**) Dissected tumor

neuromonitoring (this is usually done at about 1 cm above and 1 cm below the tumor to exclude the potential existence of small satellite tumors within the same fascicle).

- Vascular supply is usually at the proximal pole.
- Tumor is removed as a single mass whenever possible. In large tumors, intracapsular enucleation or debulking with the ultrasonic aspirator may be helpful.
- Tumor capsule is excised at the end of the procedure.

Fluorescein-guided surgery, coupled with intraoperative neurophysiological monitoring, should be implemented in plexiform neurofibromas, to achieve maximally safe resection, considering both the risks of postoperative deficit and the malignant transformation of the residual tumor [31]. General anesthesia with short-acting muscle relaxants is essential for reliable intraoperative monitoring. Continuous monitoring of the functional integrity of peripheral nerve during surgery is expected to lead to better functional preservation with the use of the vagus nerve stimulation electrodes (initially designed for thyroid surgery) [32]. Regional anesthetic blocks, if used in distal tumors, will also interfere with intraoperative EMG; therefore, they should be avoided.

The common complications related to the surgery of neurofibromas (apart from the neurological deficits) are mild and include localized pain, bleeding, scarring, and local infection.

16.12 Outcome and Prognosis

Neurofibromas are benign tumors. Functional preservation is possible in about 80% of cases after complete resection of sporadic neurofibromas and in 65–70% of cases associated with NF1. The resultant neurological deficit is usually mild and may be compensated with physiotherapy [33].

Local recurrence is extremely rare when complete excision of the lesion is performed, at least for several years [23]. Malignant transformation occurs exceedingly rarely, usually in the setting of neurofibromatosis and affecting deeply situated tumors. Even in the setting of neurofibromatosis, malignant transformation occurs in not more than 5–10% of patients [21]. It is most common in large, plexiform neurofibromas, followed by other deep neurofibromas associated with NF1, followed by cutaneous NF1-associated neurofibromas. The rate of malignant transformation is extremely low in non-NF1-associated neurofibromas [14].

Acknowledgments None.

Funding Disclosure None.

Conflict of Interest The authors have nothing to disclose, nor conflicts of interest related to this article, and the contents of this manuscript have not been previously published.

References

1. July J, Guha A. Peripheral nerve tumors. In: Grisold W, Soffietti R, editors. Neuro-oncology part II, Handbook of clinical neurology, vol. 105. Elsevier; 2012. p. 665–74. https://doi.org/10.1016/b978-0-444-53502-3.00016-1.
2. Muir D, Neubauer D, Lim IT, Yachnis AT, Wallace MR. Tumorigenic properties of neurofibromin-deficient neurofibroma Schwann cells. Am J Pathol. 2001;158:501–13. https://doi.org/10.1016/S0002-9440(10)63992-2.
3. Fugleholm K. The surgery of peripheral nerves (including tumors). Handb Clin Neurol. 2013;115:781–802. https://doi.org/10.1016/B978-0-444-52902-2.00045-X.
4. Louis DN, International Agency for Research on Cancer, Wiestler OD, Ohgaki H. WHO classification of tumours of the central nervous system. 2016; vol. 1. International Agency for Research on Cancer.
5. Woodruff JM. Pathology of tumors of the peripheral nerve sheath in type 1 neurofibromatosis. Am J Med Genet. 1999;89:23–30. https://doi.org/10.1002/(sici)1096-8628(19990326)89:1<23::aid-ajmg6>3.0.co;2-#.
6. Ortonne N, Wolkenstein P, Blakeley JO, Korf B, Plotkin SR, Riccardi VM, Miller DC, Huson S, Peltonen J, Rosenberg A, Carroll SL, Verma SK, Mautner V, Upadhyaya M, Stemmer-Rachamimov A. Cutaneous neurofibromas: current clinical and pathologic issues. Neurology. 2018;91:S5–S13. https://doi.org/10.1212/WNL.0000000000005792.
7. van Zuuren EJ, Posma AN. Diffuse neurofibroma on the lower back. J Am Acad Dermatol. 2003;48:938–40. https://doi.org/10.1067/mjd.2003.141.

8. Hassell DS, Bancroft LW, Kransdorf MJ, Peterson JJ, Berquist TH, Murphey MD, Fanburg-Smith JC. Imaging appearance of diffuse neurofibroma. AJR Am J Roentgenol. 2008;190:582–8. https://doi.org/10.2214/AJR.07.2589.
9. Schaefer IM, Fletcher CD. Malignant peripheral nerve sheath tumor (MPNST) arising in diffuse-type neurofibroma: clinicopathologic characterization in a series of 9 cases. Am J Surg Pathol. 2015;39:1234–41. https://doi.org/10.1097/PAS.0000000000000447.
10. Brandwein-Gensler MS, Mahadevia P, Gnepp DR. Chapter 5—nonsquamous pathologic diseases of the hypopharynx, larynx, and trachea. In: Gnepp DR, editor. Diagnostic surgical pathology of the head and neck. 2nd ed. Philadelphia: W.B. Saunders; 2009. p. 309–411. https://doi.org/10.1016/B978-1-4160-2589-4.00005-X.
11. Tchernev G, Chokoeva AA, Patterson JW, Bakardzhiev I, Wollina U, Tana C. Plexiform neurofibroma: a case report. Medicine. 2016;95:e2663. https://doi.org/10.1097/MD.0000000000002663.
12. Dorsi MJ, Belzberg AJ. Chapter 203—peripheral nerve tumors of the extremities. In: Quiñones-Hinojosa A, editor. Schmidek and sweet operative neurosurgical techniques. 6th ed. Philadelphia: W.B. Saunders; 2012. p. 2319–27. https://doi.org/10.1016/B978-1-4160-6839-6.10203-5.
13. Rodriguez FJ, Folpe AL, Giannini C, Perry A. Pathology of peripheral nerve sheath tumors: diagnostic overview and update on selected diagnostic problems. Acta Neuropathol. 2012;123:295–319. https://doi.org/10.1007/s00401-012-0954-z.
14. Ud Din N, Ahmad Z, Abdul-Ghafar J, Ahmed R. Hybrid peripheral nerve sheath tumors: report of five cases and detailed review of literature. BMC Cancer. 2017;17:349. https://doi.org/10.1186/s12885-017-3350-1.
15. Sandberg K, Nilsson J, Soe Nielsen N, Dahlin LB. Tumours of peripheral nerves in the upper extremity: a 22-year epidemiological study. Scand J Plast Reconstr Surg Hand Surg. 2009;43:43–9. https://doi.org/10.1080/02844310802489079.
16. Zheng H, Chang L, Patel N, Yang J, Lowe L, Burns DK, Zhu Y. Induction of abnormal proliferation by nonmyelinating Schwann cells triggers neurofibroma formation. Cancer Cell. 2008;13:117–28. https://doi.org/10.1016/j.ccr.2008.01.002.
17. Fanburg-Smith JC. Chapter 10—nerve sheath and neuroectodermal tumors. In: Folpe AL, Inwards CY, editors. Bone and soft tissue pathology. Philadelphia: W.B. Saunders; 2010. p. 193–238. https://doi.org/10.1016/B978-0-443-06688-7.00011-0.
18. Campian J, Gutmann DH. CNS tumors in neurofibromatosis. J Clin Oncol. 2017;35:2378–85. https://doi.org/10.1200/jco.2016.71.7199.
19. Bienkowski M, Furtner J, Hainfellner JA. Chapter 32—clinical neuropathology of brain tumors. In: Kovacs GG, Alafuzoff I (eds) Handbook of clinical neurology, vol 145. Elsevier, 2018. p. 477–534. https://doi.org/10.1016/B978-0-12-802395-2.00032-8.
20. Karamchandani JR, Nielsen TO, van de Rijn M, West RB. Sox10 and S100 in the diagnosis of soft-tissue neoplasms. Appl Immunohistochem Mol Morphol. 2012;20:445–50. https://doi.org/10.1097/PAI.0b013e318244ff4b.
21. Billings SD, Goldblum JR. Chapter 13—soft tissue tumors and tumor-like reactions. In: Busam KJ, editor. Dermatopathology. Philadelphia: W.B. Saunders; 2010. p. 499–564. https://doi.org/10.1016/B978-0-443-06654-2.00013-5.
22. Yeh I, Vemula SS, Mirza SA, McCalmont TH. Neurofibroma-like spindle cell melanoma: CD34 fingerprint and CGH for diagnosis. Am J Dermatopathol. 2012;34:668–70. https://doi.org/10.1097/DAD.0b013e318244819a.
23. Tonsgard JH, Yamini B, Frim DM. Chapter 48—surgical management of neurofibromatosis types 1 and 2. In: Quiñones-Hinojosa A, editor. Schmidek and sweet operative neurosurgical techniques. 6th ed. Philadelphia: W.B. Saunders; 2012. p. 581–7. https://doi.org/10.1016/B978-1-4160-6839-6.10048-6.
24. Kakkar C, Shetty CM, Koteshwara P, Bajpai S. Telltale signs of peripheral neurogenic tumors on magnetic resonance imaging. Indian J Radiol Imaging. 2015;25:453–8. https://doi.org/10.4103/0971-3026.169447.
25. Salamon J, Mautner VF, Adam G, Derlin T. Multimodal imaging in neurofibromatosis type 1-associated nerve sheath tumors. Rofo. 2015;187:1084–92. https://doi.org/10.1055/s-0035-1553505.
26. Wasa J, Nishida Y, Tsukushi S, Shido Y, Sugiura H, Nakashima H, Ishiguro N. MRI features in the differentiation of malignant peripheral nerve sheath tumors and neurofibromas. AJR Am J Roentgenol. 2010;194:1568–74. https://doi.org/10.2214/ajr.09.2724.
27. Campbell R. Chapter 58—ultrasound of soft tissue masses. In: Allan PL, Baxter GM, Weston MJ, editors. Clinical ultrasound. 3rd ed. Edinburgh: Churchill Livingstone; 2011. p. 1109–25. https://doi.org/10.1016/B978-0-7020-3131-1.00058-4.
28. Reynolds DL Jr, Jacobson JA, Inampudi P, Jamadar DA, Ebrahim FS, Hayes CW. Sonographic characteristics of peripheral nerve sheath tumors. AJR Am J Roentgenol. 2004;182:741–4. https://doi.org/10.2214/ajr.182.3.1820741.
29. Rasulic L. Current concept in adult peripheral nerve and brachial plexus surgery. J Brachial Plex Peripher Nerve Inj. 2017;12:e7–e14. https://doi.org/10.1055/s-0037-1606841.
30. Dombi E, Baldwin A, Marcus LJ, Fisher MJ, Weiss B, Kim A, Whitcomb P, Martin S, Aschbacher-Smith LE, Rizvi TA, Wu J, Ershler R, Wolters P, Therrien J, Glod J, Belasco JB, Schorry E, Brofferio A, Starosta AJ, Gillespie A, Doyle AL, Ratner N, Widemann BC. Activity of Selumetinib in neurofibromatosis type 1-related plexiform neurofibromas. N Engl J Med. 2016;375:2550–60. https://doi.org/10.1056/NEJMoa1605943.

31. Vetrano IG, Saletti V, Nazzi V. Fluorescein-guided resection of plexiform neurofibromas: how I do it. Acta Neurochir. 2019;161:2141–5. https://doi.org/10.1007/s00701-019-04038-5.
32. Saponaro-González Á, Pérez-Lorensu PJ. Novel approach to continuous neurophysiological monitoring during surgery of peripheral nerve tumors. Surg Neurol Int. 2017;8:184. https://doi.org/10.4103/sni.sni_414_16.
33. Kim DH, Murovic JA, Tiel RL, Moes G, Kline DG. A series of 397 peripheral neural sheath tumors: 30-year experience at Louisiana State University Health Sciences Center. J Neurosurg. 2005;102:246–55. https://doi.org/10.3171/jns.2005.102.2.0246.

Perineuriomas

17

Christine Brand and Gregor Antoniadis

Perineurioma is a rare tumor entity. Children and young adults are particularly affected [1]. There is no gender difference in the frequency of occurrence [2]. The tumor mainly affects the large nerves of both the upper and lower extremities with equal distribution [2]. Due to the gradual course of the disease, the diagnosis is usually made late, if at all [3].

17.1 Symptoms

Typically, a motor mononeuropathy exists. The patients show a slowly progressive paralysis with muscular atrophy (see Fig. 17.1), but only in rare cases is there a sensory deficit.

Pain is often absent. The symptoms are said to be caused by compression of the axons due to the increase in neoplastic tissue [4].

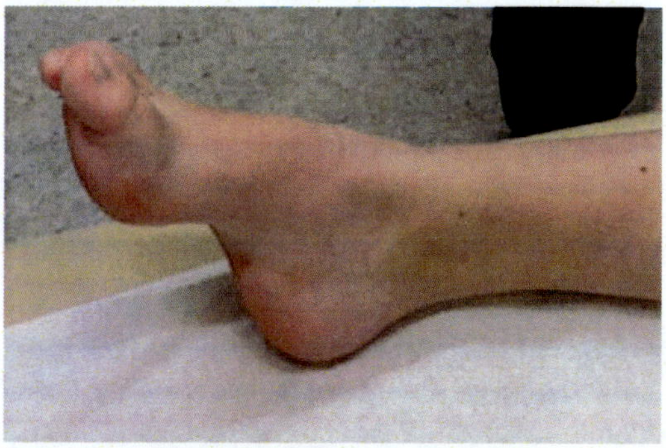

Fig. 17.1 Neurogenic clubfoot as a result of a perineurioma of the right sciatic nerve

17.2 Pathology

Perineuriomas are considered benign nerve tumors. They can occur within a nerve (intraneural) or manifest extraneurally as a soft tissue tumor. However, these rarely have a direct relationship to the nerve. Subtypes are the sclerosing and the reticular perineurioma. The malignant perineurioma is very rare and originates exclusively from extraneural perineuriomas [1]. Intraneural perineuriomas, on the other hand, do not undergo malignant transformation and are very slow growing. Perineuriomas are associated with anomalies of chromosome 22, in particular monosomy or deletion of the 22q11–q13.1 bands [5].

Macroscopically, perineurioma appears as a distinct hardening and spindle-like thickening

C. Brand
Department of Neurosurgery, Munich Clinic Bogenhausen, Munich, Germany

G. Antoniadis (✉)
Peripheral Nerve Surgery Unit, University of Ulm, Hospital Guenzburg, Guenzburg, Germany
e-mail: gregor.antoniadis@uni-ulm.de

F. Guedes et al. (eds.), *Diagnostic Assessment and Treatment of Peripheral Nerve Tumors*,
https://doi.org/10.1007/978-3-030-77633-6_17

of the affected nerve section. Histological findings are long, thin tumor cells with bipolar cytoplasmic processes with wavy or tapering nuclei [1]. The perineurioma cells infiltrate the endoneurium of the affected fascicle and form concentric whorls of perineural cells (pseudo-onion bulbs) around the nerve fiber. Immunohistochemically, a positive reaction to the epithelial membrane antigen (EMA) is, by definition, observed [6]. The perineurioma cells show no expression of the Schwann cell marker S-100. Claudin-1 and GLUT, however, are often expressed. Mitosis can occur, but necrosis is absent, as a rule [1].

17.3 Diagnostic

The gold standard in perineurioma diagnostics is MRI (ideally 3 Tesla). MRI shows long-distance enlargement of fascicles within the affected nerves and an intense, homogeneous gadolinium enhancement [3, 7, 8] (see Figs. 17.2 and 17.3). Affected fascicles appear isointense on T1- and hyperintense on T2-weighted images [3, 7, 8]. Due to its characteristic appearance, perineurioma can be distinguished from the most common differential diagnosis (chronic inflammatory demyelinating polyneuropathy/mononeuropathy) on MRI [3]. The high-resolution ultrasound can describe the extent of the tumor relatively precisely just like the MRI [9]. Both methods are also used in follow-up care [10]. In electrophysiological studies, amplitude reductions, conduction blocks, as well as denervation signs may occur in EMG.

17.4 Therapy Options

The therapy of perineuriomas is not undisputed. Due to the small number of cases, general recommendations are not available. As there is usually no complete loss of function of the affected nerve, there is a risk of functional impairment through surgery.

However, the risk of malignancy does not seem to exist [4].

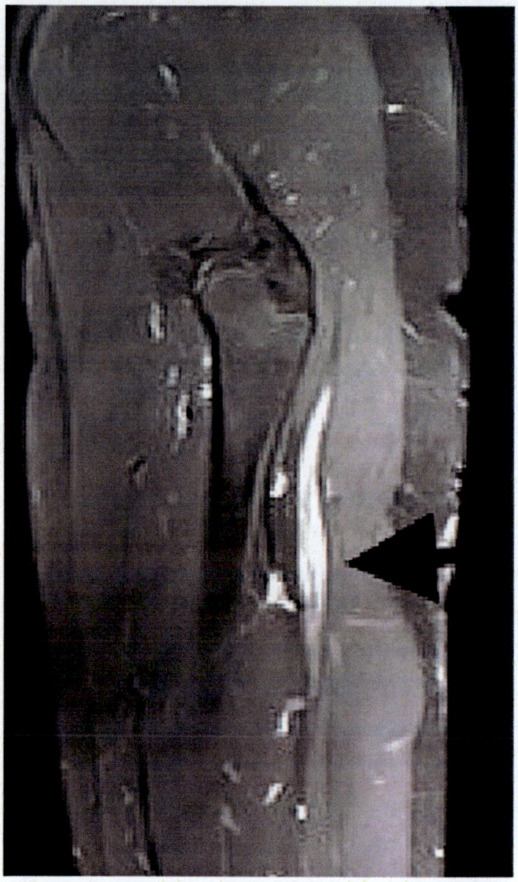

Fig. 17.2 Example of an intraneural perineurioma of the right sciatic nerve (arrow) in MRI (sagittal) after application of gadolinium

In addition to the possibility of merely observing the tumor by performing regular imaging and electrophysiological examinations, there is the alternative of surgical therapy. Here, too, various surgical strategies are available.

In order to confirm the diagnosis, at least one biopsy of an affected and non-functional fascicle should be taken [11] (see Figs. 17.4 and 17.5). Based on the theory that the axons are compressed by the tumor cells, a decompression of the fascicle by an epineurotomy makes sense, even though there are not yet studies to date able to demonstrate its effectiveness.

Another possibility is the complete resection of the tumor with subsequent reconstruction by nerve grafting [3, 4, 10, 12]. The resection

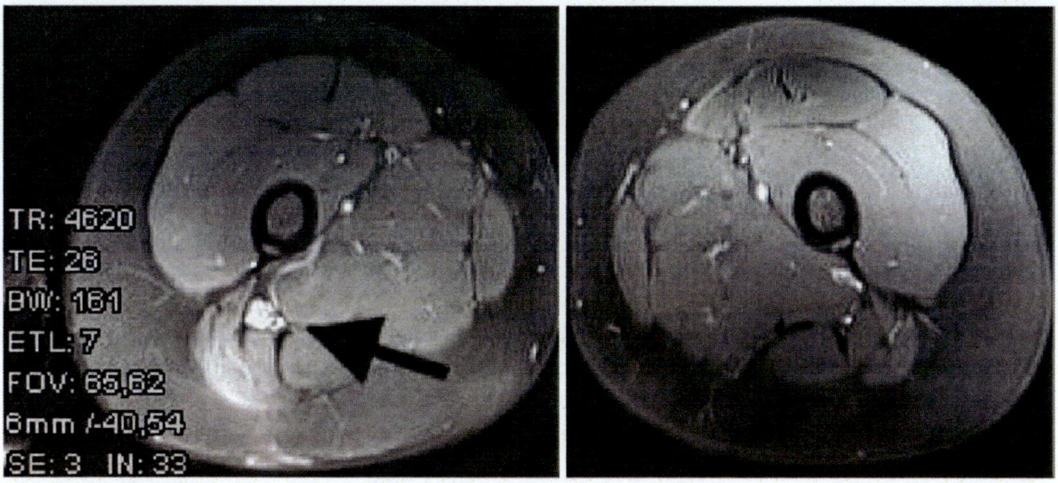

Fig. 17.3 Intraneural perineurioma of the right sciatic nerve (arrow) in MRI (axial) after application of gadolinium

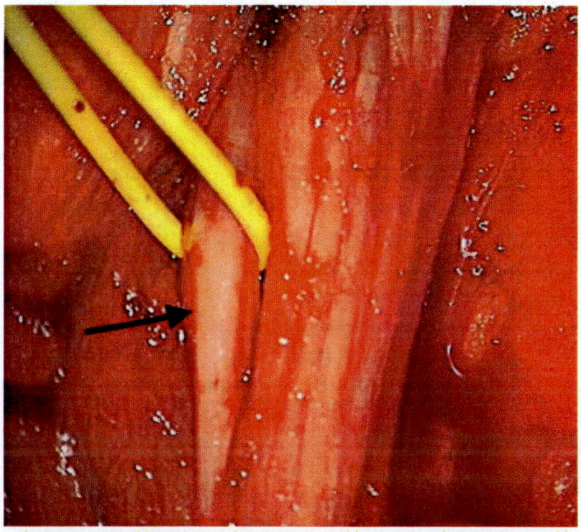

Fig. 17.4 Thickened, non-functional fascicle of the sciatic nerve (arrow) before biopsy

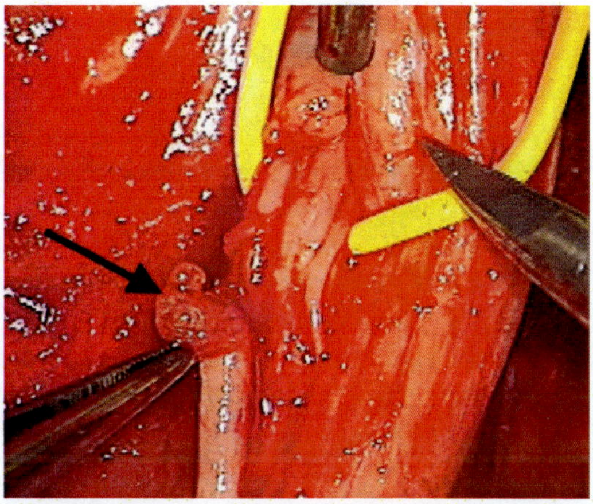

Fig. 17.5 Thickened, non-functional fascicle of the sciatic nerve (arrow) after biopsy

margins must be tumor-free to prevent re-spreading. For this, the possibility of a frozen section analysis must be available [10]. However, the presence of further tumor cells at other sites within the nerve cannot be ruled out either intraoperatively or by imaging. A complete resection of the tumor can therefore not be guaranteed. In addition, it should be noted that a complete loss of function after resection of the tumor and subsequent transplantation is initially very likely.

A third option is a tendon transfer to improve the reduced motor function. The tendon transfer can be performed in combination with or without tumor resection. Also, in certain cases, a distal nerve transfer might be possible to restore function, for example, distal anterior interosseous nerve to ulnar motor transfer if the tumor involves the proximal ulnar nerve.

Regardless of the surgical method, the surgical microscope and intraoperative nerve stimulation as well as micro-instruments should be used intraoperatively. The high-resolution ultrasound for planning the skin incision and showing the tumor extent can be helpful. The determination of the nerve conduction velocity can also be useful.

As a rule, it is not necessary to install a drainage system. We recommend elastic wrapping of the corresponding extremity. The bandage should be changed after 2 h. If no transplantation has been performed, the extremity can be mobilized immediately [10].

17.5 Results

Long-term data are not available due to the small number of studies with low case numbers. Mauermann et al. describe in a study of 23 patients with confirmed perineurioma that no significant progress was observed within 45 months. Based on these data, they favor a conservative approach [11]. In a retrospective study with 20 patients, Wilson et al. were able to show that intraneural perineuriomas rarely gain length on MRI. In addition, they do not spread to other nerves [8]. Restrepo et al. do not consider a biopsy to be necessary in the case of characteristic MRI findings with a suitable clinical course and symptoms and recommend regular follow-up examinations [3]. Gruen et al., however, performed a complete resection of the tumor with subsequent transplantation in 15 patients [13]. Ultimately, a therapy concept must be worked out individually after weighing all risks with the patient concerned.

17.6 Follow-Up Treatment

After diagnosis, we recommend the next checkup 3 months later. In addition to a current 3 Tesla MRI with gadolinium, an electrophysiological examination should be performed. If worsening of symptoms should occur, the therapy regime must be re-evaluated.

References

1. Macarenco RS, Ellinger F, Oliveira AM. Perineurioma: a distinctive and underrecognized peripheral nerve sheath neoplasm. Arch Pathol Lab Med. 2007;131:625–36.
2. Alkhaili J, Cambon-Binder A, Belkheyar Z. Intraneural perineurioma: a retrospective study of 19 patients. Pan Afr Med J. 2018;30:275. https://doi.org/10.11604/pamj.2018.30.275.16072.
3. Restrepo CE, Amrami KK, Howe BM, Dyck PJB, Mauermann ML, Spinner RJ. The almost-invisible perineurioma. Neurosurg Focus. 2015;39:E13. http:thejns.org/doi/abs/10.3171/2015.6.FOCUS15225
4. Boyanton BL, Jones JK, Shenaq SM, Hicks MJ, Bhattacharjee MB. Intraneural perineurioma: a systemic review with illustrative cases. Arch Pathol Lab Med. 2007;131:1382–92. https://doi.org/10.1043/1543-2165.
5. Emory TS, Scheithauer BW, Hirose T, Wood M, Onofrio BM, Jenkins RB. Intraneural perineurioma. A clonal neoplasm associated with abnormalities of chromosome 22. Am J Clin Pathol. 1995;103(6):696–704.
6. Ariza A, Bilbao JM, Rosai J. Immunohistochemical detection of epithelial membrane antigen in normal perineurial cells and perineurioma. Am J Surg Pathol. 1988;12(9):678–83.
7. Wilson TJ, Howe BM, Stewart SA, Spinner RJ, Amrami KK. Clinicoradiological features of intraneural perineuriomas obviate the need for tissue diagnosis. J Neurosurg. 2018;129(4):1034–40. https://doi.org/10.3171/2017.5.JNS17905.
8. Wilson TJ, Amrami KK, Howe BM, Spinner RJ. Clinical and radiological follow-up of intraneural perineuriomas. Neurosurgery. 2019;85(6):786–92. https://doi.org/10.1093/neuros/nyy476.
9. Koenig RW, Pedro MT, Heinen CPG, Schmidt T, Richter H-P, Antoniadis G, Kretschmer T. High-resolution ultrasonography in evaluating peripheral nerve entrapment and trauma. Neurosurg Focus. 2009;26:E13. https://doi.org/10.3171/FOC.2009.26.2.E13.
10. Kretschmer T, Antoniadis G, Assmus H. Nervenchirurgie Trauma, Tumor, Kompression. 1st ed. Berlin: Springer; 2014.
11. Mauermann ML, Amrami KK, Kuntz NL, Spinner RJ, Dyck PJ, Bosch EP, et al. Longitudinal study of intraneural perineurioma—a benign, focal hypertrophic neuropathy of youth. Brain. 2009;132:2265–76. https://doi.org/10.1093/brain/awp169.
12. Scheller C, Richter HP, Scheuerle A, Kretschmer T, König RW, Antoniadis G. Intraneural perineuriomas; a rare entity. Clinical, surgical and neuropathological details in the management of these lesions. Zentralbl Neurochir. 2008;69(3):134–8. https://doi.org/10.1055/s-2008-1077081.
13. Gruen JP, Mitchell W, Kline DG. Resection and graft repair for localized hypertrophic neuropathy. Neurosurgery. 1998;43:78–83.

Non-neurogenic Tumoral and Pseudotumoral Lesions Affecting Peripheral Nerve

18

Tomas Marek, Kimberly K. Amrami, and Robert J. Spinner

18.1 Non-neurogenic Tumoral and Pseudotumoral Lesions

Non-neurogenic entities affecting peripheral nerves consist of a heterogeneous group of lesions including ganglion cysts, adipose lesions of nerve, neuromuscular choristomas, and many others. Common features may include neuropathy from mass effect and the benign nature of most of them; others may be infiltrative and malignant. Clinical presentations differ vastly among these lesions. Some of them can include overgrowth or undergrowth in the territory of the affected nerve.

18.2 Benign Lesions

18.2.1 Ganglion Cysts

Ganglion cysts affecting peripheral nerves are relatively common non-neurogenic tumoral lesions often presenting with neuropathy due to compression or entrapment of the affected nerve. These lesions can be intraneural as well as extraneural.

18.2.1.1 Intraneural Ganglion Cyst

Intraneural ganglion cysts are mucinous lesions of benign character occurring within the epineurium. The most commonly affected nerve is the common peroneal nerve at the level of superior tibiofibular joint. Other nerves and sites are reported in the medical literature including the ulnar at the elbow or wrist, tibial at the knee or ankle, and many others [1].

The pathogenesis of intraneural ganglion cysts has long been controversial with many theories proposing possible explanations. In recent years, the articular theory has become widely accepted [2] with many published articles supporting it [3]. In fact, this theory has been shown to play an important role in the pathogenesis of other similar conditions such as an adventitial cysts affecting arteries and veins [4]. In this theory, an articular branch serves as a conduit through which synovial (joint) fluid penetrates into nerve from a neighboring joint; propagation is determined by pressures and pressure fluxes.

MRI is the imaging modality of choice for diagnosis [5, 6]. These lesions are best appreciated on T2-weighted images but more completely characterized after the administration of intravenous contrast. All of these cysts arise from joint(s), but the identification of the individual joint connection can be challenging. The desired

T. Marek · R. J. Spinner (✉)
Department of Neurologic Surgery, Mayo Clinic, Rochester, MN, USA
e-mail: spinner.robert@mayo.edu

K. K. Amrami
Department of Radiology, Mayo Clinic, Rochester, MN, USA

F. Guedes et al. (eds.), *Diagnostic Assessment and Treatment of Peripheral Nerve Tumors*,
https://doi.org/10.1007/978-3-030-77633-6_18

technical parameters of the MRI examination, including in-plane resolution and slice thickness, field of view, and the use of 3D imaging, should be taken into account when planning the study in order to optimize the probability of seeing what often are very subtle joint connections. Because these cysts are associated with articular branches of nerve, they typically follow a recurrent pathway that can look like a "J" or even a "U." This pattern is commonly seen in intraneural cysts affecting the deep branch of the peroneal nerve at the superior tibiofibular joint (Fig. 18.1).

Treatment of the intraneural ganglion cysts should be focused on identifying and disconnecting the joint connection. After exposing the affected nerve, all nerve branches of the affected nerve should be clearly marked with vessel loops. The cyst can be decompressed but need not to be resected. The joint connection is disconnected to prevent recurrence of the lesion. In select cases, the joint connection can be difficult to identify due to anatomical reasons. At the superior tibiofibular joint, the joint can be ablated with or without joint disconnection [2].

Outcomes post-surgery are in general very positive with return of function soon after the procedure. If a lesion is treated long after symptoms occurred (several months, years), atrophic changes in affected muscles can be permanent, and long-standing rehabilitation is necessary.

18.2.1.2 Extraneural Ganglion Cyst

Extraneural ganglion cysts are mucinous lesions which develop from a synovial joint and secondarily cause extrinsic compression; the capsular defect does not involve the articular branch. MRI plays an important role in the diagnosis as in the diagnosis of the intraneural ganglion cysts by identifying both the origin and extent of the cyst and the specific nerve affected. Treatment of these lesions consists of resection of the cyst and/or repair of the defect in the synovium or addressing the joint connection or abnormality. Outcomes are very positive in the majority of the cases; however, recurrence of the lesion can occur if the origin of the cyst at the joint is not addressed.

18.2.2 Adipose Lesions of Peripheral Nerve

In recent years, much advancement has been done in the understanding of the pathophysiology, natural history, and genetics of adipose lesions affecting peripheral nerves. This group, once considered quite homogeneous, ranges vastly in the clinical presentation, management, and outcomes and therefore can be envisioned as a spectrum of lesions. This group consists of intraneural and extraneural lipomas and lipomatosis of nerve. In some cases, a clear delineation between typical examples can be blurred [7, 8].

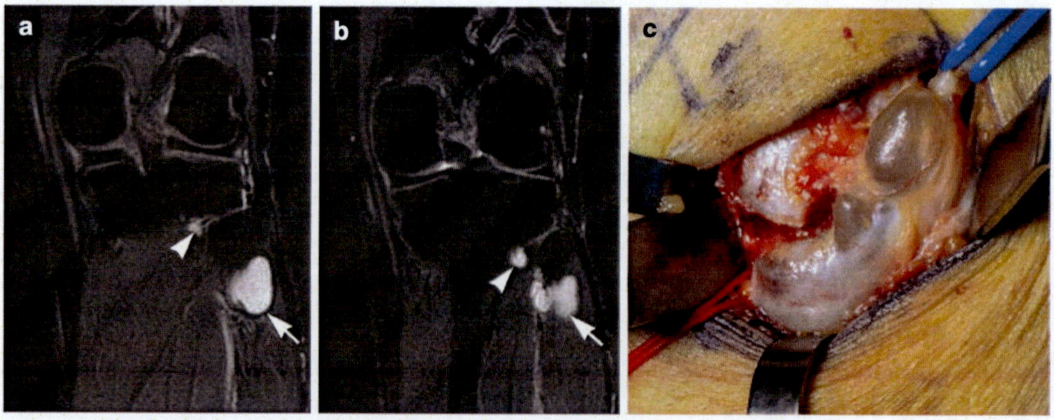

Fig. 18.1 MRI of a peroneal intraneural ganglion cyst and operative photo. (**a, b**) Serial T2-weighted FS (fat-saturated) MR images showing an intraneural ganglion cyst (arrow) and its joint connection (arrowhead) to the superior tibiofibular joint. (**c**) Operative photo of the intraneural ganglion cyst. The articular branch is marked with a red vasoloop. The common peroneal nerve is marked with a blue loop

18.2.2.1 Intraneural Lipoma

Intraneural lipomas are relatively rare adipose lesions of nerve and can be characterized as an encapsulated lipomatous mass within the epineurium of the affected nerve. These lesions are probably underreported [8]. They most commonly affect the median nerve at the wrist; however, many other locations besides the median nerve have been reported including ulnar, radial, posterior interosseous, common peroneal, superficial peroneal, brachial plexus, sciatic, and tibial nerves [8].

Patients with these lesions usually present with symptoms of compressive neuropathy. Diagnosis of these lesions is most commonly confirmed using MRI. Ultrasonography can be also useful; however, this modality does not provide as much diagnostic information as MRI, especially if a neural structure with deep location is affected (e.g., lumbosacral plexus). Intraneural lipomas have high signal intensity on T1-weighted MRI sequence, the same signal as, for example, subcutaneous fat, with suppression of the fatty elements of the lesions with techniques such as STIR (short tau inversion recovery) imaging or frequency-specific fat suppression [8] (Fig. 18.2a).

Recently, intraneural lipomas have been subclassified into two subgroups: encapsulated and hybrid intraneural lipomas. The first group is typically resected without much difficulty. On imaging, these lesions appear as a high-intensity signal encapsulated mass within the epineurium, and a capsule can often be identified around the lesion on MRI. The goal of the treatment should be total resection to achieve nerve decompression. During surgery, the epineurium is dissected, and the lesion "pops out." If such a lesion is an incidental finding, no immediate action is usually necessary, and follow-up is recommended. The other group (i.e., hybrid lesions) has been shown to demonstrate variable degree of interdigitating fat between the fascicles. This makes such lesions more difficult to dissect, and typically a more meticulous approach is needed to resect the lesion completely [8] (Fig. 18.2b).

On histopathological examination, these lesions consist predominantly of fat [8]; however, lesions consisting of mixed tissues (i.e., adipose and fibrous [9], adipose and cartilaginous [10], and adipose and eosinophilic cells with hyaline matrix [11]) have been reported. No intraneural lipoma has ever been associated with nerve-territory overgrowth, which is in contrast to lipomatosis of nerve. Overall intraneural lipomas have good clinical outcomes post-surgery with complete recovery in the majority of cases without lesion relapse.

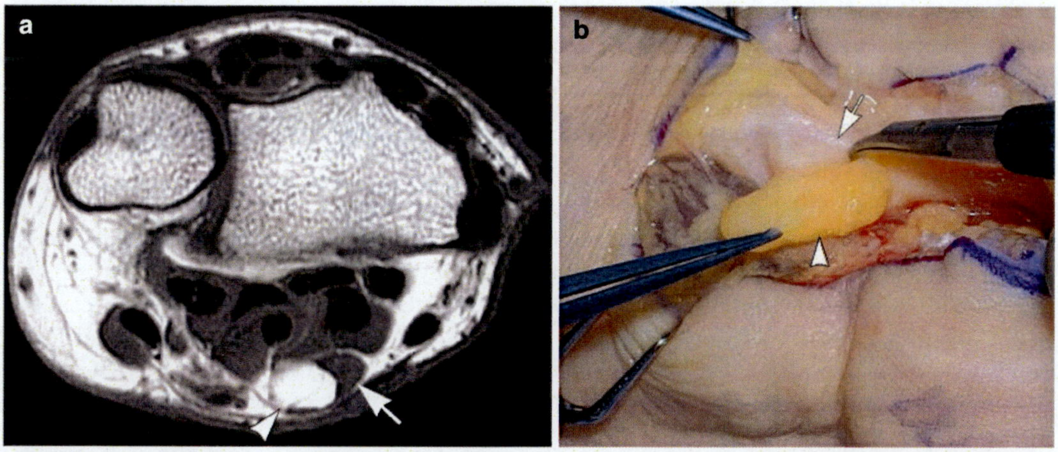

Fig. 18.2 Intraneural lipoma. (**a**) Axial T1-weighted MR image showing an intraneural lipoma (arrowhead) within the epineurium of the median nerve (arrow) at the wrist. The intraneural lipoma compressed the median nerve and caused neuropathy in this particular case. (**b**) Operative photo of the same patient as in (**a**). Intraneural lipoma (arrowhead) was easily resected after dissecting the epineurium of the median nerve (arrow)

18.2.2.2 Extraneural Lipoma

Extraneural lipomas arise outside of the epineurium and cause compressive neuropathy secondarily. Extraneural lipomas can arise as a stand-alone lesion. However, these lesions may also be associated with lipomatosis of nerve (LN), typically occurring in the territory of the same nerve (see below) [7]. MRI is utilized in the diagnosis of these lesions as well both to identify and characterize the lipoma and determine which nerve is affected. The aim of treatment is to decompress the affected nerve to improve symptoms. These lesions typically do not relapse, unless when associated with LN or in the case of incomplete resection. In such cases, they might regrow [7, 12].

18.2.2.3 Lipomatosis of Nerve

Lipomatosis of nerve (LN) is another part of the spectrum of adipose lesions affecting nerves. Unlike intra- and extraneural lipomas, LN is a fascinating pathology with a relatively broad spectrum of clinical presentations. It is characterized by abundant fibro-adipose tissue within the epineurium that splays the individual fascicles apart with interposed fat. In about 62%, there is associated nerve-territory overgrowth [12].

LN is reported much more frequently than other adipose lesions of nerve; however, confusion in terminology surrounds this entity. The term lipomatosis of nerve was proposed by WHO in 2002 [13]; however, many other terms are used in the medical literature. One of the most commonly used ones (even though outdated) is fibrolipomatous hamartoma followed by lipofibromatous hamartoma, neural fibrolipoma, and others [12]. When massive nerve-territory overgrowth is present, the term macrodystrophia lipomatosa is often utilized. This terminology inconsistency creates confusion among physicians, and one can think that each term is reserved for a different entity despite all being one pathology with different phenotypes.

LN presents early in life. Most patients typically present with symptoms in their first decade due to the LN. Family history is negative in all cases. The presenting symptoms range from compressive neuropathy (including sensory and/or motor deficit) to associated nerve-territory overgrowth, sometimes leading to massive deformities. Men and women are affected equally. A slight predominance of right-sided lesions has been reported [12]. The most commonly affected nerve is the median at the wrist; however, any other nerve can be affected. Interestingly LN does not occur or extend intradurally [14].

The diagnosis of LN can be established solely based on imaging features which have been long considered pathognomonic. The lesion is best appreciated on a T1-weighted MRI sequence, as are all other adipose lesions of nerve. On the axial plane, the abundant adipose tissue dispersed between nerve fascicles creates the so called co-axial cable-like appearance. On the longitudinal plane, the appearance is often referred to as spaghetti-like (Fig. 18.3). Similar features can be also appreciated using ultrasonography. These pathognomonic features obviate the need for a diagnostic biopsy which should be reserved only for very unclear cases with atypical features [15, 16].

One of the hallmark of LN is associated nerve-territory overgrowth which is present in about 62% of cases [12]. Overgrowth can affect soft tissue and bony structures. This can be very subtle and only present as small skin lesions [7] to very massive overgrowth leading to substantial deformities [7, 17]. Soft tissue overgrowth includes skin lesions [7], subcutaneous lipomas [7], deep extraneural lipomas [7], and muscle lipomatosis [17]. Overgrowth of osseous structures can cause dramatic deformities which can result in movement restrictions of the affected body part (Fig. 18.4). Ostechondromas might also occur as a part of the nerve-territory overgrowth features [18].

Recent genetic studies associated somatic activating PIK3CA mutations with various overgrowth syndromes, including LN. The exact pathophysiological mechanism remains unknown [19]. Interestingly, recent work identified PIK3CA mutations in LN cases irrespective of overgrowth status (i.e., mutation present in cases with and without overgrowth), suggesting that other factors are necessary for overgrowth to develop [20]. The type of nerve affected by LN seems to also play an important role in LN-associated overgrowth and might be one of

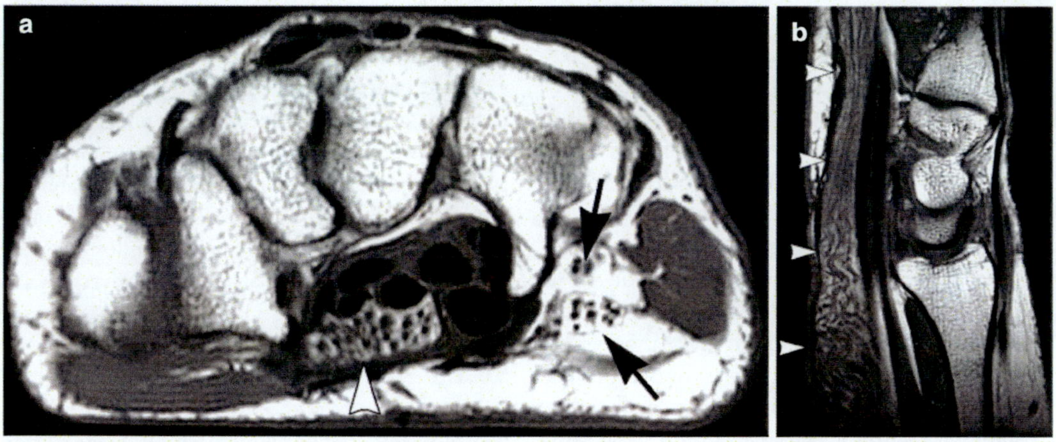

Fig. 18.3 Pathognomonic MRI of lipomatosis of nerve (LN). (**a**) Axial T1-weighted MR image demonstrating pathognomonic MRI features of LN affecting the median nerve (arrowhead) as well as the ulnar nerve and its branches (arrows) at the wrist. The so-called co-axial cable-like appearance can be appreciated in both the median and ulnar nerves. (**b**) T1-weighted MR image of the same patient as in (**a**) showing the so-called spaghetti-like appearance of the median nerve (arrowheads) in the longitudinal plane

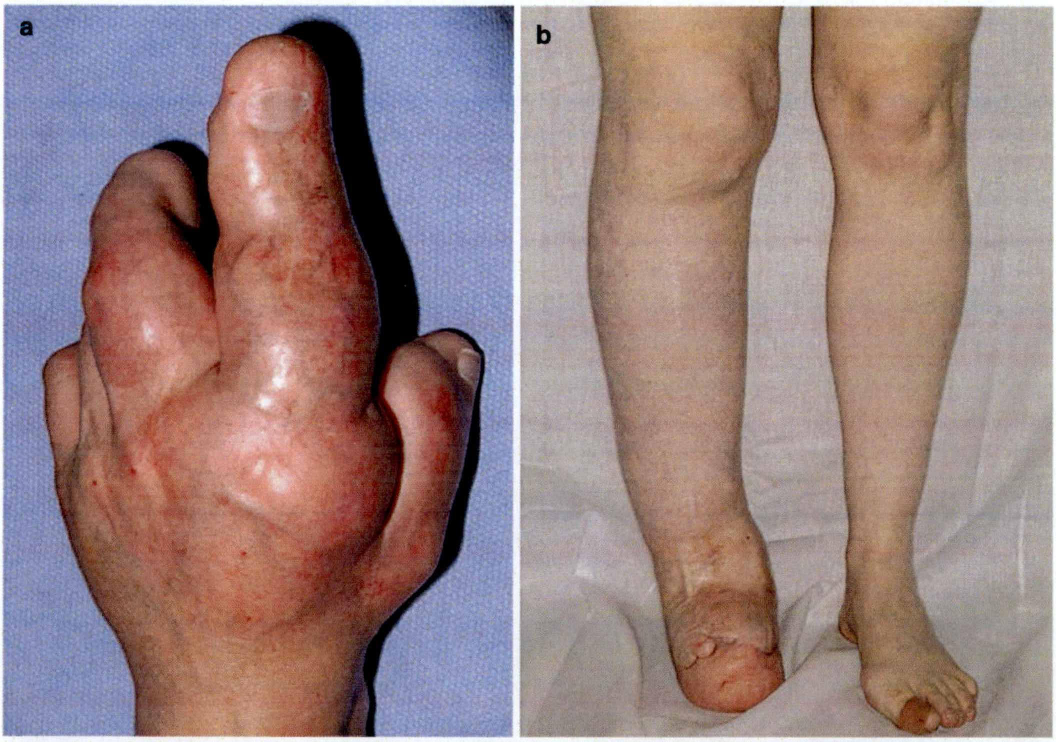

Fig. 18.4 Clinical photographs of two patients with lipomatosis of nerve and associated nerve-territory overgrowth. (**a**) A patient with LN of median nerve who has associated nerve-territory overgrowth in the distribution of the median nerve. (**b**) A patient with LN of the right lumbosacral plexus and the right sciatic nerve with massive overgrowth affecting the right lower limb

the missing pieces of the pathogenesis puzzle. Cases where only the so-called predominant sensory nerves were involved were found to be free of associated overgrowth. This is in contrast to cases with affected motor (mixed) nerves where overgrowth is present in the majority of cases. Some sort of unknown growth factor or signaling might explain this observation [21].

The treatment of LN is symptomatic as no therapy to prevent overgrowth exists. Treatment approaches vary depending on presenting symptoms and the presence and degree of overgrowth. Cosmesis is also a very important factor when planning the surgery. Nerve decompression is the treatment of choice when compressive neuropathy is the predominant feature. This is a carpal tunnel release in the majority of cases as median nerve LN is the most common site involved. Other relatively common sites of decompression are the common peroneal nerve at the fibular neck and ulnar nerve at the elbow. Extraneural lipoma(s), associated with LN, might be another reason for compressive neuropathy. Resection of the lesion is recommended in such cases. When massive overgrowth is present, soft tissue debulking procedures along with bone reduction surgeries might be pursued. In many cases, especially in children and the adolescent population, the overgrowth is often progressive and recurrent. It is not uncommon for patients to undergo several debulking procedures. Amputation surgeries can be considered as well to improve function. Several reports of nerve resection and grafting exist, however, with mixed results. This modality remains controversial [22].

None of the LN cases reported in the medical literature has ever been reported to undergo malignant transformation. This is very important as patients can be assured about the benign nature of this condition [22]. Some cases, however, require repeated procedures. This can be both for recurrent compressive neuropathy and recurrent overgrowth.

18.2.3 Neuromuscular Choristoma

Neuromuscular choristoma (NMC) is a rare peripheral nerve lesion which is characterized by the presence of heterotopic muscle tissue within the nerve. Typically it affects major nerves with the sciatic nerve being the most commonly affected one [23].

NMC may be associated with undergrowth in the territory of the affected nerve [23]. This usually affects both bony and soft tissue structures. Another common feature is progressive neuropathy. MRI features of NMC include fusiform enlargement of the affected nerve with a combination of fatty and soft tissue elements. The soft tissue elements have signal characteristics of skeletal muscle and are generally easily differentiated from soft tissue elements seen in liposarcoma (Fig. 18.5). Subtle enhancement after administration of gadolinium contrast is common, similar to the muscle; however, visualizing the enhancement depends to some degree on the imaging techniques

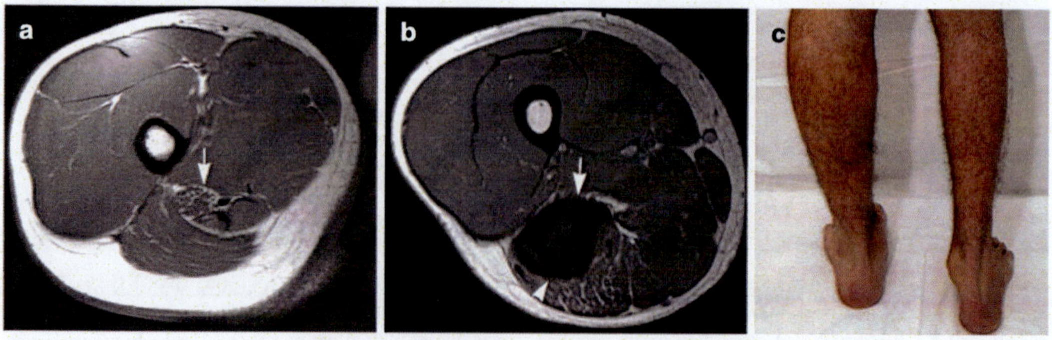

Fig. 18.5 MRI and clinical images of a patient with NMC. (**a**) Axial T1-weighted MR image showing NMC of the right sciatic nerve (arrow) in the upper thigh. The lesion has similar signal intensity as the surrounding muscles. (**b**) Axial T1-weighted MR image of the same patient showing interval development of a desmoid-type fibromatosis (arrowhead) after surgery. Sciatic nerve (arrow) is located anterior to the desmoid lesion. (**c**) Clinical photograph of the same patient showing undergrowth of the right leg

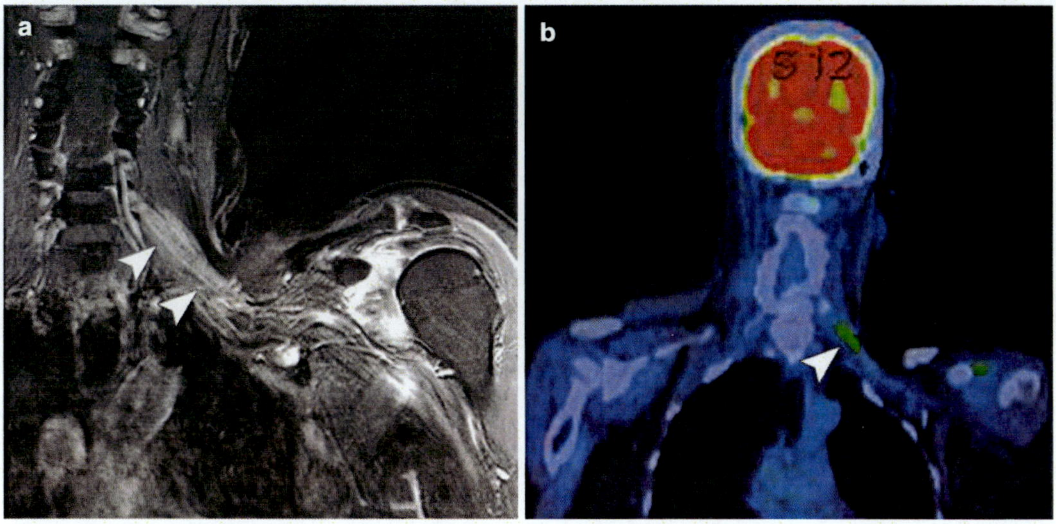

Fig. 18.6 Perineural spread of breast cancer to the brachial plexus. (**a**) Coronal T1-weighted fat-saturated SPGR (spoiled gradient recalled) acquisition post-gadolinium image shows fusiform enlargement and enhancement of the left brachial plexus (arrowheads). The diagnosis of breast cancer was confirmed with biopsy. (**b**) Coronal FDG (fluorodexoyglucose) PET (positron emission tomography)/CT (computerized tomography) image of the same patient as in A shows FDG avidity in the left brachial plexus, supporting the diagnosis of malignancy

and may not always be appreciated. Generally the lesions contain less than 50% of fat which distinguishes these lesions from LN and intraneural lipomas [24] (Fig. 18.6). Patients with diagnosis of NMC can develop associated desmoid-type fibromatosis either spontaneously or more commonly as a response to intervention such as surgery or even a biopsy. The desmoid component is often progressive and recurrent and can cause significant worsening of the symptoms [25]. Mutations of the catenin beta 1 gene (CTNNB1) have been identified in about 85% of the NMC cases with associated desmoid-type fibromatosis [26].

The treatment of NMC is controversial. Once identified and characterized with MRI, the lesion should be followed, and surgery should be pursued only with significant progression of symptoms associated with the development of desmoid-type fibromatosis [26].

18.3 Malignant Lesions

18.3.1 Perineural Spread of Cancers

Perineural spread (PNS) is a relatively uncommon metastasis mechanism when compared to other routes of metastasis such as hematogenous, lymphatic or direct, contiguous spread of a malignant tumor. In recent years, however, PNS has become more commonly appreciated as one of the ways of tumor spread and should be included in the differential diagnoses when appropriate.

Perineural invasion (PNI) plays an important role in the pathogenesis of PNS [27]. PNI should not be confused, however, with PNS as an invasion of a nerve does not necessarily lead to PNS. These two terms are often confusing in the medical literature. The propagation of a tumor along the nerve itself is probably a combination of a “route of the least resistance” and neurotropism [28].

The most common cancers that tend to demonstrate PNS are malignancies of the head and neck [29], breast [30], and skin [31] and various pelvic malignancies including prostate, bladder, vaginal, and rectal [32]. PNS can occur after many years of initial diagnosis and for this reason is oftentimes not suspected as the source of the patient’s symptoms. Reports of cases presenting 10 or more years after the treatment of primary tumors are not uncommon. This feature of delayed presentation can make the diagnosis very challenging as other potential sources of pain and other symptoms are often considered and acted on before the definitive diagnosis of PNS is made. PNS is often incorrectly diagnosed as radiation induced neuropathy. In the case of tumor involving the brachial plexus leading to hand and arm pain, this can lead to interventions such as carpal and cubital tunnel release and even cervical laminectomies before PNS is considered as the source of symptoms.

Imaging is an important tool in establishing the diagnosis of PNS. MRI and PET are the modalities of choice. MR imaging can demonstrate fusiform enlargement of the affected nerve; however, the nerve might have normal appearance on non-contrast sequences. Nodular appearance of the nerve and the so-called skip lesions can be appreciated as well [32]. When gadolinium-based contrast is utilized, the nerve usually demonstrates enhancement which is often nodular or mass-like extending along the nerve. PET imaging with FDG (or, in the case of prostate cancer, choline) tracer can be used to confirm the diagnosis but in cases involving nerves can show less avid uptake [33] (Fig. 18.6). For this reason, the radiologist evaluating such studies should be experienced in peripheral nerve imaging as changes on PET can be very subtle and identifying abnormal patterns might be challenging. Awareness of the possibility of PNS based on the clinical history is the most critical aspect of evaluating and treating these patients.

The next step in diagnosis is biopsy to prove or disprove the suspected diagnosis. An image-guided targeted approach is always preferred. Depending on the site of involvement, the biopsy can be of major neural structures [34] or a distal branch when possible [35]. Treatment should then be directed based on the exact diagnosis and can include radiation therapy, chemotherapy, biologic treatment, and/or surgery.

18.3.2 Peripheral Neurolymphomatosis

Neurolymphomatosis of peripheral nerves can be a rare manifestation of a known lymphoma; however, isolated nerve involvement has also been reported. Patients present with neuropathy and/or pain. The diagnosis can be oftentimes challenging. MRI and FDG-PET are very important imaging tools.

MRI usually demonstrates nerve enlargement, but the appearance is variable and can merely show mild T2 hyperintensity without enlargement or, alternatively, more tumefactive, mass-like lesions [36]. PET can show uptake of FDG tracer, but this depends to some degree on the size of the nerves involved and the extent of the nerve involvement (Fig. 18.7). If the nerve

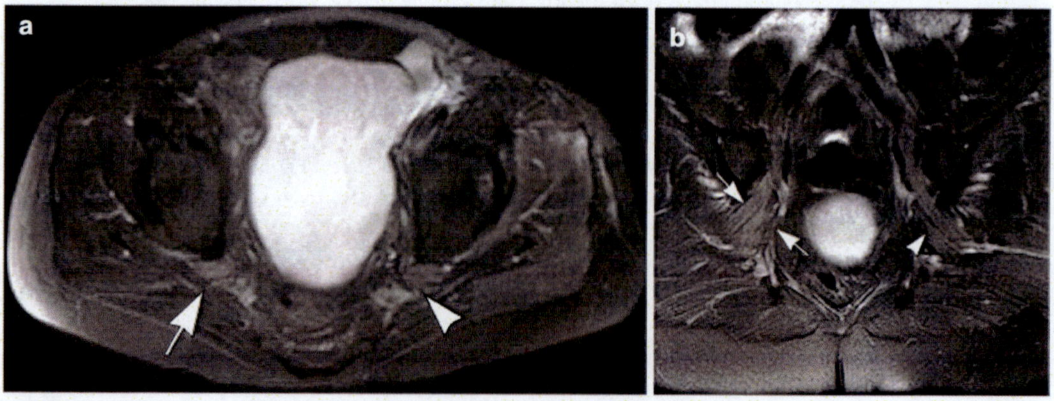

Fig. 18.7 MRI of neurolymphomatosis. (**a, b**) Axial and oblique coronal T2 fast spin echo images with fat suppression showing the enlarged, hyperintense, and indistinct right sciatic nerve (arrows) in a patient with biopsy-proven neurolymphoma. The left side is normal (arrowheads)

involvement is the sole manifestation of lymphoma, targeted biopsy should then be pursued to confirm the diagnosis followed by appropriate treatment [37].

18.4 Miscellaneous Non-neurogenic Tumoral and Pseudotumoral Lesions

18.4.1 Chronic Inflammatory Demyelinating Polyneuropathy (CIDP)

CIDP is an inflammatory disease affecting peripheral nerves predominantly in proximal locations; however, distal locations can be affected too. The patients usually present with progressive weakness which develops over several weeks. When only distal nerve involvement is present, it is often referred to as distal acquired demyelinating symmetric neuropathy (DADS). The exact pathogenesis of CIDP is not known; however, autoimmune processes are thought to be the underlying cause, resulting in demyelination. Patients with CIDP can have predominantly sensory or predominantly motor deficits [38].

The diagnosis is established using EMG, MRI, and biopsy. MRI can demonstrate enlargement of the affected nerves which are hyperintense on fluid-sensitive sequences but rarely show significant enhancement after contrast. The enlargement can give this pathology a tumor-like appearance which has been confused with plexiform neurofibromas in some cases (Fig. 18.8). The "classic" appearance of smoothly enlarged nerves with T2 hyperintensity and little or no enhancement in the appropriate clinical setting is nearly pathognomonic of this entity. If there are equivocal imaging findings, a targeted biopsy can be performed, but this should be reserved for cases where the diagnosis is ambiguous. CIDP is treated with intravenous immune globulin, corticosteroids, or plasmapheresis [39]. Follow-up imaging may not change even with successful response to treatment.

18.4.2 Amyloidosis

Amyloidosis is an umbrella term covering relatively wide spectrum of diseases which all have in common deposition of an abnormal amyloid protein. This leads to damage and impairment of the function of the organ systems/tissue where the amyloid is deposited. Peripheral nerve is one such site; however, isolated nerve involvement is very rare with only a few cases reported in the literature [40].

The patients present with progressive neuropathy. MRI should be the imaging modality of choice. The affected nerves demonstrate diffuse fascicular enlargement, often with a nodular or irregular appearance. Mass-like lesions have also been reported. The lesions are typically hypointense on T1- and hyperintense on T2-weighted sequences with irregular enhancement after contrast which helps to distinguish this from lesions such as CIDP [40]. Targeted nerve (fascicular) biopsy can confirm the diagnosis.

18.5 Conclusion

The heterogeneous group of non-neurogenic tumoral and pseudotumoral lesions affecting peripheral nerve includes many pathologic entities. The diagnosis of these lesions might be challenging at times due to their rarity. Imaging, especially MRI, is an important part of the diagnostic process as many of the lesions have characteristic imaging features. Targeted biopsy might be necessary to establish the final diagnosis; however, in select cases, such as NMC, this should be avoided. The treatment should be tailored for each individual case and should always be as conservative as possible.

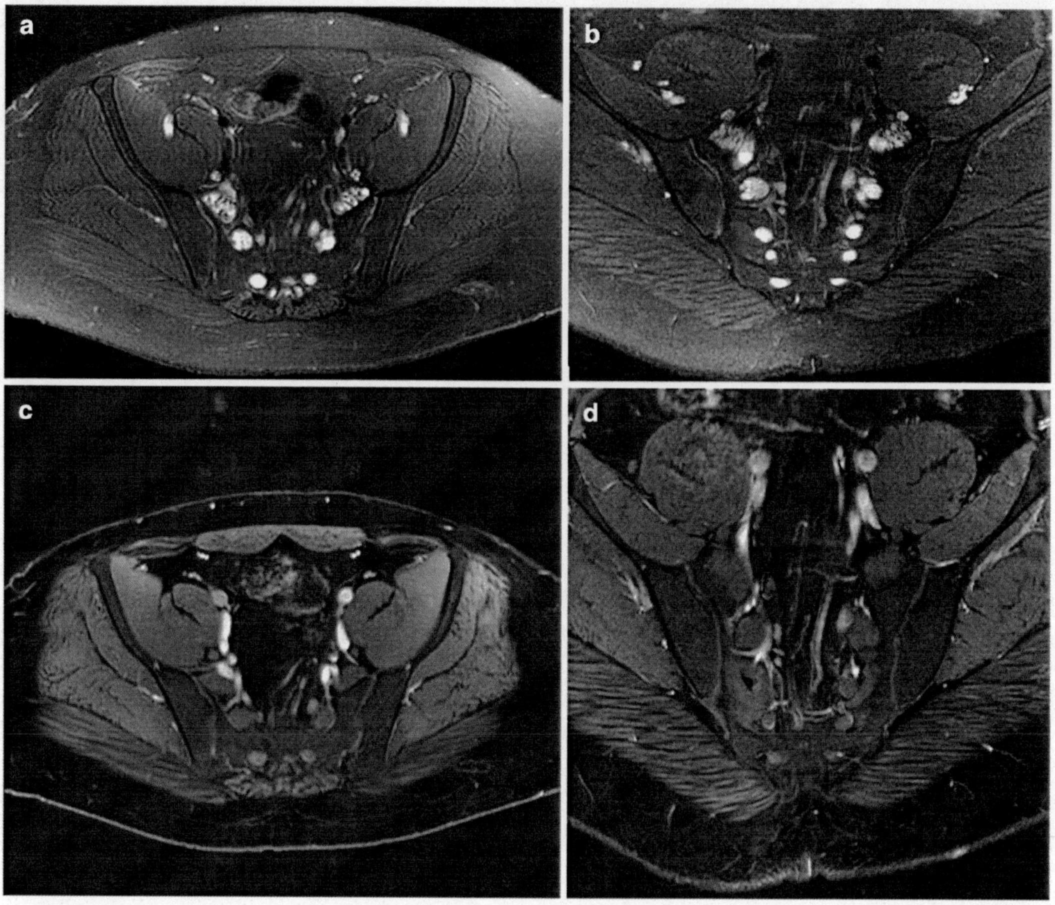

Fig. 18.8 MRI of CIDP. (**a**, **b**) Axial and oblique coronal T2-weighted fast spin echo MR images with fat suppression showing the enlarged and hyperintense nerves of the lumbosacral plexus and femoral nerves. (**c**, **d**) Corresponding post-contrast T1-weighted spoiled gradient recalled (SPGR) images with fat suppression showing the lack of contrast enhancement, characteristic of CIDP

References

1. Desy NM, Wang H, Elshiekh MA, et al. Intraneural ganglion cysts: a systematic review and reinterpretation of the world's literature. J Neurosurg. 2016;125(3):615–30.
2. Spinner RJ, Atkinson JL, Tiel RL. Peroneal intraneural ganglia: the importance of the articular branch. A unifying theory. J Neurosurg. 2003;99(2):330–43.
3. Spinner RJ, Atkinson JL, Scheithauer BW, et al. Peroneal intraneural ganglia: the importance of the articular branch. Clinical series. J Neurosurg. 2003;99(2):319–29.
4. Prasad N, Amrami KK, Winn J, Spinner RJ. Cystic adventitial disease in the popliteal artery with a joint connection to the superior tibiofibular joint: radiological evidence to support the unifying articular theory. Clin Anat. 2015;28(8):957–9.
5. McCarthy CL, McNally EG. The MRI appearance of cystic lesions around the knee. Skeletal Radiol. 2004;33(4):187–209.
6. Shahid KR, Spinner RJ, Skinner JA, et al. Evaluation of intraneural ganglion cysts using three-dimensional fast spin echo-cube. J Magn Reson Imaging. 2010;32(3):714–8.
7. Spinner RJ, Scheithauer BW, Amrami KK, Wenger DE, Hebert-Blouin MN. Adipose lesions of nerve: the need for a modified classification. J Neurosurg. 2012;116(2):418–31.
8. Marek T, Amrami KK, Mahan MA, Spinner RJ. Intraneural lipomas: institutional and literature review. Acta Neurochir. 2018;160(11):2209–18.

9. Teles AR, Finger G, Schuster MN, Gobbato PL. Peripheral nerve lipoma: case report of an intraneural lipoma of the median nerve and literature review. Asian J Neurosurg. 2016;11(4):458.
10. Kamble P, Vanan K, Mohanty SS, Rathod T, Sahay A. Intraneural lipoma with cartilagenous metaplasia of median nerve. J Case Rep. 2017;7(3):303–5.
11. Park SE, Lee JU, Ji JH. Intraneural chondroid lipoma on the common peroneal nerve. Knee Surg Sports Traumatol Arthrosc. 2011;19(5):832–4.
12. Marek T, Spinner RJ, Syal A, Mahan MA. Strengthening the association of lipomatosis of nerve and nerve-territory overgrowth: a systematic review. J Neurosurg. 2019;132(4):1286–94.
13. Fletcher C, Unni K, Mertens F. World Health Organisation classification of tumours. In: Pathology and genetics: tumours of soft tissue and bone. Lyon: IARC Press; 2002.
14. Marek T, Mahan MA, Carter JM, Amrami KK, Atkinson JL, Spinner RJ. Can lipomatosis of the nerve occur or extend intradurally? World Neurosurg. 2019;129:e555–60.
15. Marom EM, Helms CA. Fibrolipomatous hamartoma: pathognomonic on MR imaging. Skeletal Radiol. 1999;28(5):260–4.
16. Mahan MA, Niederhauser BD, Amrami KK, Spinner RJ. Long-term progression of lipomatosis of nerve. World Neurosurg. 2014;82(3–4):492–9.
17. Marek T, Howe BM, Amrami KK, Taunton MJ, Spinner RJ. Unrecognized lipomatosis of the femoral nerve and nerve-territory overgrowth. Clin Anat. 2018;31(8):1210–4.
18. Mahan MA, Amrami KK, Spinner RJ. Sciatic nerve lipomatosis and knee osteochondroma. J Neurosurg. 2013;119(4):934.
19. Keppler-Noreuil KM, Rios JJ, Parker VE, et al. PIK3CA-related overgrowth spectrum (PROS): diagnostic and testing eligibility criteria, differential diagnosis, and evaluation. Am J Med Genet A. 2015;167A(2):287–95.
20. Blackburn PR, Milosevic D, Marek T, et al. PIK3CA mutations in lipomatosis of nerve with or without nerve territory overgrowth. Mod Pathol. 2020;33(3):420–30.
21. Marek T, Mahan MA, Carter JM, Amrami KK, Benarroch EE, Spinner RJ. Lipomatosis of nerve and overgrowth: is there a preference for motor (mixed) vs. sensory nerve involvement? Acta Neurochir. 2019;161(4):679–84.
22. Marek T, Spinner RJ, Syal A, Wahood W, Mahan MA. Surgical treatment of lipomatosis of nerve: a systematic review. World Neurosurg. 2019;128:587–592.e582.
23. Kumar R, Howe BM, Amrami KK, Spinner RJ. Neuromuscular choristoma of the sciatic nerve and lumbosacral plexus: an association with nerve-territory undergrowth in the pelvis affecting soft tissue and bone. Acta Neurochir. 2014;156(5):1041–6.
24. Niederhauser BD, Spinner RJ, Jentoft ME, Everist BM, Matsumoto JM, Amrami KK. Neuromuscular choristoma: characteristic magnetic resonance imaging findings and association with post-biopsy fibromatosis. Skeletal Radiol. 2013;42(4):567–77.
25. Stone JJ, Prasad NK, Laumonerie P, et al. Recurrent desmoid-type fibromatosis associated with underlying neuromuscular choristoma. J Neurosurg. 2018;131(1):175–83.
26. Lazar AJ, Tuvin D, Hajibashi S, et al. Specific mutations in the beta-catenin gene (CTNNB1) correlate with local recurrence in sporadic desmoid tumors. Am J Pathol. 2008;173(5):1518–27.
27. Kayahara M, Nakagawara H, Kitagawa H, Ohta T. The nature of neural invasion by pancreatic cancer. Pancreas. 2007;35(3):218–23.
28. Brown IS. Pathology of perineural spread. J Neurol Surg B Skull Base. 2016;77(2):124–30.
29. Badger D, Aygun N. Imaging of perineural spread in head and neck cancer. Radiol Clin North Am. 2017;55(1):139–49.
30. Laumonerie P, Capek S, Amrami KK, Dyck PJ, Spinner RJ. Targeted fascicular biopsy of the brachial plexus: rationale and operative technique. Neurosurg Focus. 2017;42(3):E9.
31. Marek T, Howe BM, Amrami KK, Spinner RJ. Perineural spread of nonmelanoma skin cancer to the brachial plexus: identifying anatomic pathway(s). World Neurosurg. 2018;114:e818–23.
32. Capek S, Howe BM, Amrami KK, Spinner RJ. Perineural spread of pelvic malignancies to the lumbosacral plexus and beyond: clinical and imaging patterns. Neurosurg Focus. 2015;39(3):E14.
33. Stone JJ, Adamo DA, Khan DZ, et al. Multimodal imaging aids in the diagnosis of perineural spread of prostate cancer. World Neurosurg. 2019;122:e235–40.
34. Capek S, Amrami KK, Dyck PJ, Spinner RJ. Targeted fascicular biopsy of the sciatic nerve and its major branches: rationale and operative technique. Neurosurg Focus. 2015;39(3):E12.
35. Marek T, Stone JJ, Amrami KK, Spinner RJ. Targeted nerve biopsy: a technique in evolution. Clin Anat. 2018;31(8):1200–4.
36. Capek S, Hebert-Blouin MN, Puffer RC, et al. Tumefactive appearance of peripheral nerve involvement in hematologic malignancies: a new imaging association. Skeletal Radiol. 2015;44(7):1001–9.
37. DeVries AH, Howe BM, Spinner RJ, Broski SM. B-cell peripheral neurolymphomatosis: MRI and (18)F-FDG PET/CT imaging characteristics. Skeletal Radiol. 2019;48(7):1043–50.
38. Mathey EK, Park SB, Hughes RA, et al. Chronic inflammatory demyelinating polyradiculoneuropathy: from pathology to phenotype. J Neurol Neurosurg Psychiatry. 2015;86(9):973–85.
39. Dalakas MC. Medscape. Advances in the diagnosis, pathogenesis and treatment of CIDP. Nat Rev Neurol. 2011;7(9):507–17.
40. McKenzie GA, Broski SM, Howe BM, et al. MRI of pathology-proven peripheral nerve amyloidosis. Skeletal Radiol. 2017;46(1):65–73.

19 Malignant Peripheral Nerve Sheath Tumors

Fernando Guedes, Gabriel Elias Sanches, Stephanie Bulhões, Ana Caroline Siquara-de-Sousa, and Karin Soares Gonçalves Cunha

19.1 Introduction

Peripheral nerves may be subject to the development of different types of malignant tumors, the most common being the malignant peripheral nerve sheath tumors (MPNST), with up to 50% arising in the setting of neurofibromatosis type 1 (NF1) [1–3]. In this chapter, the features and management of these aggressive tumors will be discussed. Nonetheless, there are some rare malignant tumors to affect peripheral nerves, and we provide a brief overview of them below.

19.1.1 Malignant and Melanotic Schwannoma

Schwannomas are peripheral nerve sheath tumors (PNST) that in rare occasions may undergo malignant transformation. Vestibular schwannomas have been shown to undergo malignant transformation into MPNST after radiation therapy [4]. Melanotic schwannomas, on the other hand, although usually benign, may also present with an aggressive behavior (Fig. 19.1). They are usually located along the paraspinal sympathetic chain and the gastrointestinal tract and may be also misdiagnosed as malignant melanomas [4–8].

19.1.2 Ewing Sarcoma

Ewing sarcoma is the second most frequent osseous tumor to present in pediatric patients, and it may also arise from soft tissues, including rarely peripheral nerves. They have a probable origin from mesodermal or neural crest-derived cell types, and given their initially insidious clinical course, with the absence of B symptoms (i.e., moderate fever and night sweat), they may be diagnosed very late in the progression of the disease. Lastly, intraneural Ewing sarcomas may be indifferentiable from PNST on clinical and imaging grounds [9–13].

19.1.3 Desmoid Tumors and Desmoplastic Small Round Cell Tumors (DSRCT)

Desmoid tumors are neoplasms characterized by proliferation of fibroblasts. Although benign, they may have an often unpredictable clinical course. Rarely they arise from or in close

F. Guedes (✉) · G. E. Sanches · S. Bulhões
Division of Neurosurgery, Department of Surgery, Gaffrée e Guinle University Hospital, School of Medicine, Federal University of Rio de Janeiro State (UNIRIO), Rio de Janeiro, RJ, Brazil

A. C. Siquara-de-Sousa · K. S. G. Cunha
Department of Pathology, Antônio Pedro University Hospital, School of Medicine, Fluminense Federal University (UFF), Niterói, RJ, Brazil

F. Guedes et al. (eds.), *Diagnostic Assessment and Treatment of Peripheral Nerve Tumors*,
https://doi.org/10.1007/978-3-030-77633-6_19

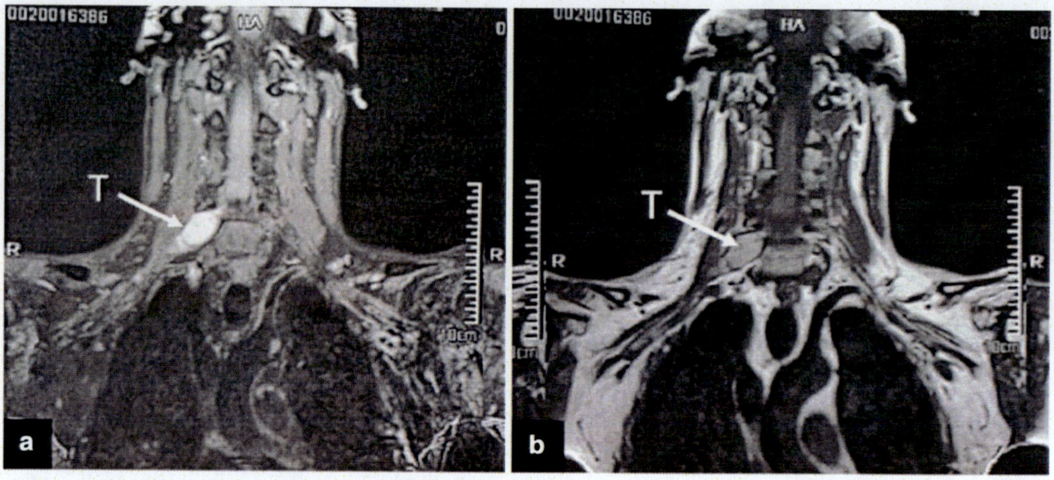

Fig. 19.1 A 50-year-old male patient presenting with a later diagnosed melanotic schwannoma. (**a**) Coronal T2-weighted MRI with fat suppression without contrast and (**b**) coronal T1-weighted MRI without contrast of a lesion affecting roots C7–C8. *T* tumor

proximity to peripheral nerves [14–16]. There is no consensus concerning their management in these instances, and treatment should be individualized. Nonetheless, given their high local recurrence rates, some authors advocate that radical surgical excision is usually recommended [14].

DSRCT are rare tumors with an aggressive behavior and a poor 5-year survival rate of 15% [17]. Although they usually present as a large abdominal or pelvic mass, there have been few reports of DSRCT affecting the brachial plexus. Similar to desmoid tumors, there is not a consensus as to how to manage these neoplasms. Some authors have employed complete resection, whereas others, subtotal resection with preservation of neurological function and adjuvant chemotherapy and local radiotherapy [17–19].

19.1.4 Metastases

Metastases may also rarely affect peripheral nerves. There have been reports of intraneural growth of different neoplasms such as melanomas, lymphomas, and adenocarcinomas. Management is invariably dependent of the metastasis histotype and may include surgical resection and adjuvant treatment [20].

19.1.5 MPNST

By definition, the term MPNST includes any malignant tumor that arises from or differentiates toward cells intrinsic to the peripheral nerve sheath, excluding tumors of epineurial soft tissue and endoneurial tumors originating from the peripheral nerve vasculature [21]. This term was introduced by the World Health Organization (WHO) to replace other older and confusing terminologies used for this tumor, such as malignant neurilemmoma, neurofibrosarcoma, and neurogenic sarcoma [22–25]. Although MPNST may originate from any peripheral nerve sheath cell, there is histological, immunohistochemical, ultrastructural, and genetic evidence that most MPNST originate from Schwann cells or their precursors [21, 26, 27].

MPNST are classified as soft tissue sarcomas, i.e., a soft tissue malignant neoplasm. Soft tissue is defined as a non-epithelial extra-skeletal tissue of the body exclusive of the reticuloendothelial system, glia, and supporting tissue of various parenchymal organs [28]. Therefore, it includes the peripheral nervous system since tumors arising from nerves present as soft tissue masses and pose similar problems in differential diagnosis and therapy [28]. Nevertheless, embryologically, soft tissues are derived from mesoderm, although they may have contribution from neuroectoderm [28].

MPNST are quite rare neoplasms and represent only 5% of all soft tissue sarcomas [21, 27, 29]. MPNST may appear de novo (from a normal nerve) or arise from the malignant transformation of a benign neural lesion, especially a neurofibroma, which usually happens in NF1 individuals [30]. Localized as well as diffuse neurofibromas which may occur sporadically or in association with NF1 do not possess a malignant potential [21]. On the other hand, plexiform neurofibromas, which are a distinct clinical and histological variant, are the most common precursors of MPNST [21]. Plexiform neurofibromas tend to affect sizable nerves and occur in NF1 individuals, but there are a few reports in individuals with no NF1 features [31–34]. Plexiform neurofibromas occur in 25–50% of NF1 individuals, and 5% of them transform into MPNST [35–37]. Localized intraneural neurofibromas, which are tumors that grow within peripheral nerves and are outlined by a fibrous border derived from the epineurium, may also undergo malignant change, but this occurs less frequently compared with plexiform neurofibromas [21, 38]. Rapid increase in size and unexplained pain (especially at rest) are considered signs and symptoms of malignant transformation of neurofibromas [30, 35, 39]. Most MPNST arise in association with large nerve trunks, including the sciatic nerve, brachial plexus, and sacral plexus. Consequently, the most common anatomical locations are the upper and lower limbs and the trunk [29]. Few cases occur in the head and neck region [28].

It has been shown, in several series, that up to 50% of the cases occur in individuals with neurofibromatosis 1 (NF1), an autosomal-dominant genetic syndrome caused by mutations in the *NF1* gene and that a small portion of MPNST arises secondary to radiotherapy, after a latency period, often 10–15 years after radiation [1–3, 40–45]. Nonetheless, MPSNT is the most common malignant neoplasm that occurs in NF1 with a prevalence of 4.6–16%, while in the general population, its prevalence is only 0.001% [27, 46–48].

Many studies have shown that the presence of NF1 has a negative influence on other clinical features of MPNST, such as local recurrences, metastases, tumor size, and survival, although there is still controversy on this matter [44, 46, 47, 49–56]. Nonetheless, a meta-analysis conducted in 2012, with >1800 patients, showed that survival was poorer in NF1 patients when considering studies from 1962 to 2012 [57].

MPNST appear to affect men and women equally, although some studies showed a slight predilection for females, whereas two large studies showed the opposite [46, 49, 55, 58–60]. MPNST are typically neoplasms of adulthood, commonly occurring between 20 and 50 years of age. In NF1, these tumors are usually diagnosed at an earlier age (28–36 years) compared with those that occur sporadically (40–44 years) [23, 43, 46, 58, 61, 62]. However, a large study from the Mayo Clinic found that 12.8% of cases of MPNST occurred in children 16 years of age or younger [63]. This study showed that most MPNST in the pediatric population arose in association with NF1 and had a contiguous neurofibromatosis component [63]. Another large study based on the "Surveillance, Epidemiology, and End Results" (SEER) program database identified 1315 MPNST, and 128 of these cases (9.7%) were pediatric. The significant predictors of survival for pediatric tumors were sex (males had better survival), race (non-Hispanic black ethnicity had worse survival), and radiation therapy, while for adult cases, these predictors were not significant for MPNST survival. When only cases of recurrence of MPNST in children were selected in a study of 73 patients younger than 21 years old, the factors with the greatest impact on prognosis were the degree of initial invasion of the neoplasm, time to recurrence, and complete surgical resection (the latter, the same conclusion as Friedrich et al. in MPNST of NF1-affected children) [64, 65].

Amirian et al., in their study based on the SEER database, identified that tumors located in the "trunk" and presenting higher grades were negatively correlated with survival. This study, however, was not able to discern among patients with or without a diagnosis of NF1 [58]. A nationwide cohort study conducted in the Netherlands demonstrated on multivariate analysis, in 741 patients diagnosed with non-retroperitoneal MPNST, that the following patients' and tumors' characteristics had a negative impact on overall survival (OS): diagnosis of NF1, older age (>60 years old), R2 (macroscopically positive) margins on resection, large (>5 cm), and deep-seated tumors. Indeed, R2 margins, larger size, deep location, as well as higher histological grade have been described as negatively influencing both disease-specific survival (DSS) and OS in different studies [1, 3, 44, 45, 66].

19.2 History of MPNST

MPNST have had many names in the history of medical literature, such as "neurofibrosarcoma," "neurogenic sarcoma," and "neurosarcoma" [40, 67–72]. This clinicopathological entity has always been studied in the context of soft tissue tumors, as the identification of its peculiarities in contrast to other sarcomas is indeed very recent. The first reports that distinguish MPNST from other sarcomas, as well as describe some of its clinical properties, probably date from the nineteenth-century German literature. Some surgeons at that time were aware of the individuality of this tumor, and of interest is the fact that in the late 1880s, Fedor Krause showed that MPNST are often related to NF1 (at the time called von Recklinghausen's disease) and that apparent metastases in these patients were actually new tumors. This observation was one of the first insights in that NF1 increases the odds of developing one or more MPNST [73]. Later, in the beginning of the twentieth century, surgeons such as Fleming and Marvin also started to show the individuality of MPNST, based on its histological and clinical characteristics [74–76]. In 1931, Stewart and Copeland acknowledged that MPNST were different among themselves, naming a subset with less aggressive histological characteristics "low-grade neurosarcomas." At the time, they inferred that these tumors also possessed an unfavorable prognosis, although it is not clear if the tumors they referred to were actually ones that we would now call "low-grade" [67].

Today, the World Health Organization still classifies MPNST as sarcomas but, in its latest series of books *WHO Classification of Tumours*, recognizes that the cell of origin is probably a precursor of Schwann cells, as well as the existence of a subset of this tumor, called low-grade MPNST. This subset exhibits a remarkably different clinical course, which allows for a less aggressive surgical approach and for the preservation of structures and function, resulting in a much better prognosis [29].

19.3 Diagnostic Criteria

Since MPNST have histopathological features reminiscent of other spindle cell sarcomas, their histopathological features may not allow diagnosis when analyzed in isolation [21]. The widely accepted criteria for the diagnosis of MPNST are described in Table 19.1, and at least one of these criteria must be present to establish the diagnosis.

Table 19.1 Diagnostic criteria for malignant peripheral nerve sheath tumor [21]

The tumor must meet at least one of the following criteria:
1. Originate from a peripheral nerve
2. Originate from a benign peripheral nerve sheath tumor (neurofibroma, schwannoma, pheochromocytoma, or ganglioneuroma/ganglioneuroblastoma)
3. Develop in a patient with NF1 and exhibit the same histopathological features as most MPNST that originate from the nerves
4. Develop in patients without NF1 but exhibit the same histopathological features of most MPNST and show immunohistochemical and/or ultrastructural characteristics of differentiation into Schwann cells or perineural cells

19.4 Oncogenesis and Genetic Profile of Malignant Peripheral Nerve Sheath Tumors

Loss of heterozygosity of the *NF1* gene has been demonstrated by several authors in NF1-associated MPNST as well as sporadic MPNST [43]. Although mutation of the two alleles of the *NF*1 gene is believed to be sufficient for the emergence of neurofibromas, many studies have shown that the development of MPNST is a multistep process, with not only biallelic inactivation of the *NF1* gene but also other molecular changes [72, 77–81]. However, the mechanisms involved in the oncogenesis of these tumors are still poorly understood.

Compatible with a disease caused by a mutation in a tumor suppressor gene, the development of neoplasms in individuals with NF1 occurs when the two alleles of the *NF1* gene are mutated.

19.4.1 *NF1* Gene

The *NF1* gene is located at chromosome locus 17q11.2 and is considered a tumor suppressor [80]. It encodes a protein called neurofibromin that is expressed in a variety of cells including neurons, Schwann cells, astrocytes, oligodendrocytes, keratinocytes, adrenal medullary cells, and leukocytes [35].

To date, the only region of neurofibromin that has a well-defined and well-known function is the region encoded in the central portion of the *NF1* gene [82, 83]. This region is homologous to the catalytic domain of the GTPase-activating protein (GAP) and is known as the GAP-related domain (GRD). GAP is a protein that has the function of inactivating Ras protein. Because neurofibromin has the GAP homologous region, it also functions to inactivate the Ras protein [82, 84].

Ras proteins are members of the G protein superfamily and represent a converging point of many cell signaling pathways [85]. They are transiently activated in response to various extracellular signals, such as growth factors, cytokines, hormones, and neurotransmitters, which stimulate tyrosine kinase receptors [85]. Ras proteins are activated when bound to GTP (Ras-GTP) and inactivated when bound to GDP (Ras-GDP).

In the cell, there are two classes of signaling proteins that regulate Ras protein activity, influencing the transition between its active (Ras-GTP) and inactive (Ras-GDP) states. Nucleotide guanine-releasing proteins (GNRP) stimulate the loss of GDP and subsequent activation of cytoplasm GTP, thereby activating Ras [86, 87]. GAP protein, as well as neurofibromin, in turn, interacts with Ras-GTP, increasing the GTP hydrolysis rate in GDP, inactivating Ras [35]. When activated, Ras proteins play an important role in activating the MAP kinase signaling pathway, which is important in controlling proliferation, differentiation, cell survival, and apoptosis [85, 88]. Other pathways are also activated by Ras, such as the phosphatidylinositol 3-kinase (PI3-k) and the phospholipase C signaling pathway [89, 90]. In cells with mutations in both alleles of the *NF1* gene, neurofibromin is defective or absent, and therefore increased levels of Ras-GTP occur, which leads to tumor development.

To explain the occurrence of NF1-associated and sporadic MPNST, since the *NF1* gene is a tumor suppressor, the "two-hit" hypothesis of oncogenesis of retinoblastoma proposed by Knudson can be used as follows [91]:

Two mutations (hits), involving both alleles of *NF1*, are required to produce neurofibromas and MPNST. In NF1 individuals, in all cells, with exception of patients with mosaic NF1, one defective allele of the *NF1* gene is inherited (germline mutation: the first hit), and the other allele is normal. Neurofibroma develops when the normal NF1 allele is mutated in Schwann cells or their precursor as a result of a spontaneous somatic mutation (the second hit). In case of MPNST, beyond *NF1* mutations, other molecular alterations are needed. In sporadic cases of neurofibroma and MPNST, both normal NF1 alleles must undergo somatic mutation in the same Schwann cell or their precursors (two hits). Of course, the probability of this event is lower and explains why neurofibromas and MPNST are less common in the general population than in NF1 individuals.

19.4.2 Other Molecular Changes in MPNST

Mutation in the *TP53* gene is one of the most common molecular abnormalities found in MPNST [81, 92, 93]. Consistent with the role of the *TP53* gene in MPNST development, experimental animals that harbor mutations in both *NF1* alleles and *TP53* mutations develop MPNST [84, 94, 95].

Beyond *NF1* and *TP53* mutations, most MPNST exhibit *CDKN2A* mutations [96, 97]. *CDKN2A* deletion is possibly an early event in the development of MPNST, occurring during progression of MPNST from an atypical neurofibroma [96]. Over the past few decades, several other growth factors and their receptors have been suggested as candidates for promoting the development of MPNST and neurofibromas, such as epidermal growth factor (EGF) and hepatocyte growth factor (HGF), among others [98–101].

Inactivation of the polycomb repressive complex 2 (PRC2), as a result of mutually exclusive inactivating mutations of its constituents EED and SUZ12, is observed in the majority of MPNST [96, 97, 102–104]. PRC2 is composed of EED, SUZ12, EZH1, and EZH2; this complex is related to epigenetic silencing by post-translational modification of histones through di- and tri-methylation of Lys27 of histone H3 (H3K27me2/3) [102, 105, 106]. Therefore, PRC2 inactivation leads to loss of methylation at H3K27. It has been suggested that PRC2 inactivation potentiates the effects of NF1 mutations by amplifying Ras-driven transcription through effects on chromatin [107].

Cytogenetic studies have shown complex karyotypes in MPNST [108]. In a study with 51 MPNST, significant loss was observed in the chromosomal regions 1p3, 9p1, 9p2, 11p1, 11q1, 11q2, 12q2, 17p1, 18p1, 18q1-q2, 19p1, 22q1, X, and Y. Gain of chromosomal material was found in chromosome 7, especially 7q1. Most involved breakpoints were 1p13, 1q21, 7p22, 9p11, 17p11, 17q11, and 22q11 [108, 109].

19.5 Macroscopic Features

MPNST macroscopy depends on its origin [21]. Those that originate from a nerve present as fusiform to globular lesions and range from white and firm to soft and yellow lumps, depending on the absence or presence of necrosis [21, 29, 46]. Those MPNST that originate from a neurofibroma may be macroscopically inapparent or multifocal. Therefore, sectioning of the entire plexiform neurofibroma is recommended [21, 29].

Most tumors are larger than 5 cm and appear as well-circumscribed lesions surrounded by a pseudocapsule of varying sizes formed by the compaction and invasion of adjacent soft tissues, as well as reactive fibrosis [21, 28, 29, 46]. Generally, heterologous elements, when present, are not macroscopically identifiable, and extensive macroscopic representation is required to define the appropriate histological grade [21].

Most MPNST arise deeply, from a major nerve under the superficial fascia, along its course, forming a large fusiform, globoid, or eccentric mass. The consistency varies from soft and fleshy to hard, and the cut surface may be cream-colored or gray. Areas of necrosis and hemorrhage are common and may be extensive [21, 28, 29, 43].

High-grade tumors (of which definition is presented below) tend to present as expansile or globular masses, of soft consistency, measuring >10 cm, entirely unencapsulated and infiltrating surrounding structures [21, 28, 29].

It is very important to identify a nerve of origin and recognize if it overlays or enters the tumor. It also must be observed if the nerve is thickened proximally and distally to the main mass, as it suggests the spread of the neoplasm along the epineurium and perineurium. Given the natural growth of MPNST within nerve fascicles, frozen sections to verify proximal and distal nerve margins may be useful [21, 28].

19.6 Histopathological Features

Most MPNST have highly cellular spindle cell proliferation [21]. Tumor cells usually have hyperchromatic nuclei, are mitotically active, and have a mild amount of weakly eosinophilic cytoplasm with indistinct borders [21, 110]. Tumor cell nuclei usually have rounded or more tapered ends, but in most cases are not pointed [21, 29]. In less cellular areas, the nuclei have a wavy or comma-like appearance similar to normal Schwann cells [28, 29]. The neoplastic cells may be arranged in large fascicles, but there is great variation. Densely cellular fascicles alternate with hypocellular, myxoid zones, where parallel orientation of cells is absent [28]. In some cases, a "herringbone" pattern may be seen [21]. Some tumors may have nodular or spiral cell arrangement (Fig. 19.2a). The latter suggests rudimentary tactoid differentiation [28]. Nuclear palisading, as observed in Antoni A areas of schwannomas, is rare in MPNST and was observed in only 6.7% of the 120 cases studied by Ducatman et al. [46]. In fact, these tumors may show a very heterogeneous microscopic appearance [43].

Most MPNST are high-grade neoplasms, and most have an abrupt transition from low- to high-grade areas (Fig. 19.2b) [46]. High-grade MPNST show prominent nuclear atypia, mitotic indices >10/10 high-power fields (HPFs) (Fig. 19.2c), and, frequently, tumor necrosis [111]. Areas of geographic necrosis with or without pseudopalisade are seen in approximately 50–75% of all cases of MPNST (Fig. 19.3a, b) [21, 29]. Low-grade MPNST may be defined as Schwann cell neoplasms with no necrosis and at least two of the following features: hypercellularity, loss of neurofibroma architecture, cytologic atypia and mitotic index between 3 and 9 mitoses/10 HPFs (Fig. 19.3c) [111]. In the study by Ducatman et al. [46], only 18% of the cases were classified as low-grade lesions.

Intermediate lesions between neurofibromas and MPNST in NF1 patients have been classified as "atypical neurofibromatous neoplasm of unknown biological potential" (ANNUBP). ANNUBP may be defined as having the same aforementioned histological characteristics of a low-grade MPNST but with a lower mitotic index between 1/50 HPFs and 3/10 HPFs [111].

In general, soft tissue tumors, measuring <5 cm in diameter and superficial, should be excised en bloc, and biopsy is not required. Peripheral nerve sheath tumors (PNSTs) are an exception, and resection should not be performed en bloc in order to preserve the nerve [27]. For larger masses, the main biopsy problem is microscopic evaluation, as it shows a small amount of the tumor that can be very heterogeneous. Evaluation of several criteria is required to determine the diagnosis of MPNST, tumor architecture, mitosis, necrosis, myxoid areas, etc., and it

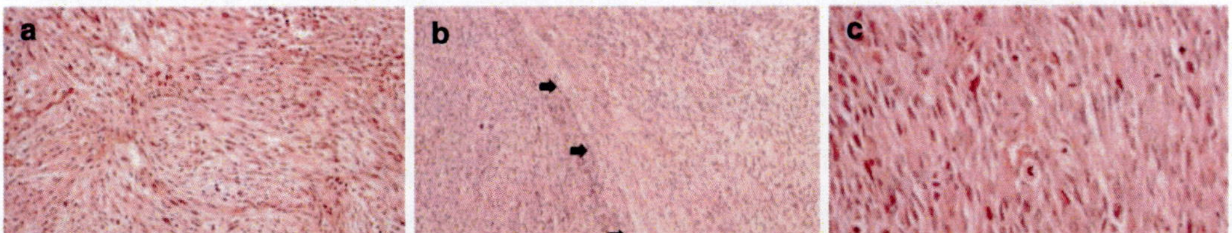

Fig. 19.2 (a) Hematoxylin and eosin, 200×: high-grade MPNST with cells in nodular arrangement. (b) Hematoxylin and eosin, 100×: MPNST with an abrupt transition between low- and high-grade areas (arrows). (c) Hematoxylin and eosin, 400×: high-grade MPNST with evident mitosis

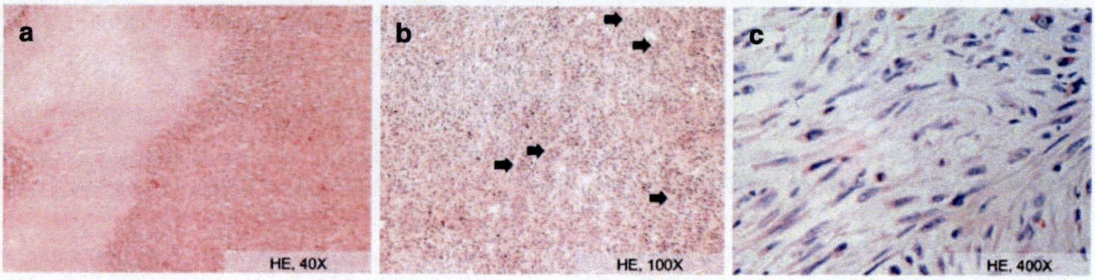

Fig. 19.3 (a) Hematoxylin and eosin, 40×: high-grade MPNST exhibiting geographic necrosis. (b) Hematoxylin and eosin, 100×: high-grade MPNST with palisade of neoplastic cells (arrows). (c) Hematoxylin and eosin, 400×: low-grade MPNST with a slight increase in cellularity, increase in nuclear size, and hyperchromatism

is usually not possible to evaluate them all on one biopsy [27]. However, it is important to try to answer the following questions: Is it a neoplasm? Is it malignant? Is it low-grade or high-grade? Is there an adequate amount of tissue to make other tests? If a variant of MPNST is suspected, the analysis may be arduous. Also, most MPNST have shown an abrupt change from low- to high-grade areas, and low-grade areas are similar to many other soft tissue tumors surrounding the nerves, such as fibrosarcomas [46, 106, 112]. Thus, the tumor may be classified as low-grade on a biopsy specimen, and, when analyzed in the complete specimen, it is a high-grade one. Therefore, even if made by an experienced pathologist with complete tumor resection, the definitive diagnosis can be challenging [106]. Biopsies can be more effective if analyzed or reviewed by experienced pathology sites [27]. There is no preferred method for biopsy, but a few studies indicate that open biopsy is more accurate than core needle biopsy, even though it has a higher rate of complication, including contamination of surrounding tissue with neoplastic cells. Additionally, fine-needle aspiration has been shown to be the least effective technique [113, 114].

19.6.1 Histopathological Grading

The primary purpose of histopathological graduation is to separate malignant neoplasms associated with a good prognosis from tumors with a poor prognosis [115]. Moreover, the value of any histopathological grading system is related not only to the ability to predict patient survival but also to identify patients who may benefit from adjuvant therapy [115]. Due to the relative rarity of sarcomas, the study of large groups of individual tumor types is problematic [115]. Therefore, the histopathological graduation systems of sarcomas are not histotype specific [115]. Currently, the two most commonly used systems for histopathological grading of sarcomas are the NCI (National Cancer Institute) and the FNCLCC (Fédération Nationale des Centres de Lutte Contre le Cancer) systems [54, 116].

The NCI system was proposed in 1984 and is based on a study of 163 patients with soft tissue sarcomas treated at the NCI [117]. In this study, six histopathological factors were analyzed (histopathological type, mitosis, necrosis, pleomorphism, cellularity, and presence of matrix). In NCI system, tumors were classified into three grades (Table 19.2).

The FNCLCC system was also proposed in 1984 and was based on a study of 155 soft tissue sarcomas [118]. Seven histopathological characteristics were evaluated: degree of tumor differentiation, cellularity, presence of atypical nuclei and giant tumor cells, mitotic activity, necrosis, and vascular embolus. Multivariate statistical analysis identified three independent prognostic factors: tumor differentiation, mitotic index, and degree of tumor necrosis. In this system, a score is independently assigned to each parameter, and the degree is obtained by summing the three scores as in Table 19.3.

Table 19.2 *National Cancer Institutes* (NCI) system for sarcoma graduation [117]

Grade	Histopathological parameter
Grade 1	Well-differentiated liposarcoma
	Myxoid liposarcoma
	Subcutaneous myxoid malignant fibrous histiocytoma
	Well-differentiated malignant hemangiopericytoma (with <1 mitosis over 10 high-power fields)
	Well-differentiated fibrosarcoma (with <6 mitoses per 10 high-power fields)
	Well-differentiated leiomyosarcoma (less than 6 mitoses per 10 high-power fields)
	MPNST (neurofibroma-type) with less than 6 mitoses per 10 high-power fields
	Myxoid chondrosarcoma with no mitotic activity
Grade 2	Any sarcoma that is not included in grade 1 and has ≤15% necrosis
Grade 3	Extra-skeletal Ewing's sarcoma/PNET (peripheral neuroectodermal tumor)
	Extra-skeletal osteosarcoma
	Chondrosarcoma mesenchymal
	Malignant triton tumor
	Any other grade 1 sarcoma with >15% necrosis[a]

[a]Based on microscopic examination only

In 2001, a study performed with 1240 patients with sarcomas aimed to evaluate the predictive value of the FNCLCC system for metastasis [119]. Although the histologic grade appeared as an independent predictor of metastasis development in most histologic types of soft tissue sarcomas, it did not occur in patients with MPNST. In contrast, in another study, comparing NF1-associated vs. sporadic MPNST, histopathological grade based on the FNCLCC system did not correlate with prognosis or outcome in NF1-associated MPNST [120]. On the other hand, FNCLCC grading parameters were useful for the evaluation of sporadic MPNST.

Therefore, since sarcomas represent a heterogeneous group of neoplasms which differ widely in their potential biological behavior and, moreover, MPNST are of neuroectodermal origin, more studies with a large series of cases should be performed to evaluate the value of the current grading systems in patients with MPNST and maybe propose a new grading system specifically for this tumor. Moreover, due to the differences in clinical behavior of sporadic and NF1-associated MPNST, they should be studied and compared as different groups of tumors.

Table 19.3 FNCLCC histopathological grading system (*Fédération Nationale des Centres de Lutte Contre le Cancer*) [118]

Tumor differentiation	
Score 1	
Sarcomas resembling normal adult mesenchymal tissue (e.g., low-grade leiomyosarcoma)	
Score 2	
Sarcomas for which the histopathological type is right (e.g., myxoid liposarcoma)	
Score 3	
Embryonal or undifferentiated sarcomas, dubious sarcomas, synovial sarcomas, osteosarcomas, primitive neuroectodermal tumors	
Mitosis count	
Score 1	0–9 mitoses per 10 high-power fields
Score 2	10–19 mitoses for 10 high-power fields
Score 3	≥20 mitoses per 10 high-power fields
Tumor necrosis	
Score 0	Without necrosis
Score 1	<50%
Score 2	≥50%
Histopathological grade	
Grade 1	Total score 2 and 3
Grade 2	Total score 4 and 5
Grade 3	Total score 6, 7, and 8

19.6.2 Immunohistochemical Characteristics

When MPNST does not originate in patients with NF1, has no evidence of origin from a nerve, nor arises from the transformation of a benign neural tumor, immunohistochemistry (IHC) plays an important role in diagnosing this neoplasm [21, 29, 62].

Since S-100 protein is expressed by Schwann cells, IHC screening for this protein is widely used for neural tumors. Nevertheless, immunopositivity for S-100 is not seen in all MPNST; it is found in 30–70% of the cases and depends on tumor grade [21, 29]. Widespread S-100 expression is usually seen in low-grade MPNST, but in high-grade tumors, S-100 immunostaining, when present, is usually focal and limited to a small number of cells [21, 121, 122]. The lack of S-100 immunoreactivity observed in many high-grade MPNST probably reflects the low degree of tumor differentiation [21, 29, 121]. Since synovial sarcomas can also express S-100, immunopositivity for this protein must be interpreted with caution [123].

Schwann cells also express CD57 (Leu-7), and therefore, positivity for this protein confirms the neural origin of MPNST. Nevertheless, like S-100 protein, expression of CD57 in MPSNTs is also variable. Therefore, the use of both anti-S-100 and anti-CD57 antibodies maximizes the identification MPNST [61]. Moreover, only a subset of MPNST express other neuronal markers such as SOX10 or glial fibrillary acidic protein (GFAP) [29, 43, 124]. Depending on the degree of differentiation, MPNST may be positive for collagen type 4 and laminin [21]. MPNST are also immunoreactive for vimentin, but the use of this immunomarker for the diagnosis of MPNST is of little validity since it is expressed in virtually all soft tissue tumors [21].

Immunopositivity for p53 protein occurs in the majority of MPNST [52, 125–127]. Loss of neurofibromin expression is commonly observed in both NF1-associated and sporadic MPNST, while it is retained in other spindle cell tumors [124, 128]. H3K27me3 loss may also serve as a useful diagnostic marker in the distinction of MPNST from other benign and malignant spindle cell neoplasms, although it shows low sensitivity in low-grade and modest sensitivity in intermediate-grade tumors [106, 112, 129, 130]. MPNST with perineural differentiation are immunopositive for epithelial membrane antigen (EMA).

19.6.3 Differential Histopathological Diagnosis

The histopathological spectrum of MPNST presents great variability, being more varied than any other soft tissue sarcoma [21, 46, 62]. The histopathological differential diagnosis of conventional MPNST includes several spindle cell malignancies, such as fibrosarcoma, leiomyosarcoma, spindle cell melanoma, monophasic synovial (spindle cell sarcoma), and malignant fibrous histiocytoma [21, 29, 46].

Fibrosarcoma should be considered in the differential diagnosis of MPNST, especially when the latter presents a fasciculate growth pattern. However, MPNST often exhibit more specific characteristics of neural origin, including a larger proportion of longer, slender spindle cells in a less remarkable fascicular pattern [21, 28]. Also, spiral and palisade tumor cell arrangements are favorable characteristics for MPNST diagnosis. Besides, MPNST feature a more prominent myxoid matrix and high- and low-grade transition areas. Cartilaginous metaplasia is more frequent in MPNST than in fibrosarcomas. In fibrosarcoma, bizarre cells and multinucleated giant ones are rarely observed. The immunopositivity for S-100 and CD57, found in many MPNST, helps differentiate both lesions, as fibrosarcomas are immunonegative for them [21, 28].

The fasciculate pattern of certain MPNST may also confuse them with single-phase synovial sarcoma and leiomyosarcoma [62]. However, monophasic synovial sarcoma contains a more uniform fasciculate pattern and presents more crowded cells with larger and more symmetrical nuclei. There is also a lack of neural differentiation characteristics often present in MPNST [21, 28]. Synovial sarcoma stroma typically presents bands of dense collagen of various thicknesses, irregularly distributed, and occasional calcifications. About 50% of synovial sarcomas have cells that express cytokeratin and EMA, which are not commonly seen in MPNST [21, 62]. Approximately one-quarter of synovial sarcomas present S-100 protein immunopositivity [21, 28, 62].

As for leiomyosarcoma, for Enzinger and Weiss [28], this differentiation can be done without major difficulties. Leiomyosarcoma cells have a more abundant distinct eosinophilic cytoplasm with spindle nuclei, more rounded ends ("cigar" type), and occasional juxtanuclear vacuoles [21, 28, 62]. Leiomyosarcomas may sometimes have immunoreactivity for the S-100 protein [21, 28]. Usually, leiomyosarcomas are immunopositive for muscle markers, which is not the case with MPNST, except for MPNST that present heterologous differentiation into rhabdomyosarcoma [28, 62].

MPNST differentiation from spindle cell melanoma can be difficult, especially since both can express the S-100 protein. Melanoma cells are generally more pleomorphic and have evident nucleoli and nuclear pseudo-inclusions [62]. In contrast to MPNST, S-100 protein immunopositivity is strong and diffuse [21]. MPNST does not express HMB45, tyrosinase, melan A, or keratin, as melanomas do [21, 29, 131].

Histopathological differentiation of low-grade MPNST from ANNUBP and cellular or atypical neurofibromas is important. Cellular neurofibroma is a term used for rare neurofibromas with hypercellularity but without mitotic activity, cytologic atypia, or loss of neurofibroma architecture [111]. ANNUBP has the same histopathological features of low-grade MPNST but with a lower mitotic index (>1/50 HPF and <3/10 HPF) [111]. Atypical neurofibromas are those with only nuclear atypia and can be sporadic or NF1-associated [111]. The presence of focal or more pronounced nuclear atypia in a neurofibroma should not be worrisome for malignancy when there is no increased mitotic activity [111]. Nuclear atypia may include nuclear enlargement two- to threefold or more, hyperchromatism, irregular chromatin distribution, and multinucleated or "bizarre cells" [111]. These features are interpreted as "degenerative atypias," and, analogous to the term ancient schwannoma, the term "ancient neurofibroma" may be used in these cases [111].

The Ki-67 antigen, an immunohistochemical marker widely used in the study of cell proliferation, has been of great value in differentiating low-grade MPNST from neurofibromas. Ki-67 immunostaining has been reported in 5% to 65% of MPNST cells, while neurofibromas typically have less than 5% of immunopositive cells [125]. It has also been suggested that the p53 protein IHC demonstration supports the diagnosis of MPNST [125, 132].

19.7 Histopathological Variants

19.7.1 Epithelioid Variant

The ability of MPNST to undergo mesenchymal or epithelial differentiation is well known [62]. In addition to the usual fusiform components, MPNST can be composed, in part, by cells with large, polygonal, or round nuclei, resembling epithelial cells, being known as epithelioid variant (Fig. 19.4) [28, 133, 134]. The nuclei have one or occasionally more than one evident nucleoli [133, 134]. Certain authors use the name epithelioid MPNST (MPNSTE) for those tumors that are predominantly or exclusively composed of epithelioid cells. Approximately 5–17% of MPNST are epithelioid in nature [28, 43, 131, 133, 135]. Unlike other MPNST, this variant is rarely (in less than 2% of cases) associated with NF1 [134, 136].

Most MPNSTE represent high-grade neoplasms, but cases of low-grade MPNSTE have been reported [136]. Regarding immunohisto-

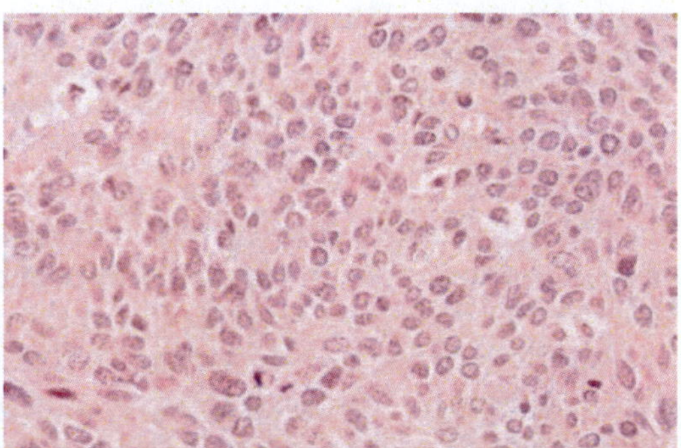

Fig. 19.4 Hematoxylin and eosin, 400×: epithelioid MPNST

chemical findings, approximately 80% of MPNSTE express S-100 protein in the cytoplasm and nucleus in a diffuse and strong form [21, 28, 29]. In some cases, cytokeratin or EMA expression may occur [21].

The histopathological features of MPNSTE are similar to other lesions. Amelanotic melanoma and clear cell sarcoma (or malignant soft tissue melanoma) can be differentiated from MPNST by the absence of a melanin marker such as HMB45 [21, 29, 131]. Also, the presence of the junctional component is useful for differentiating melanoma from MPNST [131]. Exclusion of carcinoma can be done by immunopositive for S-100 and, in most cases, by the absence of cytokeratin and EMA immunoexpression in MPNSTE. Epithelioid sarcoma differs by increased cytoplasm density and dense collagen stroma and lack of myxoid matrix. Besides, epithelioid sarcoma has no immunopositivity for S-100 protein and a positive cytokeratin reaction [21].

19.7.2 Divergent Differentiation

About 12–15% of MPNST have heterologous elements, and this is believed to occur due to divergent heterologous differentiation [21, 60, 131]. Most heterologous mesenchymal elements, when present in MPNST, are malignant and include areas of rhabdomyosarcoma, chondrosarcoma, osteosarcoma, and rarely angiosarcoma [21, 43].

Heterologous differentiation in rhabdomyosarcoma is most frequently observed in MPNST, and these tumors are termed "malignant triton tumors" [21, 28, 137]. The presence of muscle elements in these tumors occurs by neoplastic Schwann cell metaplasia [21]. Malignant triton tumors can occur in patients with and without NF1 [28, 29, 137]. Histopathologically, among the spindle cells, cells resembling those of the embryonic rhabdomyosarcoma are seen; they are round, with prominent central and hyperchromatic nucleus and with abundant eosinophilic cytoplasm [21, 137]. The distribution of rhabdomyoblasts is focal in most cases [137].

The morphological suspicion of rhabdomyosarcoma differentiation can be confirmed by immunopositivity for desmin, myogenin, muscle-specific antigen (HHF35), myoglobin, and alpha-sarcomeric actin [21, 62, 137]. Areas of additional mesenchymal or epithelial differentiation (multidirectional differentiation) can be observed in 15% of malignant triton tumors [21]. The two main lesions that make differential diagnosis with this variant of MPNST are rhabdomyosarcoma and leiomyosarcoma. Studies have shown that rhabdomyosarcomas can express S-100 protein, as well as leiomyosarcomas, presenting more difficulty in the differentiation of these lesions from MPNST. The presence of cells with classic rhabdomyosarcomatous characteristics and immunoreactivity to myoglobin and sarcomeric alpha-actinin are sufficient to rule out the diagnosis of leiomyosarcoma [62].

19.8 Clinical Considerations

As previously stated, MPNST has a strong correlation with NF1, such that around 50% of these tumors arise in this setting. Therefore, the presence of clinical signs compatible with NF1 should be thoroughly investigated, as patients with NF1 have been shown, in some studies, to present worse prognosis as well as higher rates of local recurrence and metastases, which must all be taken into account in the decision-making process [44, 46, 47, 49–52, 54, 55].

Pain must be carefully evaluated in patients with PNT, as benign tumors are generally painless or the pain is established in a slow, gradual manner. In malignant lesions, though, the noxious experience occurs prematurely and progresses very rapidly, usually worsening at night, thus halting the ability of the patients to sleep and take care of his/her own hygiene and activities of daily living. The presence of nocturnal pain or even continuous pain which increases over short periods of time (1, 2 months) must be interpreted as a red flag for the possibility of malignant transformation [138].

Tumors with diameters over 3 or 4 cm, with the following characteristics (especially when subfascial) should alert to possible malignancy: fast growth, hard consistency, pain at percussion or spontaneous, possible traversing of joints, and which are not mobile laterally. In some cases, the tumor may present spontaneous bleeding [138]. Schwabe et al. demonstrated how clinical parameters could be used in conjunction with imaging findings and proposed positive (PPV) and negative predictive values (NPV) for the presence of pain, mass growth, and neurological symptoms. However, the prevalence of MPNST in relation to all tumors in their studies is around 50%, so these findings should be applied judiciously as the calculated PPVs and NPVs might be different from what would be applicable in common practice [139]. Also, benign tumors usually do not cause motor deficits, therefore, when facing a patient with a PNT, in which a progressive motor deficit is established, accompanied by the aforementioned characteristics, this should also raise suspicion of malignancy.

19.9 Complementary Exams

19.9.1 Magnetic Resonance Imaging (MRI)

The crucial complementary exam for the proper study of a presumed MPNST is the MRI, with and without contrast, in which the following features must be evaluated in order to guide decision: the anatomic site and location of the lesion (comprehending not only the neural element of origin but also its neighboring anatomy) and evaluation of its relationship to soft tissue, vascular, osseous, and visceral structures. MRI T1 sequence without contrast is usually not accurate to distinguish the lesion from adjacent tissue. On the other hand, T2 sequence, short T1 inversion recovery (STIR) sequences, as well as sequences with contrast are valuable to discern the lesion from adjacent structures (Fig. 19.5) [140]. MRI alone cannot tell with certainty if a lesion is indeed a MPNST. However, imaging features that raise suspicion of malignancy are intratumoral hemorrhage, involvement or invasion of the surrounding soft tissue, the presence of perilesional muscular edema, heterogeneity, intratumoral necrosis, irregular margins, and larger size of the tumor (Fig. 19.6a) [141–145]. In addition, low values of apparent diffusion coefficient (ADC) ($<1.1 \times 10^{-3}$ mm/s^2) on diffusion-weighted imaging (DWI) also indicate malignancy with high sensitivity and specificity [146, 147], and new techniques, such as the diffusion tensor imaging (DTI), may help evaluate the relationship of the tumor with the fascicles of the nerve of origin (typically, MPNST present with partial of total disruption of fascicles) [148] (Fig. 19.6b).

19.9.2 Computed Tomography (CT)

Although the standard imaging exam for presumed MPNST is the MRI, CT is also able to evaluate the size of the lesion and its relationship to neighboring structures. Its utility in differentiating the lesion from its surrounding soft tissue is limited. However, CT may assist in cases in which the tumor infiltrates osseous structures or promotes bone remodeling.

19.9.3 Positron Emission Tomography (PET)

PET, particularly ^{18}F-FDG PET/CT (fluorodeoxyglucose positron emission tomography), is useful to predict malignancy with high sensitivity and can help in the decision of whether or not to perform biopsy [139, 143, 144, 149–155] (Fig. 19.6c). ^{18}F-FDG PET/CT may also be used in order to assess for metastatic lesions and to guide percutaneous biopsies into hypermetabolic areas of the tumor. A summary of the sensitivity and specificity of ^{18}F-FDG PET, as well as of the SUVmax cutoff point adopted in different studies, is provided in Table 19.4.

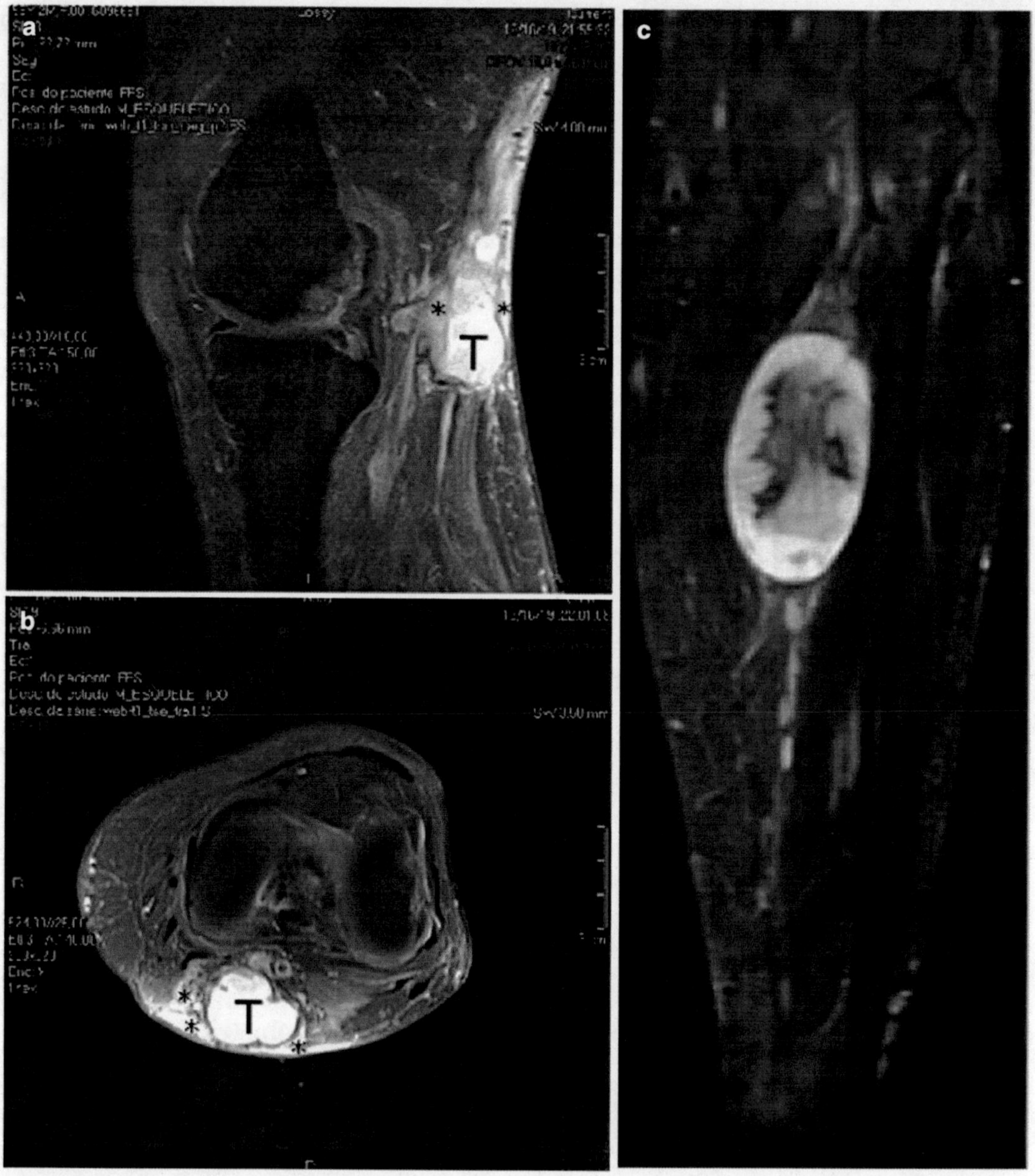

Fig. 19.5 Sagittal (**a**) and axial (**b**) T1-weighted MRI with contrast of a female, 55 years old, non-NF1 patient presenting with excruciating pain in the left leg. The tumor arises from the left tibial nerve. Note the extension of the lesion (>10 cm in the proximal-distal axis), its heterogeneity, and the peritumoral edema. *T* tumor, * peritumoral edema. The final histopathological diagnosis was of a high-grade MPNST. (**c**) STIR MRI with contrast of a male, 23 years old, NF1 patient presenting with pain in the left leg and M4 flexion of the foot. The lesion arises from the left tibial nerve. Note that the lesion is large (>5 cm) and heterogeneous. The final histopathological diagnosis was of a benign neurofibroma

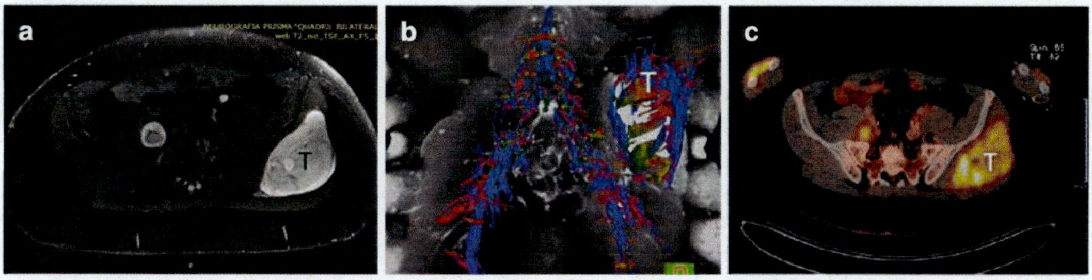

Fig. 19.6 (a) Axial T2-weighted MRI with contrast showing a large lesion inside the substance of the left gluteus medius muscle in a NF1 patient, probably arising from a branch of the inferior gluteal nerve (133 × 115 × 57 mm). Note the contrast enhancement, heterogeneity of the lesion, areas of cystic degeneration, and discrete perilesional edema. *T* tumor. (b) Diffusion tensor imaging (DTI) MRI in the same case demonstrating the relationship with the fascicles of the nerve of origin. *T* tumor. (c) Axial 18FDG-PET CT of the same lesion with a high SUVmax of 8.2. *T* tumor

Table 19.4 Quantitative studies on the predictiveness of ^{18}F-FDG PET for the discrimination of benign peripheral nerve sheath tumors and MPNST in NF1 patients

Author	Number of patients with NF1	Number of lesions	Method	SUVmax cutoff point	Sensitivity	Specificity
Cardona et al. [149]	13	25	^{18}F-FDG PET/ (CT + MRI)	1.8	100	83
Warbey et al. [150]	69	85	^{18}F-FDG PET/CT	3.5	97	87
Benz et al. [151]	13 out of 34	40	^{18}F-FDG PET/CT	6.1	94	91
Tsai et al. [152]	35	27	^{18}F-FDG PET/CT	4	100	94
Derlin et al. [143]	31	75	^{18}F-FDG PET/CT	3.5	100	74.4
Combemale et al. [153]	113	145	^{18}F-FDG PET/CT	T/L* < 1.5	97	76
Chirindel et al. [154]	41	93	^{18}F-FDG PET/CT	4.3	96	93
Salamon et al. [144]	36	36	^{18}F-FDG PET/CT	5.5	95	85
Broski et al. [155]	23 out of 38	43	^{18}F-FDG PET/ (CT + MRI)	6.1	90	78
Schwabe et al. [139]	41	70	^{18}F-FDG PET/CT	5.3	91.2	70

T/L (tumor/liver uptake ratio)

19.9.4 High-Resolution Ultrasonography (HRUS)

HRUS may also be useful in superficial lesions (i.e., extremities), but it is heavily dependent on the experience of the operator. On HRUS, MPNST usually appear as hypo- to isoechoic heterogeneous masses, with unclear margins. Sometimes, hypoechoic cystic components may occur, and round hypoechoic satellites can be seen in the tumor. Vascularization is also usually higher than what is expected for benign PNT [156–158].

19.9.5 Electrophysiological Studies

Electrodiagnostic studies consist of nerve conduction studies (NCS) and needle electromyography (EMG) and may help identify MPNST. In general, benign PNT do not generate neurological deficit. Therefore, the presence of denervation on electroneuromyography (ENMG) is highly suggestive of a more aggressive lesion. These exams are also able to identify subclinical lesions and possible concomitant neuropathies (i.e., diabetic polyneuropathy) that may confound the diagnostic workup [140]. EMG may also identify myokymic discharges, differentiating post-radiation from tumoral plexopathy, as it is only present in the former [159]. Intraoperative electrophysiological monitoring is also important when operating plexual tumors, mainly in the sacral region [160].

19.10 Preoperatory Biopsy

It is important to stress that tumors that are presumed to be benign ought not to be biopsied, given the risk of nerve injury that may cause neurological deficit and/or may initiate or increase pain [161–163]. On the other hand, potentially malignant lesions, according to the aforementioned clinical and imaging criteria, must have a preoperative biopsy.

Biopsy should be performed in an image-guided percutaneous fashion (CT, MRI, HFUS, or PET) by a radiologist. Core needle biopsy should be the preferred technique, as it is usually able to provide a reliable preoperative diagnosis [122, 164, 165]. Some surgeons opt to perform incisional biopsies in quadrants, as a more representative sample of the tumor is obtained. However, the risk of spillage of neoplastic cells must be considered and thoroughly avoided. The decision of which of these techniques should be employed is still a matter of debate, although our policy is to perform core needle image-guided biopsy in the majority of cases. If malignancy is confirmed, the needle tract must be excised along with the lesion during the definitive surgical procedure. Analysis of the collected material must always be performed by a specialized neuropathologist. Given the complexity of neural sheath tumor's histological features, the intraoperative frozen section biopsy diagnosis is often not confirmed after the evaluation of the entire lesion.

The first step after the identification of the probably malignant lesion is to stage it. This is troublesome concerning MPNST, as no staging system has yet been tailored to reliably stratify the risk to these patients. We therefore rely on The American Joint Committee on Cancer Staging System for Soft Tissue Sarcoma updated in 2017 (AJCC 8) [166]. Indeed, recent data seems to validate its use for prognostic purposes in head and neck MPNST, although this does not yet hold true to trunk and extremities' lesions [167]. As stated above, the FNCLCC histopathological grading parameters are also useful for the evaluation of sporadic MPNST, but not for those arising in the setting of NF1 [120].

19.11 Adjuvant Therapy

Although the level of evidence is not high and prospective studies are yet to be performed, adjuvant radiation therapy has been shown to be effective in achieving local control, as demonstrated by a consensus achieved by a group of clinicians and scientists [145, 168]. However, some studies diverge over its efficacy in improving overall survival [24, 169–171]. Neoadjuvant radiotherapy may also help in local control, although further studies are necessary to demonstrate its impact in overall survival [172]. There is still no pharmacological treatment for MPNST, although several drugs have shown promising results in preclinical trials [173]. Nonetheless, selumetinib has been shown, in a phase 2 trial, to decrease the size of inoperable plexiform neurofibromas in NF1 patients, thus apparently halting their progression into MPNST [174].

19.12 Surgical Considerations

Patients should be referred to a center specialized in the treatment of PNT whenever they are considered, after clinical and imaging evaluation, to harbor potential MPNST. An important aspect of this treatment is the participation of clinical and surgical oncology experts, as well as radiotherapists, clinical geneticists, and specialized neuropathology consultation. All patients should pass a routine thoracic and abdominal screening with CT in order to verify the presence of secondary lesions. A complete clinical and laboratory evaluation also must be done, and the case must be discussed in a multidisciplinary fashion.

Surgical decision should be made utilizing the aforementioned clinical and imaging criteria and the preoperative biopsy result. From a practical standpoint, for all lesions considered to be MPNST, complete resection of the tumor with negative margins is the cornerstone of treatment. This is unfeasible in several occasions, without major deficits, depending on the location and volume of the lesion [175].

The surgeon must trace clear preoperative plans, although he/she must be prepared to face unexpected findings, even with good preoperative indicators of the tumor's histological type. The patient is operated under general anesthesia, without the use of neuromuscular blocking agents and/or tourniquets, as they interfere in intraoperative neurophysiological monitoring. The surgery of MPNST follows the steps of a wide approach to the lesion, using an incision that will be centered over the tumor, along the anatomical track of the nerve, with wide margins, as it reduces the risk of damaging superficial nerve structures and provides good exposure of the nerve from which the tumor arises (Fig. 19.7) [161, 176, 177]. The surgeon should palpate the tumor before and during exposure as it may aid in surgical trajectory, and US may help localize non-palpable tumors [178]. Linear incisions should not cross joints. It is preferable to design curved incisions following cutaneous grooves. Constant evaluation of the presence of other peripheral nerves in proximity of the tumor is important, for they may be damaged by transection, retraction, and suture, resulting in pain and/or deficits [179]. During dissection, which should be performed under the surgical microscope or magnifying loupes/glasses, the surgeon must avoid at all cost the rupture of the tumoral capsule. Using neurophysiological techniques to assess functional or silent areas of the nerve of origin and at the tumor surface, the surgeon can define the true extent of the lesion [177]. The surgeon should observe frequently the distal musculature during stimulation or perform evoked EMG to evaluate the viability of fascicles. The relationship of the tumor with its vascular supply, its consistency, and the possibility of tissue invasion should be all evaluated. Dissection is conducted parallelly to the nerve and tumor. The proximal and distal poles of the nerve of origin

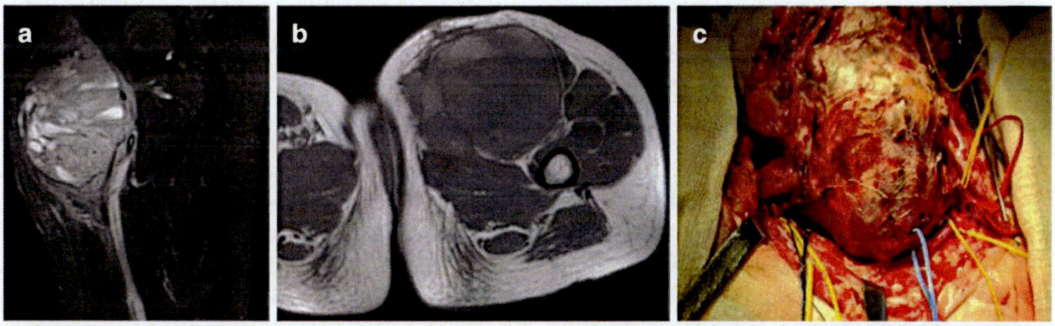

Fig. 19.7 Female, 16 years old, non-NF1, presenting with large mass in the anterior aspect of the left thigh, with intense pain and no motor deficit. A preoperatory biopsy was conducted elsewhere and was inconclusive. (**a**) Sagittal STIR MRI with contrast and (**b**) axial T1-weighted MRI without contrast showing a very large lesion arising from a branch of the left femoral nerve (>16 cm in the proximal-distal axis). Note that the tumor is heterogeneous and presents areas of cystic degeneration. (**c**) Complete exposition of the tumor during surgical resection along with the nerve of origin (branch of the femoral nerve). The final histopathological diagnosis was of a high-grade MPNST

should be exposed and isolated with vessel loops, and the lesion dissected from all surrounding soft tissue (360°) and isolated with cottonoids embedded in saline solution. Any traction of the nerve and tumor should be avoided. Small vessels that enter or leave the tumoral mass are coagulated with bipolar device in low set. Any other major vessel can be isolated and protected with cottonoids.

After exposure of the tumoral mass and isolation of the nerve of origin, without penetrating the tumor capsule, a decision should be taken to sacrifice or not the nerve of origin. This is a critical decision the surgeon must take, and it should be based in some previous information he or she must have in advance:

- Clinical and imaging information
- Result of preoperative biopsy
- Discussion of the case with patient and family

Patients harboring MPNST confirmed via preoperative biopsy should generally have the nerve of origin sacrificed, since the goal of MPNST surgery is to obtain gross total resection (GTR) and guarantee a surgical safe margin. The definition of what is such a margin is still evolving during the limb preservation era. Many surgeons state that the nerve of origin should be indeed sacrificed when the lesion is confirmed to be a MPNST, guaranteeing resection of proximal and distal segments of the nerve devoid of malignant infiltration (Fig. 19.8) [176, 180–182]. Also, all the compromised soft tissue around the tumor must be resected until negative margins are found, as negative margin status has been shown to improve overall survival both in the setting of NF1 and in sporadic cases [2, 169, 183]. We consider a negative margin of 2 cm, 360° around the tumor, to be adequate [70]. Nonetheless, GTR has been shown to be significantly less likely to be achieved in MPNST, when compared to its benign counterparts (OR = 0.22) [184].

In cases in which the preoperative biopsy was inconclusive, the surgeon may opt to repeat it or to proceed to surgery and conduct an intraoperative biopsy in quadrants, with care not to spill tumoral cells. Needless to say, a neuropathologist with experience in PNT is vital in order to arrive at the correct diagnosis. This fact is extremely important because the decision to continue with the surgical procedure or to stop it and wait for the final diagnosis will depend on the conclusion of the neuropathologist. This critical issue for the decision-making process is often unreliable, mainly in large tumors which may present different grades of malignancy in different regions of the mass. It is generally not advisable to proceed to an aggressive technique based on the frozen section diagnosis. We thus usually close the incision and wait for the definitive pathology result.

Some surgeons decide, after sacrificing a nerve compromised by MPNST, to reconstruct the gap with nerve grafts or sometimes to proceed to distal nerve transferences [185–187]. However, it is important to point out that:

1. If the patient has NF1, there is a risk that the graft will also be compromised by the disease.
2. If the patient should be submitted to radiotherapy for the malignant lesion, probably the graft will not survive or the transference will not function.

Nevertheless, these are some possibilities that should be kept in mind in patients with low-grade MPNST or even BPNST in which some motor deficit developed after surgery.

In lesions presenting in the brachial or lumbosacral plexus, the need for negative margins should be analyzed in a very specific way. What means a negative margin in such regions? Should the surgeon resect vascular elements and most of the plexus together with the tumor mass? Clearly in this type of situation, a case-by-case decision should be made. This is important because the decision taken may result in the complete functional disabling of the limb. In proximal high-grade limb tumors without metastatic spread, or in a setting that after resection of the lesion, the limb would

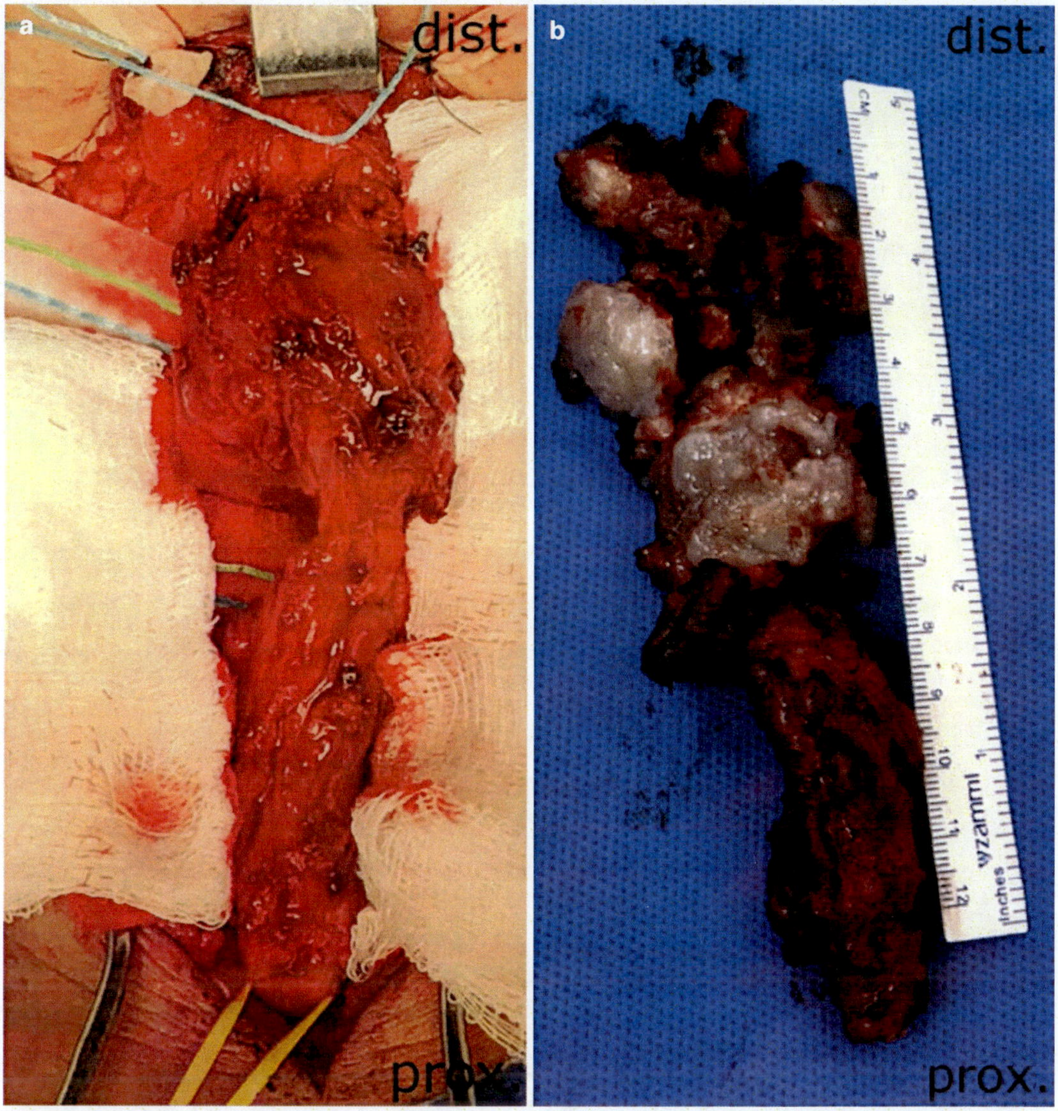

Fig. 19.8 Female, 55 years old, non-NF1 patient presenting with excruciating pain in the left leg. (**a**) Exposition of the lesion arising from the left tibial nerve. (**b**) Photograph of the lesion and of the apparently healthy proximal and distal poles of the nerve after resection of the tumor and sacrifice of the nerve of origin. The final histopathological diagnosis was of a high-grade MPNST

become useless, amputation is considered by some [188, 189]. Nonetheless, amputation appears to be associated with higher rates of postoperative complications (up to 44%), including phantom limb pain; it also causes a huge negative impact in quality of life and has not been shown to improve survival, when compared to other techniques [187, 190, 191]. Figure 19.9 shows an unfavorable evolution of a high-grade MPNST.

It is important to stress that the aforementioned principles for the treatment of MPNST also hold true for the pediatric population. We found, in a small series of surgically treated pediatric patients for MPNST in our institution, that the following symptoms should be taken as

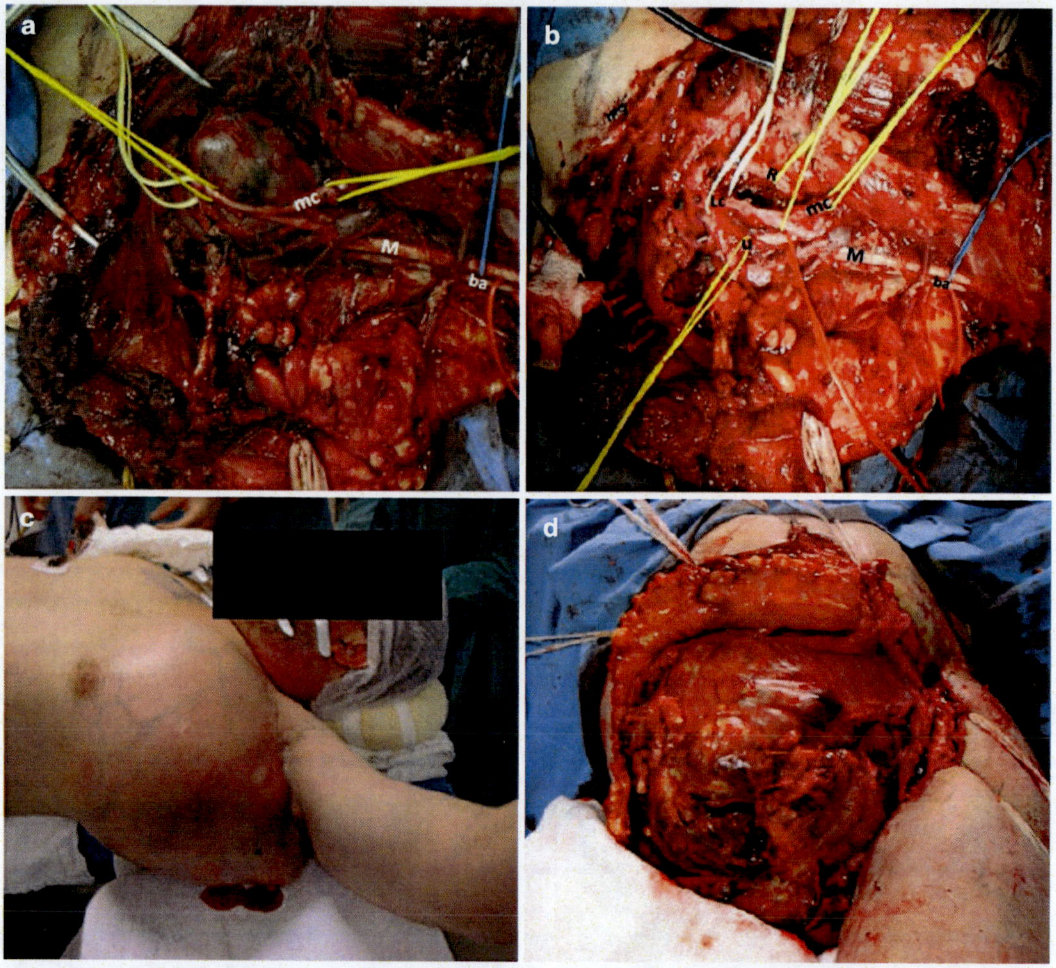

Fig. 19.9 Male, 31 years, non-NF1 patient presenting with a solitary mass in the left infraclavicular brachial plexus with intense pain and no neurological deficit. A preoperative biopsy was inconclusive. (**a**) Wide exposure of the infraclavicular and axillar region on the left, with visualization of the tumor and dissection of neural and vascular elements without rupture of the tumoral capsule: *mc* musculocutaneous nerve, *M* median nerve, *ba* brachial artery. (**b**) Surgical aspect after resection of the lesion: *Lc* lateral cord of the brachial plexus, *R* radial nerve, *u* ulnar nerve, *mc* musculocutaneous nerve, *M* median nerve, *ba* brachial artery. The excisional biopsy confirmed the diagnosis of a high-grade MPNST. The patient was referred to clinical oncology and underwent radio- and chemotherapy. After 1 year, he was surgically approached again due to local recurrence. Section of the plexus was not an option because of the patient's desire. (**c**) After 1 year and 9 months from the first operation, the patient returned with a large local recurrence, presenting with pain and cutaneous lesions due to infiltration of the tumor. (**d**) Exposition of the lesion. Amputation was not considered, given the thoracic invasion by the mass. The patient died 3 months after the last surgery due to bilateral pulmonary metastases

red flags for possible malignancy: pain, even with subtle onset; growth of the lesion; refusal to perform normal activities of daily living, such as bathing; and refusal in permitting that the region where the lump lays is touched. For high-grade lesions, the surgical goal is the same: to achieve gross total resection with wide margins [13].

19.12.1 ANNUBP and Low-Grade MPNST

Whenever a tumor is considered to be a MPNST upon clinical and imaging criteria and the preoperatory biopsy result, the lesion should be approached as a high-grade MPNST until proven otherwise. Any preoperative diagnosis of an ANNUBP or low-grade MPNST should be evaluated with care, and it should only be considered trustworthy in order to justify a less aggressive approach if it is given by a neuropathologist experienced in PNT. Nonetheless, the literature is showing a tendency to support less invasive approaches to these lesions. Bernthal et al. demonstrated, in low-grade MPNST (at the time classified as having <5 mitoses/10HPF), a disease-specific survival (DSS) of 100% after a median follow-up of 47 months after surgery, independently of margin status [175]. It is not clear, however, how many of these lesions would now be termed ANNUBP (<3 mitoses/10HPF). Watson et al. showed a DSS of 100% after a follow-up of 5 years in 12 patients with low-grade MPSNT; 4 patients presented R1 (microscopically positive ≤1 mm) or R2 (macroscopically positive) surgical margins [192]. Nelson et al. presented a series of 16 surgically treated atypical neurofibromas, ANNUBP, and low-grade MPNST in which a safe marginal resection technique was conducted with overall little morbidity and no recurrence after a median follow-up of 2.45 years [193]. Positive surgical margins, subtotal resection of the tumor, and preservation of the nerve of origin of the mass are some accepted goals by certain clinicians in the surgical process for low-grade lesions (Fig. 19.10). Differently from high-

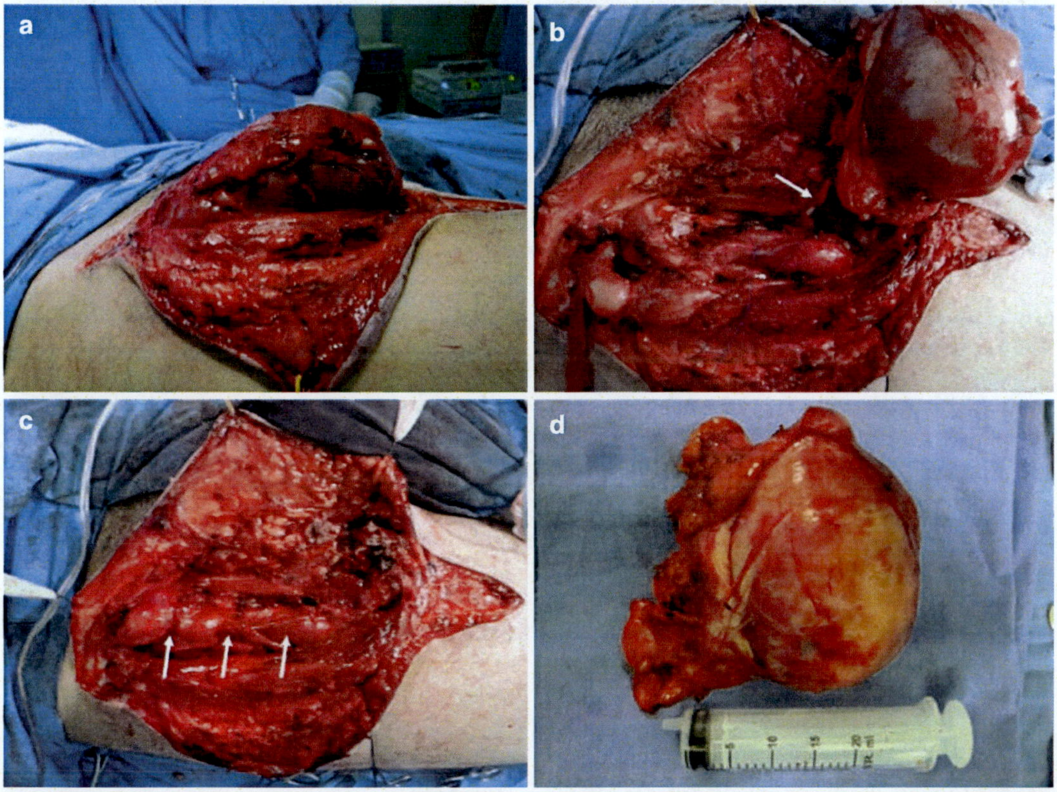

Fig. 19.10 Male, 37 years old, NF1, presenting with a large mass in the anterior aspect of the right thigh. The patient presented excruciating pain in the thigh and medial aspect of the leg, without neurological deficit. A preoperative biopsy was conducted elsewhere and was inconclusive. **(a)** Exposition of the large tumor arising from the branch of femoral nerve to the vastus medialis. **(b)** Resection of the tumor in block, white arrow indicates the branch from which the tumor arises. **(c)** Surgical aspect after tumor removal, white arrows indicate the femoral nerve with the typical plexiform aspect of NF1. **(d)** Tumor resected in one block along with the nerve of origin. The final histopathological diagnosis was of a low-grade MPNST

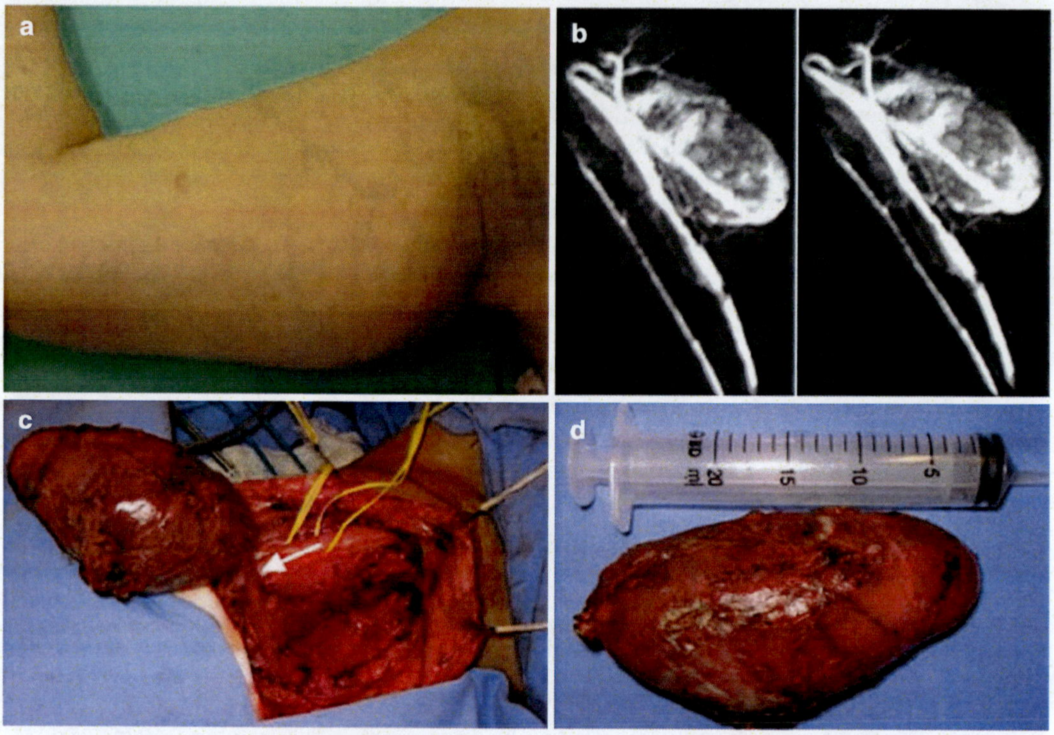

Fig. 19.11 Female, 28 years old, NF1 patient presenting with a mass in the right arm with pain and no neurological deficit. (**a**) Large mass in the medial aspect of the right arm presenting with spontaneous pain. (**b**) Angio-CT of the tumor. Note that it is highly vascularized. (**c**) Surgical resection of the lesion. White arrow indicates the nerve of origin (medial cutaneous nerve of the arm). (**d**) The tumor was resected in block without rupture of the tumoral capsule (>20 cm in its longest axis). The final histopathological diagnosis was of a low-grade MPNST

grade MPNST, it is possible to reach long survival without metastatic spread with this policy in low-grade MPNST (Fig. 19.11) [175, 192]. It is necessary, though, that further studies are conducted, in order to consolidate our understanding about this difference in prognosis and the possibility of a less aggressive approach for these premalignant and low-grade lesions [175, 192, 193].

19.13 Conclusion

MPNST comprise a group of very rare and aggressive tumors, and NF1 predisposes the patient to their development. Each case should be discussed along with a multidisciplinary team. This includes the peripheral nerve surgeon, clinical and surgical oncology experts, radiotherapists, clinical geneticists, and neuropathologists. The diagnosis should be made by the conjunction of clinical aspects, imaging exams, and preoperatory histopathology. Further studies are necessary in order to improve the diagnostic accuracy of non-invasive imaging exams. To date, however, ^{18}F-FDG PET/CT and DWI are the best non-invasive tools to evaluate for malignancy. It is crucial not to biopsy lesions with clinical and imaging characteristics that do not denote malignancy. Preoperative biopsy should be performed in an image-guided core needle fashion, although some may use fine-needle aspiration cytology as well. Sometimes an incisional in quadrants biopsy may also be used, but utmost care must be taken not to spill neoplastic cells in the field.

For high-grade MPNST, surgery should be as aggressive as possible, aiming at total resection of the lesion, which implies the sacrifice of the nerve of origin. In some regions (i.e., brachial and lumbosacral plexus), this is not always possible. For low-grade MPNST, which represent the minority of these lesions, it is possible to strive for both a complete resection and preservation of function. It is of the utmost importance to have a pathologist with experience in PNT to analyze the material during preoperative and transoperative biopsy studies and after the definitive surgical procedure. Other treatment modalities such as radiotherapy and chemotherapy have had controversial results. Yet, radiotherapy is used for local recurrence control.

References

1. Stucky C-CH, Johnson KN, Gray RJ, Pockaj BA, Ocal IT, Rose PS, et al. Malignant peripheral nerve sheath Tumors (MPNST): the Mayo Clinic experience. Ann Surg Oncol. 2012;19:878–85.
2. Anghileri M, Miceli R, Fiore M, Mariani L, Ferrari A, Mussi C, et al. Malignant peripheral nerve sheath tumors: prognostic factors and survival in a series of patients treated at a single institution. Cancer. 2006;107:1065–74.
3. LaFemina J, Qin L-X, Moraco NH, Antonescu CR, Fields RC, Crago AM, et al. Oncologic outcomes of sporadic, neurofibromatosis-associated, and radiation-induced malignant peripheral nerve sheath tumors. Ann Surg Oncol. 2013;20:66–72.
4. Seferis C, Torrens M, Paraskevopoulou C, Psichidis G. Malignant transformation in vestibular schwannoma: report of a single case, literature search, and debate. J Neurosurg. 2014;121:160–6.
5. Woodruff JM, Selig AM, Crowley K, Allen PW. Schwannoma (Neurilemoma) with malignant transformation a rare, distinctive peripheral nerve tumor. Am J Surg Pathol [Internet]. 1994;18. https://journals.lww.com/ajsp/Fulltext/1994/09000/Schwannoma__Neurilemoma__with_Malignant.3.aspx
6. Alexiev BA, Chou PM, Jennings LJ. Pathology of melanotic schwannoma. Arch Pathol Lab Med. 2018;142:1517–23.
7. Keskin E, Ekmekci S, Oztekin O, Diniz G. Melanotic schwannomas are rarely seen pigmented tumors with unpredictable prognosis and challenging diagnosis. Case Rep Pathol. 2017;2017:1–4.
8. Ida CM, Scheithauer BW, Yapicier Ö, Carney JA, Wenger DE, Inwards CY, et al. Primary schwannoma of the bone: a clinicopathologic and radiologic study of 17 cases. Am J Surg Pathol. 2011;35:989–97.
9. Grünewald TGP, Cidre-Aranaz F, Surdez D, Tomazou EM, de Álava E, Kovar H, et al. Ewing sarcoma. Nat Rev Dis Primer. 2018;4:5.
10. Mohan AT, Park DH, Jalgaonkar A, Alorjani M, Aston W, Briggs T. Intra-neural Ewing's sarcoma of the upper limb mimicking a peripheral nerve tumour. A report of 2 cases. J Plast Reconstr Aesthet Surg. 2011;64:e153–6.
11. Mitchell BD, Fox BD, Viswanathan A, Mitchell AH, Powell SZ, Cech DA. Ewing sarcoma mimicking a peripheral nerve sheath tumor. J Clin Neurosci. 2010;17:1317–9.
12. Lavorato A, Titolo P, Vincitorio F, Cofano F, Garbossa D. Intraneural Ewing sarcoma of fibular nerve: case report, radiologic findings and review of literature. World Neurosurg. 2019;123:212–5.
13. Guedes F, Brown RS, Torrão-Junior FJL, Barbosa DAN, de Andrade Gagheggi Ravanini G, RMP A. Pediatric peripheral nerve tumors: clinical and surgical aspects. Childs Nerv Syst. 2019;35:2289–97.
14. Siqueira MG, Tavares PL, Martins RS, Heise CO, Foroni LHL, Bordalo M, et al. Management of desmoid-type fibromatosis involving peripheral nerves. Arq Neuropsiquiatr. 2012;70:514–9.
15. Juliette O, Florentius K, Francis N, Macharia BN, Neema M. Desmoid tumour of the brachial plexus. Case Rep Surg. 2013;2013:1–4.
16. Alman B, Attia S, Baumgarten C, Benson C, Blay J-Y, Bonvalot S, et al. The management of desmoid tumours: a joint global consensus-based guideline approach for adult and paediatric patients. Eur J Cancer. 2020;127:96–107.
17. Miwa S, Kitamura S, Shirai T, Hayashi K, Nishida H, Takeuchi A, et al. Desmoplastic small round cell tumour successfully treated with caffeine-assisted chemotherapy: a case report and review of the literature. Anticancer Res. 2010;30:3769–74.
18. Mathys J, Vajtai I, Vögelin E, Zimmermann DR, Ozdoba C, Hewer E, et al. Desmoplastic small round cell tumor: a rare cause of a progressive brachial plexopathy. Muscle Nerve. 2014;49:922–7.
19. Guedes-Corrêa JF, Amorim RP, da Costa Pereira Pereira MR, RSV C, Costa FD, de Souza Bianchi B, et al. Multimodal treatment of an extremely rare desmoplastic small round cell tumor primary to the brachial plexus—A case report and review of literature. Surg Neurol Int. 2019;10:140.
20. Strom T, Kleinschmidt-DeMasters BK, Donson A, Foreman NK, Lillehei KO. Rare nerve lesions of non–nerve sheath origin: a 17-year retrospective series. Arch Pathol Lab Med. 2009;133:12.
21. Antonescu CR, Scheithauer BW, Woodruff JM. Tumors ot the peripheral nervous system. Silver Spring: ARP Press; 2013.
22. Kleihues P, Burger PC, Scheithauer BW. Histological typing of tumours of the central nervous system [Internet]. Berlin: Springer; 1993. http://public.ebookcentral.proquest.com/choice/publicfullrecord.aspx?p=3095845
23. Wanebo JE, Malik JM, VandenBerg SR, Wanebo HJ, Driesen N, Persing JA. Malignant peripheral nerve sheath tumors. A clinicopathologic study of 28 cases. Cancer. 1993;71:1247–53.

24. Kar M, Deo SVS, Shukla NK, Malik A, DattaGupta S, Mohanti BK, et al. Malignant peripheral nerve sheath tumors (MPNST)—clinicopathological study and treatment outcome of twenty-four cases. World J Surg Oncol. 2006;4:55.
25. Scheithauer BW. Development of the WHO classification of tumors of the central nervous system: a historical perspective. Brain Pathol. 2009;19:551–64.
26. Carroll SL, Ratner N. How does the Schwann cell lineage form tumors in NF1? Glia. 2008;56:1590–605.
27. Fisher C, Montgomery E, Thway K. Biopsy interpretation of soft tissue tumors. Philadelphia: Wolters Kluwer/Lippincott Williams & Wilkins Health; 2011.
28. Enzinger FM, Weiss SW, editors. Soft tissue tumors. 6th. ed. St. Louis: Mosby; 2014.
29. Weltgesundheitsorganisation. WHO classification of tumours of the central nervous system. Revised 4th ed. Louis DN, Ohgaki H, Wiestler OD, Cavenee WK, editors. Lyon: International Agency for Research on Cancer; 2016.
30. Burger PC, Scheithauer BW, Vogel FS. Surgical pathology of the nervous system and its coverings. 3rd ed. New York: Churchill Livingstone; 1991.
31. Marocchio LS, Oliveira DT, Pereira MC, Soares CT, Fleury RN. Sporadic and multiple neurofibromas in the head and neck region: a retrospective study of 33 years. Clin Oral Investig. 2007;11:165–9.
32. Spinner RJ, Scheithauer BW, Perry A, Amrami KK, Emnett R, Gutmann DH. Colocalized cellular schwannoma and plexiform neurofibroma in the absence of neurofibromatosis. J Neurosurg. 2007;107:435–9.
33. Levy Bencheton A, Mallet S, Rojat Habib M-C, Figarella-Branger D, Sigaudy S, Grob J-J, et al. [Isolated late-onset plexiform neurofibroma in the absence of neurofibromatosis]. Ann Dermatol Venereol. 2010;137:301–4.
34. Atkins NK, Stensby JD, Gaballah AH. Lumbosacral plexiform neurofibroma: a rare case in an adult without neurofibromatosis type I. Skeletal Radiol [Internet]. 2019 [cited 2019 Dec 1]. http://link.springer.com/10.1007/s00256-019-03281-2
35. Friedman JM, Riccardi VM, editors. Neurofibromatosis: phenotype, natural history, and pathogenesis. 3rd ed. Baltimore: Johns Hopkins University Press; 1999.
36. Korf BR. Plexiform neurofibromas. Am J Med Genet. 1999;89:31–7.
37. Packer RJ, Gutmann DH, Rubenstein A, Viskochil D, Zimmerman RA, Vezina G, et al. Plexiform neurofibromas in NF1: toward biologic-based therapy. Neurology. 2002;58:1461–70.
38. Woodruff JM. Pathology of tumors of the peripheral nerve sheath in type 1 neurofibromatosis. Am J Med Genet. 1999;89:23–30.
39. Strike SA, Puhaindran ME. Nerve tumors of the upper extremity. Clin Plast Surg. 2019;46:347–50.
40. Ducatman BS, Scheithauer BW. Postirradiation neurofibrosarcoma. Cancer. 1983;51:1028–33.
41. Evans DGR, Birch JM, Ramsden RT, Sharif S, Baser ME. Malignant transformation and new primary tumours after therapeutic radiation for benign disease: substantial risks in certain tumour prone syndromes. J Med Genet. 2006;43:289–94.
42. Scheithauer BW, Erdogan S, Rodriguez FJ, Burger PC, Woodruff JM, Kros JM, et al. Malignant peripheral nerve sheath tumors of cranial nerves and intracranial contents: a clinicopathologic study of 17 cases. Am J Surg Pathol. 2009;33:325–38.
43. Thway K, Fisher C. Malignant peripheral nerve sheath tumor: pathology and genetics. Ann Diagn Pathol. 2014;18:109–16.
44. Miao R, Wang H, Jacobson A, Lietz AP, Choy E, Raskin KA, et al. Radiation-induced and neurofibromatosis-associated malignant peripheral nerve sheath tumors (MPNST) have worse outcomes than sporadic MPNST. Radiother Oncol. 2019;137:61–70.
45. Zou C, Smith KD, Liu J, Lahat G, Myers S, Wang W-L, et al. Clinical, pathological, and molecular variables predictive of malignant peripheral nerve sheath tumor outcome. Ann Surg. 2009;249:1014–22.
46. Ducatman BS, Scheithauer BW, Piepgras DG, Reiman HM, Ilstrup DM. Malignant peripheral nerve sheath tumors. A clinicopathologic study of 120 cases. Cancer. 1986;57:2006–21.
47. Evans DGR, Baser ME, McGaughran J, Sharif S, Howard E, Moran A. Malignant peripheral nerve sheath tumours in neurofibromatosis 1. J Med Genet. 2002;39:311–4.
48. Uusitalo E, Leppävirta J, Koffert A, Suominen S, Vahtera J, Vahlberg T, et al. Incidence and mortality of neurofibromatosis: a total population study in Finland. J Invest Dermatol. 2015;135:904–6.
49. D'agostino AN, Soule EH, Miller RH. Primary malignant neoplasms of nerves (malignant neurilemomas) in patients without manifestations of multiple neurofibromatosis (Von Recklinghausens's disease). Cancer. 1963;16:1003–14.
50. Sordillo PP, Helson L, Hajdu SI, Magill GB, Kosloff C, Golbey RB, et al. Malignant schwannoma—clinical characteristics, survival, and response to therapy. Cancer. 1981;47:2503–9.
51. Zhou H, Coffin CM, Perkins SL, Tripp SR, Liew M, Viskochil DH. Malignant peripheral nerve sheath tumor: a comparison of grade, immunophenotype, and cell cycle/growth activation marker expression in sporadic and neurofibromatosis 1-related lesions. Am J Surg Pathol. 2003;27:1337–45.
52. Cunha KSG, Caruso AC, de Faria PAS, da Silva LE, Pires ARC, Geller M, et al. Malignant peripheral nerve sheath tumors: clinicopathological aspects, expression of p53 and survival. Clinics. 2012;67:963–8.
53. Porter DE, Prasad V, Foster L, Dall GF, Birch R, Grimer RJ. Survival in malignant peripheral nerve sheath tumours: a comparison between sporadic and neurofibromatosis type 1-associated tumours. Sarcoma. 2009;2009:1–5.

54. Le Guellec S, Decouvelaere A-V, Filleron T, Valo I, Charon-Barra C, Robin Y-M, et al. Malignant peripheral nerve sheath tumor is a challenging diagnosis: a systematic pathology review, immunohistochemistry, and molecular analysis in 160 patients from the French Sarcoma Group database. Am J Surg Pathol. 2016;40:896–908.
55. Martin E, Coert JH, Flucke UE, Slooff W-BM, Ho VKY, van der Graaf WT, et al. A nationwide cohort study on treatment and survival in patients with malignant peripheral nerve sheath tumours. Eur J Cancer. 2020;124:77–87.
56. de Vasconcelos RAT, Coscarelli PG, Alvarenga RP, Acioly MA. Malignant peripheral nerve sheath tumor with and without neurofibromatosis type 1. Arq Neuropsiquiatr. 2017;75:366–71.
57. Kolberg M, Holand M, Agesen TH, Brekke HR, Liestol K, Hall KS, et al. Survival meta-analyses for >1800 malignant peripheral nerve sheath tumor patients with and without neurofibromatosis type 1. Neuro Oncol. 2013;15:135–47.
58. Amirian ES, Goodman JC, New P, Scheurer ME. Pediatric and adult malignant peripheral nerve sheath tumors: an analysis of data from the surveillance, epidemiology, and end results program. J Neurooncol. 2014;116(3):609–16. https://doi.org/10.1007/s11060-013-1345-6.
59. Cashen DV, Parisien RC, Raskin K, Hornicek FJ, Gebhardt MC, Mankin HJ. Survival data for patients with malignant schwannoma. Clin Orthop. 2004:69–73.
60. Hruban RH, Shiu MH, Senie RT, Woodruff JM. Malignant peripheral nerve sheath tumors of the buttock and lower extremity. A study of 43 cases. Cancer. 1990;66:1253–65.
61. Wick MR, Swanson PE, Scheithauer BW, Manivel JC. Malignant peripheral nerve sheath tumor. An immunohistochemical study of 62 cases. Am J Clin Pathol. 1987;87:425–33.
62. Stasik CJ, Tawfik O. Malignant peripheral nerve sheath tumor with rhabdomyosarcomatous differentiation (malignant triton tumor). Arch Pathol Lab Med. 2006;130:1878–81.
63. Ducatman BS, Scheithauer BW, Piepgras DG, Reiman HM. Malignant peripheral nerve sheath tumors in childhood. J Neurooncol. 1984;2:241–8.
64. Friedrich RE, Hartmann M, Mautner VF. Malignant peripheral nerve sheath tumors (MPNST) in NF1-affected children. Anticancer Res. 2007;27:1957–60.
65. Bergamaschi L, Bisogno G, Manzitti C, D'Angelo P, Milano GM, Scagnellato A, et al. Salvage rates and prognostic factors after relapse in children and adolescents with malignant peripheral nerve sheath tumors. Pediatr Blood Cancer. 2018;65:e26816.
66. Valentin T, Le Cesne A, Ray-Coquard I, Italiano A, Decanter G, Bompas E, et al. Management and prognosis of malignant peripheral nerve sheath tumors: the experience of the French Sarcoma Group (GSF-GETO). Eur J Cancer. 2016;56:77–84.
67. Stewart FW, Copeland MM. Neurogenic sarcoma. Am J Cancer. 1931;15:1235.
68. Quick D, Cutler M. Neurogenic sarcoma: a clinical and pathological study. Ann Surg. 1927;86:810–29.
69. Guttman MR, Simon MU. Neurofibrosarcoma of the facial nerve involving the tympanomastoid. AMA Arch Otolaryngol. 1951;54:162–6.
70. Angelov L, Davis A, O'Sullivan B, Bell R, Guha A. Neurogenic sarcomas: experience at the University of Toronto. Neurosurgery. 1998;43:56–64.
71. Storm FK, Eilber FR, Mirra J, Morton DL. Neurofibrosarcoma. Cancer. 1980;45:126–9.
72. Gonzalez-Gomez P, Bello MJ, Arjona D, Alonso ME, Lomas J, De Campos JM, et al. Aberrant CpG island methylation in neurofibromas and neurofibrosarcomas. Oncol Rep. 2003;10:1519–23.
73. Krause, F.: Sammlung klrnischer Vortrage (Volkmann), 1887; N. 293–294, Leipzig.
74. Flemming LN, Marvin FW. Familial fibromyxomata of the peripheral nerves. Surg Gynec Obst. 1917;24:287.
75. McGlannan A. J Alumni Assoc Coll Phys Surg. 1911;14:97.
76. Bloodgood JC. Tr Am Burg Assoc. 1909;27:384.
77. Eisenbarth I, Beyer K, Krone W, Assum G. Toward a survey of somatic mutation of the NF1 gene in benign neurofibromas of patients with neurofibromatosis type 1. Am J Hum Genet. 2000;66:393–401.
78. Karube K, Nabeshima K, Ishiguro M, Harada M, Iwasaki H. cDNA microarray analysis of cancer associated gene expression profiles in malignant peripheral nerve sheath tumours. J Clin Pathol. 2006;59:160–5.
79. Kluwe L, Friedrich RE, Mautner VF. Allelic loss of the NF1 gene in NF1-associated plexiform neurofibromas. Cancer Genet Cytogenet. 1999;113:65–9.
80. Serra E, Puig S, Otero D, Gaona A, Kruyer H, Ars E, et al. Confirmation of a double-hit model for the NF1 gene in benign neurofibromas. Am J Hum Genet. 1997;61:512–9.
81. Lévy P, Vidaud D, Leroy K, Laurendeau I, Wechsler J, Bolasco G, et al. Molecular profiling of malignant peripheral nerve sheath tumors associated with neurofibromatosis type 1, based on large-scale real-time RT-PCR. Mol Cancer. 2004;3:20.
82. Shen MH, Harper PS, Upadhyaya M. Molecular genetics of neurofibromatosis type 1 (NF1). J Med Genet. 1996;33:2–17.
83. Le LQ, Parada LF. Tumor microenvironment and neurofibromatosis type I: connecting the GAPs. Oncogene. 2007;26:4609–16.
84. Vogel KS, Klesse LJ, Velasco-Miguel S, Meyers K, Rushing EJ, Parada LF. Mouse tumor model for neurofibromatosis type 1. Science. 1999;286:2176–9.
85. Campbell SL, Khosravi-Far R, Rossman KL, Clark GJ, Der CJ. Increasing complexity of Ras signaling. Oncogene. 1998;17:1395–413.
86. Alberts B, Bray D, Lewis J, Raff M, Roberts K, Watson JD. Biologia molecular da célula. Artes Médicas: Porto Alegre; 1997.

87. Alberts B. Molecular biology of the cell. 6th ed. Garland Science, Taylor and Francis Group: New York; 2015.
88. Kolch W. Meaningful relationships: the regulation of the Ras/Raf/MEK/ERK pathway by protein interactions. Biochem J. 2000;351(Pt 2):289–305.
89. Rodriguez-Viciana P, Warne PH, Dhand R, Vanhaesebroeck B, Gout I, Fry MJ, et al. Phosphatidylinositol-3-OH kinase as a direct target of Ras. Nature. 1994;370:527–32.
90. Kelley GG, Reks SE, Ondrako JM, Smrcka AV. Phospholipase C(epsilon): a novel Ras effector. EMBO J. 2001;20:743–54.
91. Kumar V, Abbas AK, Aster JC, editors. Robbins and Cotran pathologic basis of disease. 9th ed. Philadelphia: Elsevier/Saunders; 2015.
92. Mawrin C, Kirches E, Boltze C, Dietzmann K, Roessner A, Schneider-Stock R. Immunohistochemical and molecular analysis of p53, RB, and PTEN in malignant peripheral nerve sheath tumors. Virchows Arch Int J Pathol. 2002;440:610–5.
93. Upadhyaya M, Han S, Consoli C, Majounie E, Horan M, Thomas NS, et al. Characterization of the somatic mutational spectrum of the neurofibromatosis type 1 (NF1) gene in neurofibromatosis patients with benign and malignant tumors. Hum Mutat. 2004;23:134–46.
94. Berghmans S, Murphey RD, Wienholds E, Neuberg D, Kutok JL, Fletcher CDM, et al. tp53 mutant zebrafish develop malignant peripheral nerve sheath tumors. Proc Natl Acad Sci U S A. 2005;102:407–12.
95. Cichowski K, Shih TS, Schmitt E, Santiago S, Reilly K, McLaughlin ME, et al. Mouse models of tumor development in neurofibromatosis type 1. Science. 1999;286:2172–6.
96. Beert E, Brems H, Daniëls B, De Wever I, Van Calenbergh F, Schoenaers J, et al. Atypical neurofibromas in neurofibromatosis type 1 are premalignant tumors. Genes Chromosomes Cancer. 2011;50:1021–32.
97. Lee W, Teckie S, Wiesner T, Ran L, Prieto Granada CN, Lin M, et al. PRC2 is recurrently inactivated through EED or SUZ12 loss in malignant peripheral nerve sheath tumors. Nat Genet. 2014;46:1227–32.
98. Carroll SL, Stonecypher MS. Tumor suppressor mutations and growth factor signaling in the pathogenesis of NF1-associated peripheral nerve sheath tumors: II. The role of dysregulated growth factor signaling. J Neuropathol Exp Neurol. 2005;64:1–9.
99. DeClue JE, Heffelfinger S, Benvenuto G, Ling B, Li S, Rui W, et al. Epidermal growth factor receptor expression in neurofibromatosis type 1-related tumors and NF1 animal models. J Clin Invest. 2000;105:1233–41.
100. Holtkamp N, Atallah I, Okuducu A-F, Mucha J, Hartmann C, Mautner V-F, et al. MMP-13 and p53 in the progression of malignant peripheral nerve sheath tumors. Neoplasia. 2007;9:671–7.
101. Rao UN, Sonmez-Alpan E, Michalopoulos GK. Hepatocyte growth factor and c-MET in benign and malignant peripheral nerve sheath tumors. Hum Pathol. 1997;28:1066–70.
102. Kehrer-Sawatzki H, Mautner V-F, Cooper DN. Emerging genotype–phenotype relationships in patients with large NF1 deletions. Hum Genet. 2017;136:349–76.
103. Anderson WJ, Hornick JL. Immunohistochemical correlates of recurrent genetic alterations in sarcomas. Genes Chromosomes Cancer. 2019;58:111–23.
104. Korfhage J, Lombard DB. Malignant peripheral nerve sheath tumors: from epigenome to bedside. Mol Cancer Res. 2019;17:1417–28.
105. Margueron R, Reinberg D. The polycomb complex PRC2 and its mark in life. Nature. 2011;469:343–9.
106. Hornick JL. Limited biopsies of soft tissue tumors: the contemporary role of immunohistochemistry and molecular diagnostics. Mod Pathol. 2019;32:27–37.
107. De Raedt T, Beert E, Pasmant E, Luscan A, Brems H, Ortonne N, et al. PRC2 loss amplifies Ras-driven transcription and confers sensitivity to BRD4-based therapies. Nature. 2014;514:247–51.
108. Plaat BE, Molenaar WM, Mastik MF, Hoekstra HJ, te Meerman GJ, van den Berg E. Computer-assisted cytogenetic analysis of 51 malignant peripheral-nerve-sheath tumors: sporadic vs. neurofibromatosis-type-1-associated malignant schwannomas. Int J Cancer. 1999;83:171–8.
109. Kim A, Stewart DR, Reilly KM, Viskochil D, Miettinen MM, Widemann BC. Malignant peripheral nerve sheath tumors state of the science: leveraging clinical and biological insights into effective therapies. Sarcoma. 2017;2017:7429697.
110. Bilgic B, Ates LE, Demiryont M, Ozger H, Dizdar Y. Malignant peripheral nerve sheath tumors associated with neurofibromatosis type 1. Pathol Oncol Res. 2003;9:201–5.
111. Miettinen MM, Antonescu CR, Fletcher CDM, Kim A, Lazar AJ, Quezado MM, et al. Histopathologic evaluation of atypical neurofibromatous tumors and their transformation into malignant peripheral nerve sheath tumor in patients with neurofibromatosis 1—a consensus overview. Hum Pathol. 2017;67:1–10.
112. Lu VM, Marek T, Gilder HE, Puffer RC, Raghunathan A, Spinner RJ, et al. H3K27 trimethylation loss in malignant peripheral nerve sheath tumor: a systematic review and meta-analysis with diagnostic implications. J Neurooncol. 2019;144:433–43.
113. Rougraff BT, Aboulafia A, Biermann JS, Healey J. Biopsy of soft tissue masses: evidence-based medicine for the musculoskeletal tumor society. Clin Orthop Relat Res. 2009;467:2783–91.
114. Traina F, Errani C, Toscano A, Pungetti C, Fabbri D, Mazzotti A, et al. Current concepts in the biopsy of musculoskeletal tumors. J Bone Joint Surg Am. 2015;97:e7.
115. Kilpatrick SE. Histologic prognostication in soft tissue sarcomas: grading versus subtyping or both?

A comprehensive review of the literature with proposed practical guidelines. Ann Diagn Pathol. 1999;3:48–61.
116. Fletcher CDM, Unni KK, Mertens F, Weltgesundheitsorganisation, International Agency for Research on Cancer, editors. Pathology and genetics of tumours of soft tissue and bone; [the WHO classification of tumours of soft tissue and bone presented in this book reflects the views of a working group that convened for an editorial and consensus conference in Lyon, France, April 24–28, 2002]. Lyon: IARC Press; 2002.
117. Costa J, Wesley RA, Glatstein E, Rosenberg SA. The grading of soft tissue sarcomas. Results of a clinico-histopathologic correlation in a series of 163 cases. Cancer. 1984;53:530–41.
118. Trojani M, Contesso G, Coindre JM, Rouesse J, Bui NB, de Mascarel A, et al. Soft-tissue sarcomas of adults; study of pathological prognostic variables and definition of a histopathological grading system. Int J Cancer. 1984;33:37–42.
119. Coindre JM, Terrier P, Guillou L, Le Doussal V, Collin F, Ranchère D, et al. Predictive value of grade for metastasis development in the main histologic types of adult soft tissue sarcomas: a study of 1240 patients from the French Federation of Cancer Centers Sarcoma Group. Cancer. 2001;91:1914–26.
120. Hagel C, Zils U, Peiper M, Kluwe L, Gotthard S, Friedrich RE, et al. Histopathology and clinical outcome of NF1-associated vs. sporadic malignant peripheral nerve sheath tumors. J Neurooncol. 2007;82:187–92.
121. Hu S-W, Lin W-C, Tsai H-J, Chien S-H, Tsai K-B. Immunoprofiles in malignant peripheral nerve sheath tumor: three case reports and literature review. Kaohsiung J Med Sci. 2006;22:135–42.
122. Ogose A, Hotta T, Morita T, Higuchi T, Umezu H, Imaizumi S, et al. Diagnosis of peripheral nerve sheath tumors around the pelvis. Jpn J Clin Oncol. 2004;34:405–13.
123. Miettinen M. Modern soft tissue pathology: tumors and non-neoplastic conditions (Cambridge Medicine). In: Miettinen M (editor). 1st ed. Cambridge University Press; 2010.
124. Pekmezci M, Reuss DE, Hirbe AC, Dahiya S, Gutmann DH, von Deimling A, et al. Morphologic and immunohistochemical features of malignant peripheral nerve sheath tumors and cellular schwannomas. Mod Pathol. 2015;28:187–200.
125. Kindblom LG, Ahldén M, Meis-Kindblom JM, Stenman G. Immunohistochemical and molecular analysis of p53, MDM2, proliferating cell nuclear antigen and Ki67 in benign and malignant peripheral nerve sheath tumours. Virchows Arch Int J Pathol. 1995;427:19–26.
126. Halling KC, Scheithauer BW, Halling AC, Nascimento AG, Ziesmer SC, Roche PC, et al. p53 expression in neurofibroma and malignant peripheral nerve sheath tumor. An immunohistochemical study of sporadic and NF1-associated tumors. Am J Clin Pathol. 1996;106:282–8.
127. McCarron KF, Goldblum JR. Plexiform neurofibroma with and without associated malignant peripheral nerve sheath tumor: a clinicopathologic and immunohistochemical analysis of 54 cases. Mod Pathol. 1998;11:612–7.
128. Reuss DE, Habel A, Hagenlocher C, Mucha J, Ackermann U, Tessmer C, et al. Neurofibromin specific antibody differentiates malignant peripheral nerve sheath tumors (MPNST) from other spindle cell neoplasms. Acta Neuropathol (Berl). 2014;127:565–72.
129. Schaefer I-M, Fletcher CD, Hornick JL. Loss of H3K27 trimethylation distinguishes malignant peripheral nerve sheath tumors from histologic mimics. Mod Pathol. 2016;29:4–13.
130. Martinez AP, Fritchie KJ. Update on peripheral nerve sheath tumors. Surg Pathol Clin. 2019;12:1–19.
131. Allison KH, Patel RM, Goldblum JR, Rubin BP. Superficial malignant peripheral nerve sheath tumor: a rare and challenging diagnosis. Am J Clin Pathol. 2005;124:685–92.
132. Watanabe T, Oda Y, Tamiya S, Kinukawa N, Masuda K, Tsuneyoshi M. Malignant peripheral nerve sheath tumours: high Ki67 labelling index is the significant prognostic indicator. Histopathology. 2001;39:187–97.
133. Lodding P, Kindblom LG, Angervall L. Epithelioid malignant schwannoma. A study of 14 cases. Virchows Arch A Pathol Anat Histopathol. 1986;409:433–51.
134. Tsuchiya D, Takamura H, Saito K, Kashiwa H, Maeda K, Yamashita H. Immunohistochemical diagnosis of a rare case of epithelioid malignant peripheral nerve sheath tumor with multiple metastases. Jpn J Ophthalmol. 2004;48:565–9.
135. Laskin WB, Weiss SW, Bratthauer GL. Epithelioid variant of malignant peripheral nerve sheath tumor (malignant epithelioid schwannoma). Am J Surg Pathol. 1991;15:1136–45.
136. Yamaguchi U, Hasegawa T, Hirose T, Chuman H, Kawai A, Ito Y, et al. Low grade malignant peripheral nerve sheath tumour: varied cytological and histological patterns. J Clin Pathol. 2003;56:826–30.
137. Rekhi B, Jambhekar NA, Puri A, Agrawal M, Chinoy RF. Clinicomorphologic features of a series of 10 cases of malignant triton tumors diagnosed over 10 years at a tertiary cancer hospital in Mumbai, India. Ann Diagn Pathol. 2008;12:90–7.
138. Guedes-Corrêa JF, Barbosa DAN. Critical correlation between clinical presentation, imaging and type of peripheral nerve sheath tumors: a surgical approach. World Neurosurg. 2015;84:598.
139. Schwabe M, Spiridonov S, Yanik EL, Jennings JW, Hillen T, Ponisio M, et al. How effective are noninvasive tests for diagnosing malignant peripheral nerve sheath tumors in patients with neurofibromatosis type 1? Diagnosing MPNST in NF1 patients. Sarcoma. 2019;2019:4627521.

140. Siqueira MG, Martins RS, Teixeira MJ. Management of brachial plexus region tumours and tumour-like conditions: relevant diagnostic and surgical features in a consecutive series of eighteen patients. Acta Neurochir. 2009;151:1089–98.
141. Matsumine A, Kusuzaki K, Nakamura T, Nakazora S, Niimi R, Matsubara T, et al. Differentiation between neurofibromas and malignant peripheral nerve sheath tumors in neurofibromatosis 1 evaluated by MRI. J Cancer Res Clin Oncol. 2009;135:891–900.
142. Wasa J, Nishida Y, Tsukushi S, Shido Y, Sugiura H, Nakashima H, et al. MRI features in the differentiation of malignant peripheral nerve sheath tumors and neurofibromas. Am J Roentgenol. 2010;194:1568–74.
143. Derlin T, Tornquist K, Münster S, Apostolova I, Hagel C, Friedrich RE, et al. Comparative effectiveness of 18F-FDG PET/CT versus whole-body MRI for detection of malignant peripheral nerve sheath tumors in neurofibromatosis type 1. Clin Nucl Med. 2013;38:e19–25.
144. Salamon J, Mautner V, Adam G, Derlin T. Multimodal imaging in neurofibromatosis type 1-associated nerve sheath tumors. RöFo. 2015;187:1084–92.
145. James AW, Shurell E, Singh A, Dry SM, Eilber FC. Malignant peripheral nerve sheath tumor. Surg Oncol Clin N Am. 2016;25:789–802.
146. Well L, Salamon J, Kaul MG, Farschtschi S, Herrmann J, Geier KI, et al. Differentiation of peripheral nerve sheath tumors in patients with neurofibromatosis type 1 using diffusion-weighted magnetic resonance imaging. Neuro Oncol. 2019;21:508–16.
147. Ahlawat S, Blakeley JO, Rodriguez FJ, Fayad LM. Imaging biomarkers for malignant peripheral nerve sheath tumors in neurofibromatosis type 1. Neurology. 2019;93:e1076.
148. Ahlawat S, Chhabra A, Blakely J. Magnetic resonance neurography of peripheral nerve tumors and tumorlike conditions. Neuroimaging Clin N Am. 2014;24:171–92.
149. Cardona S, Schwarzbach M, Hinz U, Dimitrakopoulou-Strauss A, Attigah N, Mechtersheimer G, et al. Evaluation of F18-deoxyglucose positron emission tomography (FDG-PET) to assess the nature of neurogenic tumours. Eur J Surg Oncol. 2003;29:536–41.
150. Warbey VS, Ferner RE, Dunn JT, Calonje E, O'Doherty MJ. [18F]FDG PET/CT in the diagnosis of malignant peripheral nerve sheath tumours in neurofibromatosis type-1. Eur J Nucl Med Mol Imaging. 2009;36:751–7.
151. Benz MR, Czernin J, Dry SM, Tap WD, Allen-Auerbach MS, Elashoff D, et al. Quantitative F18-fluorodeoxyglucose positron emission tomography accurately characterizes peripheral nerve sheath tumors as malignant or benign. Cancer. 2010;116:451–8.
152. Tsai LL, Drubach L, Fahey F, Irons M, Voss S, Ullrich NJ. [18F]-Fluorodeoxyglucose positron emission tomography in children with neurofibromatosis type 1 and plexiform neurofibromas: correlation with malignant transformation. J Neurooncol. 2012;108:469–75.
153. Combemale P, Valeyrie-Allanore L, Giammarile F, Pinson S, Guillot B, Goulart DM, et al. Utility of 18F-FDG PET with a semi-quantitative index in the detection of sarcomatous transformation in patients with neurofibromatosis type 1. PLoS One. 2014;9:e85954.
154. Chirindel A, Chaudhry M, Blakeley JO, Wahl R. 18F-FDG PET/CT qualitative and quantitative evaluation in neurofibromatosis type 1 patients for detection of malignant transformation: comparison of early to delayed imaging with and without liver activity normalization. J Nucl Med. 2015;56:379–85.
155. Broski SM, Johnson GB, Howe BM, Nathan MA, Wenger DE, Spinner RJ, et al. Evaluation of 18F-FDG PET and MRI in differentiating benign and malignant peripheral nerve sheath tumors. Skeletal Radiol. 2016;45:1097–105.
156. Gruber H, Glodny B, Bendix N, Tzankov A, Peer S. High-resolution ultrasound of peripheral neurogenic tumors. Eur Radiol. 2007;17:2880–8.
157. Telleman JA, Stellingwerff MD, Brekelmans GJ, Visser LH. Nerve ultrasound in neurofibromatosis type 1: a follow-up study. Clin Neurophysiol. 2018;129:354–9.
158. Pedro MT, Antonidias G, Scheuerle A, et al. Intraoperative high-resolution ultrasound and contrast-enhanced ultrasound of peripheral nerve tumors and tumorlike lesions. Neurosurg Focus. 2015;39(3):E5.
159. Simmons Z. Electrodiagnosis of brachial plexopathies and proximal upper extremity neuropathies. Phys Med Rehabil Clin N Am. 2013;24:13–32.
160. Guedes-Correa JF, Torrao F, De Souza Moreira CA, Amorim RMP. The importance of intraoperative neurophysiological monitoring for resection of lumbosacral plexus tumors. Neurol Psychiatry Brain Res. 2018;28:7–12.
161. Kim DH, Murovic JA, Tiel RL, Kline DG. Operative outcomes of 546 Louisiana State University Health Sciences Center peripheral nerve tumors. Neurosurg Clin N Am. 2004;15:177–92.
162. Carrino J, Khurana B, Ready J, Silverman S, Winalski C. Magnetic resonance imaging-guided percutaneous biopsy of musculoskeletal lesions. J Bone Joint Surg Am. 2007;89:2179–87.
163. Levi AD, Ross AL, Cuartas E, Qadir R, Temple HT. The surgical management of symptomatic peripheral nerve sheath tumors. Neurosurgery. 2010;66:833–40.
164. Brahmi M, Thiesse P, Ranchere D, Mognetti T, Pinson S, Renard C, et al. Diagnostic accuracy of PET/CT-guided percutaneous biopsies for malignant peripheral nerve sheath tumors in neurofibromatosis type 1 patients. PLoS One. 2015;10:e0138386.
165. Pianta M, Chock E, Schlicht S, McCombe D. Accuracy and complications of CT-guided core needle biopsy of peripheral nerve sheath tumours. Skeletal Radiol. 2015;44:1341–9.

166. Amin MB, Edge S, Greene F, Byrd DR, Brookland RK, Washington MK, Gershenwald JE, Compton CC, Hess KR, et al. (Eds.). AJCC cancer staging manual. 8th ed. Springer International Publishing: American Joint Commission on Cancer; 2017.
167. Mowery A, Clayburgh D. Malignant peripheral nerve sheath tumors: analysis of the national cancer database. Oral Oncol. 2019;98:13–9.
168. Ferner RE, Gutmann DH. International consensus statement on malignant peripheral nerve sheath tumors in neurofibromatosis. Cancer Res. 2002;62(5):1573–7.
169. Wong WW, Hirose T, Scheithauer BW, Schild SE, Gunderson LL. Malignant peripheral nerve sheath tumor: analysis of treatment outcome. Int J Radiat Oncol. 1998;42:351–60.
170. Kahn J, Gillespie A, Tsokos M, Ondos J, Dombi E, Camphausen K, et al. Radiation therapy in management of sporadic and neurofibromatosis type 1-associated malignant peripheral nerve sheath tumors. Front Oncol. 2014;4:324.
171. Sloan L, Terezakis SA, Blakeley JO, Slobogean B, Kleinberg LR. Long-term outcomes of radiation therapy (RT) in the management of malignant peripheral nerve sheath tumors (MPNST) in patients with neurofibromatosis type 1 (NF1). Int J Radiat Oncol Biol Phys. 2018;102:e474–5.
172. Bishop AJ, Zagars GK, Torres KE, Bird JE, Feig BW, Guadagnolo BA. Malignant peripheral nerve sheath tumors: a single institution's experience using combined surgery and radiation therapy. Am J Clin Oncol. 2018;41:465–70.
173. Prudner BC, Ball T, Rathore R, Hirbe AC. Diagnosis and management of malignant peripheral nerve sheath tumors: current practice and future perspectives. Neurooncol Adv [Internet]. 2019 [cited 2020 Mar 3]. https://doi.org/10.1093/noajnl/vdz047.
174. Gross AM, Wolters PL, Dombi E, Baldwin A, Whitcomb P, Fisher MJ, et al. Selumetinib in children with inoperable plexiform neurofibromas. N Engl J Med. 2020;382:1430–42.
175. Bernthal NM, Putnam A, Jones KB, Viskochil D, Randall RL. The effect of surgical margins on outcomes for low grade MPNSTs and atypical neurofibroma: outcomes of intermediate nerve sheath Tumors. J Surg Oncol. 2014;110:813–6.
176. Gachiani J, Kim D, Nelson A, Kline D. Surgical management of malignant peripheral nerve sheath tumors. Neurosurg Focus. 2007;22:1–8.
177. Tiel R, Kline D. Peripheral nerve tumors: surgical principles, approaches, and techniques. Neurosurg Clin N Am. 2004;15:167–75.
178. Russell SM. Preserve the nerve: microsurgical resection of peripheral nerve sheath tumors. Neurosurgery. 2007;61(3 Suppl):113–8.
179. Spinner RJ. Complication avoidance. Neurosurg Clin N Am. 2004;15:193–202.
180. Das S, Ganju A, Tiel RL, Kline DG. Tumors of the brachial plexus. Neurosurg Focus. 2007;22:1–6.
181. Goertz O, Langer S, Uthoff D, Ring A, Stricker I, Tannapfel A, Steinau H-U. Diagnosis, treatment and survival of 65 patients with malignant peripheral nerve sheath tumors. Anticancer Res. 2014;34:777–83.
182. Perrin RG, Guha A. Malignant peripheral nerve sheath tumors. Neurosurg Clin N Am. 2004;15:203–16.
183. Dunn GP, Spiliopoulos K, Plotkin SR, Hornicek FJ, Harmon DC, Delaney TF, et al. Role of resection of malignant peripheral nerve sheath tumors in patients with neurofibromatosis type 1. J Neurosurg. 2013;118:142–8.
184. Guha D, Davidson B, Nadi M, Alotaibi NM, Fehlings MG, Gentili F, et al. Management of peripheral nerve sheath tumors: 17 years of experience at Toronto Western Hospital. J Neurosurg. 2018;128:1226–34.
185. Garozzo D. Peripheral nerve tumors in neurofibromatosis 1: an overview on management and indications for surgical treatment in our experience. Neurol India. 2019;67(Supplement):S38–44.
186. Dorsi M, Belzberg A. Chapter 23. Peripheral nerve tumours of the extremities. In: Schmidek and Sweet, editor. Operative neurosurgical tehniques. Elsevier; 2012. pp. 2319–2327.
187. Gortz O, Langer S, Uthoff D, Ring A, Strcker I, Tannapfel A, et al. Diagnosis, treatment and survival of 65 patients with malignant peripheral nerve sheath tumors. Anticancer Res. 2014;34:777–84.
188. Smith HG, Thomas JM, Smith MJF, Hayes AJ, Strauss DC. Major amputations for extremity soft-tissue sarcoma. Ann Surg Oncol. 2018;25:387–93.
189. Stevenson MG, Musters AH, Geertzen JHB, van Leeuwen BL, Hoekstra HJ, Been LB. Amputations for extremity soft tissue sarcoma in an era of limb salvage treatment: local control and survival. J Surg Oncol. 2018;117:434–42.
190. Williard WC, Collin C, Casper ES, Hajdu SI, Brennan MF. The changing role of amputation for soft tissue sarcoma of the extremity in adults. Surg Gynecol Obstet. 1992;175:389–96.
191. Daigeler A, Lehnhardt M, Khadra A, Hauser J, Steinstraesser L, Langer S, Goertz O, Steinau HU. Proximal major limb amputations—a retrospective analysis of 45 oncological cases. World J Surg Oncol. 2009;7:15. Published online 2009 Feb 9.
192. Watson KL, Al Sannaa GA, Kivlin CM, Ingram DR, Landers SM, Roland CL, et al. Patterns of recurrence and survival in sporadic, neurofibromatosis type 1-associated, and radiation-associated malignant peripheral nerve sheath tumors. J Neurosurg. 2017;126:319–29.
193. Nelson CN, Dombi E, Rosenblum JS, Miettinen MM, Lehky TJ, Whitcomb PO, et al. Safe marginal resection of atypical neurofibromas in neurofibromatosis type 1. J Neurosurg. 2019:1–11.

20 Management of Brachial Plexus Tumors

Sophie Y. Su, Martijn J. A. Malessy, Line G. Jacques, and Eric L. Zager

20.1 Clinical Presentation

Patients with brachial plexus tumors (Table 20.1) can present with variable symptoms ranging from an asymptomatic, palpable mass to focal or radiating pain and sensory or motor deficits. Huang and colleagues found that pain was the most common presenting symptom followed by sensory changes and weakness. Severe pain was typically associated with malignant features [1]. Important features to note on history and physical exam include the size and location of the mass, its mobility, pain at rest, with movement, or on palpation, paresthesia or dysesthesia, and association with other findings such as characteristic café au lait spots, axillary freckling, other masses, or cutaneous neurofibromas [2, 3]. Tumors that affect the C8-T1 lower roots can present with an ipsilateral Horner syndrome, classically described as ptosis, anhidrosis, and miosis. Additionally, due to the proximity of the brachial plexus to the subclavian artery and vein, vascular changes such as a weak pulse, discolored, swollen, or cool limb can occur from mass effect.

Table 20.1 Common brachial plexus tumors [1–3]

Peripheral nerve sheath tumors (PNSTs)	
Benign	Schwannoma
	Neurofibroma
	Perineurioma
Malignant	MPNSTs (formerly referred to as malignant schwannoma, neurogenic sarcoma, and neurofibrosarcoma)
Peripheral non-neural sheath tumors (PNNSTs)	
Benign	Lipoma
	Hemangioma
	Desmoid tumor
	Ganglioneuroma
	Meningioma
	Osteochondroma
Malignant	Metastasis (breast, pulmonary, lymphoma, melanoma)
	Pancoast tumor
	Sarcomas (fibrosarcoma, synovial sarcoma, osteosarcoma)

20.2 Diagnostic Evaluation

20.2.1 Radiographic Imaging

Diagnostic imaging studies, such as MRI (Figs. 20.1 and 20.2) and ultrasound (Fig. 20.3a–c), are indispensable to denote the relationship of the lesion to the surrounding nerves and vascular

S. Y. Su · E. L. Zager (✉)
Department of Neurosurgery, Perelman School of Medicine, University of Pennsylvania, Philadelphia, PA, USA
e-mail: Eric.Zager@uphs.upenn.edu

M. J. A. Malessy
Department of Neurosurgery, Leiden University Medical Center, Leiden, The Netherlands

L. G. Jacques
Department of Neurosurgery, University of California at San Francisco, San Francisco, CA, USA

F. Guedes et al. (eds.), *Diagnostic Assessment and Treatment of Peripheral Nerve Tumors*,
https://doi.org/10.1007/978-3-030-77633-6_20

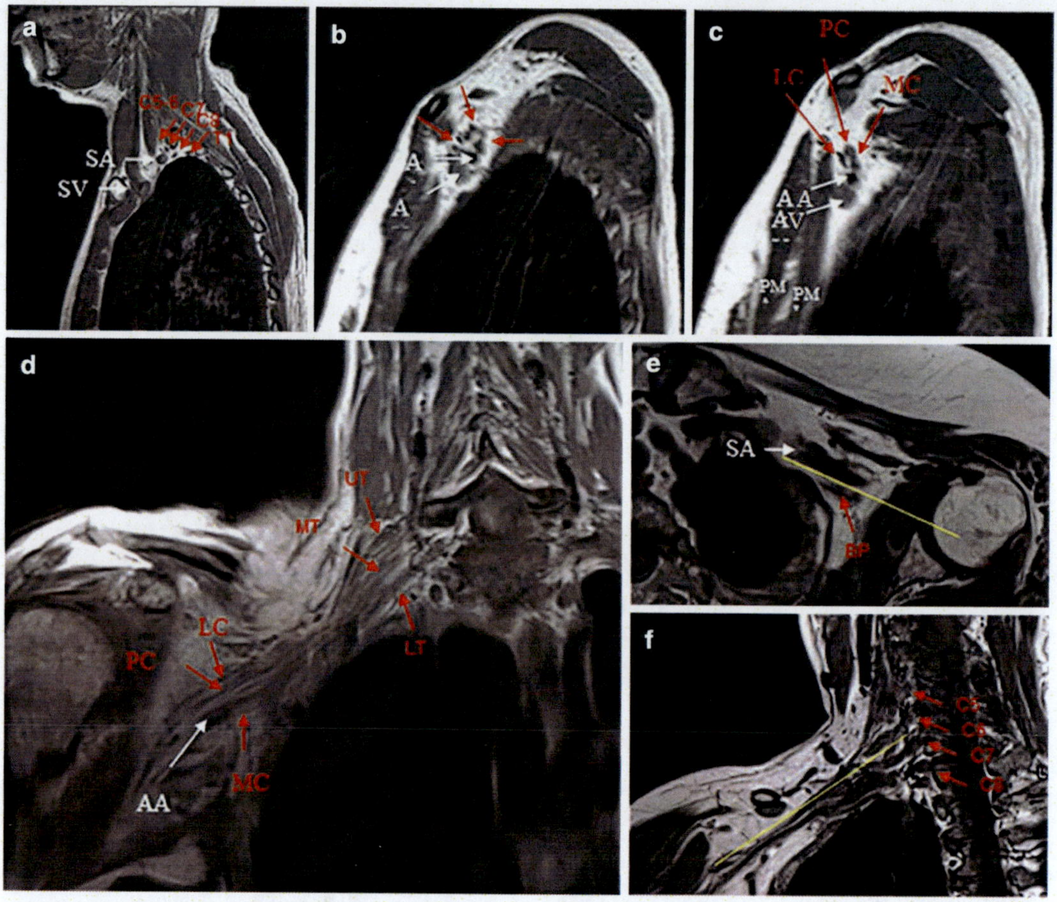

Fig. 20.1 MRI of brachial plexus anatomy. T1-weighted images with a sagittal view demonstrating spinal nerves (**a**) (*red arrows*) in the interscalene triangle, (**b**) divisions (*red arrows*) in the retroclavicular space, and (**c**) cords (*red arrows*). Coronal view (**d**) demonstrates trunks outside the interscalene triangle and cords surrounding the axillary artery. Axial view (**e**) shows the relationship of the subclavian artery to the brachial plexus, best visualized on the oblique coronal plane (**f**) which can visualize most of the roots (*red arrows*) and distal elements of the plexus. The *yellow line* demarcates the oblique axial plane to visualize the entire plexus. *AA* axillary artery, *AV* axillary vein, *LC* lateral cord, *LT* lower trunk, *MC* medial cord, *MT* middle trunk, *PC* posterior cord, *PMA* pectoralis major muscle, *PMI* pectoralis minor muscle, *SA* subclavian artery, *SV* subclavian vein, *UT* upper trunk. (Reproduced from, Mikityansky et al. 2012)

structures. Plain X-rays and CT are useful in some cases to evaluate for bony changes secondary to lesions adjacent to the spine, causing foraminal enlargement or vertebral body erosion. Patients in whom malignant lesions are suspected undergo chest and abdominal CT scans or PET studies [4]. CT of the chest with 3D reconstruction can be helpful for patients with tumor involving C8-T1 to determine the position and relationship of the first rib to the tumor. However, MRI has long been considered the preferred imaging modality for brachial plexus tumors [5], providing details on location, margins, and adjacent structures (Figs. 20.1 and 20.2). Short T1 inversion recovery (STIR) sequences and contrast sequences are particularly useful in characterizing nerve sheath tumors from adjacent structures [6]. Abnormal findings on MRI include loss of fat planes along the plexus, diffuse or nodular enlargement of the plexus, T2 hyperintensity, or T1 contrast enhancement (Fig. 20.2a, b) [7]. Unfortunately, these findings can all be

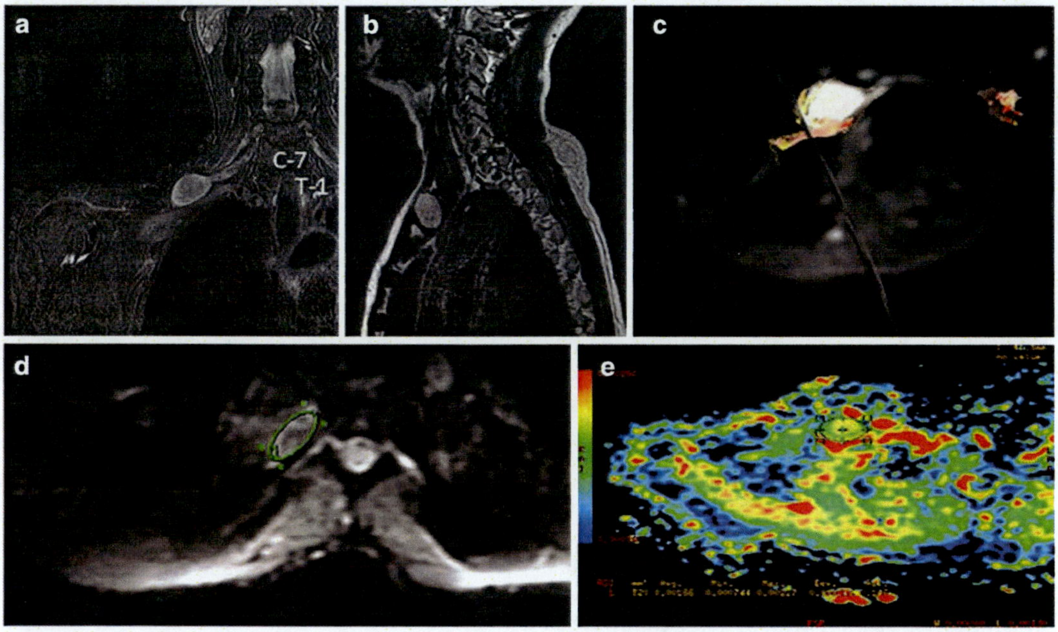

Fig. 20.2 Specialized MRI sequences of the brachial plexus. MRI coronal (**a**) view shows a well-defined 3 × 2 cm ovoid T2 hyperintense mass in the right interscalene triangle. The C7 nerve root is enlarged, and contiguous with the mass. T1-weighted post-contrast image (**b**) shows enhancement of the mass. The C7 nerve fibers are shown by DTI (**c**) to be splayed both dorsally and ventrally around the mass. MRI with region of interest (*green circle*) (**d**) shows an ADC value to be 1.7×10^{-3} mm²/s (**e**), which is indicative of a less aggressive tumor

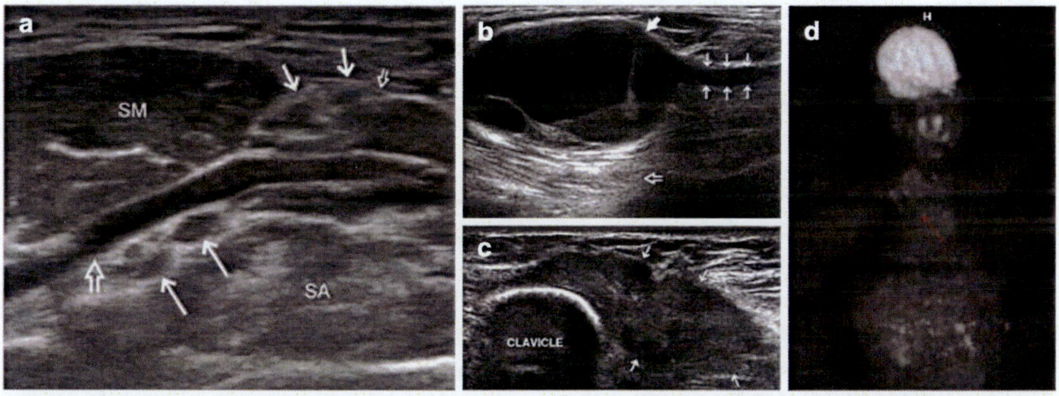

Fig. 20.3 Supplementary imaging modalities of the brachial plexus. Transverse view of ultrasound at the outlet of the interscalene triangle showing normal anatomy (**a**). Posterior scapular artery (*open arrow*) separates the middle and lower trunk (*long arrows*) from the divisions of the upper trunk (*short arrows*). The small suprascapular nerve marked by *small open arrow*. Longitudinal view of ultrasound showing large nerve sheath tumor (**b**) (*thick arrow*) arising from the upper trunk (*thin arrows*) of the brachial plexus. The trunk is thickened and in continuity with the tumor. The tumor has marked cystic degeneration with hyperintensity posteriorly (*open arrow*). Transverse view of ultrasound (**c**) showing solid, well-defined metastatic deposit (arrows) from breast cancer located posterior to clavicle. The brachial plexus is indistinguishable from the metastasis. PET scan (**d**) showing mild FDG avidity (*red arrow*) corresponding to a mass at the pulmonary apex and base of the right neck. *SA* scalenus anterior, *SM* scalenus medius. (**a–c** are reproduced from Griffith et al. 2018)

found in lesions as different as benign and malignant peripheral nerve sheath tumors (PNSTs), metastatic disease, or post-radiation neuritis [8]. While no MRI sequence can definitely distinguish a benign from malignant PNST, features on MRI that suggest more malignant lesions include heterogeneous contrast enhancement, irregular margins and perilesional edema, bony destruction, necrosis, and hemorrhage [3, 7]. Additionally, low values of apparent diffusion coefficient (ADC) on MRI favor malignant lesions, and higher values favor benign lesions (Fig. 20.2d, e) [8]. MRA or CTA may also add important information regarding tumor relationships with major vascular structures.

Plain MRI T1 sequences, however, may not distinguish a benign nerve lesion from other soft tissue lesions. Additionally, standard MRI is limited in differentiating tumor and normal nerve structures. Diffusion tensor tractography (DTT) is a relatively new MRI technique that has been able to improve the specificity of MRI in differentiating tumor and normal nerve structures. Previously used to track degeneration and regeneration of nerves, there are groups that have evaluated the utility of DTT in peripheral nerve tumors [9, 10]. DTT can provide valuable information about the relationship of normal nerve fascicles to PNSTs and improve preoperative planning (Fig. 20.2c). However, DTT is limited for lesions that are close to large vessels or lesions that extensively split nerve fibers [10]. Furthermore, applying DTT to smaller lesions or intralesional nerves may yield less accurate imaging [9].

For patients with breast cancer who have received radiation, radiation plexopathy is a condition that can be clinically difficult to discern from an infiltrative, metastatic plexus lesion [6, 11, 12]. MRI and PET-CT, in such a case, can be useful in distinguishing tumor from radiation fibrosis. Particularly, positron emission tomography (PET) (Fig. 20.3d) would show increased uptake in metastatic plexopathy or a malignant nerve sheath lesion, whereas it would have decreased uptake in radiation plexopathy [13]. The finding of myokymia on electromyography (EMG), while rare, may also indicate radiation plexopathy [12].

Another useful advanced imaging technique is magnetic resonance neurography (MRN) which uses STIR sequences to selectively image spinal and peripheral nerves and enable better characterization of the nerves [14, 15]. MRN can detect fascicle enlargement and perilesional edema. High signal intensity in nerve fascicles on MRN correlates to abnormal findings on electromyography (EMG) and nerve conduction studies (NCS) [16]. MRN can be beneficial when standard MRI and EMG studies are inconclusive. Du et al., in particular, found that MRN can be useful in detecting brachial plexus tumors in patients who had received prior radiation to the plexus and differentiate among metastasis, radiation-induced tumors, and radiation-induced fibrosis [15].

20.2.2 High-Resolution Ultrasound

High-resolution ultrasonography (HRU) for the brachial plexus is a technically complex but a reliable and cost-effective method to visualize individual nerves and lesions in the plexus. Technical considerations of HRU include a good understanding of the anatomy and an understanding of the technology to work with the patient's body habitus. The spinal nerves can be first identified based on morphology of the transverse process and then traced out to the trunks in the supraclavicular fossa (Fig. 20.3a) [17]. The cords and proximal nerves can be identified in the infraclavicular fossa. Normal brachial plexus features include homogeneous and hypoechoic appearance of the nerves as tubular structures in the longitudinal view and oval structures on axial view [17]. A benign nerve sheath tumor appears as a hypoechoic, well-defined ovoid mass along the parent nerve (Fig. 20.3b). Unfortunately, while HRU can localize the nerve sheath tumors, it cannot reliably distinguish between benign schwannomas and neurofibromas. Typically, schwannomas may be more eccentrically located lesions, while neurofibromas often consist of multiple lesions [18]. During ultrasound assessment, paresthesia with either pain or numbness may be elicited with pressure from the transducer [19]. A metastatic lesion on ultrasound also appears as a well-defined, hypoechoic mass but generally will be larger and hyperemic and have an irregular margin (Fig. 20.3c). Segmental neural thickening may also be present suggesting metastatic infiltration of adjacent nerves. This is in contrast to radiation fibrotic plexopathy which shows more diffuse disease as well as thickened and stiff soft tissue [19].

One unique diagnostic application of ultrasound is evaluation for diaphragmatic paralysis or paresis in situations where there is concern for damage to the phrenic nerve due to mass effect or an intraneural lesion. In cases of paralysis, ultrasound can show either absent diaphragmatic motion or paradoxical movement of the hemidiaphragm where inspiration causes cranial movement and expiration causes caudal movement [20]. Phrenic nerve function can also be assessed with fluoroscopic sniff test during which the movements of the hemidiaphragms are observed with inspiration and expiration [21].

There are caveats in relying on ultrasound for diagnosis. First, the quality of the study is operator-dependent and necessitates that the operator understands the anatomy and potentially subtle findings [22]. There can be anatomical variation, especially in the relationship of the upper trunk to the anterior scalene muscle [19]. Secondly, the choice of US probe affects resolution or depth. Probes with higher frequency will provide more optimal imaging with improved resolution but at the cost of depth penetration [23]. Lapegue et al. recommends using a high-frequency probe with at least 10 MHz [17]. Alternatively, Griffith et al. recommend changing the transducer to assess different areas of the brachial plexus depending on the patient's habitus, depth of the brachial plexus, and ability of the transducer to access the area of interest [19]. Ultrasound is limited in its visualization of the nerve roots located in the neural foramina and visualization of the lower nerves at C8 and T1 if the patient has a short neck [24].

HRU does have the advantage of spatial resolution compared to other imaging modalities. Using ultrasound, nerves can be characterized over a long distance and also dynamically [17]. HRU also has a Doppler component which allows evaluation of the vascular structures relative to the nerves [24]. Additionally, HRU is much more cost-effective compared to MRI [22]. When patients have contraindications to MRI such as implants or claustrophobia, HRU can become valuable in assessing brachial plexus lesions [24].

20.2.3 Electrodiagnostic Studies

Standard electrophysiologic studies include needle electromyography (EMG) and nerve conduction studies (NCS) which can evaluate the functional integrity of sensory and motor nerves. Needle EMG records electrical activity from muscle fibers both at rest and during contraction. The potentials generated by the muscle fibers, called motor unit action potentials (MUAPs), are evaluated by their appearance, size, duration, and firing pattern to gain information about the functional integrity of the nerves. EMG is able to obtain information on proximal muscles where NCS recordings cannot be done. In particular, needle EMG is helpful in localizing lesions along the brachial plexus although a nerve that is severely compromised is easier to localize than one that is partially or mildly affected [25]. EMG or NCS can also determine the severity of impairment or reveal subclinical deficits of involved nerves that do not have a clinical correlate [1, 6].

Nerve conduction studies can measure electrical activity of either motor or sensory nerves by detecting a sensory nerve action potential (SNAP) or a compound muscle action potential (CMAP) due to activation of cutaneous sensory nerves or muscle fibers distal to the site of stimulation. Gradually increased voltages are applied to activate axons and to induce a SNAP or CMAP. Information such as the area, amplitude, duration, latency, and conduction time of sensory and motor nerves can be obtained. Focal tumors can cause a conduction block, which is a CMAP reduction and is considered to be one of the most reliable signs of compressive neuropathy [26].

The primary utility of electrodiagnostic studies is to confirm a clinical diagnosis or to help localize lesions when the clinical exam or imaging is non-localizing [27]. Additionally, EMG can differentiate non-cancerous pathology as radiation plexopathy has characteristic myokymia and fasciculation potentials [4, 28]. However, given that most electrodiagnostic studies will be normal with a benign tumor, these studies should not replace the history and/or examination of a patient. Unfortunately, EMG and NCS cannot detect pure sensory nerve root pathologies, and the information measured on motor units can depend on length of symptoms [15]. Electrodiagnostic studies can also identify other neuropathic conditions that may cloud the clinical picture, such as a generalized sensorimotor polyneuropathy, entrapment neuropathy, or a discrete radiculopathy. In general, electrodiagnostic studies are not mandatory in the evaluation of brachial plexus tumors. However, we consider intraoperative neuromonitoring to be an essential component of operative resection of most plexus tumors.

20.2.4 Role of Biopsy

The role of biopsy for brachial plexus lesions largely depends on whether the lesion is thought to be malignant or benign [6]. If a lesion is thought to be a malignant peripheral nerve sheath tumor (MPNST) (by both clinical and imaging criteria), there are stronger arguments for a needle biopsy. Patients who present with severe pain, rapidly enlarging masses, and progressive neurological deficits have a presumed malignancy and require expedited tissue sampling for planning a multimodality treatment regimen. Unfortunately, there is still an overlap between radiographic findings of a malignant versus benign peripheral nerve tumor. Tissue evaluation by histology is the only definitive way to confirm malignancy, which would then affect further management [4, 6]. A metastatic workup is recommended to gauge extent of disease [29].

Biopsy, in patients with suspected MPNSTs, can be performed either as a fine-needle aspiration (FNA) or percutaneous core biopsy. Open biopsy is considered by some to be a contraindication for MPNSTs as biopsy can lead to seeding of tumor cells into the surrounding tissue. FNA and core biopsies are more limited in tissue sampling but significantly less invasive. FNA can only obtain individual cells for histocytology, while a core biopsy allows for a larger sample. The downsides of biopsies are that they occasionally have a low yield as sensitivity is not high, functional nerves or vessels can be damaged, and/or resultant scarring can only make subsequent surgeries more difficult [3, 4, 6, 30]. However, for patients with MPNSTs, biopsy-confirmed diagnosis can allow for appropriate counseling and discussion of the necessary surgical approach and pre- and post-surgical management. On the other hand, most authors do not recommend needle or incisional biopsy for BPNSTs as biopsy is often extremely painful, leading to neuropathic pain or functional nerve damage, scarring, and loss of tissue planes that can make subsequent operations more difficult and less successful [29, 31]. Furthermore, in the case of a heterogeneous tumor, a biopsy could lead to a sampling error [4].

20.3 Surgical Management

20.3.1 Indications

Detailed preoperative evaluation, selection of patients, and timing of surgery for patients who are diagnosed with tumors of the brachial plexus are key in achieving good outcomes and avoiding complications. An important factor in management of brachial plexus tumors depends on a careful history and physical examination. Relevant factors in the history include growth rate of the lesion, development or progression of symptoms such as pain and neurologic deficits, prior radiation therapy, and family history or personal history of other diseases such as neurofibromatosis [1, 29]. Unfortunately, very little data exists on the natural history of peripheral nerve tumors and the rates of malignant transformation. While the incidence of MPNSTs has ranged from 0.001 to 4% in patients without neurofibromatosis-1 (NF1) [32, 33], the risk of malignancy in patients with NF1 increases up to 13% [33]. Furthermore, malignant lesions are more likely to present with severe pain and rapidly progressive neurologic symptoms. As such, clinical indications for surgery include increase in symptoms such as pain, paresthesia or weakness, growth of the lesion to over 3 cm in diameter, other radiographic indicators of possible malignancy, and the patient's concern for malignancy [3, 29]. If a tumor grows slowly but remains asymptomatic, these lesions are monitored conservatively with serial radiographic imaging [3]. In the case of patients with NF1, also known as von Recklinghausen disease, surgery may be offered even when lesions are small given that surgery for larger lesions can be more complicated [29]. Additionally, the threshold for surgery for neurofibromas associated with NF1 is lower as these lesions have a 10–15% risk of malignant transformation [2].

In discussing surgery, beyond the standard risks of anesthesia, postoperative infections, or wound complications, patients with PNSTs are at risk for new neurologic deficits or worsening neurologic dysfunction. In a series by Donner et al., 11% of patients developed worse motor deficits, 15% developed new motor deficits, and 10% developed painful paresthesia [34]. Risk factors that predispose to a postoperative neurodeficit include tumor size, proximal tumor location, history of NF1, prior biopsy or surgery, and preoperative irradiation [35]. Frank discussion and detailed counseling of the potential complications are mandatory with each patient prior to surgery. The alternatives of continued conservative management or empiric radiation therapy must also be presented.

20.4 Surgical Approaches

Surgical approaches to lesions of the brachial plexus depend primarily on location of the lesion in relationship to the clavicle and the involved segment(s) of the brachial plexus. Preoperatively, the surgeon should discuss the goals of nerve monitoring with both the anesthesiologist and the electrophysiologist for the best possible neuromonitoring and to ensure that the appropriate muscles will be sampled with the electrodes.

20.4.1 Anterior Approach

The most common surgical approach is anteriorly, either supra- or infraclavicular approach (Figs. 20.4 and 20.5) with rates up to 72.7% in Huang et al. [1]. For the anterior approach, the patient is supine on the operating table with the ipsilateral base of the neck and shoulder blade elevated by pads and the head turned to the contralateral side. For a supraclavicular lesion, the arm is placed alongside the body and draped so that the arm and hand can be moved and observed for muscle contractions following stimulation. For an infraclavicular lesion that extends into the axilla, the arm can be placed in abduction.

The anterior supraclavicular approach is most useful for lesions of the spinal nerves, trunks, and divisions of the brachial plexus (Fig. 20.4). Either a transverse incision parallel to the clavicle or L-shaped incision is made over the posterior triangle of the neck (Fig. 20.4d). Supraclavicular nerves and major veins are preserved as much as possible during transection of the platysma, development of subplatysmal flaps, and mobilization laterally of the supraclavicular fat pad. The lateral border of the sternocleidomastoid muscle is retracted medially and may be partly divided from the clavicle inferiorly to enhance exposure if needed. Care should be taken not to damage the supraclavicular medial nerve. The posterior belly of omohyoid can be retracted but may also be divided to enhance visualization and retraction. Under omohyoid lies the phrenic nerve within the thin fascia anterior to the anterior scalene muscle. The phrenic nerve travels in an oblique manner from lateral to medial position and is stimulated to confirm its identity, with brisk contraction of the hemidiaphragm. The crossing of the phrenic nerve with the lateral border of the anterior scalene muscle is a reliable landmark for the identification of spinal nerve C5, which runs just below. When bleeding is encountered around the phrenic

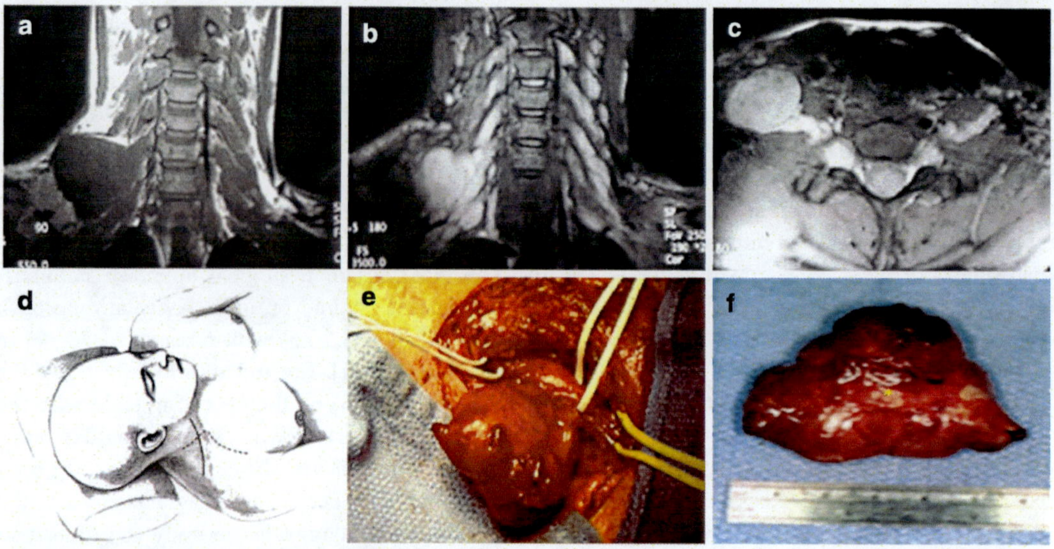

Fig. 20.4 Anterior supraclavicular approach. MRI showing T1 coronal (**a**), T2 coronal (**b**), and T2 axial (**c**) scans of a supraclavicular plexiform neurofibroma. A transverse incision parallel to clavicle (**d**, *solid line*) marks the most cosmetic incision for a supraclavicular approach, whereas the dotted line represents an incision for a combined supraclavicular and infraclavicular approach. Intraoperative resection (**e**) shows the neurofibroma extending from the nerve fibers (*yellow loops*). The resected lesion (**f**) is shown with an enlarged solitary nerve fiber (*). (**d** is reproduced from Kline et al. 2001)

nerve, either gentle tamponade or judicious, low-current bipolar coagulation with constant irrigation should be used to prevent thermal injury. Due to the presence of a tumor, brachial plexus elements may have a different course. Generally, lateral and posterior to the anterior scalene muscle will be the trunks of the brachial plexus surrounded by a fat pad. Typically, the first component of the brachial plexus that is encountered is the C5 spinal nerve [36]. Careful dissection around the upper nerves is needed to protect the long thoracic nerve, which lies posterior to C6, and the suprascapular nerve, which arises laterally from the distal upper trunk. To gain access to the lower spinal nerves and/or lower trunks, a portion of the anterior scalene muscle must be excised.

The anterior infraclavicular approach is targeted for lesions involving the cords of the brachial plexus and terminal nerves to the upper extremity (Fig. 20.5). The incision is made below the clavicle along the deltopectoral groove (Fig. 20.5b, c). We usually preserve the cephalic vein within this groove. The deltoid and pectoralis major muscles need to be separated and retracted (Fig. 20.5d), while the pectoralis minor muscle is typically transected at the coracoid process. Alternatively, the different elements can be dissected free through a transpectoral approach, working superior and inferior to the pectoralis minor. After exposure of pectoralis minor, transection of the muscle will expose the axilla and the cord level of the brachial plexus (Fig. 20.5e–g) [37]. The lateral cord is typically encountered first in the infraclavicular space. The terminal branches of the lateral cord include the musculocutaneous nerve to coracobrachialis, biceps and brachialis muscles, and the lateral cord contribution to the median nerve. The latter can be traced distally to the median nerve and then later used to identify the medial cord. The axillary artery is palpated and mobilized for control as needed. The posterior cord is dissected if involved with the lesion and is located lateral to the lateral cord but in a deeper plane. Typically, in the presence of a tumor, all the involved neural elements must

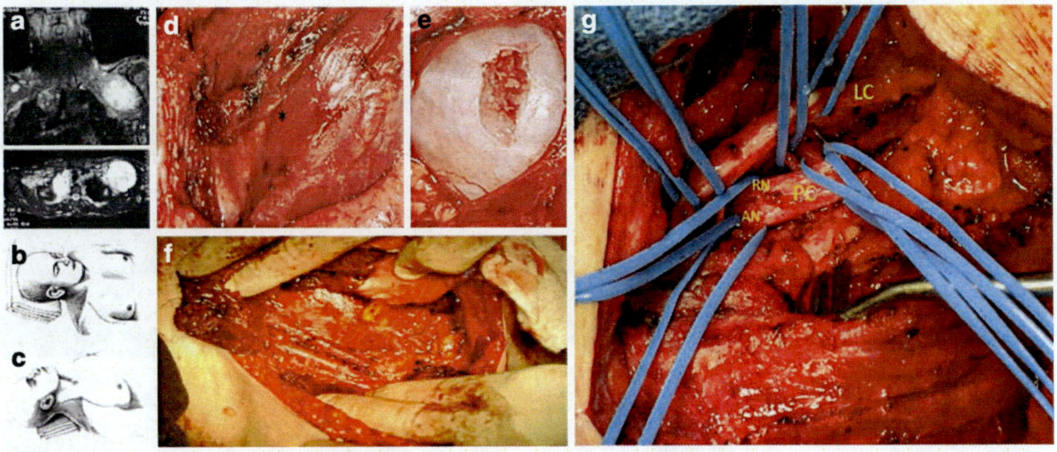

Fig. 20.5 Anterior infraclavicular approach. Coronal and axial views of T1-weighted, post-contrast MRI (**a**) showing an infraclavicular neurofibroma in a patient with NF1. The incision is made below the clavicle along the deltopectoral groove (**b**) or can be extended above the clavicle (**c**) for a combined approach. (**d**) The pectoralis major muscle (*) needs to be retracted, while pectoralis minor is transected to visualize the lesion (**e**), axillary vessels (**f**) or brachial plexus (**g**). *LC* lateral cord, *PC* posterior cord, *RN* radial nerve, *AN* axillary nerve. (**b** and **c** are reproduced from Kline et al. 2001)

be dissected out to reveal anatomical relationships before each element can be identified, both by anatomic inspection and electrical stimulation. Upon closure of the infraclavicular approach, the pectoralis minor muscle can be repaired if dissected, but does not require reapproximation. In contrast, the pectoralis major muscle must always be reapproximated if transected, although it is rarely required.

Major complications from the anterior approach can include injury to adjacent neural or vascular structures. The phrenic nerve is commonly encountered en route to the brachial plexus, and transient phrenic palsy may occur. We prefer not to loop or retract this delicate nerve and always keep it within view while dissecting. Excessive manipulation, traction, or inadvertent sharp, blunt, or coagulation injury to elements of the brachial plexus can cause new or worsened motor and/or sensory deficits postoperatively. Notably, injury to nerves from the tumor itself or iatrogenic injury from surgery can lead to postoperative complex regional pain syndrome (CRPS) with worsening of pain and changes in appearance, temperature, and sensation of the extremity [38]. Bleeding intraoperatively or development of a postoperative hematoma can occur due to the abundance of traversing vessels. Injury to the subclavian artery or vein can lead to severe hemorrhage, and an intraoperative consult to vascular surgery may rarely be needed for repair. On the left side, injury to the thoracic duct or its tributaries may result in a chylous effusion that on rare occasions may require a chest tube, wound re-exploration, or endovascular embolization [39]. With rare cases of anomalous lymphatic drainage, this may occur on the right side as well. Lastly, pleural injury can lead to a pneumo-, hemo-, or chylothorax. A pleural injury can be investigated by filling the surgical site with saline and asking the anesthesiologist to perform a Valsalva maneuver to assess for an air leak.

20.4.2 Posterior Approach

The posterior subscapular approach is an alternative surgical approach to the brachial plexus (Fig. 20.6). Indications for this approach include lesions involving proximal roots and spinal nerves of the lower levels (i.e., C8 or T1) or lower trunk lesions that extend into the chest

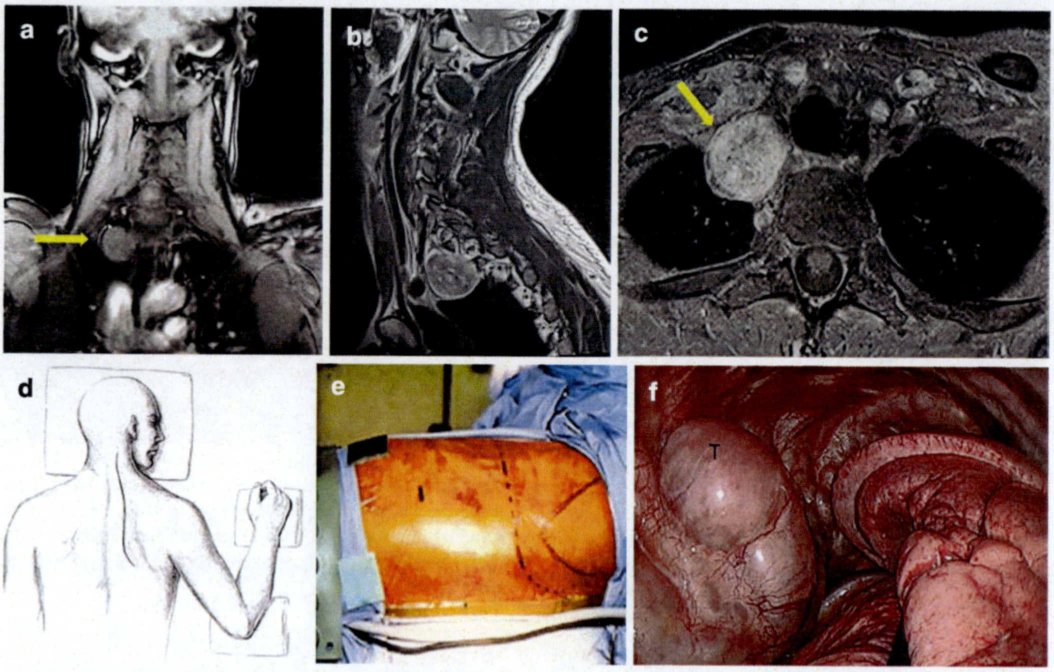

Fig. 20.6 Variety of surgical approaches for the lower trunk. Coronal (**a**), sagittal (**b**), and axial (**c**) MRI showing an enlarging paraspinal nerve sheath tumor involving the lower trunk of the brachial plexus. In this location, this lesion may be approached through the posterior subscapular approach (**d**). Alternatively, the minimally invasive modification of this posterior approach may be used to minimize muscle dissection by centering incision over the first rib and confirmed with fluoroscopy. Some surgeons would choose the trap-door incision shown in Fig. 20.7. This region may also be approached thoracoscopically with the assistance of thoracic surgery (**e**) for direct visualization of a tumor (*T*) (**f**, image courtesy of Dr. Pechet from UPenn Department of Thoracic Surgery). We were able to resect this lesion completely without deficit through an anterior supraclavicular approach. (**d** is reproduced from Kline et al. 2001)

(Fig. 20.6a–c) [40]. It is particularly useful for patients with lesions that have a dumbbell-shape with both an intra- and extraforaminal component [41]. Additionally, the posterior approach may be preferred for patients with prior radiation to the neck or anterior chest, prior neck surgery, bony abnormalities (cervical ribs or large C7 transverse processes), or morbid obesity [42, 43].

The patient is positioned prone with chest rolls and padding on all pressure points [42, 43]. The ipsilateral arm is flexed forward at the shoulder and elbow and placed on a padded Mayo stand so that the height of the arm can be lowered below the operating table to externally rotate the scapula (Fig. 20.6d) [41–43]. Recently, Crutcher et al. described a minimally invasive modification of the posterior subscapular approach which likely reduces the morbidity of the exposure through the paraspinal muscles [42]. The skin incision is made centered over the posterior aspect of the first rib, halfway between the medial border of the scapula and the spinous processes [42]. The trapezius muscle is the first muscle encountered under which lies levator scapulae, rhomboid minor, and rhomboid major in a cranial to caudal fashion. When dissecting through these muscles, it is important to divide away from the medial edge of the scapula to avoid the dorsal scapular nerve and ascending branch of the transverse cervical artery [44]. Deep to the rhomboid minor is the posterior chest wall and T1 costotransverse joint which can be used as a reference point for resection. The extent of bony resection to improve visualization depends on the pathology. Scalene muscles and intercostal muscles need to be dissected off the cranial and caudal sides of the rib, respectively, to clear the rib prior to resection. With the posterior and middle scalene muscles dissected off the transverse processes, the lower spinal nerves and trunk will be exposed. Tracking the spinal nerves medially and retraction of the paraspinous muscles will reveal the intraforaminal course of the roots [41]. The dissection can be extended cranially up to the C7 spinal nerve or even caudally down to the third rib [42].

While the posterior approach can expose proximal segments such as the intraforaminal roots, the surgery does require more muscle dissection [41]. Complications from this approach can include a winged scapula from muscle dissection or injury to the long thoracic nerve, injury to phrenic nerve or brachial plexus, cervical spine instability, and pneumo- or hemothorax [41, 42]. To minimize the risk of a winged scapula, it is key to close the muscles in anatomic layers. To prevent either pneumo- or hemothorax, pleural rents can be evaluated by filling operative cavity with saline and asking the anesthesia team to perform a Valsalva maneuver. Pleural rents can be repaired primarily, and hemostasis can be achieved with bipolar cautery. A chest tube can be placed in the operative field, as needed [43]. From the posterior approach, fortunately, major vessels lie deep to the brachial plexus. The vertebral artery lies anterior to the nerve roots, while the subclavian artery is anterior and inferior to the lower trunk of the brachial plexus [41].

20.5 Unique Approaches

20.5.1 Combined

Larger tumors that span a significant portion of the brachial plexus can be approached through a combined technique or transclavicular approach, using incisions of both the supra- and infraclavicular approaches. For lesions involving the plexus posterior to the clavicle, anterior-inferior clavicular mobilization can be performed. The clavicle can be wrapped with moist sponges and retracted either cranially or caudally depending on access needs [36].

20.5.2 Transclavicular

Occasionally, retraction of the clavicle may not be sufficient, and complete visualization of the entire brachial plexus is necessary. In such cases, a transclavicular approach can be used to access the supra-, retro-, and infraclavicular aspects of the brachial plexus. An oblique vertical incision is made along the posterior border of the sternocleidomastoid that curves posteriorly parallel to the clavicle before extending into the deltopectoral groove [45]. Osteotomy of the middle third of the clavicle is performed after which the subclavius muscle and suprascapular vessels are dissected. Tumors involving the divisions of the brachial plexus can then be exposed [46]. The clavicle can then be realigned with screws and a plate that is typically pre-contoured to fit the S-shape anatomy of the clavicle [45].

20.5.3 Thoracic Surgery-Assisted Procedures

Video-assisted thoracoscopic surgery (VATS), performed by thoracic surgery, has been proposed as an alternative surgical corridor to the proximal lower nerve roots and trunks (Fig. 20.6e). The endoscopic camera allows direct visualization of the thoracic apex and the presence of any lesions (Fig. 20.6f).

A trap-door approach (Fig. 20.7) involving a partial sternotomy/thoracotomy may be needed for lesions involving tumors located in the C8-T1 inferior trunk trajectory. Commonly used by thoracic surgery to gain access to the lesions invading or abutting the brachiocephalic and subclavian vessels, these same vessels unfortunately can affect resectability [47].

20.6 Surgical Technique

Regardless of the approach, certain strategies are key in minimizing neural complications. Surgery is not performed under paralytics so that intraoperative nerve stimulation can be performed to gauge the functional status of the nerve. Planning

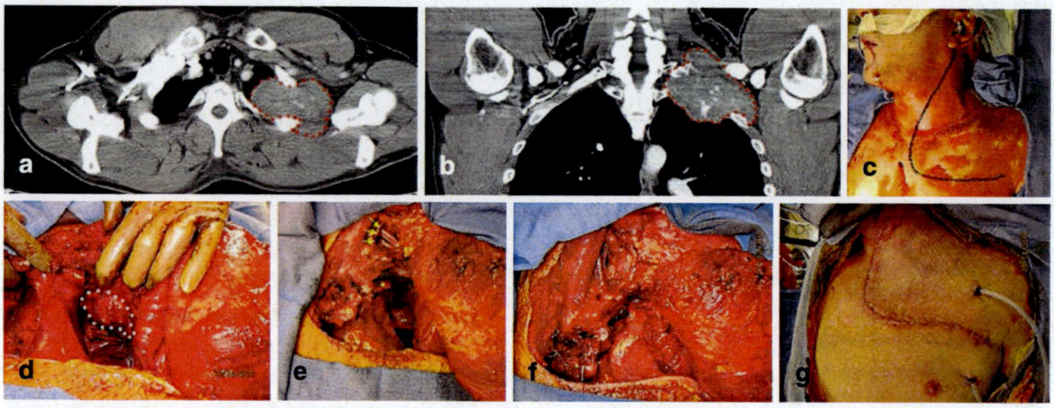

Fig. 20.7 Unique surgical approaches: trap-door incision. Axial and coronal CT scans (**a**, **b**) demonstrate a chondrosarcoma (*outlined in red*) arising from the first two ribs and involving the lower trunk of the brachial plexus. Incision (**c**) demarcating trap-door approach for thoracosternotomy and neck dissection with thoracic surgery. The tumor (*outlined in white*) is visualized after lung deflation (**d**). Exposure of the brachial plexus trunks (*yellow arrows*) above clavicle (**) with the mediastinum below and rib resection (*) after tumor resection (**e**). View of the surgical cavity (**f**) after repair of the manubrium and lung re-expansion. Final skin closure (**g**) for trap-door approach

of the skin incision is crucial with manual palpation and ultrasound to minimize the length but still allow for adequate exposure of normal nerves proximal and distal to the lesion. PNSTs can integrate layers of nerve fascicles into a pseudocapsule of connective tissue that is distinct from the true schwannoma capsule of the tumor. Identifying the pseudocapsule is crucial as the first step in the resection of a schwannoma. Stone and Spinner identify the boundary between the pseudocapsule and true tumor capsule by relying on color differences where the pseudocapsule appears grayish white in contrast to the yellow appearance of the true capsule [35]. Accurate identification of this border can facilitate the subsequent intraneural dissection and tumor enucleation while preserving nerve integrity and function. Repetitive nerve stimulation also plays an important role in identifying motor (but not sensory) nerve fascicles along the pseudocapsule and a safe zone for dissection.

20.6.1 Gross Total Versus Subtotal Resection

Gross total resection is the goal for treatment of benign brachial plexus tumors without neurologic compromise [1]. Schwannomas typically displace most surrounding nerve fascicles which can be dissected free and preserved, thus aiding in complete removal of the schwannoma. In BPNST, tumors need not be resected en bloc. For larger lesions, internal debulking, occasionally with the CUSA, decreases the tension on the overlying and outstretched fascicles. Thereby, the risk of an iatrogenic traction injury to the fascicles while developing the plane with the tumor is diminished. Neurofibromas, on the other hand, can have multiple fascicles entering the tumor or incorporated into the capsule. Plexiform neurofibromas can have more infiltrative features and are inseparable from important nerve fibers, necessitating a subtotal resection and leaving residual tumor to preserve function [6]. Nonplexiform neurofibromas, similar to schwannomas, can usually be completely resected with sparing of the parent nerve [30].

Benign non-neural peripheral nerve sheath tumors (BNNPNSTs), such as lipomas, hemangiomas, and desmoid tumors, are extrinsic lesions that grow adjacent to the brachial plexus and cause symptoms through compression. However, these lesions can adhere to or invade into the epineurium, making complete resection extremely difficult without associated neurologic compro-

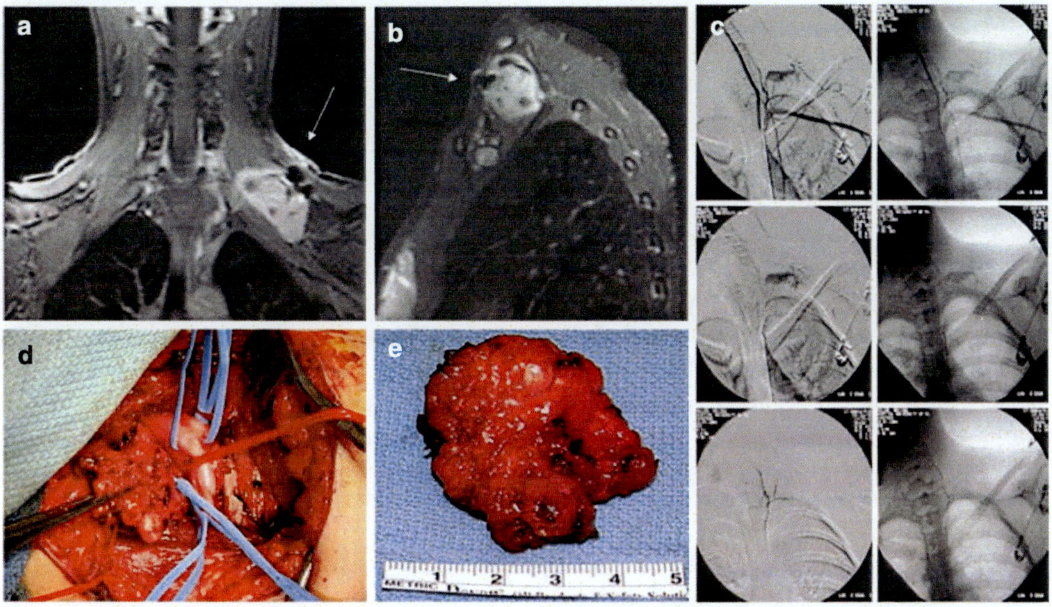

Fig. 20.8 Unique tumors of the brachial plexus: Hemangioma. T1-weighted coronal (**a**) and sagittal (**b**) MRI sequences showing a left brachial plexus hemangioma with homogeneous contrast enhancement (*arrow*). Digital subtraction angiography (**c**) which revealed a vascular tumor with intratumor aneurysm with multiple feeding vessels. Post-embolization imaging revealed reduced flow to the lesion. Subsequent surgery through anterior supraclavicular approach (**d, e**) revealed the vascular mass displacing the trunks of the brachial plexus. (Reproduced from Ranalli et al. 2009)

mise [2]. Lipomas can be incompletely resected and still allow for relief of symptoms. Hemangiomas may be extremely vascular, and, in some cases, preoperative angiography and embolization may be needed to allow safe resection (Fig. 20.8) [28]. More commonly, complete resection of BNNPSNTs is not necessary, and decompression and/or neurolysis of the brachial plexus is sufficient to improve symptoms [2].

For MPNSTs, the best chances for patient survival involve aggressive, complete en bloc tumor resection and adjacent tissue preceded or followed by radiation therapy. However, while MPNSTs can invade the nerve and cause neurologic impairment, full resection is often difficult or impossible to achieve depending on the location along the brachial plexus. Occasionally, MPNSTs extend into the neural foramen requiring a posterior approach first, with laminectomy and intradural section of the involved root filaments. Subsequently, the resection is continued in the supine position with an anterior approach of the extraforaminal tumor mass. Complete resection can lead to significant functional and neurovascular loss. Amputation of the limb is a surgical option that comes with high morbidity when wide excision is not possible and patients already have compromised limb function [4]. For MPNSTs of the distal brachial plexus, amputation would entail removal of the scapula, clavicle, and shoulder along with transection and ligation of the subclavian vessels [4]. While limb amputation has been cited to decrease local recurrence rates, more studies are finding no survival difference in limb amputation compared to a limb-sparing approach. As such, more surgeons are approaching MPNSTs with the goals of wide local resection of the tumor, decompression of the neural elements, and pre- or postoperative radiation and/or chemotherapy [2, 4, 48, 49]. Surgical management for metastatic disease to the brachial plexus tends to be more individualized depending on severity of symptoms and extent of systemic metastases [2]. Similar to

MPNSTs, surgical approach for malignant non-neural sheath tumors must also be individualized, with en bloc resection if possible, but subtotal resection for nerve decompression may be appropriate in certain cases [2, 4].

20.6.2 Nerve Grafts

Nerve reconstruction may be necessary in cases where resection of a brachial plexus tumor requires sectioning of a functional nerve fascicle or an iatrogenic injury occurred to a parent nerve during resection of a benign PNST. An autologous nerve graft may be interposed to mitigate any deficit. Patients will have best results if grafting occurs at the time of tumor resection and no later than 6 months after injury [50]. An exception to this rule is for plexiform neurofibromas. While the lesion is technically benign, it has a relatively higher risk of malignant transformation and also grows both circumferentially and along the length of the parent nerve. As such, graft repair is more controversial for this diagnosis.

When the diagnosis is MPNST, some authors argue that nerve grafts are relatively contraindicated given that tumor can spread along the graft and there is a higher rate of graft failure. Furthermore, patients with MPNSTs usually undergo postoperative radiation which reduces the chance of functional nerve recovery [50]. Unfortunately, the prognosis of this aggressive tumor is typically so poor that effective re-innervation is not possible for many patients with MPNSTs [6]. However, there are cases in which nerve reconstruction, especially distal nerve transfers, is a reasonable approach following resection of a MPNST.

There are general principles necessary to optimize graft healing. The nerve graft should not be under tension. It is important that the graft covers the entire caliber of the nerve stump and that the proximal and distal stumps are healthy, tumor-free tissues [50]. Kretschmer et al. even recommend sending frozen sections of the stumps to confirm tumor-free margins prior to grafting [50].

The sural nerve is the most common nerve graft donor. In patients with systemic diseases such as NF1, the sural nerve may also be a site of tumor burden and should be assessed [50]. The sural nerve is more easily accessible when the patient is positioned for a posterior approach; however, the leg can be positioned internally rotated and flexed at the knee and hip so that the posterolateral calf is exposed. Plexus reconstruction with distal nerve transfers can also be considered in certain cases, especially when the nerve stumps are not in optimal condition following tumor resection.

20.7 Intraoperative Adjuncts

20.7.1 Ultrasound

Intraoperative ultrasound (IUS) was first used by Fornage to look at the appearance of peripheral nerves under ultrasound and validated by Gofeld in cadaveric studies [51]. IUS can be helpful in incision planning, localizing lesions that are small or deep, minimizing surgical exploration, and confirming resection of all lesions in cases of multiple tumors [23]. Additionally, IUS can help in understanding complex anatomy where large tumors distort normal anatomy and mask the location of important vasculature such as the subclavian vessels. Lastly, in the case of multifocal tumors, resection of one lesion may alter the surgical area so that the other tumors become hidden. IUS can then be helpful to localize the remnant tumors.

20.7.2 Intraoperative Neuromonitoring

Intraoperative neuromonitoring (IONM) can involve electromyography (EMG) to record compound muscle action potentials (CMAPs), nerve action potentials (NAPs), motor evoked potentials (MEPs), and somatosensory evoked potentials (SSEPs). The main purpose of IONM includes differentiating lesional from normal nerve fascicles and preventing iatrogenic injury from surgery. Although the techniques for stimulating and recording intraoperatively are similar to preoperative electrodiagnostic studies, special stimulating and recording electrodes may be necessary, and resultant data can be more varied due to anesthesia and the challenging electrical environment in the OR [26].

Direct nerve stimulation through monopolar or bipolar electrodes can help identify nerve from other tissues especially when the lesion has distorted normal anatomy. Multiple types of data are typically recorded including MEPs, SSEPs, NAPs from the nerve, or CMAPs from the distal muscles. It is important to stimulate at multiple sites within the surgical field to help define baseline nerve function and to characterize areas of damage [26]. Nerve stimulation with absent or low-amplitude NAP recordings may suggest nonfunctional fascicles that can be sacrificed to optimize tumor resection [52]. Otherwise, nerve stimulation allows surgeons to map out the path of functional nerve fascicles along the surface of the lesion. While malignant lesions may invade into nerves, benign lesions typically displace adjacent functional nerves and fascicles. As such, direct stimulation is an important intraoperative adjunct to identify and preserve normal nerve function during resection [3, 53]. Schwannomas, for example, often have one or a few nonfunctional nerve fascicles entering and leaving the lesion. These fascicles can be identified with stimulation and sacrificed for gross total resection. In contrast, neurofibromas often have more functional nerve fascicles adherent to the tumor capsule and within the tumor itself, and repetitive stimulation may thus dictate tumor debulking and capsule residual along the nerves [3, 31]. Electrophysiology thus allows intraoperative real-time decision-making on the extent of resection to minimize a functional deficit [30].

For tumors that have an intraforaminal component and the proximal segment of nerves cannot be stimulated, motor evoked potentials or sensory evoked responses are an alternative to measure nerve response. MEPs are evoked through transcranial electrical stimulation and recorded from the target muscle. SSEPs record the response of the brain or spinal cord to sensory fiber stimulation and can assist with localizing lesions in the sensory system [37, 54]. Changes in MEPs and/or SSEPs may indicate injury to the parent nerve and if severe enough may prompt a surgeon to consider nerve grafting to ameliorate any functional deficit. More often, these modalities serve as reassurance to the surgeon that the plexus elements remain functional throughout the tumor resection.

20.7.3 Frozen Histology

Intraoperative tumor histology is key as many malignant PNSTs are not identified until the time of surgery, unless a prior biopsy was performed. Waiting intraoperatively for pathology to process, frozen sections is important as subsequent operative strategies are dependent on the diagnosis and become complicated with a malignant diagnosis. However, we generally do not make irreversible nerve-sacrificing decisions based on a frozen section diagnosis alone. It is preferable to close the incision and wait for permanent pathology to make management decisions in cases of malignancy. If aggressive tumor resection is opted by the patient, frozen sections are also important in evaluating the extent of invasion of nearby structures and determination of tumor-free margins, as patients with clean margins have improved disease-free survival [2].

20.8 Postoperative Considerations

Historically, after anterior approaches to the brachial plexus, the arm was placed in a sling for 4–6 weeks [36]. Now postoperatively, patients typically do not have any physical restrictions, and early mobilization is encouraged to preserve range of motion. Early motion with passive and active range of motion can actually help decrease the formation of adhesions to the surrounding tissue [36]. An exception occurs for surgeries involving nerve repair where limitations on mobilization are recommended to avoid tension on the repair site for 3 weeks with gradual return of mobilization.

Long-term patients with MPNSTs require serial screening for potential relapse. Patients who had subtotal resection of even benign lesions need to be monitored for growth. Particularly for patients with a genetic predisposition such as NF1, monitoring for malignant transformation of residual lesions is needed. Lastly, for patients who had preexisting motor deficits or developed new postoperative dysfunction, occupational and physical therapy can be beneficial to maximize functional status.

20.9 Alternatives to Surgery

Stereotactic radiosurgery, particularly the frameless CyberKnife system, has been investigated for use in treating benign paraspinal PNSTs with demonstrations of safety and efficacy [55, 56]. Shin and colleagues evaluated radiosurgery in both benign and malignant spinal neurogenic tumors and found that radiosurgery provided a 95.4% local control rate in benign tumors [57]. Other studies have replicated similar or better local control rates [55, 58]. Further studies are needed to determine benefit of single or multi-session radiation and the prescribed dose needed for symptom resolution.

Surgical resection nonetheless is usually considered the treatment of choice for benign peripheral nerve tumors given that most lesions are well-circumscribed and surgery can provide a cure with gross total resection. However, stereotactic radiosurgery may be favored as a treatment modality for patients who are poor surgical candidates due to advanced age or serious medical comorbidities. Additionally, radiosurgery can be beneficial for patients with multiple peripheral lesions due to genetic conditions such as neurofibromatosis, difficult to access lesions, or recurrent lesions [59].

Patients with MPNSTs are recommended to undergo radiotherapy given evidence that radiation can reduce local recurrence [60]. Chemotherapy, on the other hand, has not been proven to be beneficial. MPNSTs are thought to be poorly responsive to chemotherapy so it is given only in patients with systemic metastasis [2]. Chou and colleagues demonstrate the challenging nature of treating MPNSTs as they found adjuvant therapy with radiation, chemotherapy, or combination had no significant influence on recurrence or survival [61]. Some sarcomas and Pancoast tumors, however, represent the types of non-neural malignant tumors for which induction chemoradiotherapy is initiated 4–6 weeks prior to surgery. Induction chemoradiotherapy can significantly shrink tumor size and burden making subsequent surgery more likely to preserve nerve function [62].

References

1. Huang JH, Zaghloul K, Zager EL. Surgical management of brachial plexus region tumors. Surg Neurol. 2004;61:372–8.
2. Das S, Ganju A, Tiel RL, Kline DG. Tumors of the brachial plexus. Neurosurg Focus. 2007;22:1–6.
3. Desai KI. Primary benign brachial plexus tumors: an experience of 115 operated cases. Neurosurgery. 2012;70:220–33.
4. Gachiani J, Kim D, Nelson A, Kline D. Surgical management of malignant peripheral nerve sheath tumors. Neurosurg Focus. 2007;22:1–8.
5. Kichari JR, Hussain SM, Den Hollander JC, Krestin GP. MR imaging of the brachial plexus: current imaging sequences, normal findings, and findings in a spectrum of focal lesions with MR-pathologic correlation. Curr Probl Diagn Radiol. 2003;32:88–101.
6. Siqueira MG, Martins RS, Teixeira MJ. Management of brachial plexus region tumours and tumour-like conditions: relevant diagnostic and surgical features in a consecutive series of eighteen patients. Acta Neurochir. 2009;151:1089–98.
7. Bowen BC, Pattany PM, Saraf-Lavi E, Maravilla KR. The brachial plexus: normal anatomy, pathology, and MR imaging. Neuroimaging Clin N Am. 2004;14:59–85.
8. Yuh EL, Jain Palrecha S, Lagemann GM, Kliot M, Weinstein PR, Barbaro NM, Chin CT. Diffusivity measurements differentiate benign from malignant lesions in patients with peripheral neuropathy or plexopathy. AJNR Am J Neuroradiol. 2015;36:202–9.
9. Schmidt M, Kasprian G, Amann G, Duscher D, Aszmann OC. Diffusion tensor tractography for the surgical management of peripheral nerve sheath tumors. Neurosurg Focus. 2015;39:1–6.
10. Cage TA, Yuh EL, Hou SW, Birk H, Simon NG, Noss R, Rao A, Chin CT, Kliot M. Visualization of

nerve fibers and their relationship to peripheral nerve tumors by diffusion tensor imaging. Neurosurg Focus. 2015;39:1–6.

11. Kori SH, Foley KM, Posner JB. Brachial plexus lesions in patients with cancer: 100 cases. Neurology. 1981;31:45–50.
12. Kori SH. Diagnosis and management of brachial plexus lesions in cancer patients. Oncol Williston Park N. 1995;9:756–60; discussion 765
13. Ahmad A, Barrington S, Maisey M, Rubens RD. Use of positron emission tomography in evaluation of brachial plexopathy in breast cancer patients. Br J Cancer. 1999;79:478–82.
14. Filler AG, Kliot M, Howe FA, Hayes CE, Saunders DE, Goodkin R, Bell BA, Winn HR, Griffiths JR, Tsuruda JS. Application of magnetic resonance neurography in the evaluation of patients with peripheral nerve pathology. J Neurosurg. 1996;85:299–309.
15. Du R, Auguste KI, Chin CT, Engstrom JW, Weinstein PR. Magnetic resonance neurography for the evaluation of peripheral nerve, brachial plexus, and nerve root disorders. J Neurosurg. 2010;112:362–71.
16. Gupta R, Villablanca PJ, Jones NF. Evaluation of an acute nerve compression injury with magnetic resonance neurography. J Hand Surg. 2001;26:1093–9.
17. Lapegue F, Faruch-Bilfeld M, Demondion X, Apredoaei C, Bayol MA, Artico H, Chiavassa-Gandois H, Railhac J-J, Sans N. Ultrasonography of the brachial plexus, normal appearance and practical applications. Diagn Interv Imaging. 2014;95:259–75.
18. Hung EHY, Griffith JF. Pitfalls in ultrasonography of soft tissue tumors. Semin Musculoskelet Radiol. 2014;18:79–85.
19. Griffith JF. Ultrasound of the brachial plexus. Semin Musculoskelet Radiol. 2018;22:323–33.
20. Lee FC, Singh H, Nazarian LN, Ratliff JK. High-resolution ultrasonography in the diagnosis and intraoperative management of peripheral nerve lesions. J Neurosurg. 2011;114:206–11.
21. Nason LK, Walker CM, McNeeley MF, Burivong W, Fligner CL, Godwin JD. Imaging of the diaphragm: anatomy and function. Radiographics. 2012;32:E51–70.
22. Zeidenberg J, Burks SS, Jose J, Subhawong TK, Levi AD. The utility of ultrasound in the assessment of traumatic peripheral nerve lesions: report of 4 cases. Neurosurg Focus. 2015;39:E3.
23. Haldeman CL, Baggott CD, Hanna AS. Intraoperative ultrasound-assisted peripheral nerve surgery. Neurosurg Focus. 2015;39:1–4.
24. Simoni P, Ghassemi M, Le VD-M, Boitsios G. Ultrasound of the normal brachial plexus. J Belg Soc Radiol. 2017;101:1–6.
25. Mansukhani KA. Electrodiagnosis in traumatic brachial plexus injury. Ann Indian Acad Neurol. 2013;16:19–25.
26. Daube JR, Rubin DI. Nerve conduction studies. In: Aminoffs electrodiagnosis in clinical neurology. Elsevier; 2012. p. 289–325.
27. Fisher MA. Electrophysiology of radiculopathies. Clin Neurophysiol. 2002;113:317–35.
28. Simmons Z. Electrodiagnosis of brachial plexopathies and proximal upper extremity neuropathies. Phys Med Rehabil Clin N Am. 2013;24:13–32.
29. Spinner RJ, Kline DG. Surgery for peripheral nerve and brachial plexus injuries or other nerve lesions. Muscle Nerve. 2000;23:680–95.
30. Russell SM, Kline DG. Complication avoidance in peripheral nerve surgery: injuries, entrapments, and tumors of the extremities—part 2. Neurosurgery. 2006;59:ONS449–57.
31. Ball JR, Biggs MT. Operative steps in management of benign nerve sheath tumors. Neurosurg Focus. 2007;22:1–4.
32. Ducatman BS, Scheithauer BW, Piepgras DG, Reiman HM, Ilstrup DM. Malignant peripheral nerve sheath tumors. A clinicopathologic study of 120 cases. Cancer. 1986;57:2006–21.
33. Evans DGR, Baser ME, McGaughran J, Sharif S, Howard E, Moran A. Malignant peripheral nerve sheath tumours in neurofibromatosis 1. J Med Genet. 2002;39:311–4.
34. Donner TR, Voorhies RM, Kline DG. Neural sheath tumors of major nerves. J Neurosurg. 1994;81:362–73.
35. Stone JJ, Spinner RJ. Go for the gold: a "plane" and simple technique for resecting benign peripheral nerve sheath tumors. Oper Neurosurg. 2020;18(1):60–8.
36. Tender GC, Kline DG. Anterior supraclavicular approach to the brachial plexus. Neurosurgery. 2006;58:ONS360–5.
37. Jung I-H, Yoon K-W, Kim Y-J, Lee SK. Analysis according to characteristics of 18 cases of brachial plexus tumors: a review of surgical treatment experience. J Korean Neurosurg Soc. 2018;61:625–32.
38. Borchers AT, Gershwin ME. Complex regional pain syndrome: a comprehensive and critical review. Autoimmun Rev. 2014;13:242–65.
39. Chen E, Itkin M. Thoracic duct embolization for chylous leaks. Semin Interv Radiol. 2011;28:63–74.
40. Biggs MT. Posterior subscapular approach for specific brachial plexus lesions. J Clin Neurosci. 2001;8:340–2.
41. Dubuisson AS, Kline DG, Weinshel SS. Posterior subscapular approach to the brachial plexus. Report of 102 patients. J Neurosurg. 1993;79:319–30.
42. Crutcher CL 2nd, Kline DG, Tender GC. A modified, less invasive posterior subscapular approach to the brachial plexus: case report and technical note. Neurosurg Focus. 2017;42:1–4.
43. Tender GC, Kline DG. Posterior subscapular approach to the brachial plexus. Neurosurgery. 2005;57:377–81.
44. Berger A, Schaller E, Mailänder P. Brachial plexus injuries: an integrated treatment concept. Ann Plast Surg. 1991;26:70–6.
45. Zadnik M, Eglseder WAJ, Shur VB. Transclavicular approach for brachial plexus reconstruction. Tech Hand Up Extrem Surg. 2008;12:126–30.
46. Birch R, Bonney G, Marshall RW. A surgical approach to the cervicothoracic spine. J Bone Joint Surg Br. 1990;72:904–7.
47. Nomori H, Abe M, Sugimura H, Takeshi A. Twenty-five years' experience with a trap-door thoracotomy

modified with disconnection of the first rib for tumors invading the anterior superior sulcus. Ann Thorac Surg. 2014;97:1946–9.
48. Goertz O, Langer S, Uthoff D, Ring A, Stricker I, Tannapfel A, Steinau H-U. Diagnosis, treatment and survival of 65 patients with malignant peripheral nerve sheath tumors. Anticancer Res. 2014;34:777–83.
49. Perrin RG, Guha A. Malignant peripheral nerve sheath tumors. Neurosurg Clin N Am. 2004;15:203–16.
50. Kretschmer T, Antoniadis G, Heinen C, Borm W, Scheller C, Richter H-P, Koenig RW. Nerve sheath tumor surgery: case-guided discussion of ambiguous findings, appropriateness of removal, repeated surgery, and nerve repairs. Neurosurg Focus. 2007;22:1–9.
51. Gofeld M, Bristow SJ, Chiu S, Kliot M. Preoperative ultrasound-guided mapping of peripheral nerves. J Neurosurg. 2013;119:709–13.
52. Wu G, Belzberg A, Nance J, Gutierrez-Hernandez S, Ritzl EK, Ringkamp M (2019) Solutions to the technical challenges embedded in the current methods for intraoperative peripheral nerve action potential recordings. J Neurosurg:1–10.
53. Kwok K, Davis B, Kliot M. Resection of a benign brachial plexus nerve sheath tumor using intraoperative electrophysiological monitoring. Neurosurgery. 2007;60:316–21.
54. Alon M, Rochkind S. Pre-, intra-, and postoperative electrophysiologic analysis of the recovery of old injuries of the peripheral nerve and brachial plexus after microsurgical management. J Reconstr Microsurg. 2002;18:77–82.
55. Selch MT, Lin K, Agazaryan N, Tenn S, Gorgulho A, DeMarco JJ, DeSalles AAF. Initial clinical experience with image-guided linear accelerator-based spinal radiosurgery for treatment of benign nerve sheath tumors. Surg Neurol. 2009;72:668–75.
56. Bhatnagar AK, Gerszten PC, Ozhasaglu C, Vogel WJ, Kalnicki S, Welch WC, Burton SA. CyberKnife frameless radiosurgery for the treatment of extracranial benign tumors. Technol Cancer Res Treat. 2005;4:571–6.
57. Shin D-W, Sohn M-J, Kim H-S, Lee D-J, Jeon SR, Hwang YJ, Jho E-H. Clinical analysis of spinal stereotactic radiosurgery in the treatment of neurogenic tumors. J Neurosurg Spine. 2015;23:429–37.
58. Gerszten PC, Quader M, Novotny J, Flickinger JC. Radiosurgery for benign tumors of the spine: clinical experience and current trends. Technol Cancer Res Treat. 2012;11:133–9.
59. Chaudhary N, Iyer A, Chang SD. Radiosurgery for benign spine tumors and vascular malformations. In: Youmans and Winn neurological surgery. 7th ed. Elsevier. p. 272, 2250–2254.e1.
60. Wong WW, Hirose T, Scheithauer BW, Schild SE, Gunderson LL. Malignant peripheral nerve sheath tumor: analysis of treatment outcome. Int J Radiat Oncol Biol Phys. 1998;42:351–60.
61. Chou D, Bilsky MH, Luzzati A, et al. Malignant peripheral nerve sheath tumors of the spine: results of surgical management from a multicenter study. J Neurosurg Spine. 2017;26:291–8.
62. Davis GA, Knight S. Pancoast tumor resection with preservation of brachial plexus and hand function. Neurosurg Focus. 2007;22:1–8.

21 Management of Lumbosacral Plexus Tumors

Fernando Guedes, Gabriel Elias Sanches, Rosana Siqueira Brown, and Rodrigo Salvador Vivas Cardoso

21.1 Introduction

LSPT are rare and heterogeneous, such that only in the last decades there have been studies conducted to analyze these lesions as a distinct group [1]. The published material dealing specifically about LSPT in the literature is still scarce and limited to a few case series [1–3]. Some larger surgical series of peripheral nerve tumors (PNT) include LSPT in its casuistry, and some do not discriminate the location of the lesions with enough specificity in order to assess which lesions are indeed LSPT [4–12].

Lumbosacral plexopathy is less frequent than brachial plexopathy and, in opposition to the latter, is more frequently caused by non-traumatic etiologies. Lumbosacral plexopathy secondary to neoplastic infiltration has indeed been found to be around eight times more common than traumatic plexopathy [13]. Tumors may arise from the lumbosacral plexus (LSP) or damage it via direct compression and/or infiltration from nearby soft tissues or bones, or via perineural, lymphatic, or hematogenic spread [14–16].

The clinical presentation of LSPT is unspecific, usually with subacute diffuse abdominal or lumbar pain. In some instances, however, it is similar to those of radiculopathies or peripheral nerve injuries. In general, its diagnosis cannot be made solely based on clinical parameters, and imaging exams are frequently necessary [1, 13, 17, 18].

These patients will often be referred to the specialist with a concluded diagnosis or with inconclusive imaging exams that ought to be reevaluated and eventually repeated with clear specifications for the visualization of the LSP.

The prognosis of patients harboring LSPT invariably depends on the type of tumor that is causing the plexopathy, given the heterogeneity of the group of lesions that may inflict the LSP. Surgical treatment, whenever indicated, should be discussed in a multidisciplinary manner, with the general surgery, oncology, radiology, pathology, and clinical genetic teams.

21.2 Anatomical Considerations

The LSP is formed from the roots T12 to S3 and is divided into two anatomical regions: the lumbar plexus and the sacral plexus.

The lumbar plexus originates from the roots T12-L4, which bifurcate into an anterior and posterior division inside the psoas major substance and give rise to six terminal branches. The iliohypogastric, ilioinguinal (T12-L1), and genitofemoral nerves (L1-L2) provide motor and sensory innerva-

F. Guedes (✉) · G. E. Sanches · R. S. Brown
R. S. V. Cardoso
Division of Neurosurgery, Department of Surgery, Gaffrée e Guinle University Hospital (HUGG), School of Medicine, Federal University of Rio de Janeiro State (UNIRIO), Rio de Janeiro, RJ, Brazil

F. Guedes et al. (eds.), *Diagnostic Assessment and Treatment of Peripheral Nerve Tumors*,
https://doi.org/10.1007/978-3-030-77633-6_21

tion to the lower abdomen and inguinal region. The iliohypogastric and the ilioinguinal nerves are usually formed from the bifurcation of a single trunk arising from T12 to L1 roots. However, there is one common anatomic variation in which both nerves arise only from L1 ventral ramus. The genitofemoral nerve is normally formed from roots L1 to L2 and usually bifurcates into its genital and femoral branches after leaving the substance of psoas major. In some instances, however, this bifurcation occurs inside the muscle. The femoral, obturator, and lateral cutaneous nerves of the thigh arise from roots L2 to L4 and provide motor and sensorial innervation to the thigh.

The sacral plexus is formed by the ventral rami of roots L4-S4 which also bifurcate into an anterior and posterior division. S1-S4 roots arise from the ventral sacral foramina, whereas branches from L4 and L5 roots form the lumbosacral trunk, which travels medially to the obturator nerve and joins the other structures of the sacral plexus. Mainly all anterior divisions coalesce to form the tibial division of the sciatic nerve and give branches to quadratus femoris and muscles of the leg (L4-L5-S1). The pudendal nerve also arises from the anterior divisions of the roots S2-S3-S4. The posterior division, with the exception of S3 and S4, forms the fibular division of the sciatic nerve and emit the following branches: superior gluteal nerve (L4-L5-S1), inferior gluteal nerve (L5-S1-S2), and posterior cutaneous nerve of thigh (S1-S2-S3) [19, 20].

21.3 Etiology

Various types of tumors may affect the LSP. They can be classified as neurogenic or non-neurogenic, as well as in benign or malignant. The neurogenic lesions include the benign schwannomas, neurofibromas, and perineuriomas and the malignant peripheral nerve sheath tumor (MPNST). The benign non-neurogenic lesions may be tumoral, such as leiomyomas [21], or non-tumoral, such as abscesses, hematomas, and vascular or inflammatory lesions [16]. The LSP may also be affected by direct malignant invasion from many pelvic organs, such as colon, cervix, ovaries, urinary bladder, and prostate glands as well as lymphomas and retroperitoneal sarcomas [1, 16, 17, 22, 23]. Malignant infiltration from adjacent organs appears to be more common than primary tumors of the LSP [13, 24]. A summary of the most common LSPT is presented in Table 21.1.

Pelvic tumors may often be classified as retroperitoneal, and some of these also affect the LSP. They can be further classified by histopathological type, with sarcomas accounting for more than 90% (i.e., liposarcoma and leiomyosarcoma) [25, 26] or as "solid" or "cystic" concerning their appearance on imaging exams [25, 27]. Solid retroperitoneal tumors include liposarcomas, leiomyosarcomas, and lymphomas, whereas cystic masses include cystic lymphangioma, cystic teratoma, cystic mesothelioma, and others [27].

21.3.1 Benign Neurogenic Lesions

It is hard to evaluate what is the most common benign neurogenic tumor to affect the LSPT, as both neurofibromas and schwannomas are correlated to different genetic syndromes, respectively, NF1 and schwannomatosis. The variable frequency of these syndromes among different series presented in the literature may distort the available clinical and surgical findings.

Table 21.1 Common types of tumors to affect the LSP

	Neurogenic	Non-neurogenic
Benign	Schwannomas Neurofibromas Perineuriomas Ganglioneuromas	Leiomyomas Pseudo-tumoral lesions (abscesses, hematomas)
Malignant	MPNST	Metastases (colorectum, uterus, cervix, prostate, bladder) Lymphomas Sarcomas Chordomas

In one series, schwannomas accounted for 18 of 20 presented LSPT (90%), 5 of these in the setting of schwannomatosis [4]. Alderete et al. also presented a high prevalence of these tumors among LSPT: 14 out of 42 (37%). However, there is no mention in the study if some of these patients presented schwannomatosis [3].

In another surgical series, neurofibromas accounted for 30 of all 44 tumors (68%) affecting the "pelvic plexus"; 12 of these were associated with NF1 [2]. Tonsgard et al. showed, in a series of 91 CT imaging exams conducted in NF1 patients, that around 40% of these patients had neurofibromas (mostly asymptomatic) in the abdominal and pelvic region, with the sacral plexus as one of the most common sites of these lesions [28]. Furthermore, Zacharia et al. demonstrated, in a series of 43 patients with some form of abdominopelvic involvement due to NF1, that 27 (63%) presented lesions to the LSP [29].There have also been reports of perineuriomas affecting the LSP, although its occurrence is notoriously rare [30].

21.3.2 Malignant Neurogenic Lesions

MPNST are virtually the only malignant neurogenic tumors to affect the LSP. Among the possible locations for the MPNST, the LSP seems to be among the most uncommon. In a nationwide cohort study, it was reported that around 5% of MPNST (43 out of 784 tumors) were situated in the retroperitoneum, although there was no mention of how many of these were actually in the LSP [12]. Nonetheless, retroperitoneal MPNST had a significantly worse outcome, with a median survival of 1.1 years compared to 6.0 years in patients with MPNST in other locations [12]. Another large series presented a higher frequency of MPNST in "lumbosacral nerve roots": 37 out of 289 (12.8%) [31]. Porter et al. presented a similar frequency, with 9 out of 123 MPNST in the lumbosacral plexus (11%) [32]. Lafemina et al. reported, in turn, that 30 out of 105 MPNST (28.5%) presented in the abdomen or retroperitoneum, although there is no mention of the LSP in their study [8].

In several large series of surgically treated MPNST, however, there is no mention of LSP, and the tumors are only classified as presenting in the "trunk" or "core" [5–7, 9–12]. Therefore, it is difficult to evaluate the frequency of MPNST that arise from the LSP when compared to other locations.

In two surgical series of only LSPT, it was reported 2 MPNST among all 44 tumors (5%) and 8 MPNST out of all 38 cases (21%) [2, 3]. However, in a large series of surgically treated PNT, there were no cases of MPNST among the 20 LSPT presented [4]. In another series of 16 patients with LSPT, only one presented with a MPNST (6%) [33]. Lastly, in a series conducted to distinguish MPNST among other peripheral nerve sheath tumors (PNST) at the pelvis, Ogose et al. reported that 11 out of 30 lesions were MPNST (37%), but none presented in the LSP [34].

It is important to observe, however, that among all the malignant lesions that affect the LSP, MPSNT is one of the less common etiologies. Therefore, when facing a lesion with malignant characteristics, other possibilities should be considered, particularly metastases of pelvic malignant tumors (discussed ahead).

21.3.3 Non-neurogenic Benign Lesions (Tumoral and Non-tumoral)

Benign lesions originating from organs in proximity (i.e., uterus) can cause plexopathy symptoms by extrinsic compression. Leiomyomas are known to assume large proportions and have been described to cause plexopathy via compression. Ganglioneuromas have also been reported in this setting [21, 35, 36]. Some pseudo-tumoral lesions, such as psoas' hematoma, especially in the context of anticoagulation [16, 37–39], hemophilic pseudotumors [40, 41], aneurisms of the internal iliac arteries [42], isolated hypogastric artery aneurisms [43], or abscesses (Fig. 21.1) [16], can also produce neurological deficits of the LSP (or its roots) due to extrinsic compression. In the specific case of intrapsoas abscesses, signs and symptoms may also be due to the inflammatory nature of the disease.

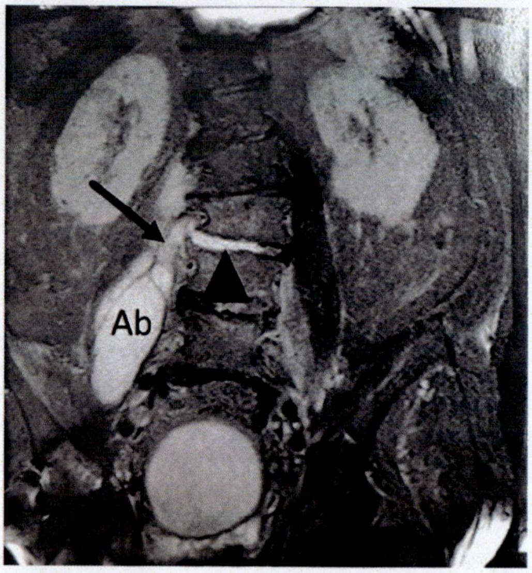

Fig. 21.1 Male, 54 years old, non-diabetic, with a previous urological surgery and vesical catheterization 2 months prior, presenting with intense lumbar pain, irradiating to the right inferior limb. Coronal T1-weighted MRI with contrast showing an intrapsoas abscess secondary to discitis. Note the abscess inside the psoas, the discitis, and the communication between the abscess and the infected disk space. The patient underwent CT-guided drainage of the abscess and antibiotics for 2 months with resolution of the case. Ab, abscess; arrowhead, discitis; arrow, communication between discitis and abscess

21.3.4 Non-neurogenic Malignant Tumors

The most common metastatic tumors to affect the LSP include colorectal adenocarcinoma, uterine and cervix malignancies, retroperitoneal sarcoma, and lymphoma (Fig. 21.2), which can directly infiltrate or cause retroperitoneal lymph node enlargement and further compression of the LPS [13, 16, 17, 33, 44]. Sarcomas appear to be indeed the most common tumor to grow in the retroperitoneal space [25, 26, 45]. It is suggested that pelvic malignant tumors, such as prostate, cervical, bladder, and rectal cancers, are able to spread retrogradely along the nerve from the end organ to the lumbosacral nerves and roots [18, 46–48]. This tendency to infiltrate along the nerve may explain why some patients with findings of diffuse plexopathy do not have radiographically demonstrable mass lesions and why in some circumstances the location of the pelvic tumor seems unrelated to the principal site of neurologic involvement. Diffuse large B-cell lymphoma, Burkitt lymphoma, Hodgkin lymphoma, and mucosa-associated lymphoid tissue (MALT) lymphomas also appear to have a propensity for the sacral plexus [18]. Retroperitoneal soft tissue sarcomas may also affect the LSP, and they usually present a worse prognosis than those located in extremities [49].

21.4 Clinical Considerations

A complete neurological examination should be conducted in patients potentially harboring LSPT. It is a common practice to use, for the systematic assessment of motor and sensory function, the British Medical Research Council (BMRC) or the Louisiana State University Health Sciences Center grading system (LSUHSC). The Visual Analogue Scale (VAS) is used for the assessment of pain.

Other components of the general physical examination may help in the diagnostic workup of LSPT. An increase in abdominal girth is usually present in patients harboring retroperitoneal tumors [50]. Also, on rectal touch, a mass can be palpated when the tumor is in the deep pelvis compromising the lower sacral plexus [18, 44].

The clinical presentation of LSPT is unspecific [51], and its diagnosis may not be possible using only clinical parameters. The literature indicates that pain is the most common symptom related to LSPT, and from our experience, all patients were referred to our service presenting some form of pain [1, 13, 17, 18]. Some authors state that its sensitivity is as high as 98%, and, given its high sensitivity, the absence of pain should prompt the investigation of other diagnoses [44]. The pain onset is usually subacute, sometimes described as a discomfort and whose location is not always correlated to the affected level of the LSP [17, 18]. The characteristic of the pain is usually aching and/or pressure-like and could be radicular, local, or referred [1]; in case of malignancy, it often worsens at night [52]. The pain is usually followed, after weeks, by motor and sensorial deficits [17, 18, 53].

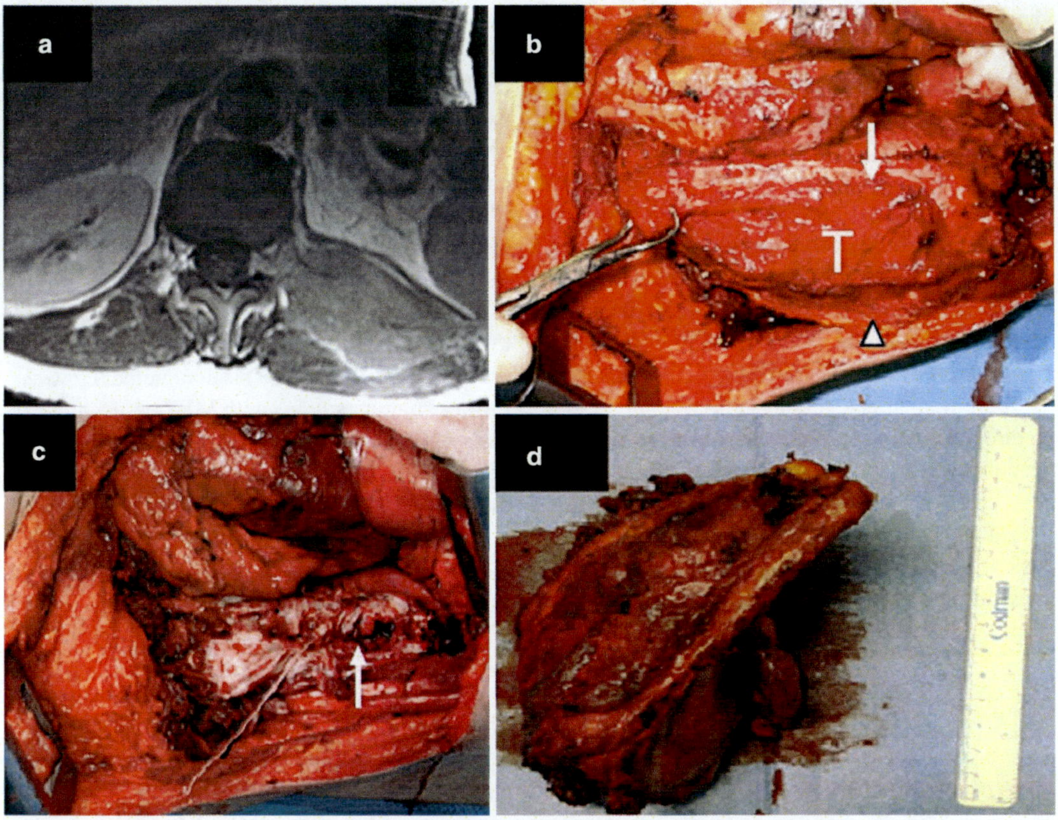

Fig. 21.2 Female, 67 years, presenting with intense lumbar pain for 3 months, with no neurological deficit. (**a**) T1-weighted MRI without contrast showing the invasion of left quadratus lumborum muscle by the tumor at level L2-L3. (**b**) Surgical exposure of the lesion. T, tumor; arrow, 11th rib; arrowhead, 12th rib. (**c**) Surgical aspect after tumor resection. It is possible to observe the cut L1 and L2 roots (arrow) to allow for radical resection of the mass. (**d**) The lesion was resected along with the 11th and 12th ribs. The final histopathological diagnosis was of a B-cell non-Hodgkin lymphoma. The lesion was solitary and the patient underwent radio- and chemotherapy. Unfortunately, she developed metastases to the pelvis and vertebral column and died 4 months after surgery

Tumors in the upper LSP (T12-L4) can cause pain in the costovertebral area, radiating to the upper thigh, whereas lesions in the lower LSP (L4-S4) are related with pain in the iliac crest, buttocks, perineum, and the posterior aspect of the thighs [17]. Some clinicians state that pain is exacerbated by lying down and alleviated by walking, and straight-leg raising test usually reproduces the same pain [53].

Jaeckle et al. summarize the sensitivity of signs and symptoms of 85 patients with malignant tumors affecting the LPS as follows: leg weakness (86%), sensory loss (73%), reflex asymmetry (64%), focal tenderness according to the topography involved (55%), positive direct and reverse straight-leg raising test (53% and 45%, respectively), leg edema (47%), rectal mass (39%), dysesthesia (15%), fasciculations (12%), and decreased sphincter tone (12%) [1]. Bowel or bladder incontinence or impotence is rarely seen, unless the plexopathy is bilateral and sacral [53]. Bilateral involvement can be present and should raise suspicion of widespread metastatic lesions [17].

Despite the low specificity of plexopathy symptoms, some important pointers may help in differentiating plexual lesions from those affecting only one root or only specific peripheral nerves. For example, if impairment of different nerves that arise from different roots is securely diagnosed (i.e., sciatic, obturator, femoral, pudendal nerves, and the cutaneous posterior nerve of the thigh), a plexopathy or polyneuropathy is more likely than a radiculopathy. The patient may also present "hot dry foot" due to damage to the retroperitoneal lumbar sympathetic nerves, which indicates a plexual lesion, rather than a radiculopathy [18, 53–55]. Additionally, involvement of gluteal nerves along with other nerves (i.e., femoral and/or sciatic nerves) indicates that there is a plexual lesion, as the superior and inferior gluteal nerves arise directly from the plexus [55].

Moreover, clinical findings may not only be due to direct neural compromise. Extrinsic mass effect on pelvic structures, such as the bladder and ureter, may cause signs and symptoms as well [29].

However, when it comes to some benign lesions, such as schwannomas and neurofibromas, they may be completely asymptomatic and detected incidentally [28, 56–58].

21.5 Complementary Exams

21.5.1 Electrophysiological Studies

Electrodiagnostic studies are useful to determine the presence of a lumbosacral plexopathy and differentiate it from other similar entities, such as radiculopathies and peripheral nerve injuries. Plexopathy is usually represented by reduction on the amplitudes on both compound action potentials and sensory nerve action potentials asymmetrically, normal or mildly reduced conduction velocities, and prolonged late response (F wave) [17, 24]. This nerve conduction study may help rule out radiculopathies. The pattern of muscle innervation may also aid in the diagnosis of a plexopathy. In addition, the presence of myokymic discharges may help rule out the hypothesis of LSPT, as it is only present in radiation plexopathy [17].

21.5.2 Computed Tomography (CT)

Imaging studies are of paramount importance for the diagnostic workup of presumed LSPT. Computed tomography (CT) may be sufficient for the diagnosis of LSPT and is especially useful when there are associated osseous lesions, be it osseous remodeling or tumor infiltration. Schwannomas can be identified by central enhancement on CT and by the target sign [34]. CT may also suggest the presence of a retroperitoneal tumor through the anterior displacement of abdominal structures, such as the aorta, due to the mass effect of the lesion [59]. In practice, tumors may be identified by CT before a magnetic resonance imaging (MRI) is conducted. However, further imaging studies with MRI are usually necessary for a better identification of the lesion and preoperative planning of surgical approach. CT may also be useful to evaluate metastatic diseases, in cases in which malignancy is suspected.

21.5.3 Magnetic Resonance Imaging (MRI)

MRI has been shown to be more sensitive than CT in the context of lumbosacral neoplastic plexopathy and should be the method of choice for presumed LSPT [23]. Magnetic resonance imaging (MRI) has great visualization of the soft tissue, being capable to clarify plexus nerve inflammation, swelling, and the presence of masses [60–64]. It is useful in distinguishing several causes of lumbosacral plexopathy, such as neoplasms (through compression or infiltration), traumatic injuries, abscesses, hematomas, diabetic lumbosacral radiculoplexus neuropathy, and even post-surgical inflammatory neuropathy [16, 17, 34, 37, 65]. MRI may also help in the evaluation of multiple lesions in patients with NF1 (Fig. 21.3a).

A specific modality of MRI called magnetic resonance neurography (MRN), which is based on the short T1 inversion recovery (STIR) sequence, is especially useful for the anatomical study of the LSP and lesions intrinsic to it [66]. Studies of neurography with 3T MRI present with promising results, being able to provide a clear view of the LSP and its peripheral branches, differentiating pathological tissue from normal, as well as evaluating their relationship with surrounding structures [66–70]. MR diffusion tensor imaging (DTI) has also been utilized in the context of PNT. This technique may aid in the evaluation of the tumor's relationship to neighboring fascicles (Fig. 21.3c) [71–73]. These qualities improve diagnostics and preoperative anatomical study.

It is not unusual that patients with complaints about the lower limb and hip (i.e., local or irradiated pain) are referred to a specialist with an inconclusive imaging study. This is because the most common causes for these symptoms are degenerative pathologies of the hip and lumbar column, as well as radiculopathies, and the imaging studies requested by physicians are often not suited to visualize the entire LSP. In such instances, a second imaging study, preferably MRI, should be conducted, with the specification that the pelvis is to be evaluated along the longitudinal axis of the LSP (from L1 vertebra to the sciatic notch) [17].

MRI may also aid to evaluate if a mass is benign or malignant. Different characteristics favor the hypothesis of malignancy, such as peritumoral edema, surrounding tissue invasion, necrosis, hemorrhage, heterogeneity and cystic changes, intratumoral lobulation, irregular or peripheral contrast enhancement, and larger proportions (>5 cm) [60–64]. Schwannomas and retroperitoneal sarcomas may develop cystic changes as well. In these cases, the presence of a smooth regular border (probably related to a capsule) may suggest a schwannoma as opposed to a malignant lesion, in which the presence of an irregular margin is more likely [74–76]. Lastly, lesions with lower apparent diffusion coefficient (ADC mean) values on diffusion weighted imaging (DWI) have been associated with malignancies with both high sensitivity and specificity in the context of PNT [77, 78].

21.5.4 Positron Emission Tomography (PET)

In cases in which malignant tumors are suspected, PET is indicated when other imaging studies are not satisfactory [16, 65]. PET has indeed been shown to differentiate benign PNT from MPNST with great sensitivity, based on the maximum standardized uptake value (SUVmax) of the lesion (Fig. 21.3b). It may also be helpful

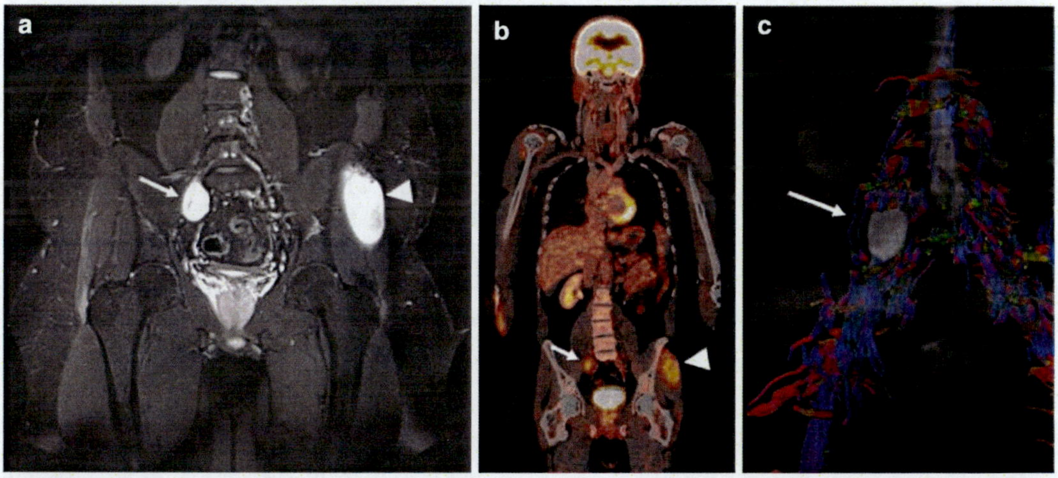

Fig. 21.3 Male, 23 years old, NF1. (**a**) Magnetic resonance neurography (MRN) and (**b**) positron emission tomography (PET-CT) demonstrating two lesions. Arrow, lesion arising from the right lumbosacral trunk (34 × 27 mm) with SUVmax of 4.8. Arrowhead, lesion inside the substance of the left gluteus medius muscle (133 × 115 × 57 mm), with a high SUVmax of 8.2. (**c**) Diffusion tensor imaging (DTI) of the lesion in the right lumbosacral trunk showing its relationship to surrounding fascicles. Arrow indicates the fascicles dislocated by the tumor

in order to evaluate the presence of distant metastases in cases in which malignancy is suspected [64, 79–82].

21.5.5 General Complementary Exams

Simple complementary exams can also aid to exclude other etiologies for lumbosacral plexopathy. Blood glucose or oral glucose tolerance tests may help evaluate the possibility of diabetes, which is a major cause of lumbosacral plexopathy. Cerebrospinal fluid analysis is also helpful in evaluating possible inflammatory or infectious disorders. Serology is also recommended when the patient has a history of insect bite (i.e., serology for *Borrelia burgdorferi*) [65].

21.5.6 Preoperative Biopsy

There is scarce documentation concerning preoperative biopsies in the lumbosacral plexus, and there is still an ongoing debate about the role of preoperative biopsy of PNT. General surgical series of MPNST do not approach the proper indications and techniques for these lesions [4, 5]. Nonetheless, for lesions intrinsic to neural elements, we recommend that only lesions presumed to be malignant are biopsied [83].

If biopsy is to be conducted, it should only be performed in an image-guided fashion, given the risks of damaging important structures of the LSP. Ogose et al. described good results using CT-guided core-needle biopsy to peripheral nerve sheath tumors (PNST) around the pelvis, three of which to the LSP, with no resulting neurological deficits [34].

21.6 Wait-and-See Approach

Not every tumor of the LSP warrants surgical treatment, especially when it comes to retroperitoneal schwannomas, which, when incidentally diagnosed, may harbor a slower-growing behavior. When an asymptomatic lesion is presumed to be a schwannoma on MRI, or after biopsy, and is not related to any genetic syndrome (NF2 or schwannomatosis), it may be managed with a "wait-and-see" approach [56, 58]. In Ogose et al.'s series of 22 retroperitoneal schwannomas conducted in this way, only 2 were lately operated [58].

These patients must be followed up with CT or MRI initially after 3–6 months of the diagnosis, then every 6 months, and then every other year [56, 58]. If the patient remains asymptomatic without interval changes on cross-sectional imaging, a further follow-up only with clinical history and examination may be considered [56].

21.7 Surgical Treatment

21.7.1 Surgical Indications

Surgery is indicated if the patient presents clinical symptoms caused by the tumor, such as the development of intense abdominal or perineal pain, lumbalgia, sciatalgia, neurological deficits, intestinal obstipation, and urinary retention or incontinence. It is also indicated whenever a tumor presents characteristics that indicate malignancy, with or without a preoperative biopsy, always considering the extent of the lesion, the presence of secondary lesions, and the general status of the patient.

The decision-making process should be tailored along with the general surgery team in order to evaluate which surgical approach should be preferred in each selected case. The aspects that should be considered in the decision are:

(a) If the tumor arises from or compresses/infiltrates the LSP
(b) The location of the tumor in the LPS, if located in the lumbar plexus, sacral plexus, or both of them, such as tumors affecting the lumbosacral trunk
(c) Its relation to surrounding structures (psoas muscles, vertebral column, major vessels, and viscera)

(d) The tumor's volume
(e) The vascularization of the tumor

21.7.2 Basic Techniques of Surgical Resection of PNT

Independently of the location of the tumor in the LSP, some steps should be followed during its exposure and resection.

During resection of the tumor, bleeding should be controlled with the usage of cottonoids embedded in warm saline solution and bipolar coagulation should be avoided. The surgeon must be ready to stop resection, in case intraoperative neurophysiological studies inform that there is an impending damage to important neurological structures. During dissection and resection of PNT, we use straight and curved micro-scissors, Penfield dissectors, and nerve hooks.

After exposure of probable schwannomas, stimulation ought to be conducted, generally at the equator of the lesion, in order to identify an electrically silent area devoid of functional fascicles. Then, the pseudocapsule (usually white-grayish and tough), but not the true capsule (usually yellowish and soft), is incised. A cleavage plain is developed in a fascicle-free corridor, and dissection is conducted circumferentially from this point to the proximal and distal poles of the tumor. Schwannomas generally arise from one or two non-functional fascicles, and the functional fascicles are generally displaced to the periphery of the lesion. This morphology facilitates their resection en bloc. After resection of the tumor, eversion of the borders of the nerve ("open book" maneuver) is conducted in order to evaluate any possible tumoral remnants inside the nerve (Fig. 21.4). In opposition to schwannomas presenting in other locations, the surgeon should not hesitate in resecting this tumor in a piecemeal fashion in the LSP, as resection en bloc may cause damage to important neurological structures (through compression/stretch) during its removal.

Neurofibromas, on the other hand, are generally more difficult to be resected en bloc, as they tend to originate from more than one fascicle and often there are functional fascicles in the intimacy of the tumor. Therefore, it is not uncommon for the resection to be conducted in a piecemeal and eventually subtotal technique, depending on information obtained via neurophysiological monitoring.

If the lesion presents characteristics of malignancy, intraoperative biopsy ought to be performed, and then a decision should be taken: to proceed to a partial resection or to stop the procedure and wait for the definitive histopathological diagnosis. In case the lesion is metastatic, the surgeon ought to avoid rupture of the tumor capsule.

21.8 Surgical Approaches

Three surgical approaches to the LSP are generally preferred, as well as some variations of these techniques depending on the extent of the tumor:

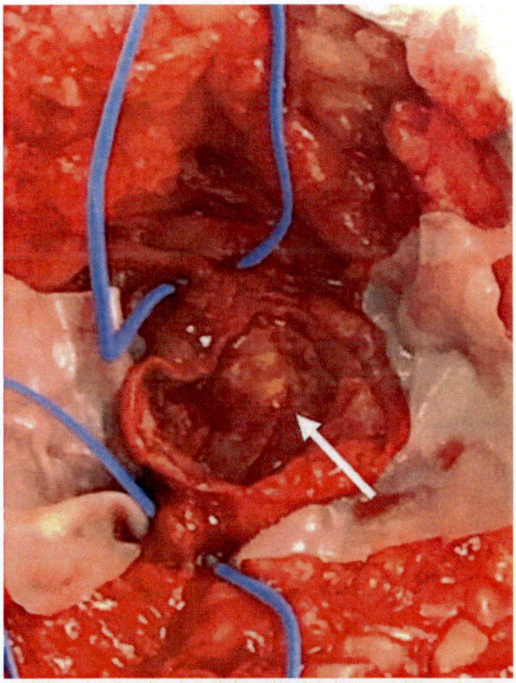

Fig. 21.4 "Open book" maneuver, consisting in eversion of the nerve's border in order to evaluate any remaining tumoral tissue. Arrow indicates a remaining portion of a schwannoma located inside the nerve

1. Dorsal approach
2. Anterolateral retroperitoneal approach (lumbotomy)
3. Anterior transabdominal approach

The access to the retroperitoneum is assisted by the general surgery team, followed later by the neurosurgery team to perform the microsurgical dissection of the LSP and resection of the tumor. Some centers have also had good results with the aid of minimally invasive techniques; this is a growing field with promising results [84–87].

In any of the following approaches, intraoperative neurophysiological monitoring should be performed. In our experience, it aided in the resection of several LSPT and reduced the incidence of complications [88].

Several techniques for the intraoperative neurophysiological monitoring are available: continuous electroencephalogram (EEG), spontaneous and evoked electromyography, and somatosensory evoked potential through stimulation of muscles and evaluation of EEG. Motor evoked potentials of different muscles should also be performed through transcranial electrical stimulation in C4-CZ and C3-CZ (related to the primary sensorimotor cortex), using the abductor digiti minimi response as a control. One should evaluate the vastus medialis bilaterally for the assessment of roots L2-L3-L4, the tibialis anterior for L4-L5-S1, the gastrocnemius for S1-S2, the abductor hallucis for L5-S1, and the external anal sphincter for S2-S3-S4 [88, 89]. These techniques provide the surgeon the security that there is no impending damage to important neurological structures and should be used whenever available. When the lesion is in the sacral plexus, however, we find this monitoring to be indispensable, because of the risks of deficit to important structures such as S2 and S3 roots that innervate the anal and urethral sphincters.

21.8.1 Dorsal Approach

The dorsal approach is useful to access proximal lesions of the lumbar plexus (T12- L1), some of which have intraforaminal components. The patient is placed in the prone position, and a dorsal incision is performed over the spinal apophysis after localization by intraoperative imaging exam (X-ray). Dissection of the paravertebral muscle is performed, and partial laminectomy and facetectomy are carried out; dissection outside the limits of the spine then follows, and it is important at this point not to compress the roots compromised by the tumor.

21.8.2 Extended Dorsal Approach

An extended dorsal approach can also be performed in order to access upper structures of the lumbar plexus. The longitudinal incision is initiated around 3 cm medially to the antero-superior iliac spine and extends to the anterior border of the 11th rib, where it extends obliquely and posteriorly until the level of the spinal apophysis of the 11th thoracic vertebra. Following the incision to the skin and subcutaneous fat, division or dissection of the aponeuroses of the external oblique muscle and of the serratus anterior muscle covering the 11th rib is performed. The sectioning of the fibers of the serratus anterior and of the latissimus dorsi muscle is then carried out. Then, the liberation of the 11th rib's periosteum is performed until it reaches the costovertebral articulation, in order to permit the resection of the aforementioned rib. At this moment, care must be taken not to damage the neurovascular bundle that follows the inferior border of the rib. The next step is the sectioning of the fibers of the external oblique, internal oblique, and transverse abdominal muscles, with caution not to enter the peritoneal cavity. Following, the removal of the 11th rib is performed, also with caution not to open the parietal pleura. In case that should happen, it must be corrected immediately. The access to the retroperitoneum is then performed through blunt dissection from the inferior pole of the initial incision, in order to expose the iliac insertion of the psoas major muscle, all the way to its superior insertion, at the level of T12-L1. After that, careful dissection of psoas major muscle fibers is conducted, and the tumor is exposed.

21.8.3 Anterolateral Retroperitoneal Approach

The anterolateral retroperitoneal approach, or lumbotomy, permits the access of the structures of the lumbar plexus, from L1 to L4/L5. The patient is positioned in an oblique position, with a cushion under the decubitus flank and with the hips and shoulders fixated to the operating table, with the contralateral hip in a 30° angle and thorax in a 60° angle in relation to the operating table; thus, the patient stays in a shape of an inverted "V" (Fig. 21.5). The ipsilateral leg must be flexed to relax the psoas muscle, as to diminish the tension over the LSP, facilitating dissection. The surgeon then positions him-/herself posteriorly to the patient. The operating field must permit that key anatomical structures, such as the last ribs and the iliac crests, are identified by palpation. The incision is performed in an oblique fashion, with the posterior half of the 12th rib as the superior point, following the lateral margin of the rectus anterior, ending in a point equidistant to the umbilicus and the pubic symphysis. Once the incision is performed on the skin and subcutaneous fat, division or dissection of the aponeurosis, the external oblique muscle, internal oblique muscle, transverse abdominal muscle, and transversalis fascia is then performed. At this moment, the surgeon must be careful not to damage the peritoneum, and if it should happen, its correction and the evaluation of any lesion to intraperitoneal organs must be done promptly. The access to the retroperitoneum is performed through blunt dissection between the adipose tissue and the psoas major muscle fascia, in order to create enough room to access the neurological structures.

In both the extended dorsal approach and in the anterolateral retroperitoneal approach, once the retroperitoneum is accessed, the auxiliary surgeon must traction the intraperitoneal content in the anterior direction, with the help of malleable retractors. In case there is necessity to move away the lumbar aorta or inferior vena cava, the ligature of the lumbar arteries or veins can be performed. As these smaller vessels are located posteriorly to the large vessels, careful maneuvers and effective ligature must be performed, as to prevent severe bleeding, which is difficult to control in this setting. In the dissection of deep planes, when trying to access the nerve roots of interest, caution must be taken not to damage the sympathetic trunk, the genitofemoral nerve, and the ureter, as they are usually not visualized from this approach. The psoas major muscle should not be cut. Instead, delicate dissection of its muscle fibers is conducted using microsurgical techniques at the point of maximum convexity over the tumor, identified by palpation. Once the delicate dissection of the psoas major muscle fibers is conducted and the tumor is visualized, its further exposure is conducted with the aid of dynamic retractors, avoiding continuous traction over the neural elements. Further dissection and exposure are then carried out with care not to damage vascular pedicles that usually arise from the posterior aspect of the lesion. If these vessels are damaged in a moment when the tumor and its vascular supply are still not adequately exposed, bleeding that is difficult to control may occur.

The synthesis of the musculoaponeurotic planes must be performed in an individualized and meticulous fashion in order to avoid the emergence of incisional hernias. In selected cases, it is possible to access nerve roots located in the crossing of the ureter with the primitive iliac vessels through an inguinotomy approach.

21.8.4 Anterior Transabdominal Approach

The anterior transabdominal approach is utilized for tumors in the lumbosacral trunk to S1-S4 levels. The approach is conducted by positioning the patient in dorsal decubitus,

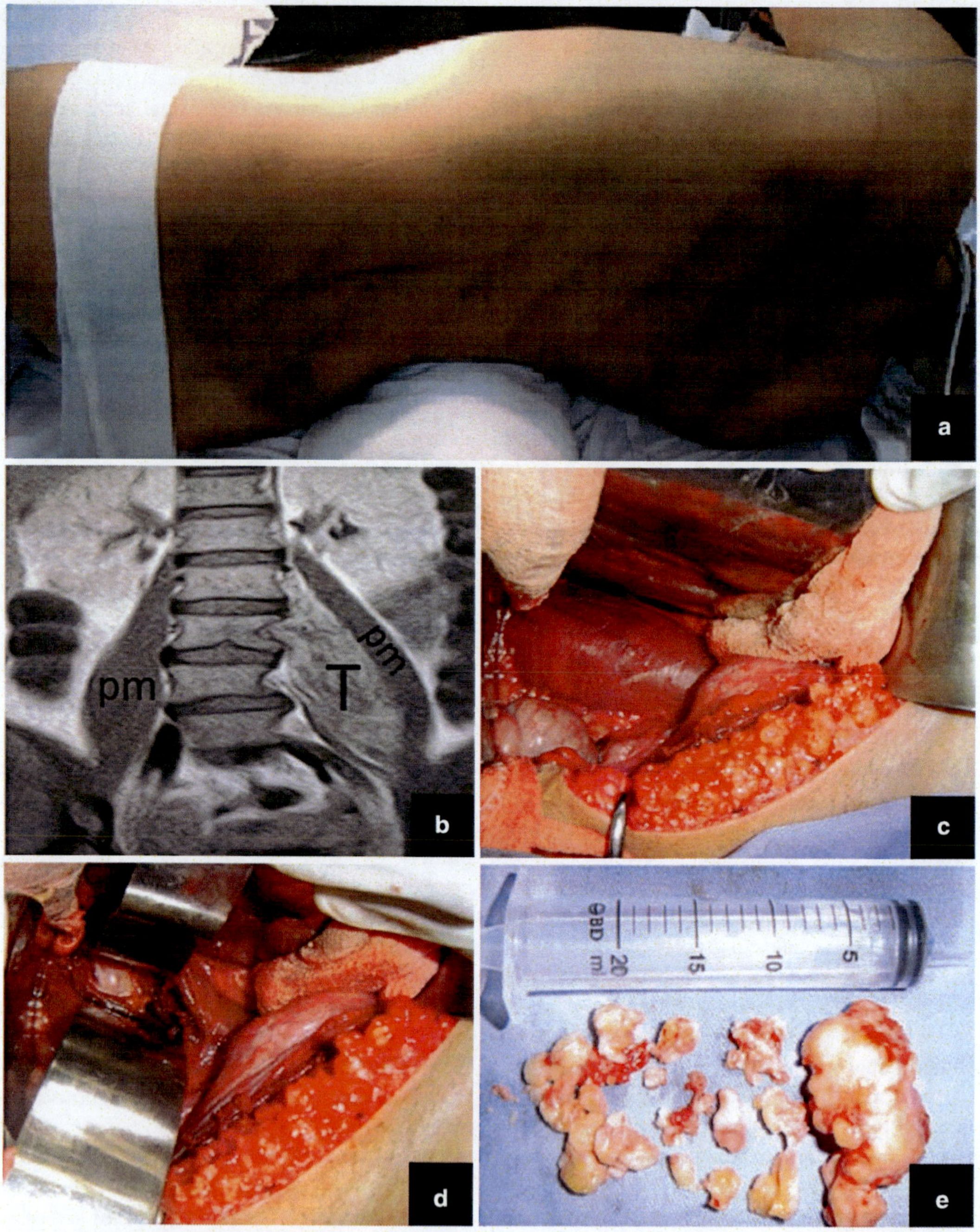

Fig. 21.5 (**a**) Positioning of the patient for the anterolateral retroperitoneal approach. (**b**) Coronal T1-weighted MRI without contrast showing a lesion inside the substance of the psoas major at levels L2-L5 (Note the "paper-thin" thickness of p.m.). *T* tumor, *pm* psoas major. (**c**) The psoas major muscle from the perspective of a lumbotomy. (**d**) Dissection of psoas major fibers (it is possible to see the tumor underneath the muscle). (**e**) The final histopathological diagnosis, after complete surgical resection, was of a schwannoma

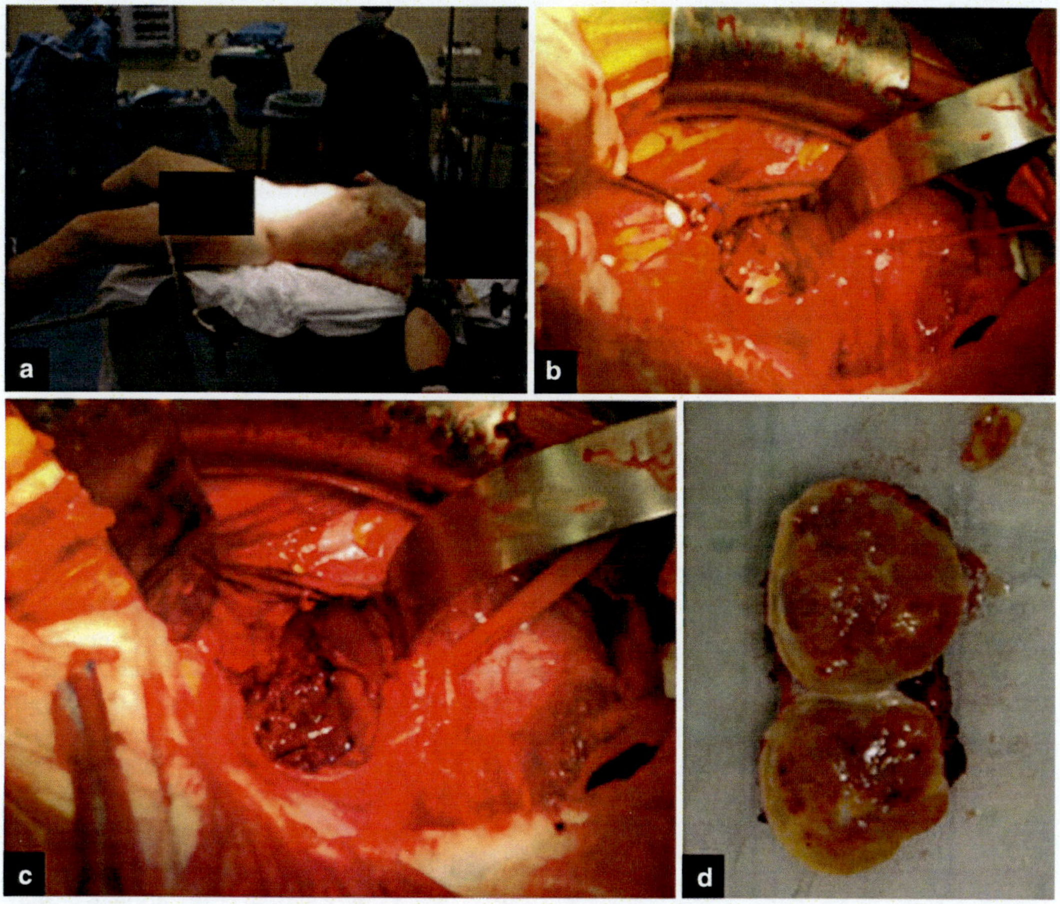

Fig. 21.6 (**a**) Positioning of the patient for the anterior transabdominal approach. The surgeon is positioned between the legs of the patient. (**b**) Exposure of the tumor deep in the ischiorectal fossa. (**c**) Surgical aspect after resection of the lesion. (**d**) The final histopathological diagnosis was of a schwannoma

and besides an indwelling bladder catheter, an orogastric catheter is also placed (Fig. 21.6). The latter should be used only during the surgical act. Then, a median vertical or a transverse (Pfannenstiel) incision is performed. The median incision is preferred and should start 2–3 cm superior to the umbilicus, or just inferior to it, and extend to the pubic symphysis, along the linea alba. In cases of previous abdominal and/or pelvic surgery, the access to the LSP through this access may be hindered. After abdominal incision is performed, the peritoneum is incised with care, avoiding damage to the intraperitoneal content, and at this point, the operating table is put in Trendelenburg position, and the intraperitoneal contents are moved in a proximal direction and maintained away from the operating field with the aid of surgical dressing. In the necessity to open the posterior peritoneum at the level of L5-S1, a ligature of the median sacral artery must be performed first. The dissection to access the nervous structures of the LPS located in the pelvis must be performed carefully in order to avoid damage to the pre-sacral plexus of parasympathetic nerves, sacral median artery, aorta, inferior vena cava, primitive iliac vessels, internal and external iliac vessels, and the ureter. Fortunately, the ureter is located laterally using this approach, helping to prevent iatrogenic lesions. The large vessels are then identified and positioned laterally. The posterior peritoneum is incised in a vertical fashion, medially to the common iliac artery. The hypogastric plexus is usually not visible from this approach as it is involved by retroperitoneal fat tissue; therefore its mobilization and dissection must be carried out with care. At this point, one should avoid using retractors, and cautery devices are forbidden during maneuvers for dissection of tumors in this area. To control small bleeders, we use bipolar coagulation at low setting and never in the neural elements. The exact location of the tumor can be assessed using digital palpation. Tumors at this level are usually supplied by branches of rectal and iliac vessels, and this approach allows for their localization and ligature. Once the ligature is concluded, the tumor is resected with care, following the same principles stated above.

21.8.5 Surgical Complications

Dafford et al. reported that weakness was the most common postoperative finding in patients. Among the 12 patients harboring NF1-associated neurofibromas in this series, demonstrable weakness after surgery occurred in 11 (92%) [2]. Alderete et al. assessed the morbidity associated with surgical excision of neurogenic tumors of the pelvis in 38 patients and reported that the most common complication was some grade of nerve paralysis, observed in 32% of the patients. Clinical evidence of postoperative nerve palsy presented more often in patients surgically treated for malignant lesions (7 of 12, 58%), when compared to those treated for benign tumors (5 of 26, 19%) [3]. Poor neurological outcomes thus seem to be related to malignant lesions and the need for wide surgical margins. However, continuous traction of neural structures during surgery may also lead to deficit. Guedes et al. reported a case in which a patient presented with a foot drop after surgery, which was probably caused by the stretch of neural structures during the removal of a sacral schwannoma [90]. Therefore, autostatic retractors should not be used when approaching the LSP.

21.9 Final Considerations

LSPT are rare, and there are only few series conducted in order to study them as a distinct group of lesions [2, 3]. Their management must be conducted in a multidisciplinary way. They most commonly cause a pressure-like subacute pain that may be present as diffuse abdominal pain, lumbar pain, radicular pain extending to the leg, or even perineal pain. They may also cause symptoms related to neurological deficits, such as leg weakness and sensory loss, related to compression of venous structures, such as leg edema, and related to compression of abdominal viscera, such as constipation and/or urinary retention. Albeit rare, autonomic involvement and urinary incontinence may also be present. MRI is of paramount importance for determining the tumor's anatomical relations to the LSPT and neighboring structures and therefore should be the imaging exam of choice.

The location of the tumor in relation to the LPS and the lumbosacral column will determine which surgical approach is preferred, and this decision should be made together with the general surgery team. Intraoperative functional assessment, multimodal evaluation, as well as microsurgical techniques should be used in order to preserve neurological function. It is not always possible to achieve a complete resection to these lesions. A suggested algorithm for aid during the decision-making process when facing a presumed LSPT is presented in Fig. 21.7 [91].

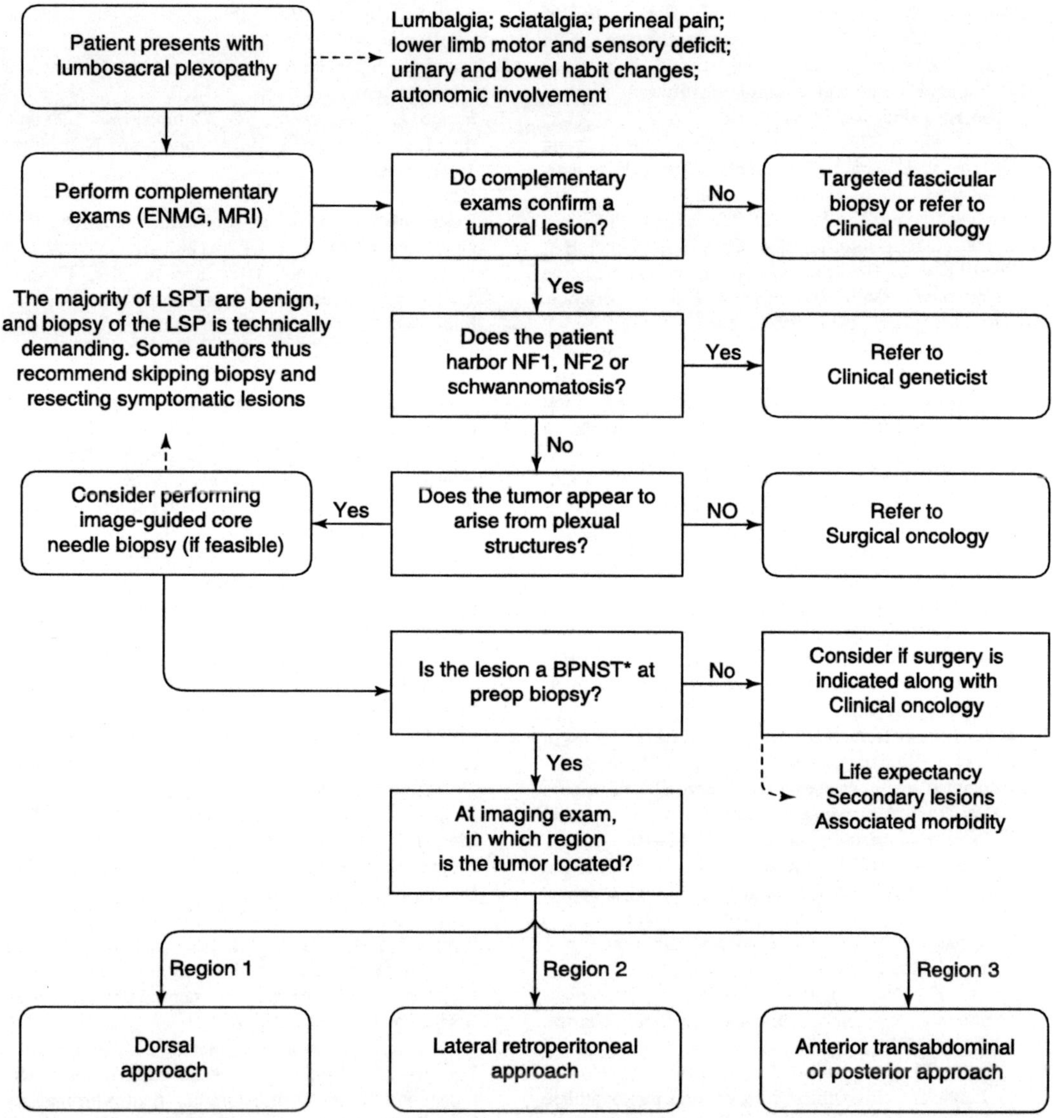

Fig. 21.7 A suggested algorithm for guidance during decision-making when facing a presumed lumbosacral plexus tumor. *LSP* lumbosacral plexus, *ENMG* electroneuromyography, *MRI* magnetic resonance imaging, *18FDG-PET/CT* [F-18] fluoro-D-glucose-positron emission tomography, *BPNST** benign peripheral nerve sheath tumor. (Reprinted by permission from [Springer Nature Customer Service Centre GmbH]: [Springer] [Acta Neurochirurgica] [Surgical Management of Symptomatic Lumbar, Sacral, and Lumbosacral Plexus Tumors: a Peripheral Nerve Unit Experience. Guedes et al.] [(c) 2021]) [91]

References

1. Jaeckle KA, Young DF, Foley KM. The natural history of lumbosacral plexopathy in cancer. Neurology. 1985;35:8–15.
2. Dafford K, Kim D, Reid N, Kline D. Pelvic plexus tumors. Neurosurg Focus. 2007;22:1–5.
3. Alderete J, Novais EN, Dozois EJ, Rose PS, Sim FF. Morbidity and functional status of patients with pelvic neurogenic tumors after wide excision. Clin Orthop. 2010;468:2948–53.
4. Guha D, Davidson B, Nadi M, Alotaibi NM, Fehlings MG, Gentili F, et al. Management of peripheral nerve sheath tumors: 17 years of experience at Toronto Western Hospital. J Neurosurg. 2018;128:1226–34.

5. Anghileri M, Miceli R, Fiore M, Mariani L, Ferrari A, Mussi C, et al. Malignant peripheral nerve sheath tumors: prognostic factors and survival in a series of patients treated at a single institution. Cancer. 2006;107:1065–74.
6. Zou C, Smith KD, Liu J, Lahat G, Myers S, Wang W-L, et al. Clinical pathological, and molecular variables predictive of malignant peripheral nerve sheath tumor outcome. Ann Surg. 2009;249:1014–22.
7. Stucky C-CH, Johnson KN, Gray RJ, Pockaj BA, Ocal IT, Rose PS, et al. Malignant peripheral nerve sheath tumors (MPNST): the Mayo Clinic experience. Ann Surg Oncol. 2012;19:878–85.
8. LaFemina J, Qin L-X, Moraco NH, Antonescu CR, Fields RC, Crago AM, et al. Oncologic outcomes of sporadic, neurofibromatosis-associated, and radiation-induced malignant peripheral nerve sheath tumors. Ann Surg Oncol. 2013;20:66–72.
9. Valentin T, Le Cesne A, Ray-Coquard I, Italiano A, Decanter G, Bompas E, et al. Management and prognosis of malignant peripheral nerve sheath tumors: the experience of the French Sarcoma Group (GSF-GETO). Eur J Cancer. 2016;56:77–84.
10. Yuan Z, Xu L, Zhao Z, Xu S, Zhang X, Liu T, et al. Clinicopathological features and prognosis of malignant peripheral nerve sheath tumor: a retrospective study of 159 cases from 1999 to 2016. Oncotarget. 2017;8:104785–95.
11. Miao R, Wang H, Jacobson A, Lietz AP, Choy E, Raskin KA, et al. Radiation-induced and neurofibromatosis-associated malignant peripheral nerve sheath tumors (MPNST) have worse outcomes than sporadic MPNST. Radiother Oncol. 2019;137:61–70.
12. Martin E, Coert JH, Flucke UE, Slooff W-BM, Ho VKY, van der Graaf WT, et al. A nationwide cohort study on treatment and survival in patients with malignant peripheral nerve sheath tumours. Eur J Cancer. 2020;124:77–87.
13. Jaeckle KA. Neurological manifestations of neoplastic and radiation-induced plexopathies. Semin Neurol. 2004;24:385–93.
14. Brejt N, Berry J, Nisbet A, Bloomfield D, Burkill G. Pelvic radiculopathies, lumbosacral plexopathies, and neuropathies in oncologic disease: a multidisciplinary approach to a diagnostic challenge. Cancer Imaging. 2013;13:591–601.
15. Ladha SS, Spinner RJ, Suarez GA, Amrami KK, Dyck PJB. Neoplastic lumbosacral radiculoplexopathy in prostate cancer by direct perineural spread: an unusual entity. Muscle Nerve. 2006;34:659–65.
16. Planner AC, Donaghy M, Moore NR. Causes of lumbosacral plexopathy. Clin Radiol. 2006;61:987–95.
17. Dyck PJB, Thaisetthawatkul P. Lumbosacral plexopathy. Continuum (Minneap Minn). 2014;20:1343–58.
18. Gwathmey KG. Plexus and peripheral nerve metastasis. Handb Clin Neurol. 2018;149:257–79.
19. Van Alfen N, Malessy MJA. Diagnosis of brachial and lumbosacral plexus lesions. Handb Clin Neurol [Internet]. Elsevier; 2013 [cited 2020 May 14]. p. 293–310. https://linkinghub.elsevier.com/retrieve/pii/B9780444529022000187
20. Standring S. Gray's anatomy: the anatomical basis of clinical practice. 2016.
21. Felice KJ, Donaldson JO. Lumbosacral plexopathy due to benign uterine leiomyoma. Neurology. 1995;45(10):1943–4.
22. Pettigrew LC, Glass JP, Maor M, et al. Diagnosis and treatment of lumbosacral plexopathies in patients with cancer. Arch Neurol. 1984;41:1282–5.
23. Taylor BV, Kimmel DW, Krecke KN, Cascino TL. Magnetic resonance imaging in cancer-related lumbosacral plexopathy. In: Mayo Clinic Proceedings 1997;72(9):823–829. Elsevier.
24. Tavee J, Mays M, Wilbourn AJ. Pitfalls in the electrodiagnostic studies of sacral plexopathies. Muscle Nerve. 2007;35:725–9.
25. Osman S, Lehnert BE, Elojeimy S, Cruite I, Mannelli L, Bhargava P, et al. A comprehensive review of the retroperitoneal anatomy, neoplasms, and pattern of disease spread. Curr Probl Diagn Radiol. 2013;42:191–208.
26. Rajiah P, Sinha R, Cuevas C, Dubinsky TJ, Bush WH Jr, Kolokythas O. Imaging of uncommon retroperitoneal masses. Radiographics. 2011;31:949–76.
27. Wee-Stekly W-W, Mueller MD. Retroperitoneal tumors in the pelvis: a diagnostic challenge in gynecology. Front Surg. 2014;1:49.
28. Tonsgard JH, Kwak SM, Short MP, Dachman AH. CT imaging in adults with neurofibromatosis-1: requent asymptomatic plexiform lesions. Neurology. 1998;50(6):1755–60.
29. Zacharia TT, Jaramillo D, Poussaint TY, Korf B. MR imaging of abdominopelvic involvement in neurofibromatosis type 1: a review of 43 patients. Pediatr Radiol. 2005;35:317–22.
30. Mauermann ML, Amrami KK, Kuntz NL, Spinner RJ, Dyck PJ, Bosch EP, Engelstad J, Felmlee JP, Dyck PJ. Longitudinal study of intraneural perineurioma—a benign, focal hypertrophic neuropathy of youth. Brain. 2009;132(8):2265–76.
31. Watson KL, Al Sannaa GA, Kivlin CM, Ingram DR, Landers SM, Roland CL, et al. Patterns of recurrence and survival in sporadic, neurofibromatosis type 1-associated, and radiation-associated malignant peripheral nerve sheath tumors. J Neurosurg. 2017;126:319–29.
32. Porter DE, Prasad V, Foster L, Dall GF, Birch R, Grimer RJ. Survival in malignant peripheral nerve sheath tumours: a comparison between sporadic and neurofibromatosis type 1-associated tumours. Sarcoma. 2009;2009:1–5.
33. Ko K, Sung DH, Kang MJ, Ko MJ, Do JG, Sunwoo H, et al. Clinical electrophysiological findings in adult patients with non-traumatic plexopathies. Ann Rehabil Med. 2011;35:807.
34. Ogose A, Hotta T, Morita T, Higuchi T, Umezu H, Imaizumi S, et al. Diagnosis of peripheral nerve sheath tumors around the pelvis. Jpn J Clin Oncol. 2004;34:405–13.

35. Lee SJ, Hong BY, Yoon JH, Kim JS, Lim SH. A lumbosacral plexopathy compressed by huge uterine myoma. Am J Phys Med Rehabil. 2018;97:e58–9.
36. Wan Z, Yin T, Chen H, Li D. Surgical treatment of a retroperitoneal benign tumor surrounding important blood vessels by fractionated resection: a case report and review of the literature. Oncol Lett. 2016;11:3259–64.
37. Conesa X, Ares O, Seijas R. Massive psoas haematoma causing lumbar plexus palsy: a case report. J Orthop Surg. 2012;20(1):94–7.
38. Klein SM, D'Ercole F, Greengrass RA, Warner D. Enoxaparin associated with psoas hematoma and lumbar plexopathy after lumbar plexus block. Anesthesiology. 1997;87(6):1576–9. https://doi.org/10.1097/00000542-199712000-00040.
39. Aveline C, Bonnet F. Delayed retroperitoneal haematoma after failed lumbar plexus block. Br J Anaesth. 2004;93(4):589–91. https://doi.org/10.1093/bja/aeh242.
40. Gebarski KS, Gebarski SS, Glazer GM, Samuels BI, Francis IR. The lumbosacral plexus: anatomic-radiologic-pathologic correlation using CT. Radiographics. 1986;6(3):401–25.
41. Nachimuthu G, Arockiaraj J, Krishnan V, Sundararaj GD. Hemophilic pseudotumor of the first lumbar vertebra. Indian J Orthop. 2014;48(6):617.
42. Wider C, Kuntzer T, Segesser L-K, Qanadli SD, Bogousslavsky J, Vingerhoets F. Bilateral compressive lumbosacral plexopathy due to internal iliac artery aneurysms. J Neurol. 2006;253(6):809–10. https://doi.org/10.1007/s00415-006-0083-5.
43. Brin BJ. Isolated hypogastric artery aneurysms. Arch Surg. 1982;117(10):1329. https://doi.org/10.1001/archsurg.1982.01380340051012.
44. Jaeckle K. Neurologic manifestations of neoplastic and radiation-induced plexopathies. Semin Neurol. 2010;30:254–62.
45. Storm FK, Mahvi DM. Diagnosis and management of retroperitoneal soft-tissue sarcoma. Ann Surg. 1991;214:2–10.
46. Hébert-Blouin M-N, Amrami KK, Myers RP, Hanna AS, Spinner RJ. Adenocarcinoma of the prostate involving the lumbosacral plexus: MRI evidence to support direct perineural spread. Acta Neurochir. 2010;152:1567–76.
47. Capek S, Howe BM, Amrami KK, Spinner RJ. Perineural spread of pelvic malignancies to the lumbosacral plexus and beyond: clinical and imaging patterns. Neurosurg Focus. 2015;39:E14.
48. Jacobs JJ, Capek S, Spinner RJ, Swanson KR. Mathematical model of perineural tumor spread: a pilot study. Acta Neurochir. 2018;160(3):655–61.
49. Stojadinovic A, Leung DHY, Hoos A, Jaques DP, Lewis JJ, Brennan MF. Analysis of the prognostic significance of microscopic margins in 2,084 localized primary adult soft tissue sarcomas. Ann Surg. 2002;235:424–34.
50. Hueman MT, Herman JM, Ahuja N. Management of retroperitoneal sarcomas. Surg Clin North Am. 2008;88:583–97.
51. Dozois EJ, Wall JCH, Spinner RJ, Jacofsky DJ, Yaszemski MJ, Sim FH, et al. Neurogenic tumors of the pelvis: clinicopathologic features and surgical outcomes using a multidisciplinary team. Ann Surg Oncol. 2009;16:1010–6.
52. Thomas JE, Cascino TL, Earle JD. Differential diagnosis between radiation and tumor plexopathy of the pelvis. Neurology. 1985;35(1):1–7.
53. Jaeckle KA. Plexopathies. In: Levin VA, editor. Cancer in the nervous system. 2nd ed. New York: Oxford University Press; 2002. p. 413–22.
54. Evans R, Watson CPN. The hot foot syndrome: Evans' sign and the old way. Pain Res Manag. 2012;17:31–4.
55. Smith S, Knight R. Clinical neurophysiology in peripheral nerve injuries. In: Surgical disorders of the peripheral nerves. London: Springer; 2010.
56. Strauss DC, Qureshi YA, Hayes AJ, Thomas M. Management of benign retroperitoneal schwannomas: a single-center experience. Am J Surg. 2011;202:194–8.
57. Li Q, Gao C, Juzi JT, Hao X. Analysis of 82 cases of retroperitoneal schwannoma. Aust N Z J Surg. 2007;77:237–40.
58. Ogose A, Kawashima H, Hatano H, Ariizumi T, Sasaki T, Yamagishi T, et al. The natural history of incidental retroperitoneal schwannomas. PLoS One. 2019;14:e0215336.
59. Chaudhari A, Desai P, Vadel M, Kaptan K. Evaluation of primary retroperitoneal masses by computed tomography scan. Int J Med Sci Public Health. 2016;5:1423.
60. James AW, Shurell E, Singh A, Dry SM, Eilber FC. Malignant peripheral nerve sheath tumor. Surg Oncol Clin N Am. 2016;25:789–802.
61. Salamon J, Mautner V, Adam G, Derlin T. Multimodal imaging in neurofibromatosis type 1-associated nerve sheath tumors. RöFo. 2015;187:1084–92.
62. Matsumine A, Kusuzaki K, Nakamura T, Nakazora S, Niimi R, Matsubara T, et al. Differentiation between neurofibromas and malignant peripheral nerve sheath tumors in neurofibromatosis 1 evaluated by MRI. J Cancer Res Clin Oncol. 2009;135:891–900.
63. Wasa J, Nishida Y, Tsukushi S, Shido Y, Sugiura H, Nakashima H, et al. MRI features in the differentiation of malignant peripheral nerve sheath tumors and neurofibromas. Am J Roentgenol. 2010;194:1568–74.
64. Derlin T, Tornquist K, Münster S, Apostolova I, Hagel C, Friedrich RE, et al. Comparative effectiveness of 18F-FDG PET/CT versus whole-body MRI for detection of malignant peripheral nerve sheath tumors in neurofibromatosis type 1. Clin Nucl Med. 2013;38:e19–25.
65. van Alfen N, Malessy MJA. Diagnosis of brachial and lumbosacral plexus lesions. Handb Clin Neurol. 2013;115:293–310.
66. Zhai H, Lv Y, Kong X, Liu X, Liu D. Magnetic resonance neurography appearance and diagnostic evaluation of peripheral nerve sheath tumors. Sci Rep. 2019;9:6939.

67. Soldatos T, Andreisek G, Thawait GK, Guggenberger R, Williams EH, Carrino JA, Chhabra A. High-resolution 3-T MR neurography of the lumbosacral plexus. Radiographics. 2013;33(4):967–87.
68. Cejas C, Escobar I, Serra M, Barroso F. High resolution neurography of the lumbosacral plexus on 3 T magnetic resonance imaging. Radiología. 2015;57(1):22–34.
69. Mürtz P, Kaschner M, Lakghomi A, Gieseke J, Willinek WA, Schild HH, Thomas D. Diffusion-weighted MR neurography of the brachial and lumbosacral plexus: 3.0 T versus 1.5 T imaging. Eur J Radiol. 2015;84(4):696–702.
70. Delaney H, Bencardino J, Rosenberg ZS. Magnetic resonance neurography of the pelvis and lumbosacral plexus. Neuroimaging Clin N Am. 2014;24(1):127–50.
71. Kasprian G, Amann G, Panotopoulos J, Schmidt M, Dominkus M, Trattnig S, et al. Peripheral nerve tractography in soft tissue tumors: a preliminary 3-tesla diffusion tensor magnetic resonance imaging study. Muscle Nerve. 2015;51:338–45.
72. Cage TA, Yuh EL, Hou SW, Birk H, Simon NG, Noss R, et al. Visualization of nerve fibers and their relationship to peripheral nerve tumors by diffusion tensor imaging. Neurosurg Focus. 2015;39:E16.
73. Bruno F, Arrigoni F, Mariani S, Patriarca L, Palumbo P, Natella R, et al. Application of diffusion tensor imaging (DTI) and MR-tractography in the evaluation of peripheral nerve tumours: state of the art and review of the literature. Acta Biomed. 2019;90:68–76.
74. Hughes MJ, Thomas JM, Fisher C, Moskovic EC. Imaging features of retroperitoneal and pelvic schwannomas. Clin Radiol. 2005;60(8):886–93.
75. Cohan RH, Baker ME, Cooper C, Moore JO, Saeed M, Dunnick NR. Computed tomography of retroperitoneal malignancies. J Comput Assist Tomogr. 1988;12:804–10.
76. Nakashima J, Ueno M, Nakamura K, Tachibana M, Baba S, Deguchi N. Differential diagnosis of primary benign and malignant retroperitoneal tumours. Int J Urol. 1997;4:441–6.
77. Well L, Salamon J, Kaul MG, Farschtschi S, Herrmann J, Geier KI, et al. Differentiation of peripheral nerve sheath tumors in patients with neurofibromatosis type 1 using diffusion-weighted magnetic resonance imaging. Neuro Oncol. 2019;21:508–16.
78. Ahlawat S, Blakeley JO, Rodriguez FJ, Fayad LM. Imaging biomarkers for malignant peripheral nerve sheath tumors in neurofibromatosis type 1. Neurology. 2019;93:e1076.
79. Ferner RE. Neurofibromatosis 1 and neurofibromatosis 2: a twenty first century perspective. Lancet Neurol. 2007;6:340–51.
80. Warbey VS, Ferner RE, Dunn JT, Calonje E, O'Doherty MJ. [18F]FDG PET/CT in the diagnosis of malignant peripheral nerve sheath tumours in neurofibromatosis type-1. Eur J Nucl Med Mol Imaging. 2009;36:751–7.
81. Benz MR, Czernin J, Dry SM, Tap WD, Allen-Auerbach MS, Elashoff D, et al. Quantitative F18-fluorodeoxyglucose positron emission tomography accurately characterizes peripheral nerve sheath tumors as malignant or benign. Cancer. 2010;116:451–8.
82. Raad R, Lala S, Allen J, Babb J, Mitchell C, Franceschi A, et al. Comparison of hybrid 18F-fluorodeoxyglucose positron emission tomography/magnetic resonance imaging and positron emission tomography/computed tomography for evaluation of peripheral nerve sheath tumors in patients with neurofibromatosis type 1. World J Nucl Med. 2018;17:241.
83. Dangoor A, Seddon B, Gerrand C, Grimer R, Whelan J, Judson I. UK guidelines for the management of soft tissue sarcomas. Clin Sarcoma Res. 2016;6:20.
84. Yang MS, Kim KN, Yoon DH, Pennant W, Ha Y. Robot-assisted resection of paraspinal Schwannoma. J Korean Med Sci. 2011;26:150–3.
85. Seo IY, Boldbaatr Y, Choi KH. Laparoscopic resection of ancient schwannoma embedded in the psoas muscle. Surg Laparosc Endosc Percutan Tech. 2011;21:e336–8.
86. Baten E, Lerut J, Kempeneers I. Hybrid open/closed resection procedure for ancient retroperitoneal Schwannoma: case report and review of the literature. Acta Chir Belg. 2016;116:289–92.
87. Freitas B, Figueiredo R, Carrerette F, Acioly MA. Retroperitoneoscopic resection of a lumbosacral plexus schwannoma: case report and literature review. J Neurol Surg A Cent Eur Neurosurg. 2018;79:262–7.
88. Guedes-Correa JF, Junior FT, Moreira CA, Amorim RM. The importance of intraoperative neurophysiological monitoring for resection of lumbosacral plexus tumors. Neurol Psychiatry Brain Res. 2018;28:7–12.
89. Krassioukov AV, Sarjeant R, Arkia H, Fehlings MG. Multimodality intraoperative monitoring during complex lumbosacral procedures: indications, techniques, and long-term follow-up review of 61 consecutive cases. J Neurosurg Spine. 2004;1(3):243–53.
90. Guedes-Corrêa JF, Basílio-de-Oliveira CA, Santos M, de Amorim RMP, Megali R. Tumores do plexo lombossacral: Relato de dois casos e revisão da literatura. Arq Bras Neurocir Braz Neurosurg. 2008;27:96–101.
91. Guedes F, Sanches GE, Brown RS, Cardoso RSV, Siquara-de-Sousa AC, Ascenção A, Iglesias AC. Surgical management of symptomatic lumbar, sacral, and lumbosacral plexus tumors: a peripheral nerve unit experience. Acta Neurochir (Wien). 2021. https://doi.org/10.1007/s00701-021-04789-0. Epub ahead of print. PMID: 33694013.

22 Management of Paraspinal Nerve Sheath Tumors

Christopher F. Dibble and Wilson Z. Ray

Abbreviations

EMG	Electromyography
MEP	Motor evoked potentials
MIS	Minimally invasive spine
MPNST	Malignant peripheral nerve sheath tumor
MRI	Magnetic resonance imaging
NF1/NF2	Neurofibromatosis
PaNST	Paraspinal nerve sheath tumor
SSEP	Somatosensory evoked potentials

22.1 Introduction

Paraspinal nerve sheath tumors (PaNST) are a complex group of pathologies that are both challenging and satisfying to treat. In this chapter we offer our recommendations for the management of PaNST as well as review of the existing literature. Overall these lesions are best approached in a multidisciplinary fashion, but surgical decision-making stands at the center of the treatment strategy, and surgical expertise and pre- and postoperative support are key drivers in outcomes. Peripheral nerve surgeons are often multidisciplinary in training already and with PaNST are further expected to extend their comfort zones to include thoracotomies and extradural/intradural dissections, operating on the cervical spine and around the cervicomedullary junction and operating on the lumbar spine in large patients, to name a few of the challenges. Neurosurgeons, because of their experience and necessary comfort with operating around the spine and spinal cord, may be uniquely well positioned to perform these cases, unlike some other areas of peripheral nerve where our orthopedics or plastics colleagues often have significant expertise in matters of the hand or limb.

A PaNST is defined as a tumor either centered lateral to the neural foramen originating from or involving the nerve sheath or with an intracanal or intraforaminal origin with a significant soft tissue component outside the spinal canal. Most PaNST originate from the sensory components of the associated nerve root, frequently at the transition zone between the central nervous system (CNS) and peripheral nervous system. This is the so-called Redlich-Obersteiner's zone where myelination source switches from oligodendrocytes to Schwann cells. There is a relatively even distribution of PaNST between the different levels of the spine, although in the past there have been suggestions that cervical or thoracic spine had an increased incidence [1].

PaNST are often referred to interchangeably as dumbbell tumors, which are defined as having

C. F. Dibble · W. Z. Ray (✉)
Department of Neurological Surgery, Washington University School of Medicine, Saint Louis, MO, USA
e-mail: RayZ@wudosis.wustl.edu

F. Guedes et al. (eds.), *Diagnostic Assessment and Treatment of Peripheral Nerve Tumors*,
https://doi.org/10.1007/978-3-030-77633-6_22

communicating intraforaminal and extraforaminal components, and about 10–15% of PaNST have this dumbbell shape [2]. To the peripheral nerve surgeon, many clinically relevant PaNST will be some form of dumbbell tumor, but for the sake of classification, it should be noted that all dumbbell tumors are PaNST, but not all PaNST are dumbbell tumors (i.e., PaNST can just be lateral to the foramen).

The differential diagnosis for paraspinal mass lesion can be quite broad, with PaNST as most likely, but also including metastases, intraforaminal synovial cysts, chordoma, sarcoid, extradural arachnoid cyst, and abscess [3]. Generally though, MRI is able to delineate whether a lesion is a PaNST, which have been estimated at about 8% of all primary tumors of the CNS [4, 5]. The majority are benign, and the differential of PaNST is relatively small, with schwannomas being the most common at 65%, followed by neurofibromas at 30% [6, 7]. Both tumors can occur at any age and are associated with neurofibromatosis 1 or 2 (NF1/NF2), and schwannomatosis, a subtype of NF [8, 9].

One particularly complex PaNST is the plexiform neurofibroma. These can be quite large and unresectable, especially in NF patients. They can undergo malignant degeneration and should be surveilled if not operable. Fortunately, they can remain stable, and patients may only suffer radicular symptoms (Fig. 22.1). Chemical and biological targets are currently under investigation for therapy of plexiform neurofibromas. Selumetinib has indeed been shown to reduce the size of inoperable plexiform neurofibromas, thus apparently stopping their progression into MPNST.

Malignant peripheral nerve sheath tumor (MPNST) is the next most common at 1–5%, [4, 5]. This disease is very aggressive and carries a poor prognosis. MPNST can occur at any age and can be associated with NF1, a history of prior radiation therapy and degeneration of existing PaNST. The clinical presentation for MPNST is typically one of severe pain, even at rest, and progressive neurological deterioration. Much less common PaNST have been described, including perineurioma, spindle cell tumors, fibrous histiocytoma, solitary fibrous tumor, paraganglioma, angiolipoma, and hemangioma [1, 10]. Finally, sympathetic chain nerve sheath tumors are a rare and usually benign PaNST in the cervical and thoracic spine [11].

Practically speaking, nerve sheath tumors can often be differentiated from other lesions preoperatively by history, physical, and imaging, but as with other aspects of medicine, it is prudent to keep a broad differential initially and investigate unusual lesions because if non-neoplastic, management is often nonsurgical. Many PaNST are associated with neurocutaneous disorders such as NF1/N2, and genetic counseling may be important for diagnosis and prognostication.

22.2 Workup

A thoughtful physical exam is a key component to workup of a PaNST, and as with many other aspects of medicine, the history often clinches the diagnosis. A thorough spine exam should be conducted, including strength, sensation to pinprick with attention to dermatomal patterns, reflexes, and gait/balance/proprioception. Myelopathy and radiculopathy should be appreciated. A family history of neurofibromatosis or other phakomatosis should be queried. If the anatomy allows, PaNST may manifest as a mobile mass with accompanying dermatomal pain. If possible to palpate a mass, a fixed or infiltrative one is more concerning than a well-circumscribed and mobile one. Attention should be paid to the spinal level of involvement in terms of the sensory level or dermatomal distribution.

22.3 Imaging and Electrodiagnostic Studies

Thorough pre-operative imaging and electrodiagnostics are critical for managing paraspinal nerve sheath tumors. In most cases, MRI with and without contrast is the gold standard for lesion characterization and surgical planning. It is sensitive, and in addition to critical information about size and location, the surgeon can appreciate intrinsic lesion characteristics suggesting the diagnosis. The relationship of the lesion to the spinal cord and nerve roots can be appreciated, as some tumors can compress or rotate the thecal sac. The location of the tumor must be understood with relation to important vascular structures, as well as the lungs or viscera.

With cervical tumors, it is especially important to appreciate the course of the vertebral arteries, as well as their contributions to cerebral vascular territories. Depending on the anatomy of the lesion, different levels of invasiveness for imaging may be warranted. In some cases inspection of the vertebral arteries on T2 sequences is sufficient. If there

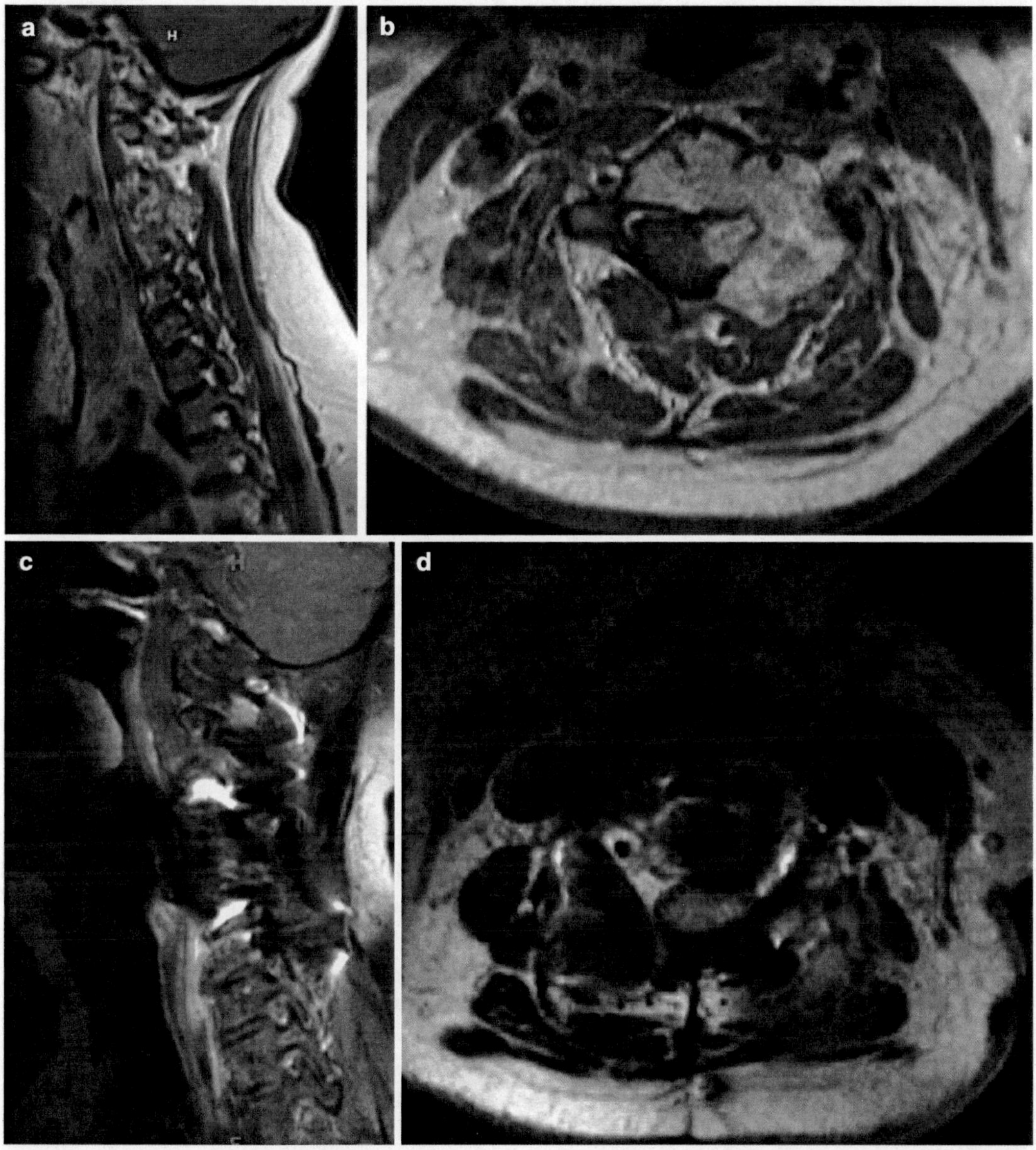

Fig. 22.1 This patient is a 56-year-old female with symptoms of progressive upper extremity weakness who was found to have what appeared to be extradural/extramedullary compressive lesion involving the C4 vertebral body and invading the left vertebral artery (**a**) and (**b**). After an extensive workup and a planned sacrifice of the left-sided vertebral body by our interventional radiology colleagues, the patient was brought for a combined anterior-posterior decompression and reconstruction (**c**–**f**). The anterior component included C4 corpectomy and then anteriorly several days later we performed C3–C6 decompression and C2–C6 fusion, with resection of large left C3 tumor. Pathology showed Schwannoma. Metallic artifact limits post operative evaluation but it was read as complete tumor resection

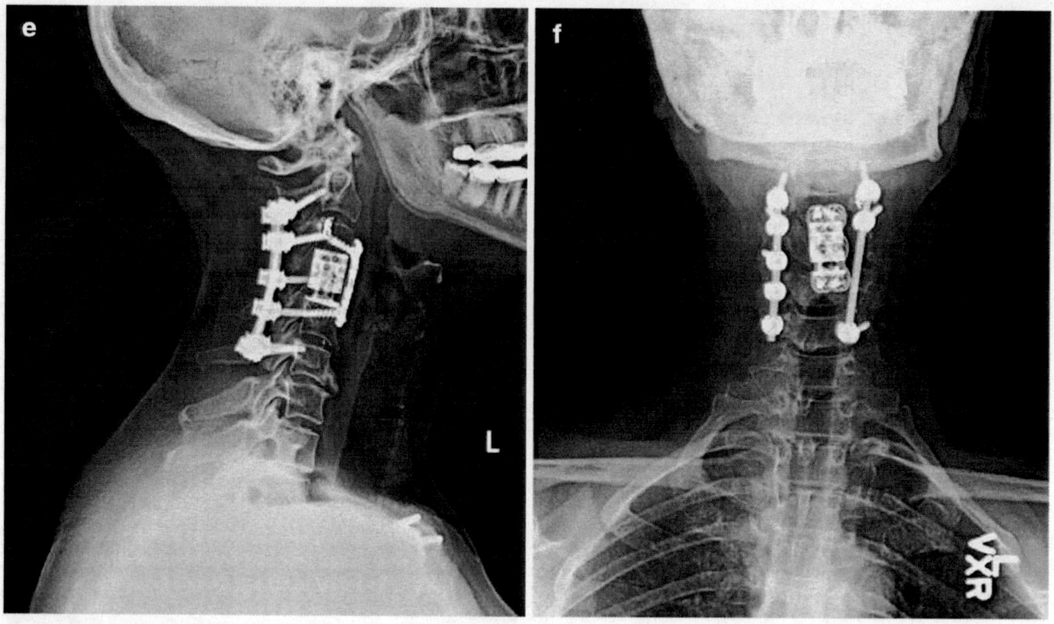

Fig. 22.1 (continued)

is higher concern for artery involvement, a CT or MR angiogram of the head and neck can be obtained. While catheter angiography is not completely without risk to the patient, it is critical in surgical planning in cases where the artery is clearly at risk or involved. Angiography also gives the opportunity for pre-operative tumor embolization or arterial sacrifice.

Schwannomas and neurofibromas, which account for the majority of paraspinal tumors, can be difficult to differentiate from each other based on imaging alone. Generally, both tumor types are hypo- or isointense on T1 and are avidly contrast enhancing [12]. They are often hyperintense and homogenous or displaying an area of central hypointensity. In most cases, paraspinal nerve sheath tumors are associated with the dorsal or sensory nerve rootlets [3, 10]. Depending on growth pattern, they can be intradural or intradural/extradural. Central location or diffuse involvement of the nerve is more suggestive of a neurofibroma, whereas eccentricity of the lesion to the nerve suggests schwannoma [13]. Radiographically, lesion size larger than 5 cm, ill-defined margins, invasion of fat planes, and peritumoral edema are concerning for MPNST [14].

Frank necrosis on MRI is concerning for a higher-grade neoplasm such as MPNST [15]. Sometimes neurogenic muscle denervation can be appreciated as T2 bright muscle edema, and diffusion MRI has recently been shown to be useful in the diagnosis of MPNST. CT scan can also be a useful adjunct in some cases. Paraspinal nerve sheath tumors, especially dumbbell tumors, can be associated with significant bony remodeling and erosion. Better appreciating the bony anatomy is also helpful for patients that will need instrumented fusion. Increased uptake in positron emission tomography (PET) can be helpful to diagnose MPNST, but benign PaNST can have significant uptake as well [16].

Electrodiagnostic testing can be a useful adjunct in the diagnosis and management of paraspinal nerve sheath tumors. In some sense electrodiagnostics are less helpful in managing these tumors than it is in the more common compressive neuropathies, in that MRI often clinches the diagnosis or dictates management because of the anatomic location of a tumor. We find them to be helpful in differentiating chronicity of tumors when there is limited imaging history. Specifically, chronic motor changes imply a slower-growing lesion, whereas fibrillations or other evidence of acute denervation is more concerning for an aggressive lesion such as MPNST [17]. As with all electrodiagnostic studies, testing is technical and is operator specific and should be both performed and interpreted by sophisticated practitioners. The tumors often involve the sensory nerve and can have disruption of sensory nerve action potentials on nerve conduction studies.

22.4 Surgical Indications

Like other aspects of nerve surgery, the decision when to intervene on a PaNST is often a matter of clinical judgment with no absolute right or wrong answer. The single most important factor favoring an operative intervention to us is development of a neurological deficit, but increasing size, worsening pain or numbness, and encroachment of other critical structures are also indications to operate. It is important to note that not all PaNST require surgical intervention. In cases where patients are not symptomatic, the mass is stable in size, and they have other surgical comorbidities. Surveillance imaging and clinical follow-up are reasonable. For small and asymptomatic tumors that are often detected incidentally, we will repeat MRI 3–6 months after the initial study to ensure short-term stability and then repeat annually to monitor for growth.

When the decision is made to move forward with treatment, it should be done in a thoughtful and multidisciplinary fashion. In some cases with NF1 and NF2, the peripheral nerve surgeon is the primary entry point for complex patients to the healthcare system, and thus we must make the initial decisions to get oncology, radiation oncology, or genetics involved. Important questions must be answered such as is tissue diagnosis needed, are there noninvasive treatment options, and is further screening warranted? It goes without saying that for some patients, this diagnosis will be the worst news of their lives so far and that they are right to be concerned about developing serious problems like neurological deficits in some cases. A knowledgeable and well-trained peripheral nerve surgeon can help these patients immensely by knowing when to operate, how to set expectations, and having good surgical outcomes from good training and adherence to common sense surgical principles.

22.5 Surgical Management

Treatment for benign PaNST is primarily surgical, with the goals of (1) providing tissue diagnosis, (2) maximal safe tumor resection, and (3) protection of key neurovascular structures and preservation of pre-operative neurological function. In general, symptomatic patients should undergo early surgery, and gross total resection of benign PaNST is often curative. There is no established role for chemotherapy. Radiation therapy, either fractionated or stereotactic, is used in select cases, usually inoperative, malignant, or recurrent tumors, although there is concern that patients with NF1/NF2 are at increased risk for radiation-induced malignancy [18, 19].

Goals of surgery should be discussed and understood by the patient, whether it is tissue diagnosis, debulking, or gross total resection. Next, consider approach, positioning, intraoperative needs, and neuromonitoring. For instance, when planning resection of a dumbbell tumor, the surgeon must consider whether the configuration represents inward extension of an epidural tumor through the neural foramen or extradural extension of an intradural tumor, because this informs whether intradural exploration will be needed.

We also think that it is a best practice to have a discussion with anesthesia colleagues about the plan for the case and any special considerations they might have. For instance, ventilation considerations if the patient needs a lung to be partially let down during an anterolateral thoracic spine approach or blood pressure management when working near the spine or the need for potentially serious transfusions if working near great vessels. It is important to keep in mind that when bony work is done, especially multilevel laminectomies or situations destabilizing the facet joints, caution must be taken to minimize the risk of the patient to develop progressive deformity. Osteoplastic laminotomies may be one way to avoid this. If the rostral or caudal facet joint is injured, instrumentation and fusion may be necessary.

22.6 Intraoperative Considerations

Usually PaNST grow concentrically around the spinal nerve root, usually the sensory root. Neurofibromas often necessitate sacrifice of the nerve root because it is an intrinsic tumor of the nerve root, whereas schwannomas can sometimes be resected without sacrificing the nerve root because they are located eccentrically concerning the involved root [20]. This sacrifice of the neurofibroma roots is often inconsequential in the sense that these nerves are usually nonfunctioning and involved with tumor already, and function has either been lost or compensated. Neurofibromas can range from well demarcated to diffuse and are associated with the epineurium. They can be more challenging to get gross total resection than with schwannomas, which rarely recur and are unlikely to undergo malignant transformation [21]. Intraoperative ultrasound can be a helpful adjuvant for tumor and abnormal tissue location, and we have used it with success as a relatively inexpensive and noninvasive diagnostic adjuvant [22].

Intraoperative neuromonitoring is an important adjunct for performing maximally safe surgery. It is our preference to use somatosensory evoked potentials (SSEP) and motor evoked potentials (MEP) in all cases with a paraspinal tumor that has intraforaminal components or is involving any CNS structures in the cervical or thoracic spine, as well as in the conus. We use electromyography (EMG) to aid in resection of tumor from functional nerve roots in the cervical, lumbar, and sacral spine. We also find that a handheld nerve stimulator can be helpful intraoperatively, especially to help delineate motor nerve roots when anatomy is challenging.

22.7 Surgical Considerations by Tumor Location

The approach for addressing paraspinal tumors should be highly tailored to the individual case. Before the critical decision of operative approach can be made, the exact size, anatomy, and imaging characteristics, along with patient-specific considerations, must all be thoroughly studied and appreciated. Pre-operative optimization is important, especially for NF1 and NF2 patients. All patients undergoing elective surgeries at our institution are evaluated by a specialized pre-operative anesthesia service, along with routine screening labs. In some cases, such as involving hand function, or myelopathy when there is significant intraforaminal extension, patients may benefit from a regimen of “pre-habilitation” or laying a foundation with physical or occupational therapists prior to undergoing surgical intervention.

22.8 Cervical Spine and Craniocervical Junction

Approaching paraspinal nerve sheath tumors in the cervical spine can be challenging, due to the presence of critical neurological and vascular structures, along with cranial nerves and territory important to the airway and feeding. Fortunately, the same workhorse techniques that spine surgeons are familiar with—the anterior paramedian “ACDF” and posterior midline approaches—are most commonly used. With a posterior approach, the bony exposure must allow complete visualization of the tumor, without having to manipulate the spinal cord or nerve roots aggressively.

Neuromonitoring can be a useful adjunct here as well as EMG. Sometimes it can be a difficult judgment whether to take an involved nerve root versus sparing it along with gross tumor. We prefer a technique of adequate but not overly aggressive soft tissue and bony exposure and then dissect the tumor as possible from normal neurological structures. A combination of instruments can be used for this, and we use Penfield and occasionally Rhoton dissectors, straight and curved micro-scissors, blunt and sharp nerve hooks, and bipolar cautery judiciously. The tumor should be debulked as necessary (with the aid of cavitron ultrasonic aspirator, if available), and overall a plane should be developed and should be peeled off of normal neurological structures as possible, working back and forth with a combination of blunt and sharp dissection and bipolar cautery. Sometimes spinal reconstruction is required postoperatively (Fig. 22.2).

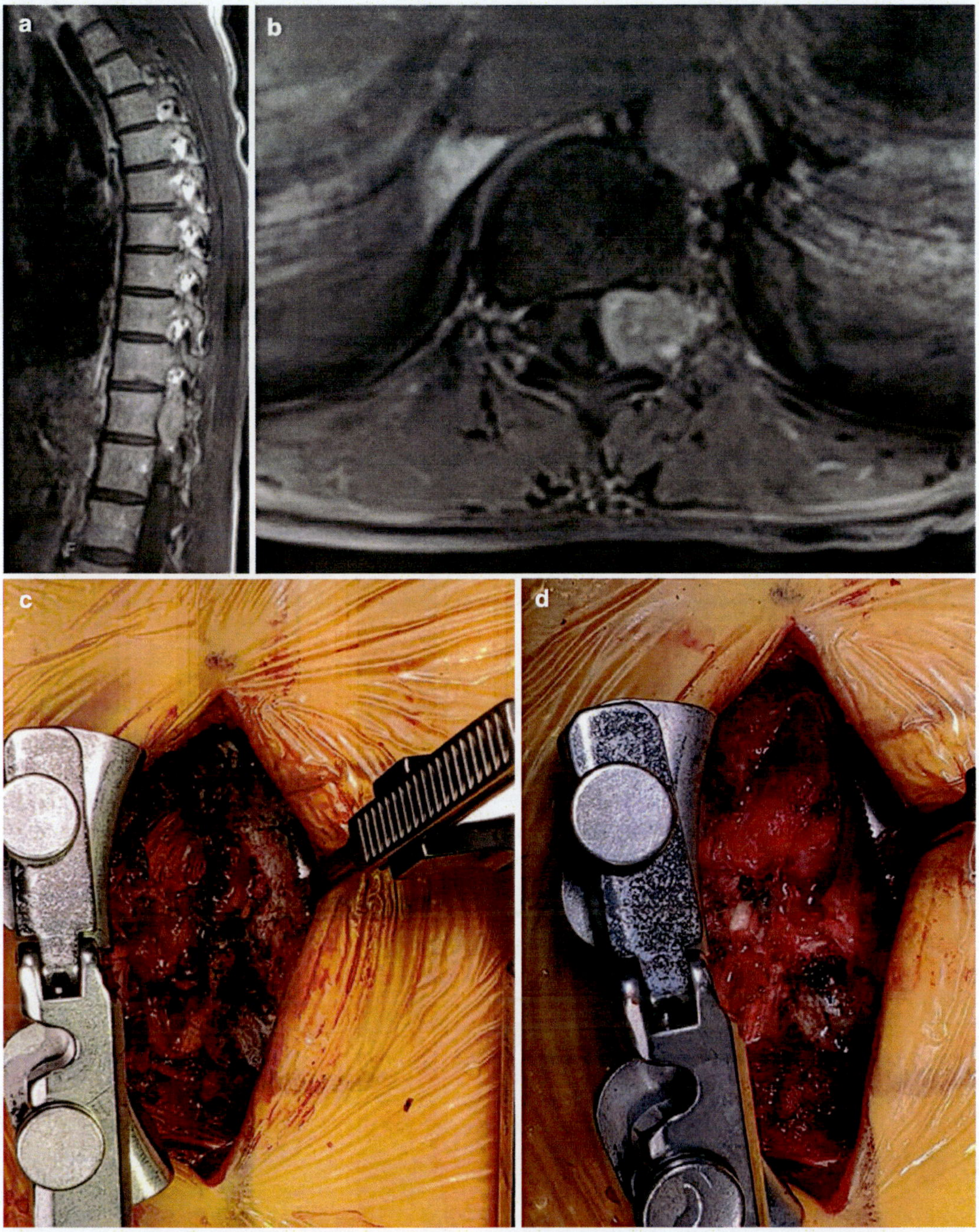

Fig. 22.2 This patient is a 50-year-old female who presented with caudal thoracic radicular pain and signs of early myelopathy. She underwent a T11–T12 laminectomy with resection of intradural extramedullary tumor, and pathology was consistent with Schwannoma. **(a)** Sagittal and then **(b)** axial pre-operative MRI demonstrates a contrast-enhancing lesion at the left T11 and T12 neural foramen, extending from within the central canal to the paraspinal space, causing spinal stenosis and mass effect on the thoracic cord. Note expansion of the neural foramen. **(c)** Intraoperative photograph demonstrating the initial bony exposure of the case, **(d)** The tumor is exposed, **(e)** Gross total resection has been achieved, with the involved nerve roots tied off with silk ties after ligation, **(f)** Closure: After thorough irrigation and immaculate hemostasis, application of a generous amount of fibrin glue, followed by layered closure and skin glue

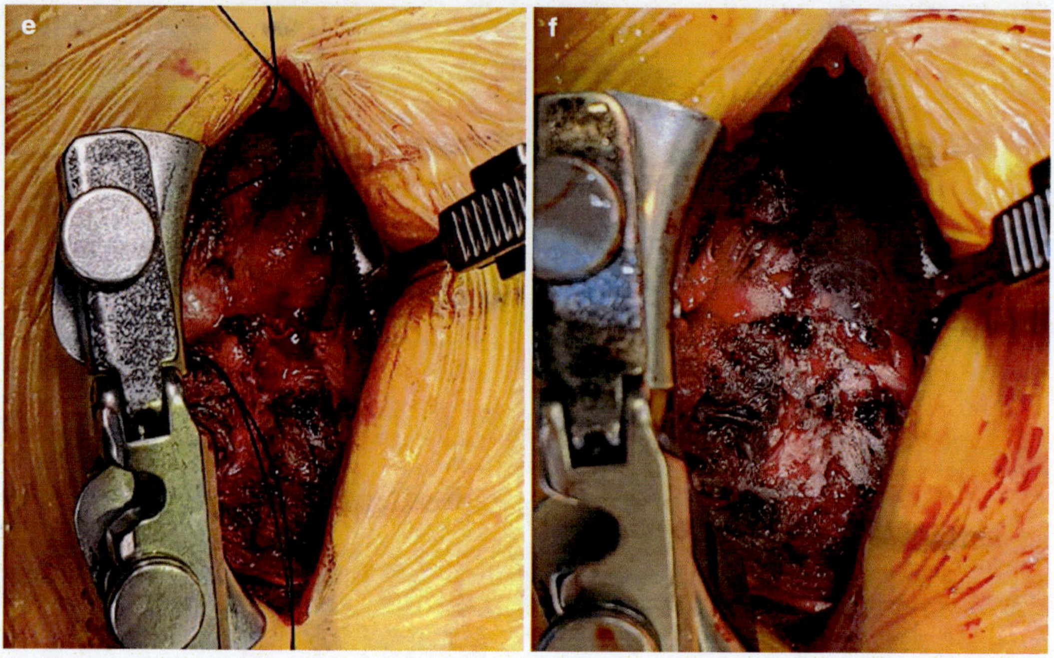

Fig. 22.2 (continued)

Any traction on the spinal cord or nerve roots should be avoided. When normal anatomy is distorted, trace from normal to pathology, use nerve stimulation, and use good surgical anatomic principles to identify midline markers and stay oriented. Maintaining midline at the craniocervical junction is critical in order to avoid injuring the vertebral arteries, as is a pre-operative appreciation of their course. Depending on the extent of the tumor and whether diagnosis is known beforehand, intraoperative pathology can be helpful in surgical decision-making. Careful hemostasis should be maintained with a combination of hemostatic agents and pressure, along with microirrigation.

Any planning of cervical approaches for tumors must take into account managing the carotid and vertebral arteries, especially around the craniocervical junction. If there is concern that the tumor is involving the artery, the anatomy and physiology of the vertebral arteries should be appreciated, and consultation may be warranted with endovascular colleagues for a potential catheter angiogram. In certain challenging cases, intentional pre-operative endovascular sacrifice of the artery may be warranted. The ability of the patient to tolerate this can be anticipated with a balloon occlusion test. Intraoperatively, the cephalad and caudal areas of the artery involved by the tumor must be exposed for control. The artery should be free by meticulous technique and protected. True vertebral artery injuries during PaNST resections are rare, and an injury should be handled in the usual fashion, which is hemostasis with hemostatic agents and pressure, followed by attempt at primary reconstruction, with or without consultation with a vascular colleague, then endovascular or surgical sacrifice. For high lesions, consultation with otorhinolaryngology specialists is recommended, especially for lesions involving the airway and/or esophagus.

22.9 Thoracic

Thoracic PaNST, which make up about 35% of cases, present their own set of challenges due to the anatomy of the ribs, lungs, and great vessels [23]. As the paraspinal portion of the tumor enlarges, it can involve the aorta, vena cava, and azygous veins. SSEP and MEP neuromonitoring is a useful adjuvant. Like the cervical spine, great care must be taken not to put traction on the spinal cord, and in fact the thoracic spinal canal is narrower than the cervical one. Unlike the subaxial cervical spine, there are no significant consequences for taking nerve roots other than dermatomal sensory loss over the ribs. Typically this is well tolerated by most patients, with the exception of the T1 nerve root, which warrants special consideration. If the paraspinal components of these tumors grow significantly, they can involve the subclavian artery. Furthermore, as a contributing root to the brachial plexus, T1 is a critical nerve for hand function [24]. If nerve roots are taken, they should be ligated with silk suture to prevent CSF leak. If destabilization occurs, such as disruption of the pars or facet complex, instrumented fusion must be considered.

The most common approaches to PaNST of the thoracic spine are the standard midline posterior, with or without paramedian exposure for costotransversectomy (Fig. 22.3). The costotransversectomy exposure is significant compared to the standard posterior one, with transverse process, medial portion of the rib and rib head, and resection of the entire costovertebral articulation. We position prone unless the tumor has significant lateral extension, in which case we will go to lateral. After sub-periosteal dissection and exposure, the proximal 3–6 cm of rib head is taken, freeing up the lateral margins of the approach corridor. A laminectomy, facetectomy, and then pediculectomy are then performed. At this point the lateral aspect of the spinal cord is exposed, and the involved nerve roots are ligated and retracted before resection of the tumor.

With the assistance of thoracic or vascular colleagues, larger, anterior, or more lateral tumors can be accessed by trans-sternal, open, mini, or endoscopic thoracotomy or a combination of these approaches. We attempt to avoid thoracotomies when possible due to the morbidity of the procedure and our familiarity with posterior and posterolateral approaches. For an excellent description of a thoracoscopic approach to a PaNST, please see Dr. Kline's 2007 article *Surgical approaches to paraspinal nerve sheath tumors* [2]. Briefly, proper endoscopic instruments are required, and the patient is positioned in lateral decubitus. Fluoroscopy is used to identify the level, and a lung is often purposefully deflated for access. Care must be taken to not injure pleura or segmental vessels. The intraforaminal portion of the tumor is resected once the tumor is debulked. Dumbbell tumors may require a combined anterior and posterior approach. If there is cord compression, however, the intraspinal component of the tumor ought to be resect first, as the priority is to decompress the spinal cord.

22.10 Lumbosacral

Lumbosacral PaNST can be challenging cases as they are more prone to grow to large sizes before being detected. Their location can also be complex in that it involves both the spinal canal and retroperitoneum. Large tumors may compress the iliopsoas and femoral nerve, iliac vessels, kidneys, ureters, and lumbosacral plexus and may require staged operations. Lumbosacral PaNST can be approached in a traditional posterior or paramedian approach or anterior retroperitoneal approaches with a paramedian or flank incision, both workhorse approaches for neurosurgeons.

For the retroperitoneal approach, we typically perform this with the help of a vascular access surgeon, in a manner similar to an anterior lumbar interbody fusion. The location of the abdominal aorta bifurcation must be appreciated, as with the inferior vena cava confluence. We have the best success with anterior access at L4-S1, but in certain cases, the anatomy will allow for access up to even L2. Great care must be taken to avoid injuring the ureter, as well as to not place too much retraction on the psoas muscle so as to avoid injuring the femoral nerve.

22.11 Minimally Invasive Surgery

Minimally invasive spine (MIS) surgery options for thoracic and lumbar PaNST management are increasingly becoming an option. Multiple case

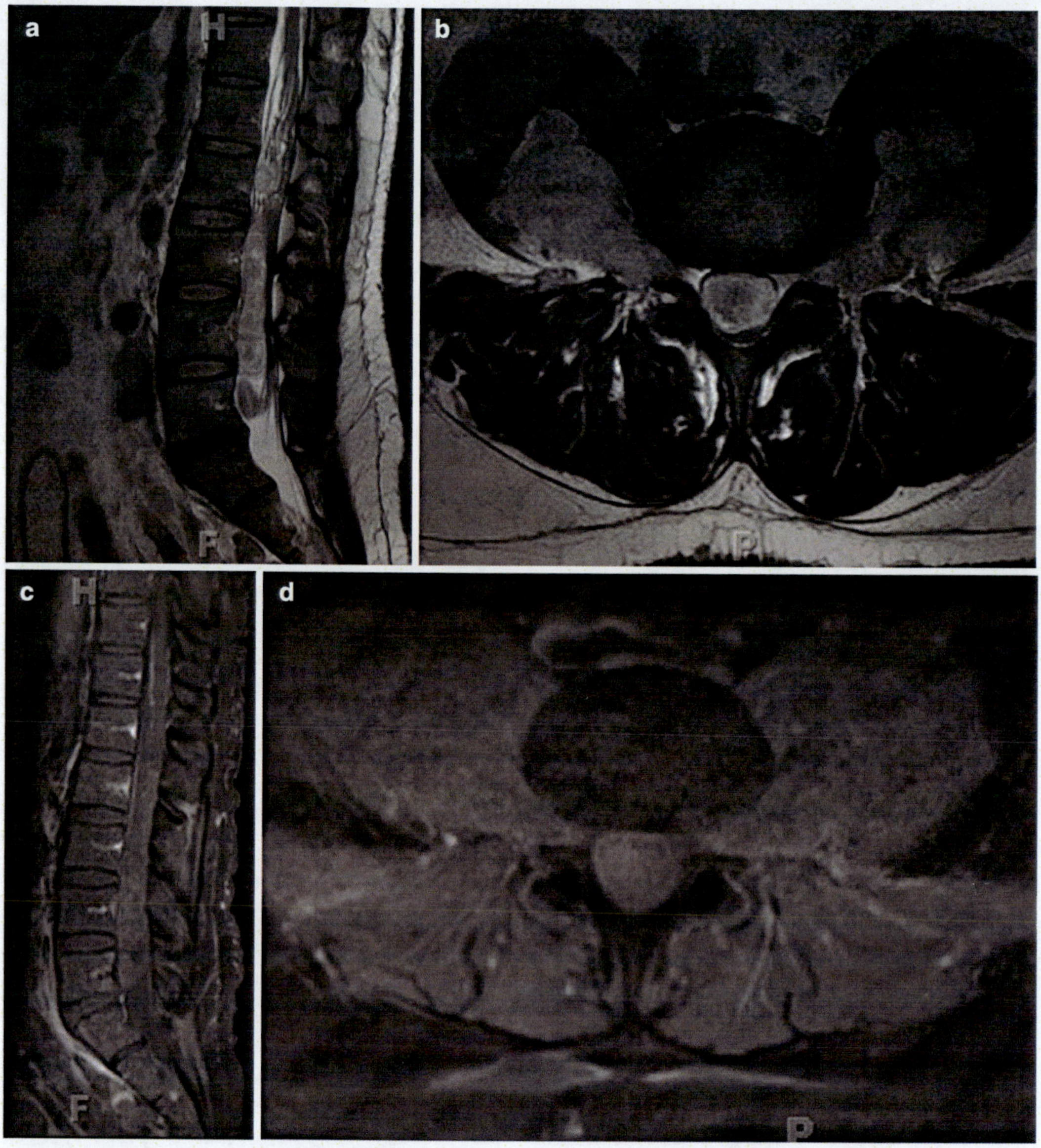

Fig. 22.3 Extensive bilateral plexiform neurofibromas in a 50-year-old male patient with NF1. He presented with radicular leg symptoms. These lesions were ultimately observed, and he remained neurologically stable. (**a**) and (**b**) show T2 non contrast sagittal and axial cuts, respectively, and (**c**) and (**d**) show contrast enhanced T1 sequences

series and literature reviews have been published recently and report successful outcomes with bony work and dumbbell tumor resection [25, 26]. The authors in these studies prefer a tubular retractor approach (either serial dilation or expandable). As long as the goals of surgery can be met with MIS surgery, in our opinion it is a reasonable option given the potential added benefits: shorter hospital stay, lower blood loss, less postoperative pain, and quicker return to function, at least as shown in spine and other areas [27]. MIS surgery is more challenging for larger tumors. This remains a developing area of neurosurgery, and as MIS surgery and navigation/robotics continue to advance, there likely may be exciting new advances for patients and surgeons.

22.12 Special Considerations for MPNST Management

MPNST is an unfortunate diagnosis as they are highly aggressive sarcomas with metastatic and local seeding potential. MPNST can arise de novo or by malignant degeneration of a benign nerve sheath tumor. They are associated with NF1, and 5% of patients with this diagnosis will go on to develop an MPNST [2, 28]. Malignant degeneration is often characterized by intense neuropathic pain and increasing growth rate and size. Pain at rest and that is only partly relieved by pharmacologic therapy are also more concerning for MPNST. It is important to have a discussion with the patient about surgical goals, because there is an argument to pursue an aggressive en bloc resection with MPNST that may leave the patient with serious postoperative morbidity. Even with maximal resection and adjuvant therapy, a 5-year survival is less than 50% [29, 30]. Some authors state that biopsy is indicated if a lesion presents clinical and imaging features that denote malignancy.

22.13 Acute Postoperative Considerations

Aftercare depends on the patient and outcome of the procedure. As with any procedure around vascular and neurological structures, a high suspicion must be maintained for reversible causes of neurological deficits, such as postoperative hematomas or hypotension. If there is a concern for hematoma, either return to the OR and immediate exploration or imaging, plus or minus vascular imaging, depends on the level of concern. Complications from resections of cervicothoracic sympathetic chain tumors include Horner's syndrome and so-called first bite syndrome, where there is pain with chewing that is worst with the first bite, related to hypersensitivity from sympathetic denervation [31]. Thoracic PaNST patients who underwent anterior or lateral approach should be watched for signs of pneumothorax or respiratory difficulty. When we do significant intradural work or have cervical durotomies, we keep patients with the head of the bed around 45° for the first 24 postoperative hours.

Drains must be watched closely, and patients should be mobilized as soon as possible. We do not routinely prescribe braces or slings unless there is serious concern for destabilization or if it is for comfort. Postoperatively, our practice is to give 24 h of antibiotic prophylaxis and start prophylactic doses of heparin or Lovenox on hospital day 1. Both postoperative and neuropathic pain can be severe, and an aggressive pain management regimen should be planned out preoperatively. In some cases, IV narcotics are helpful for acute pain. If the pain is refractory or complex, we do not hesitate to consult our pain management anesthesia colleagues for additional pharmacological strategies. While ICU care is usually not necessary, rigorous neurological checks are critical postoperatively when there is any concern and so we have a low threshold for putting a patient in a higher level of care. Some authors state that for any intradural work, the patient should be routinely monitored in the ICU overnight. Similarly, if there is a question of spinal cord injury or compression, it is important to maintain blood pressure in the postoperative period to at least 110% of normal. In these cases we will monitor patients in the ICU or stepdown unit with an arterial line and frequent neurological checks.

22.14 Adjuvant Therapy

Postoperative and non-operative treatment is dependent on pathology and extent of resection. PaNST is a surgical disease in that if a gross total resection is performed, except with MPNST, the need to adjuvant therapy is low. For MPNST and variants, chemotherapy and/or radiation may be recommended, in collaboration with oncology and radiation oncology [32, 33]. However, it is important to understand that the molecular mechanisms of MPNST (and nerve sheath tumors in general) are still being uncovered, and there is some controversy as to whether adjuvant therapies have an effect on recurrence or survival [34]. Further studies on chemo- and bio-therapeutics are ongoing. Selumetinib has indeed been shown, in a phase 2 trial, to reduce the size of inoperable plexiform neurofibromas.

22.15 Radiosurgery

The role of radiosurgery in managing PaNST is evolving and is currently without high-level evidence. Lessons learned from radiosurgical treatment of benign intradural, extramedullary nerve sheath tumors show that good local control can be achieved and patients can experience pain relief, but it is typically not associated with improved neurological symptoms like surgical decompression. Radiation-induced myelopathy is the most severe complication, ranging from 1 to 4% [35–37]. Radiation therapies continue to improve and will likely continue to be an important second-line treatment.

22.16 Outcomes and Prognosis

Prognosis is dependent on histopathology. Sporadic, solitary schwannomas overall do very well and do not have impairment of life expectancy [38]. Recurrence rate is about 5% after what was thought to be complete resection [39]. Patients with solitary neurofibromas also do well. Patients with syndromic tumors often have morbidity and mortality from the other consequences of their diseases and also can be at risk for malignant degeneration to MPNST. They are also at higher risk for recurrence. It is also important for these patients to understand that there is some evidence that they will not make as good neurological recovery after surgery [40]. With regard to myelopathy and radiculopathy, like the rest of nerve surgery, neurological outcomes are a function of length of the extent and duration of compression. Patients who have severe deficits pre-operatively are less likely to experience improvement. Most myelopathic patients experience improvement, but the vast majority do experience pain and paresthesia as well [2].

22.17 Summary and Key Points

PaNST are challenging for the peripheral nerve surgeon due to their anatomical relationship to the spinal cord, nerve roots, and major vasculature, as well as their heterogeneous presentations and ability to occur throughout the neuroaxis. The surgical approach depends on lesion relationship with spinal and paraspinal anatomy. Surgery is generally indicated for weakness, myelopathy, or intractable pain and paresthesias. It is also indicated whenever a lesion is suspected to be a MPNST. Management should take into account maximal sparing of neurological function and not creating iatrogenic spinal instability. Patients with NF1 and NF2 require complex multidisciplinary management and may benefit from adjuvant therapy. MPNST is an aggressive tumor with poor prognosis. Keys to success involve multidisciplinary workup and treatment, realistic patient expectations, and excellent surgical planning and technique. With skill and some luck, the peripheral nerve surgeon will be able to significantly improve lifespan and lifestyle for their patients with paraspinal nerve sheath tumors.

References

1. Dorsi MJ, Belzberg AJ. Paraspinal nerve sheath tumors. Neurosurg Clin N Am. 2004;15(2):217–22, vii
2. Cherqui A, et al. Surgical approaches to paraspinal nerve sheath tumors. Neurosurg Focus. 2007;22(6):E9.
3. Kim J, et al. Synovial sarcoma of the spine: a case involving paraspinal muscle with extensive calcification and the surgical consideration in treatment. Eur Spine J. 2014;23(1):27–31.
4. Ostrom QT, et al. Epidemiology of gliomas. Cancer Treat Res. 2015;163:1–14.
5. Gittleman HR, et al. Trends in central nervous system tumor incidence relative to other common cancers in adults, adolescents, and children in the United States, 2000 to 2010. Cancer. 2015;121(1):102–12.
6. el-Mahdy W, et al. Spinal intradural tumours: part I—extramedullary. Br J Neurosurg. 1999;13(6):550–7.
7. Klekamp J, Samii M. Surgery of spinal nerve sheath tumors with special reference to neurofibromatosis. Neurosurgery. 1998;42(2):279–89; discussion 289–90
8. Seppala MT, et al. Multiple schwannomas: schwannomatosis or neurofibromatosis type 2? J Neurosurg. 1998;89(1):36–41.

9. Gonzalvo A, et al. Schwannomatosis, sporadic schwannomatosis, and familial schwannomatosis: a surgical series with long-term follow-up. Clinical article. J Neurosurg. 2011;114(3):756–62.
10. Rodriguez FJ, et al. Pathology of peripheral nerve sheath tumors: diagnostic overview and update on selected diagnostic problems. Acta Neuropathol. 2012;123(3):295–319.
11. Rosner M, Fisher W, Mulligan L. Cervical sympathetic schwannoma: case report. Neurosurgery. 2001;49(6):1452–4.
12. Wasa J, et al. MRI features in the differentiation of malignant peripheral nerve sheath tumors and neurofibromas. AJR Am J Roentgenol. 2010;194(6):1568–74.
13. Beaman FD, Kransdorf MJ, Menke DM. Schwannoma: radiologic-pathologic correlation. Radiographics. 2004;24(5):1477–81.
14. Pilavaki M, et al. Imaging of peripheral nerve sheath tumors with pathologic correlation: pictorial review. Eur J Radiol. 2004;52(3):229–39.
15. Yu YH, et al. Radiological findings of malignant peripheral nerve sheath tumor: reports of six cases and review of literature. World J Surg Oncol. 2016;14:142.
16. Tovmassian D, Abdul Razak M, London K. The role of [(18)F]FDG-PET/CT in predicting malignant transformation of plexiform neurofibromas in neurofibromatosis-1. Int J Surg Oncol. 2016;2016:6162182.
17. Schwabe M, et al. How effective are noninvasive tests for diagnosing malignant peripheral nerve sheath tumors in patients with neurofibromatosis type 1? Diagnosing MPNST in NF1 patients. Sarcoma. 2019;2019:4627521.
18. Falavigna A, da Silva PG, Teixeira W. Radiotherapy-induced tumors of the spine, peripheral nerve, and spinal cord: case report and literature review. Surg Neurol Int. 2016;7(Suppl 4):S108–15.
19. Kahn J, et al. Radiation therapy in management of sporadic and neurofibromatosis type 1-associated malignant peripheral nerve sheath tumors. Front Oncol. 2014;4:324.
20. Celli P. Treatment of relevant nerve roots involved in nerve sheath tumors: removal or preservation? Neurosurgery. 2002;51(3):684–92; discussion 692
21. Woodruff JM, et al. Congenital and childhood plexiform (multinodular) cellular schwannoma: a troublesome mimic of malignant peripheral nerve sheath tumor. Am J Surg Pathol. 2003;27(10):1321–9.
22. Vasudeva VS, et al. Use of intraoperative ultrasound during spinal surgery. Global Spine J. 2017;7(7):648–56.
23. Rong HT, et al. Management of dumbbell and paraspinal tumors of the thoracic spine using a single-stage posterolateral approach: case series. Orthop Surg. 2018;10(4):343–9.
24. Ohya J, et al. Combined video-assisted thoracic surgery and posterior spinal surgery for the treatment of dumbbell tumor of the first thoracic nerve root. Asian Spine J. 2015;9(4):595–9.
25. Paullus P, et al. Minimally invasive approach to resection of paraspinal schwannoma. Neurosurg Focus. 2018;44(Video Suppl 1):V5.
26. Zairi F, et al. Minimally invasive resection of large dumbbell tumors of the lumbar spine: advantages and pitfalls. Clin Neurol Neurosurg. 2018;168:91–6.
27. Nzokou A, Weil AG, Shedid D. Minimally invasive removal of thoracic and lumbar spinal tumors using a nonexpandable tubular retractor. J Neurosurg Spine. 2013;19(6):708–15.
28. Gilder HE, et al. The implications of intradural extension in paraspinal malignant peripheral nerve sheath tumors: effects on central nervous system metastases and overall survival. J Neurosurg Spine. 2018;29(6):725–8.
29. Kolberg M, et al. Survival meta-analyses for >1800 malignant peripheral nerve sheath tumor patients with and without neurofibromatosis type 1. Neuro Oncol. 2013;15(2):135–47.
30. Wang T, et al. Malignant peripheral nerve sheath tumor (MPNST) in the spine: a retrospective analysis of clinical and molecular prognostic factors. J Neurooncol. 2015;122(2):349–55.
31. Wax MK, et al. Cervical sympathetic chain schwannoma. Laryngoscope. 2004;114(12):2210–3.
32. Grobmyer SR, et al. Malignant peripheral nerve sheath tumor: molecular pathogenesis and current management considerations. J Surg Oncol. 2008;97(4):340–9.
33. McLaughlin EJ, et al. Treatment of a malignant peripheral nerve sheath tumor and its complications through a multidisciplinary approach. J Neurosurg Pediatr. 2011;7(5):543–8.
34. Chou D, et al. Malignant peripheral nerve sheath tumors of the spine: results of surgical management from a multicenter study. J Neurosurg Spine. 2017;26(3):291–8.
35. Dodd RL, et al. CyberKnife radiosurgery for benign intradural extramedullary spinal tumors. Neurosurgery. 2006;58(4):674–85; discussion 674–85
36. Sachdev S, et al. Stereotactic radiosurgery yields long-term control for benign intradural, extramedullary spinal tumors. Neurosurgery. 2011;69(3):533–9; discussion 539
37. Gerszten PC, et al. Radiosurgery for benign intradural spinal tumors. Neurosurgery. 2008;62(4):887–95; discussion 895–6
38. Seppala MT, et al. Long-term outcome after removal of spinal schwannoma: a clinicopathological study of 187 cases. J Neurosurg. 1995;83(4):621–6.
39. Fehlings MG, et al. Risk factors for recurrence of surgically treated conventional spinal schwannomas: analysis of 169 patients from a multicenter international database. Spine (Phila Pa 1976). 2016;41(5):390–8.
40. Lenzi J, et al. Spinal nerves schwannomas: experience on 367 cases-historic overview on how clinical, radiological, and surgical practices have changed over a course of 60 years. Neurol Res Int. 2017;2017:3568359.

23 Nerve Tumors of Childhood and Infancy

Svetlana Kvint, Zarina S. Ali, Line G. Jacques, Gregory Heuer, and Eric L. Zager

23.1 Introduction

Peripheral nerves are vulnerable to a wide array of inflammatory, infiltrative, hyperplastic, degenerative, and neoplastic processes, the treatment of which depends on accurate clinical and histopathologic assessment. As they are rarely encountered in the pediatric population, peripheral nerve tumors (PNTs) often prove a diagnostic challenge in this cohort. Although many of the tumors seen in the adult population can also present in childhood, their relative contribution to morbidity is divergent between the two cohorts. In fact, lesions that dominate in adults are supplanted by lesser known but highly aggressive pathologies in children. Familiarity with the clinical presentation, diagnostic adjuncts, and therapeutic indications of pediatric PNTs is a requirement for achieving clinical success. It is the goal of this review to summarize the key features of the most commonly encountered pediatric PNTs, highlighting the key considerations in their management and recommended surgical techniques. Lesions will be presented in the context of three broad categories: benign, malignant, and reactive or hyperplastic lesions.

23.2 Epidemiology

Although they encompass a diverse pathology, PNTs are infrequently encountered in the pediatric population. When found, they are most commonly associated with genetic syndromes (Table 23.1). As a consequence of their rarity, the true incidence of pediatric peripheral nerve tumors is unknown. The available estimates of incidences are inferred from published case series reports and local and national tumor registries which are limited by grouping within the soft tissue sarcoma category. In the context of these limitations, it is estimated that soft tissue tumors account for 6–8% of all childhood neoplasia [1]. Of these, 14% are believed to arise from the peripheral nervous system [2].

Although the breadth of pathology is shared by the adult and pediatric populations, there are key differences in the relative incidences found in each population. For instance, while schwannomas and neurofibromas account for roughly 90% of all PNTs in adults, they account for less than 50% of pediatric peripheral nerve neoplasms.

S. Kvint · Z. S. Ali · E. L. Zager (✉)
Department of Neurosurgery, Perelman School of Medicine, University of Pennsylvania, Philadelphia, PA, USA
e-mail: Eric.Zager@uphs.upenn.edu

L. G. Jacques
Department of Neurosurgery, University of California at San Francisco, San Francisco, CA, USA

G. Heuer
Division of Neurosurgery, Children's Hospital of Philadelphia, Perelman School of Medicine, University of Pennsylvania, Philadelphia, PA, USA

F. Guedes et al. (eds.), *Diagnostic Assessment and Treatment of Peripheral Nerve Tumors*,
https://doi.org/10.1007/978-3-030-77633-6_23

Table 23.1 Genetic syndromes associated with peripheral nerve tumors

Syndrome	Incidence	Genetic anomaly	Associated tumors affecting peripheral nerves	Other tumors
Neurofibromatosis 1	1:4000	17q12	Neurofibromas	Gliomas
		Neurofibromin	MPNSTs	Neuroendocrine tumors
Neurofibromatosis 2	1:40,000	22q12	Schwannomas	Meningiomas
Li-Fraumeni	Rare	17p13	Neuroblastoma	Breast, lung, colon
		TP53	Rhabdomyosarcoma	Soft tissue sarcoma
Gorlin	1:57,000	9q22	Rhabdomyosarcoma	Medulloblastoma
Cowden	Rare	10q23	Soft tissue hamartomas	Cerebellar gangliocytoma
		PTEN/MMAC	Adjacent to peripheral nerves	GI polyposis
Carney's	Rare	Protein kinase A subunit a1	Melanotic schwannomas	Spotty skin pigmentation Cardiac myxoma Endocrine tumors

Additionally, as a consequence of their embryonal nature, neuroblastomas represent a large portion of childhood PNTs, with 99.5% of all peripheral neuroblastic tumors occurring in the first two decades of life and accounting for one-third of pediatric PNTs [3]. In fact, among infants, children, preteens, and young adults, the three most common tumors involving the peripheral nerves are benign neurofibromas, malignant neuroblastomas, and rhabdomyosarcomas (RMS). Taken together, these three tumors comprise almost 90% of all pediatric PNTs. Interestingly, there are distinct age-related peaks in incidence among these tumors, with neuroblastomas most common in children <2 years, rhabdomyosarcomas occurring at 2–6 years of age, and neurofibromas at 10–19 years of age with a second peak in adults at 30 years of age [4, 5].

23.3 Tumor Categories

23.3.1 Benign

23.3.1.1 Neurofibroma

In a large series, Coffin et al. showed that neurofibromas accounted for 43% of peripheral neurogenic tumors and 90% of all benign pediatric peripheral nerve sheath tumors [2]. Although a sizable portion of pediatric neurofibromas occur sporadically, 30% are associated with neurofibromatosis type 1 (NF-1) [6]. Histologically, neurofibromas are composed of Schwann cells, perineurial cells, and fibroblasts interspersed with nerve fibers, strands of collagen, and a myxoid matrix. It is the presence of intra-tumoral nerve fibers that both distinguish neurofibromas from schwannomas and accounts for the poor surgical planes within involved fascicles.

As with adult lesions, pediatric neurofibromas can be grouped into two morphological categories: fusiform and plexiform. Fusiform neurofibromas result from an isolated proliferation of neoplastic cells within the sheath of an affected nerve; resultantly, they present as a nodular swelling on gross examination (Fig. 23.1). Dermal fusiform neurofibromas are characteristic of NF-1. These lesions are rarely painful, associated with a motor deficit, or prone to malignant degeneration; however, as they usually occur in large numbers, dermal fusiform neurofibromas can be disfiguring. In contrast, comprising 90% of neurofibromas, intraneural fusiform neurofibromas—either local or diffuse—involve major peripheral nerves or a plexus. When solitary, these lesions are most commonly sporadic. However, as only 20% of syndromic lesions exhibit normal preoperative function, sensorimotor dysfunction and multiplicity of lesions are associated with a diagnosis of NF-1 [6].

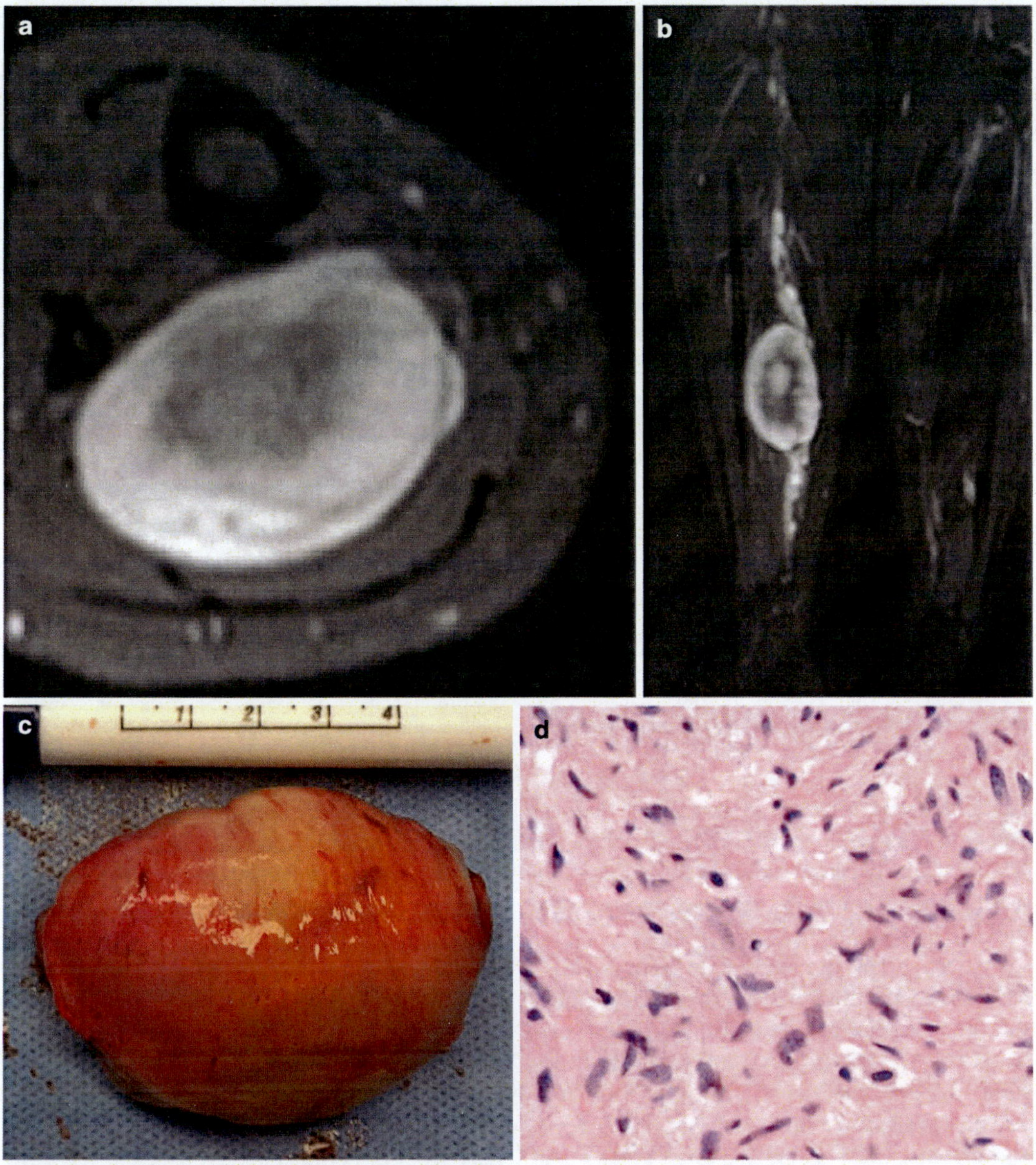

Fig. 23.1 Neurofibroma of tibial nerve in 16-year-old girl with history of NF-1, presenting with a painful, right calf mass. (**a**, **b**) Axial PD FS and coronal STIR MRI demonstrating well circumscribed mass in posterior calf. (**c**) Gross specimen. (**d**) Neoplastic Schwann cells with wavy pointed nuclei in a background of collagenous stroma

Plexiform neurofibromas, constituting the second morphologic category, are characterized by a network-like growth pattern, arising from multiple adjacent nerve fascicles and involving multiple branches of a large nerve or plexus (Fig. 23.2). "Superficial" plexiform neurofibromas present as large soft subcutaneous swellings; skin is commonly hyperpigmented and hypertrophied. Although "deeper" lesions are occult to visual inspection, their detection is facilitated by

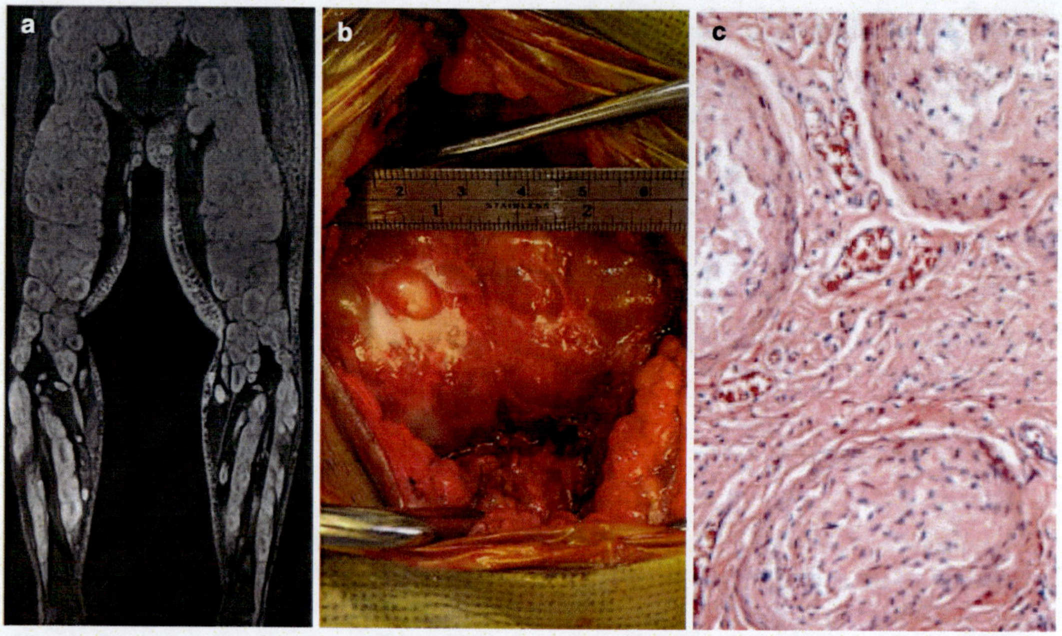

Fig. 23.2 Plexiform neurofibroma in 16-year-old male, with history of NF-1, presenting with painful and enlarging subcutaneous tumors in the proximal left thigh. (**a**) Coronal STIR MRI demonstrating extensive and innumerable plexiform neurofibroma in the pelvis and bilateral lower extremities. (**b**) Intra-operative view. (**c**) Plexiform nodules in background of neurofibromatous proliferation

the motor and sensory abnormalities that are commonly seen along the affected nerve [7]. Unlike their fusiform counterparts, plexiform neurofibromas are almost exclusively associated with NF-1 [8].

It is important to note that nondermal NF-1-associated neurofibromas—particularly those that are plexiform in morphology—are at an elevated risk for sarcomatous degeneration. It has been suggested that the relative risk of an NF-1 patient developing a malignant peripheral nerve sheath tumor (MPNST) is 133 times greater than that of the general population. The reported lifetime risk ranges from 2 to 10%; notably, for internal plexiform lesions, lifetime risk increases to 10–15% [9, 10]. Resultantly, pediatric patients with NF-1 warrant careful, long-term follow-up and aggressive intervention when malignant features arise.

23.3.1.2 Schwannoma

While schwannomas are the most common PNTs in adults, they are relatively uncommon in the pediatric population, accounting for only 5% of pediatric neurogenic tumors [2]. In fact, as a consequence of their relative rarity, pediatric patients with one or more confirmed schwannomas should be evaluated for an NF2 mutation, schwannomatosis, Carney complex, or a dominant syndrome associated with multiple schwannomas, multiple nevi, and multiple vaginal leiomyomas [11, 12]. For well-circumscribed, encapsulated masses of benign neoplastic Schwann cells, these tumors arise from a single nerve root or peripheral nerve fascicle and grow in an eccentric fashion, progressively displacing uninvolved fascicles [13]. Classically, the histology of schwannomas is biphasic; compact areas called Antoni A alternate with less compact areas called Antoni B. Cellular palisades called Verocay bodies can be seen within the Antoni A regions (Fig. 23.3). Other pathologic variants of schwannoma include plexiform, melanotic, and cellular types. As can be inferred, the melanotic subtype is characterized by an accumulation of melanin in the neoplastic cell and is associated with

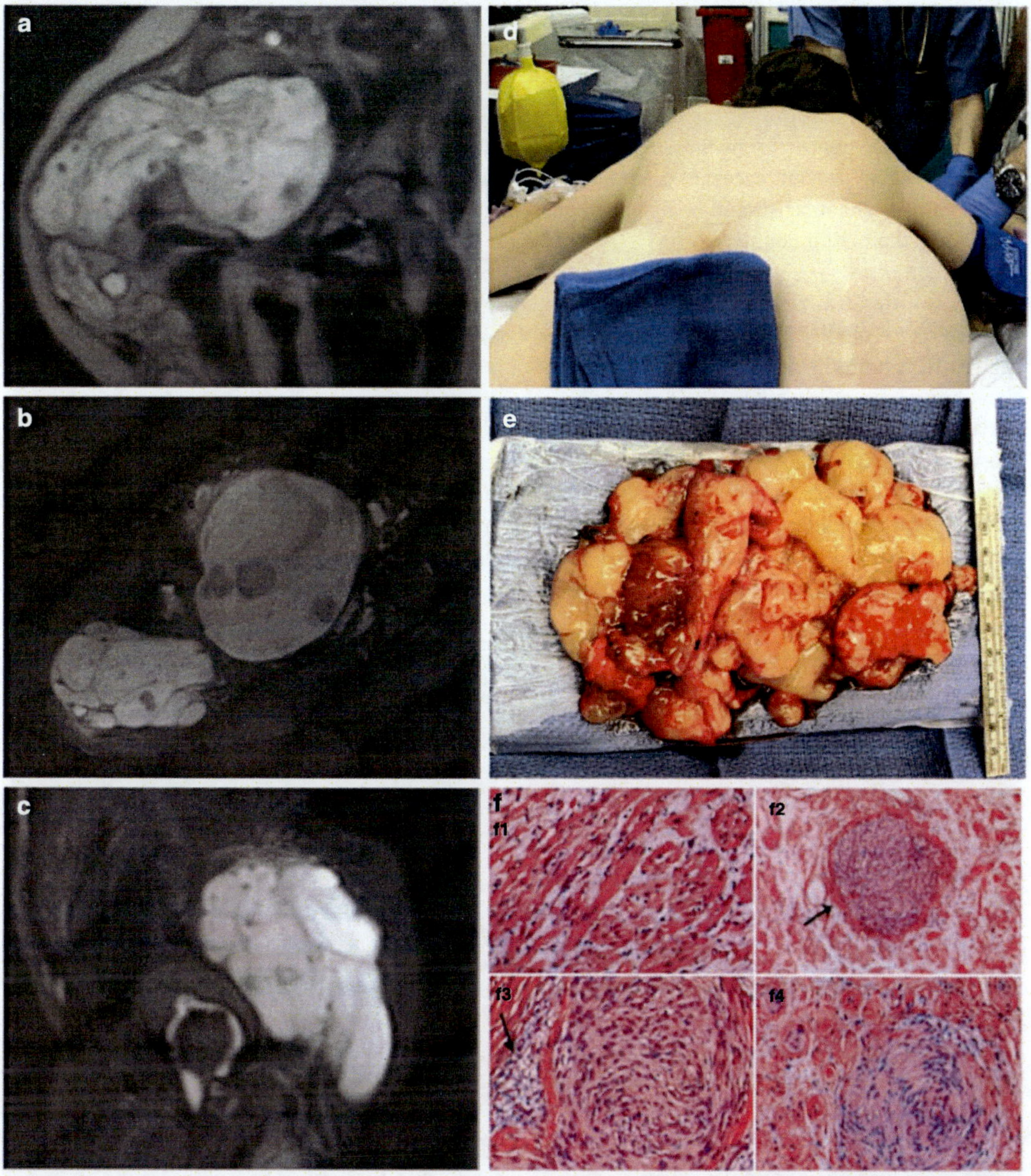

Fig. 23.3 Hybrid nerve sheath tumor—combined neurofibroma and schwannoma features—in 16-year-old girl with history of NF-1 and progressive discomfort due to mass effect. (**a–c**) Coronal, Axial and Sagittal T2-WI demonstrating a large, multi-lobular mass extending from the pelvis through the right sciatic foramen, and into the posterior aspect of the right lower extremity. (**d**) Intraoperative positioning. (**e**) Gross specimen, 8 × 12 cm. (**f**) Pathology—(1) Tumor cells with dense, eosinophilic collagen bundles resembling shredded carrots. (2) Distinct schwannoma tumorlet (arrow), surrounded by neurofibromatous elements. (3) Schwannoma tumorlets with classic compact Antoni A morphology comprising densely packed, concentric layers of Schwann cells and adjacent Antoni B areas (arrow). (4) Low-power image depicting close association of onion bulb structures with the schwannoma tumorlets

melanophages. It is distinct among the schwannoma subtypes as a consequence of its malignant potential and clear association with Carney complex [11]. Given that the biological and clinical behavior of pediatric schwannomas appears largely identical to adult cases, as a general rule, pediatric schwannomas should be managed analogously to their adult counterparts.

23.3.1.3 Perineurioma

Perineuriomas are benign tumors that are exceedingly rare in both the pediatric and adult populations, representing less than 1% of all peripheral nerve neoplasms. Although perineuriomas are most often diagnosed in the second and third decades of life, in about 50% of patients, symptoms present in childhood and adolescence [14]. The diagnostic delay is most likely due to the slowly progressive, painless loss of motor and sensory function that characterizes perineurioma (Fig. 23.4). In fact, because progressive muscle weakness is a far more common symptom than pain or sensory disturbances, the differential diagnosis of a perineurioma should be considered in any child with a motor deficit involving a single major nerve or plexus as the only meaningful symptom [15]. Composed of differentiated perineurial cells, these tumors can be classified into two main types: intraneural and extraneural soft tissue perineuriomas. Although far less common, intraneural perineuriomas are more clinically relevant as a consequence of the fact that they are far more likely to be symptomatic. Histologic examination of a cross section of an affected nerve typically shows irregularly enlarged, hypercellular nerve fascicles containing spindled perineurial cells arranged in "pseudo-onion bulb-like whorls" around one or more centrally situ-

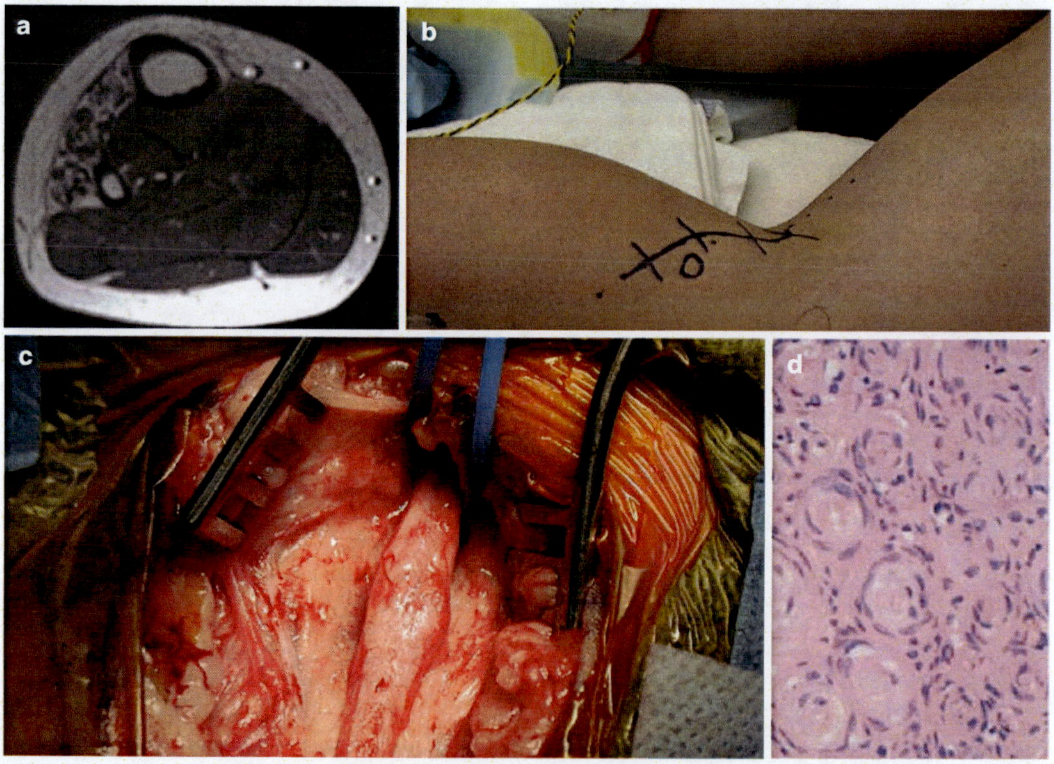

Fig. 23.4 Common peroneal nerve perineurioma in a 12-year-old male presenting with progressive, painless footdrop. (**a**) Axial T1-WI showing atrophy of anterolateral muscles of the R leg. (**b**) Intraoperative positioning and planned incision. (**c**) Intraoperative view of perineurioma involving CPN. (**d**) Section demonstrating tightly whorled cells around each individual nerve fiber, pseudo-onion bulb formation

ated Schwann cell and axons in varying stages of degeneration [16]. The clinical management of perineuriomas remains controversial on both the diagnostic and therapeutic front. Although most authors advocate a diagnostic biopsy prior to surgical intervention, a recent report by Wilson et al. largely obviated the need for tissue diagnosis by identifying a set of clinical and radiological features – Perineurioma Diagnostic Criteria – that achieved a specificity and positive predictive value of 100% for the diagnosis of perineuriomas [17]. Regardless of methodology, once a diagnosis is achieved, most authors advocate decompression and external neurolysis alone in an effort to preserve nerve function. Others prefer resection with neural grafting or end-to-end nerve repair referencing two motivators: (1) an intraneural perineurioma is a progressive condition that evolves inexorably to a total loss of nerve function, and (2) the recently recognized potential for malignant degeneration [18, 19].

23.3.1.4 Ganglioneuroma

Believed to arise from the neural crest, ganglioneuromas (GNs) represent the mature end of the range of neuroblastic tumors. They are encapsulated, slow-growing tumors that histologically consist of mature ganglion cells, satellite cells, Schwann cells, and fibrous stroma. Distinguished by the absence of immature elements, GNs are considered to be the benign counterparts of the immature neuroblastomas and undifferentiated and/or partially differentiated ganglioneuroblastomas [20]. Median age at diagnosis correlates well with the grade of differentiation among neuroblastic tumors—10 years of age for GNs. Occurring anywhere along the sympathetic nerve chain, GNs are usually asymptomatic until local mass effect is achieved. In a series of 162 patients, the most frequent symptoms leading to diagnosis were pain (34.2%), palpable tumor mass (9.3%), and reduced general condition (6.2%). Surgery alone—with an aim to relieve symptoms related to mass effect and decrease the risk of malignant transformation—is sufficient for treatment, achieves an excellent prognosis, and does not need to be radical if only minor residuals are left (e.g., <2 cm) [21].

23.3.1.5 Neurothekeoma

Neurothekeomas are poorly understood, rare, benign cutaneous tumors ascribed to neural sheath origin. With a mean age of presentation of 25 years, these tumors most commonly localize to the head, neck, and upper limb [22]. While most are slow-growing and asymptomatic, atypical neurothekeomas—characterized by large size of up to 6 cm—penetration into subcutaneous fat and/or muscle, diffusely infiltrating borders, vascular invasion, a high mitotic rate, and marked cytological pleomorphism have been described [23]. Despite these atypical features, no evidence of recurrence or metastasis has been reported in surgically treated neurothekeomas.

23.3.2 Malignant

23.3.2.1 Malignant Peripheral Nerve Sheath Tumor

MPNSTs account for 5–10% of soft tissue sarcomas [24]. Arising from the nerve sheath of peripheral nerves or from pre-existing benign nerve sheath tumors, they favor large nerve trunks—brachial plexus, sacral plexus, and sciatic nerve—but can involve any peripheral nerve [25, 26]. The presence of NF-1 is the main risk factor for MPNSTs; in fact, NF-1 patients account for more than half of MPNSTs [27]. Associated with approximately 10% of these tumors, radiation exposure is another major risk factor for the development of MPNSTs [28]. On average, radiation-associated MPNSTs occur 15 years after radiation exposure, with a range of 4–41 years [9, 29, 30].

The majority of MPNSTs present in adulthood; however, the average age of presentation is younger in the subset of MPNST patients with NF-1 [31]. Approximately 10–20% of patients with MPNSTs present during childhood [32]. In a review of 165 pediatric-age MPNST patient, Bates et al. found that adolescents between the ages of 15 and 19 exhibited a statistically higher incidence than their younger counterparts [25]. Patients usually present with a painful, growing mass and sensorimotor dysfunction in the distribution of the involved neural structures (Fig. 23.5). Tumors may

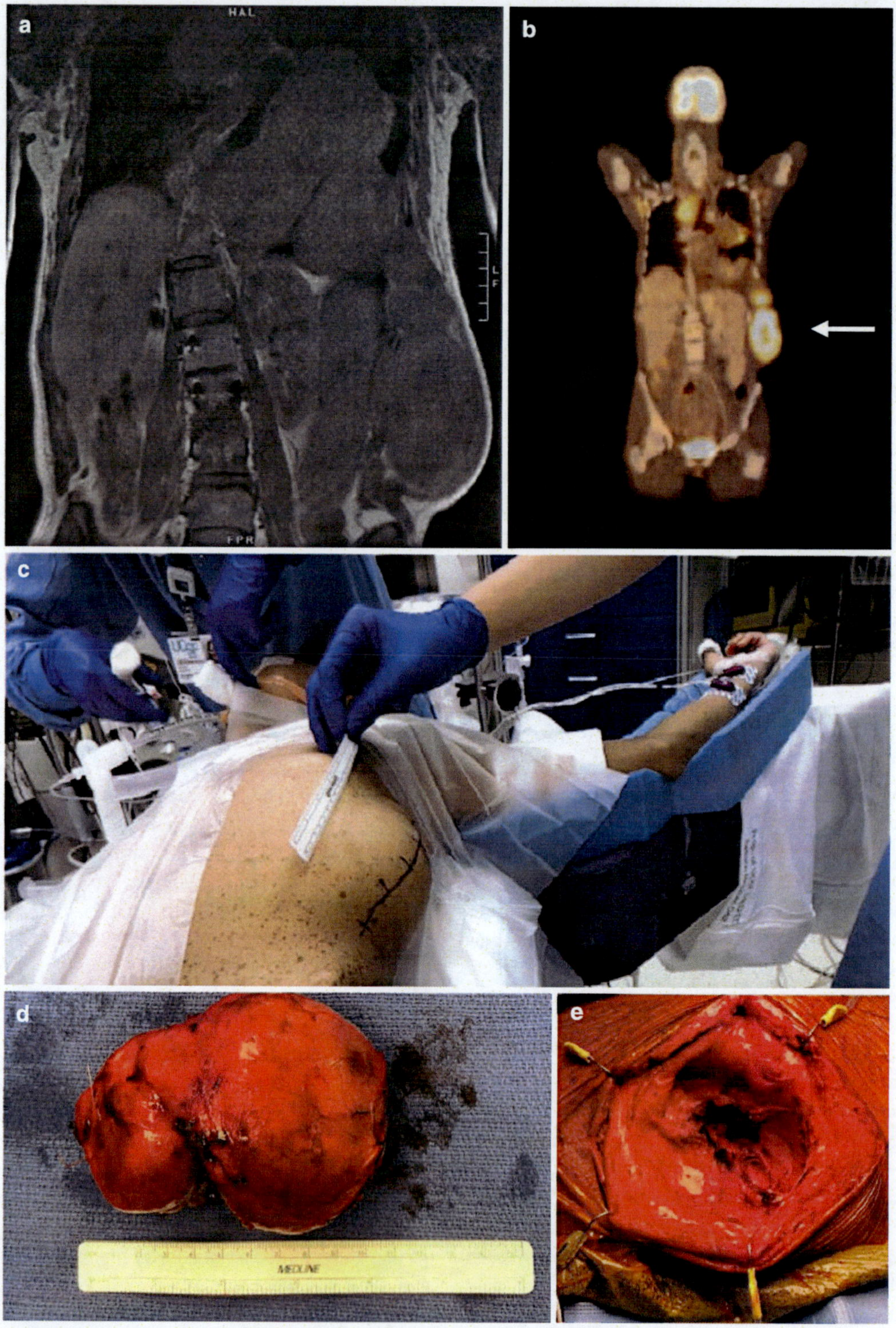

Fig. 23.5 MPNST arising in a neurofibroma presenting as a large, painful, left-sided thoraco-abdominal wall mass. (**a**) Coronal T2 MRI. (**b**) PET scan with evidence of hyper-metabolic region (arrow). (**c**) Intraoperative positioning. (**d**) Gross specimen. (**e**) Intraoperative view following resection

be single or multiple and, while favoring the trunk and extremities, can also be seen in the head and neck [9]. Regional lymph node involvement and distant metastases at the time of presentation have also been described [25, 33].

On gross examination, MPNSTs appear as firm tumors that cause fusiform enlargement of the nerve from which they originate. They have poor pseudocapsules, fail to respect tissue planes, and are locally aggressive. In fact, their malignant potential is related to their ability to infiltrate neurovascular and lymphatic structures. Histologic examination reveals high cellularity, nuclear atypia, increased perivascular cellularity, mitotically active spindle cells, as well as areas of hemorrhage and necrosis [34]. Additionally, MPNSTs can exhibit divergent differentiation into mesenchymal-derived cells—cartilage, bone, fat, etc. [35] Given these features, it is sometimes challenging to distinguish MPNSTs from other sarcomatous lesions. Differentiation often relies on the presence of NF-1 and if the histologic, immunohistochemical, or ultrastructural features are suggestive of Schwann cell differentiation. Given this histopathologic convergence, it is not surprising that, as with other soft tissue sarcomas, gross total resection with wide margins is the preferred primary treatment of MPNSTs.

23.3.2.2 Neuroblastoma

Accounting for approximately one-third of pediatric PNTs, neuroblastomas—tumors derived from primordial neural crest cells—are the most malignant of the embryonal lineage of neoplasms affecting peripheral nerves [2]. As the most common extra-cranial solid tumor in infants and children, neuroblastomas represent 8–10% of all childhood tumors and account for approximately 15% of cancer-related deaths in the pediatric population [36]. The median age at diagnosis is 22 months, with 90% of patients diagnosed before 5 years of age [37].

The clinical presentation of neuroblastomas depends on tumor size, location, degree of invasion, catecholamine secretion, and incidence of paraneoplastic syndromes. Arising from the sympathetic ganglia and adrenal medulla, primary neuroblastic tumors can localize to the cervical (5%), thoracic (15%), abdominal (25%), and pelvic regions (5%) [36]. As a consequence of patients' developmental age, neuroblastomas usually present late in their course, some with evidence of distant metastases [38]. Presenting symptoms can be constitutional in nature or attributable to mass effect: abdominal distention, respiratory distress, constipation, difficulty urinating, dysphagia, asymmetric paresis, Horner's syndrome, and thoracic outlet syndrome. In up to 15% of patients, epidural extension may result in neurological deficits such as progressive paralysis [36]. The neuroendocrine capacity of neuroblastoma, in turn, can manifest with early-onset tachycardia and hypertension. Finally, while symptomatic paraneoplastic syndromes are rare, occurring in <0.01% of *all* cancers, several have been associated with neuroblastomas: intractable diarrhea with electrolyte disturbances due to the release of vasoactive intestinal peptide (VIP), opsoclonus-myoclonus syndrome, encephalomyelitis, and/or sensory neuropathy [39–41].

Despite the management challenges inherent to a disease with the biological and clinical heterogeneity of neuroblastomas, outcomes have steadily improved over the last 30 years: 5-year survival rates rising from 52 to 74% [42]. This is attributable, at least in part, to the fact that the current clinical approach to neuroblastomas is determined by patients' risk stratification. Resultantly, it is of paramount importance that accurate staging and histopathologic classification occur prior to therapeutic intervention. Tumor size, regional invasion, and distant spread are usually assessed with CT or MRI imaging. As 90% of patients have meta-iodobenzylguanidine (MIBG)-avid tumors, MIBG scans can be used to supplement these modalities; in contrast, adjunct imaging with [18-F]-fluorodeoxyglucose positron emission tomography (FDG-PET) is recommended for patients who do not have MIBG-avid disease [43]. Because all neuroblastomas are categorized as small round blue cell tumors with Homer-Wright pseudo-rosettes and associated with mitoses, nuclear karyorrhexis, and pleomorphism, biologic stratification relies on molecular studies aimed at determining ploidy, *MYCN* amplification, and the presence of other chromosomal aberrations [44] (Table).

23.3.2.3 Ganglioneuroblastoma

Ganglioneuroblastomas (GNs) represent the intermediate stage of neuroblastic tumor differentiation. Neuroblastomas and ganglioneuroblastomas share clinical features and a malignant potential. Although this potential is higher in neuroblastomas, these lesions are grouped together for the purposes of cancer reporting, staging, and survival statistics. In contrast, ganglioneuroblastoma intermixed (GNBI), while widely seen as a malignant entity, has "maturing" histological features. The median age of diagnosis for GNBI is 5 years of age. Like GNs, GNBI tumors are usually asymptomatic until local mass effect is achieved. Once this occurs, however, the most frequent symptoms leading to diagnosis are pain, palpable tumor mass and reduced general condition. Interestingly, observational data suggest that GNBI lesions mimic GNs in their response to surgical resection. Specifically, event-free survival (EFS) and overall survival (OS) of patients with incomplete tumor resection are not inferior to that of patients with complete resection if tumor residuals were smaller than 2 cm [21].

23.3.2.4 Rhabdomyosarcoma

Accounting for 4.5% of all cases of childhood cancer, rhabdomyosarcoma (RMS) is the most common pediatric soft tissue sarcoma. Although most cases of RMS occur sporadically, the disease has been associated with familial syndromes, including Li-Fraumeni and neurofibromatosis 1 (Table). Approximately 65% of cases are diagnosed in children younger than 6 years of age; however, the incidence of RMS has a bimodal distribution, with peaks at 2–6 and 10–18 years of age. This distribution reflects the influence of the histologic subtypes of this small round blue cell tumor. Specifically, embryonal RMS diagnosis rates are highest at birth and extend through childhood before declining; in contrast, alveolar RMS diagnosis rates peak at childhood and adolescence prior to declining. The differential incidence is not the only distinguishing clinical feature of these histologic subtypes. Affecting two-thirds of RMS patients, the embryonal subtype is more likely to localize in the head and neck region; extremity involvement is less frequent. Overall prognosis for embryonal RMS is relatively good with a 5-year OS rate of 60%. Alveolar RMS, in turn, is more likely to localize in the trunk or extremities, is often associated with peripheral nerves, and has a slightly worse prognosis with a 5-year OS rate of 54%.

Patients with RMS generally present with a painless mass or with symptoms of mass effect or invasion. Most relevant to this text is the pain or weakness that is consequent to the invasion or encasement of adjacent peripheral nerves. Imaging is important in staging the disease and in evaluating tumor size, the extent of local invasion, and distant spread. Though seldom feasible, en bloc GTR and concurrent preservation of function is the goal. As such, staging is integral for determining whether neo-adjuvant therapy should be utilized prior to surgical resection in an effort to decrease tumor size and thereby decrease surgical morbidity.

23.3.2.5 Triton Tumor

As previously mentioned, MPNSTs may occasionally contain other malignant mesenchymal components, the most common of which is skeletal muscle. Malignant triton tumors (MTTs) represent the subtype of MPNSTs with this rhabdomyosarcomatous differentiation. The metaplastic theory of their origin postulates that Schwann cells, derived of neural crest cells, retain a capacity for mesenchymal differentiation during malignant transformation; furthermore, it accounts for the pluridirectional differentiation seen in 15% of MTTs [45]. In a review of 200 MTT cases, Li et al. found that 41.7% of cases occurred in patients with NF-1 [46]. While median age at diagnosis was 29, patients with NF-1 most commonly presented in the 20–39 age range, while patients without NF-1 had two peaks: the 20s and 50s. The group also showed that 1-, 2-, and 5-year survival rates were 69%, 48%, and 35%, respectively. Cox proportional hazards analysis, in turn, revealed that complete resection (hazard ratio, 0.396; $P = 0.032$) and metastases (hazard ratio, 3.188; $P = 0.004$) were associated with mortality.

23.3.3 Reactive and Hyperplastic

23.3.3.1 Neuroma

Although there is a spectrum of lesions characterized as neuromas—Morton's neuromas, Pacinian neuromas, and palisaded encapsulated neuromas—traumatic neuromas are the most common in children. Occurring at sites of nerve injury, traumatic neuromas are disorganized bundles of fascicles that occur as a consequence of misdirected axonal regeneration [47]. These lesions may present with persistent pain—sometimes limiting function—and sensory disturbances. Early diagnosis and intervention are indicated as to prevent development of a chronic pain syndrome. Conservative management includes massage and desensitization. If this fails, a trial injection of local anesthetic can aid in predicting the success of neuroma surgery [48]. When elected, surgery commonly involves neuroma excision and subsequent nerve grafting or transposition into the muscle or other tissues [49, 50]. Success with this approach is stalled by the pathophysiology that first necessitated intervention—the high likelihood that the freshly treated nerve will reform a new neuroma in its attempt to regenerate. Targeted muscle reinnervation (TMR) aims to preempt this result by co-opting a newly neuroma-free nerve to a newly divided nearby motor nerve; as such, it achieves guided entry and reinnervation of the newly denervated muscle. In a recent randomized clinical trial, when compared with conventional neurectomy, this approach to traumatic neuromas was shown to achieve a statistically significant improvement in phantom limb pain and a trend toward improved residual limb pain [51].

23.3.3.2 Intraneural Ganglion Cyst

Intraneural ganglion cysts are non-neoplastic cystic formations located within the epineurium of the peripheral nerves (Fig. 23.6). Although they can occur in relation to any peripheral nerve, the common peroneal nerve is the most commonly affected, and the fibular neck is the most frequently affected site [52]. The articular theory stipulates that intraneural ganglion cysts are a result of a pressure differential between a degenerating joint and the epineural space of an articular nerve. Presenting symptoms include sensorimotor dysfunction in the distribution of the affected nerve. Surgical management consists of disconnecting the articular branch and/or addressing the joint abnormality. Resection of the cyst is not necessary and may lead to recurrence if the joint connection remains. In many cases, clinical improvement is observed a few days after surgery and progresses steadily in subsequent months. The best results were achieved in relation to pain control; recovery of motor function is less predictable and more changeable [53].

23.3.3.3 Lipomatous Tumor

Although very prevalent lesions, lipomas rarely affect peripheral nerve. In their experience with 146 non-neural nerve sheath tumors, Kim et al. found that adipose tumors accounted for 11% of lesions [54]. Due to their slow-growing nature, adipose lesions of nerve usually present as asymptomatic or minimally symptomatic swelling; severe nerve dysfunction is seldom reported [55]. Lipomatous tumors are classified according to the presence of a diffuse (lipomatosis) or encapsulated (lipoma) lesion. This distinction is fundamental in determining a therapeutic approach. Lipomatosis consists of a diffuse interfascicular fatty tissue, with macroscopically entrapped fascicles. Resultantly, surgical management involves nerve decompression alone rather than an attempt to remove the tumor. In contrast, lipomas are encapsulated epineural masses that displace rather than surround nerve fascicles. Surgical resection via an interfascicular approach is generally safe and effective in reducing neuropathic symptoms.

23.3.3.4 Inflammatory Pseudotumor of Nerve

Inflammatory pseudotumor (IPT) is a tumor-like expansion of nerves that results from the presence of inflammatory infiltrates, interstitial fibrosis, excess vascularity, and a variable increase in lipocytes. The inflammatory infiltrates are most commonly benign lymphocytes, plasma cells, eosinophils, and histiocytes; occasionally poorly formed granulomas and multi-nucleated giant

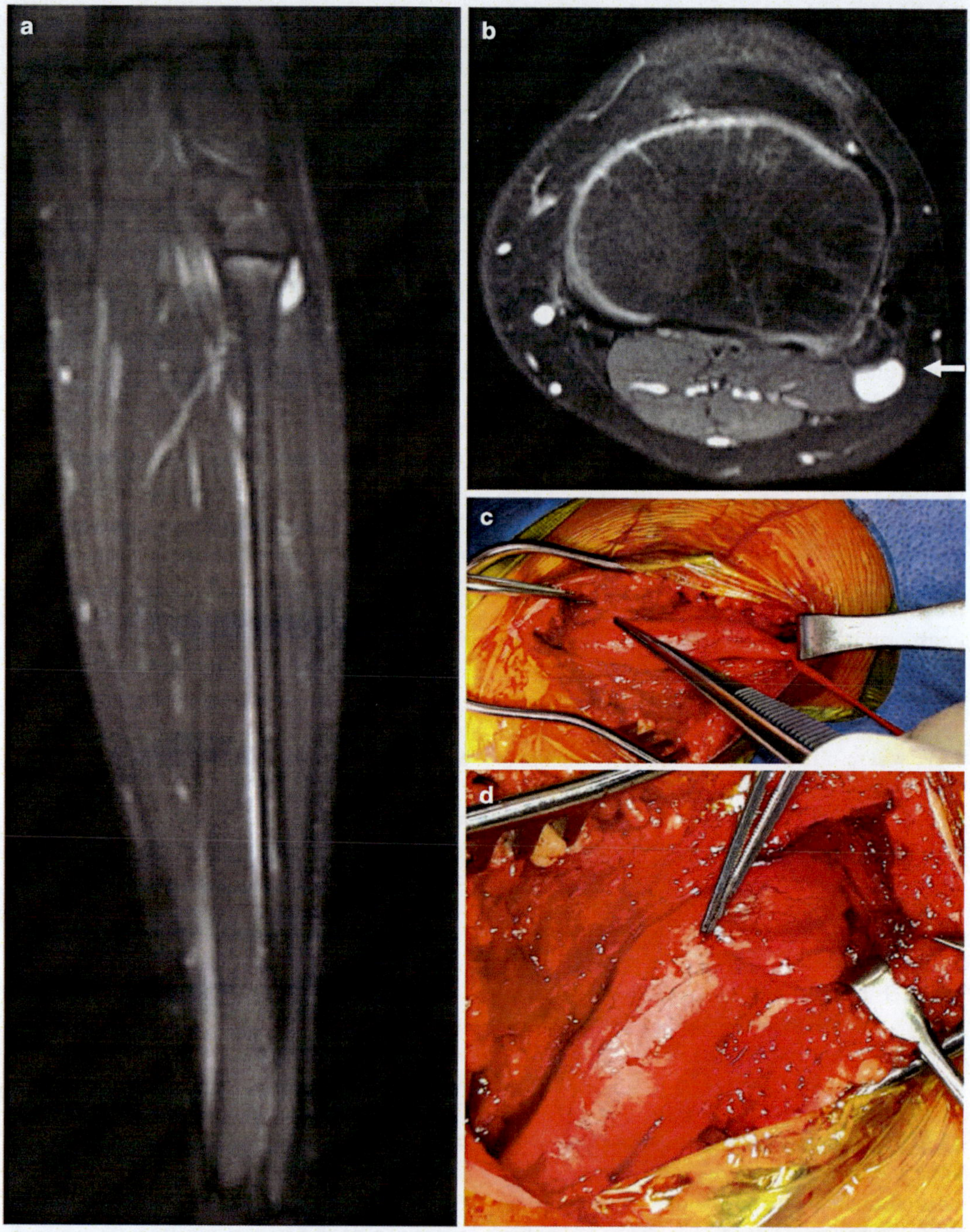

Fig. 23.6 Intraneural ganglion cyst in a 13-year-old male presenting with left foot drop, positive Tinel's at fibular head. (**a**) Coronal STIR MRI demonstrating Lesion of the left common peroneal nerve as it wraps around the fibular head. (**b**) Axial PD MRI demonstrating lesion (arrow). (**c**, **d**) Intraoperative view

cells are seen. IPT is an unusual cause of a progressive mononeuropathy, classically presenting with sensory loss, paresthesias, pain, and weakness [56]. The rate of symptom onset varies from acute to slowly progressive. Neuroimaging is not diagnostic in that it demonstrates a lesion with heterogeneous MRI signal characteristics, reflecting their mixed composition. Thus, because the growth pattern is suggestive of malignancy, biopsy is essential. Initiation of intravenous steroids is the treatment of choice once diagnosis is confirmed [57].

23.4 Clinical Presentation and Physical Exam

Pediatric PNTs most commonly present as a painless, soft tissue mass in the extremity or as an incidental finding on imaging obtained during the evaluation of an unrelated somatic complaint. The classically described signs and symptoms—a palpable/visible mass, motor palsy, sensory deficit, autonomic dysfunction, and pain—occur less frequently [58]. Regardless of their symptomatic classification, pediatric PNTs present a diagnostic challenge as a consequence of their rarity and the challenges of eliciting a history and exam from very young children. In fact, late presentation is common with malignant tumors and is often associated with advanced local invasion and distant metastases. Resultantly, although the general differential diagnosis of a soft tissue mass is extensive and includes infectious/inflammatory lesions, vascular malformations, and neoplastic lesions that arise from organs and/or soft tissues, clinical consideration of PNTs is of paramount importance in achieving early diagnosis and optimal therapeutic results.

The timely diagnosis of PNTs is often facilitated by underlying syndromic features. For example, during an evaluation of a painless mass, the clinical consideration of a neurofibroma is expedited in the setting of clinical stigmata of NF-1. Relatedly, given their origin in the sympathetic nervous system, neuroblastomas commonly present as abdominal, mediastinal, and thoracic mass lesions. Symptoms are often consequent to autonomic dysreflexia, paraneoplastic agents, local compression affecting neighboring visceral organs, and, in cases near or adjacent to the sympathetic chain, a classic Horner's triad [40].

In the absence of syndromic features, clinical diagnosis relies on detailed physical examination and imaging. Objective loss of function in the distribution of the affected nerve is relatively rare with benign PNTs. Characterized by an extremely slow rate of growth and consequent gentle stretch of involved fascicles, benign PNTs are commonly associated with well-preserved neural function—even in context of large mass lesions. In contrast, non-functioning disabling weakness is an ominous sign of malignancy [59]. In fact, the presence of any neurologic deficit predicts malignancy with a positive predictive value (PPV) of 73%. Greater degrees of neurologic deficit (i.e., motor strength less than 3/5), are exclusively seen in association with malignant tumors (PPV = 100%) [60]. Importantly, even frank deficits sometimes avoid clinical detection as a consequence of that fact that proper strength testing is onerous among young children and virtually impossible in infants. Consequently, functional asymmetry and altered progression through developmental milestones have emerged as primary clinical measures. Classic postures on clinical exam—attributable to muscle loss, atrophy, and weakness in specific muscle groups—are additional subtle indices of pathology. Myelopathy—consequent to spinal cord compression from intrinsic nerve root lesions or infiltration of neuroblastic lesions through neural foramina—is another rare but important diagnostic clue [61].

The clinical presentation of PNTs can also manifest as impaired and/or altered sensation. Children may complain of sensory loss or paresthesia in an anatomical distribution. However, even when subjective complaints are lacking, a history of inadvertent injuries to the extremities may signal that such deficits exist [59]. Pain and dysesthesia are relatively common symptoms among patients with PNTs—75% of patients report pain in some setting [59, 62]. Importantly, there is clinical utility in distinguishing whether pain is induced (i.e., the Tinel's sign) or is present at rest. Ogose et al. found that pain at rest occurred in nearly all (15/16) patients with MPNSTs but in only 5/99 (5%) patients with benign schwannomas or neurofibromas; in contrast, 94/99 (95%) of patients with benign tumors had a positive Tinel's test. As such, when compared to the induced pain of benign lesions, resting pain—caused by chemical algogens released by invasive tumor—has a 75% PPV of malignancy [60].

Clinical feature	PPV (%)
Presence of any neurological deficit	73
Severe motor deficits (MRC < 3/5)	100
Any pain	20–30
Resting pain	75

23.5 Diagnostics

23.5.1 Imaging

Although patient size and noncompliance make diagnostic imaging a challenging proposition in the pediatric population, appropriate imaging is of paramount importance in the diagnosis and management of PNTs. Because it provides unparalleled image resolution, reveals involvement of adjacent neurovascular structures, demonstrates proximal and distal lesions with equal efficacy, and can often definitively identify the nerve involved, magnetic resonance imaging (MRI) is the imaging modality of choice. In fact, MRI features can often aid in predicting the subtype of PNT present. For example, while fusiform dilation and intrafascicular growth are suggestive of neurofibromas, schwannomas are characterized by extrafascicular growth—demonstrating the "entering or exiting nerve" sign as well as displaced passerby fascicles around the capsule [63]. Additionally, although lipomas and ganglion cysts share an origin that is mainly, but not always, outside the nerve sheath, lipomas are characteristically bright on T1 and T2 signal, while ganglion cysts are bright on T2 with an origin that can be traced to a joint capsule in proximity to the nerve [64, 65].

Although definitive diagnosis invariably requires tissue sampling, several MRI features have been identified as predictive of the benign nature or malignant potential of PNTs [66]. Tumor size is a major correlate of malignancy. While median lesion size for benign PNTs ranges from 2.7 to 5.0 cm, a range of 7.5 to 9.9 cm is more characteristic of malignant PNTs. Mean size demonstrates a similar distribution with a range of 3.4 to 5.5 and 7.2 to 10 cm for benign and malignant tumors, respectively. Although Chhabra et al. cited a value of 6.1 cm, the optimal diagnostic cutoff for predicting malignancy has yet to be defined [67]. Perilesional edema, as opposed to ill-defined margins, may also be indicative of malignant potential. In a review of 41 histologically diagnosed cases, Wasa et al. observed well-defined tumor margins in most cases of MPNSTs (76%) and neurofibromas (85%), with no statistically significant difference noted between them. In contrast, perilesional edema was seen in 40% of MPNSTs and in none of the neurofibromas [68].

T1 and T2 signal intensity is similarly revealing. Seen in benign neurofibromas, the "target sign," a central hypointense region seen on T2-weighted, was absent in all cases of MPNSTs reviewed by Bhargava et al.—suggesting utility in distinguishing benign from malignant tumors [69]. In contrast, T1 heterogeneity, reflecting intratumoral cystic change, is rarely seen in neurofibromas [70]. Resultantly, this feature can assist in the differentiation of neurofibromas from MPNSTs, in which malignant transition can result in the occurrence of necrosis or hemorrhage [71]. These intratumoral changes contribute to nonhomogeneous enhancement—another suggested distinguishing feature. Ogose et al. observed that MPNSTs show peripheral enhancement on T1-weighted images, as opposed to the central enhancement seen with benign neurogenic tumors [60].

Despite these predictive features, routine MRI sequences have not demonstrated success in accurately grading tumors. In a series of 43 lesions, Broski et al. found that conventional MRI had a 62.5–81.3% sensitivity and a 94.1–100% specificity for accurately differentiating malignant from benign nerve sheath tumors [72]. Relatedly, in a series of 127 patients, Karsy et al. found that MRI-based categorization predicated on lesion characteristics on T1- and T2-weighted imaging differed from final pathology in 51% of patients; furthermore, approximately half of the MRI studies were inconclusive [73]. This circumstance has prompted some authors to advocate for the use of functional MRI techniques to augment diagnostic sensitivity [74, 75]. As a consequence of their ability to interrogate tissue microstructure, diffusion-weighted imaging (DWI) and diffusion tensor imaging (DTI) overcome the limitations of anatomic MR imaging [76] (Fig. 23.7). DWI with apparent diffusion

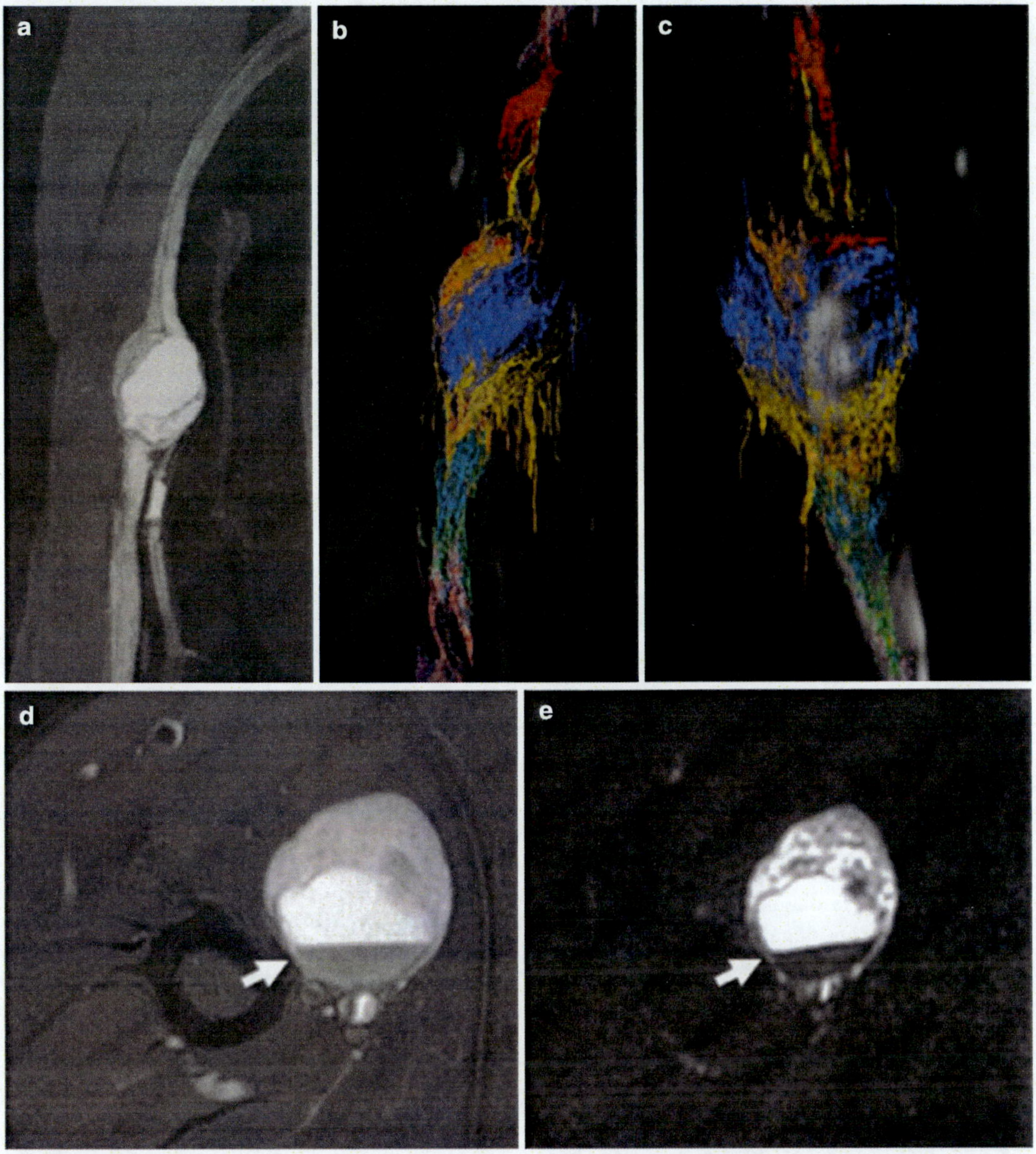

Fig. 23.7 Ancient schwannoma presenting as diffuse enlargement of the median nerve in the upper extremity. (**a**) Tumor conspicuity is readily visualized with 3D PSIF, along with central cystic changes. (**b**) DTI (0 s/mm²) with fiber tractography demonstrating peripheral location of fascicles. (**c**) Fiber tractography reveals partial absence of tracts, splayed around the cystic area. (**d–g**) Axial T2 SPAIR (**d**), DTI ($b = 0$ s/mm²) (**e**), DTI ($b = 600$ s/mm²) (**f**), and colored MD map (**g**) show fluid level due to internal hemorrhage (arrows). MD values of 1.9 and 2.8×10^{-3} mm²/s are seen in solid and cystic tumor regions, respectively, consistent with a benign lesion. Red and blue colorations represent areas of high and low diffusivity, respectively. FA of median nerve was reduced to 0.1–0.2, consistent with neuropathy. (From: Mazal, A.T., Ashikyan, O., Cheng, J. *et al.* Diffusion weighted imaging and diffusion tensor imaging as adjuncts to conventional MRI for the diagnosis and management of peripheral nerve sheath tumors: current perspectives and future directions. *Eur Radiol* **29**, 4123–4132 (2019). https://doi.org/10.1007/s00330-018-5838-8, with permission)

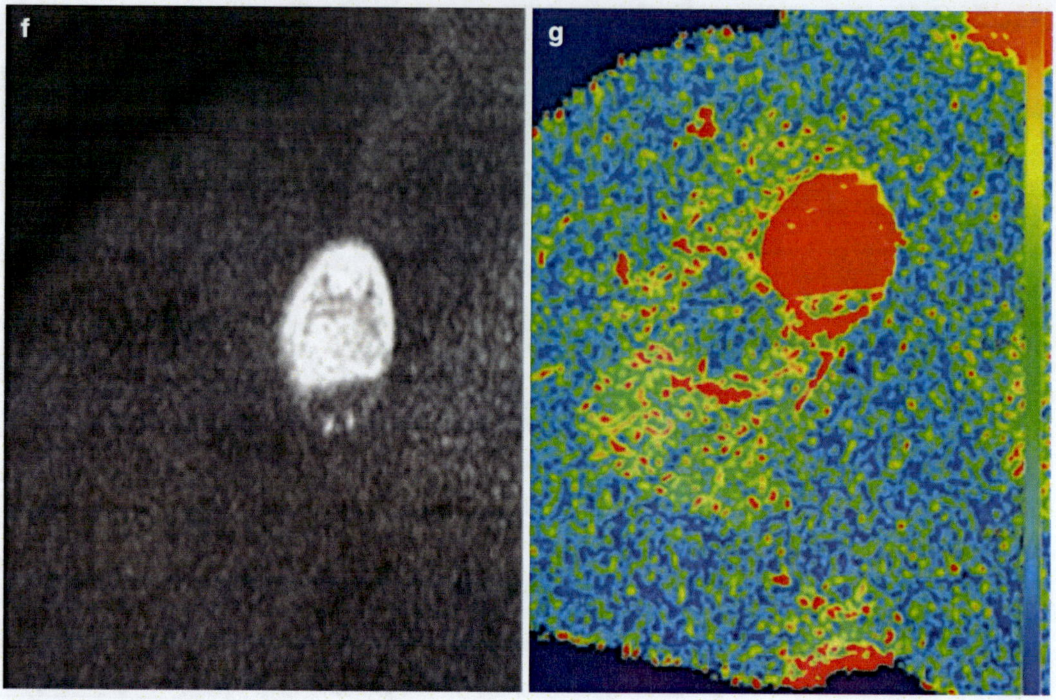

Fig. 23.7 (continued)

coefficient (ADC) mapping provides insight into tumor cellularity with low ADC values serving as markers for malignancy. In a review of 31 PNSTs, Demehri et al. found that a cutoff of ADC $<1.0 \times 10^{-3}$ mm²/s diagnosed malignancy with 100% sensitivity and negative predictive value; in contrast, ADC values $>1.0 \times 10^{-3}$ mm²/s characterized all of the reviewed neurofibromas. Relatedly, the DTI-derived functional anisotropy of invaded nerves is significantly lower than that of their contralateral counterparts [77, 78].

The utility of PET/CT as an adjunct in predicting the malignancy of PNTs has also been explored. Several groups have reported that the maximum standardized uptake value (SUV_{max}), total lesion glycolysis (TLG), and metabolic tumor volume (MTV) are significantly higher in malignant as compared to benign nerve sheath tumors [79–83]. In fact, a combination of these factors resulted in 90–100% sensitivity and 52.2–82.6% specificity for malignant peripheral nerve sheath tumors [72]. As such, MRI and PET/CT can be utilized in a complementary fashion to help triage lesions to biopsy.

Importantly, high-resolution ultrasonography (HRUS) is now emerging as a useful screening tool in the context of genetically predisposing syndromes. Shown to detect subclinical involvement of peripheral nerves, HRUS has successfully identified pathology in the context of normal nerve conduction studies (NCS) [84]. As the presence of plexiform neurofibromas and benign tumor load are risk factors for the development of MPNSTs, HRUS has utility in identifying a subgroup of patients who could benefit from frequent follow-up [85].

23.5.2 Electrodiagnostic Testing

Technically challenging in infants and young children, nerve conduction studies (NCS) and electromyography (EMG) have limited utility in the preoperative management of pediatric PNTs. As there are no neurophysiological characteristics that can differentiate between malignant and benign masses, these studies rarely contribute to diagnostic evaluation. Still, in cases where surgical intervention is deferred and monitoring elected, these modalities can be used to document baseline nerve function and evaluate for interval deterioration.

Tumor pathology	MRI imaging	SUV_{max}	DWI and DTI
Neurofibroma	Unencapsulated Fascicular sign Target sign Split fat sign Open infiltration of parent nerve Multi-fascicular involvement	Low (<2–3)	Low DWI ADC > 1.3×10^{-3} mm/s² Tracts—partial disruption
Schwannoma	Fascicular sign Target sign Split fat sign Encapsulated Cystic changes, calcification Eccentric to parent nerve One or two fascicular involvement	Low (<2–3)	Low DWI ADC > 1.3–1.5×10^{-3} mm/s² Tracts—nearly normal
Malignant peripheral nerve sheath tumor	Perilesional edema Heterogeneous or peripheral enhancement Intra-tumoral necrosis/hemorrhage Peri-tumoral enhancement Generally, >5 cm	High (>3–4)	High DWI ADC < 1.1×10^{-3} mm/s² Tracts—high-grade disruption

23.6 Indications for Intervention

23.6.1 Biopsy

There is ongoing debate about the necessity, efficacy, and safety of preoperative biopsies for the distinction between benign and malignant PNTs. While benign PNTs respond well to marginal excision, malignant PNTs require staging and a multimodal treatment approach which may include surgery, radiation therapy, and, at times, chemotherapy. Inappropriate marginal excision for histologically malignant lesions increases both the likelihood of a positive margin of excision and tumor recurrence rates. The utility of pre-surgical differentiation in guiding the appropriate surgical approach is a commonly cited argument among proponents of preoperative biopsy. Critics, in turn, cite its potential for inconclusive or inaccurate results as well as the risk of onset or worsening of pain, neurological deficits, and other complications that may prohibit future surgical excision and outcomes.

In a series of 140 cases, Levi et al. demonstrated that there was a significantly increased risk of postoperative neurologic deficits—sensory loss or motor deficits—in patients who had undergone a preoperative biopsy. In fact, patients who had undergone a previous procedure at the surgical site were 2.7 times more likely to develop postoperative neurologic deficits than those who had not ($P < 0.001$) [86]. It can only be inferred that this finding reflects the impact of compromised tissue planes—presumably the result of biopsy-induced fibrosis and/or hemorrhage—on surgical resection. New onset and exacerbation of existing neuropathic pain are other recognized complications of biopsy. Given that medications such as amitriptyline and gabapentin have been shown to be of benefit, unintentional axonal damage is the likely etiology [87].

In a series of 41 consecutive CT-guided core-needle biopsies, Pianta et al. showed that small lesion size and a close proximity between the biopsy needle and the nerve were the pain predictors of incident and exacerbated pain post-biopsy [87]. While the lesional contribution to the lesion-nerve complex is clinically immutable, advances in diffusion tensor imaging (DTI) promise to improve the safety profile of biopsy procedures [88]. A preliminary study by Schmidt et al. showed a good correlation between preoperative fascicular visualization and intraoperative anatomy [78]. Preoperative visualization of the fascicular course and integrity using fiber tractography is therefore likely to be of great value in preventing neural injury by informing pre-procedural planning.

The potential for iatrogenic injury and lifelong morbidity must be considered whenever biopsy of a PNT is proposed. Resultantly, we do not perform preoperative biopsies in cases that appear benign with respect to clinical presentation and imaging findings. In the setting of aggressive features, however, four-quadrant biopsy may be indicated.

23.6.2 Surgery

Given the histopathological heterogeneity seen in malignant PNTs, a small biopsy sample does not guarantee a representative diagnosis. Resultantly, a benign biopsy in a suspected malignant lesion should be treated with caution. The fact remains that surgical excision and pathological analysis are the only definitive means of determining malignancy. We factor this uncertainty into our clinical approach. In our practice, the treatment paradigm is founded on two major factors: (1) symptomatic or asymptomatic nature of the mass and (2) presence of clinical or imaging features concerning for a malignant diagnosis. Surgical excision is the recommended approach for symptomatic PNTs regardless of their malignant potential. The approach to asymptomatic lesions is far more nuanced:

- Clinical surveillance and interval MRI imaging at 6 months are the only recommended interventions for incidentally discovered and/or stable PNTs without high-risk imaging features.
- Surgery is the safest option for masses presenting with clinical history or imaging features concerning for malignancy.
- Regardless of imaging findings, surgical treatment is the safest option in cases of asymptomatically growing PNTs; however, small lesions that are growing slowly and remain asymptomatic are often observed [89].
- In the absence of high-risk imaging features, asymptomatic palpable or visible PNTs can be excised for cosmetic purposes and to improve quality of life.

23.7 Surgical Techniques

Although the development of chemotherapeutic agents like selumetinib—an FDA-approved kinase inhibitor for the treatment of plexiform neurofibromas—heralds an increased role for medical therapy in the management of PNTs, surgical resection remains the mainstay of therapy at this time. The surgical treatment of a PNT is dependent on its neoplastic nature and anatomic location. Although the breadth of surgical approaches seen in PNT surgery is beyond the scope of this work, the principles and techniques essential to improving symptoms, preserving neurologic function, and minimizing the chance for recurrence will be addressed as they relate to both benign and malignant pathologies [90, 91].

Regardless of the malignant potential of the target lesion, tumor location is a key determinant of surgical success. When feasible, preoperative contrasted MRI imaging should be obtained to help define the relationship between the PNT and adjacent structures. Although angiography is rarely required, it can be useful to evaluate for vascular invasion in PNTs located at the base of the neck, chest, or retroperitoneum. On rare occasions, preoperative embolization may be essential for safe resection of a vascular lesion (e.g., hemangiomas of the brachial plexus) involving neural elements [92]. Finally, CT imaging may reveal remodeling and/or compromise of adjacent bony structures, such as the spinal canal, neural foramina, or vertebral bodies.

23.7.1 Benign PNTs

Interfascicular resection is a surgical technique used to safely treat benign peripheral nerve sheath tumors through careful dissection of functional neural elements off the tumor surface; thereby, functional neural elements can be preserved, and mass enucleation permitted: [93–95]

- The surgical incision should be planned to center on the mass. Intraoperative US or preoperative US and/or MRI with markers can be used to facilitate localization if the lesion is not palpable on physical exam.
- The anesthesia technique must allow for repetitive nerve stimulation and recording.
- A longitudinal incision, following the course of the nerve, should be extended to a length

that allows access to both the proximal and distal normal segments of the affected nerve; an S- or Z-shaped path should be used across joint creases.

- Complete external neurolysis, superficial tumor exposure, and vessel loop control of the proximal and distal aspects of the normal nerve should be achieved. This allows functional fascicles streaming around the tumor in the pseudocapsule to be visualized during resection.
- Inspection of the mass surface allows for identification of a fascicle-free window. Nerve stimulation can and should be used as an adjunct to map functional nerve fibers and identify a "silent" region. Plexiform lesions—seen frequently in patients with schwannomatosis and neurofibromatosis—present a particular challenge given the presence of multiple entering and exiting fascicles.
- An epineurotomy of the tumor pseudocapsule in the "silent" region should be performed with a knife or sharp dissector in a direction parallel to the nerve fibers.
- Interfascicular dissection should be continued until the true tumor capsule is found. Once this occurs, the tumor should be circumferentially mobilized from the pseudocapsule and the fascicles running along its surface. Neuromonitoring can be utilized during this phase of the operation to decrease the incidence of fascicular injury.
- Once the tumor is free circumferentially, entering and exiting fascicles should be identified. These should be tested to ensure they are nonfunctioning prior to transection.
- Following tumor enucleation, the sides of the pseudocapsule should be spread in opposite directions and evaluated for residual tumor. If safe to do so, the remaining tumor should be removed.
- Hemostasis should be achieved with an absorbable gelatin-compressed sponge and gentle direct pressure; bipolar electrocautery should be used sparingly and only if absolutely necessary. The surgical site should then be closed in anatomical layers.

23.7.2 Malignant PNTs

For patients with a suspected or biopsy-proven malignant PNT, accurate staging and a multidisciplinary approach are crucial for directing treatment. Presently, adjuvant treatments have failed to significantly improve survival among patients with malignant PNTs. As with other soft tissue sarcomas, surgery remains the primary curative modality for operable malignant peripheral nerve sheath tumors, rhabdomyosarcomas, and neuroblastomas. The goal of surgery is gross total resection (GTR) of the tumor with histologically negative margins. When anatomically feasible, resection is accomplished by en bloc excision of the tumor along with its parent nerve. Guided by life—as opposed to limb-sparing approach, en bloc resection can result in significant functional loss—especially if the tumor's origin is within the brachial or lumbosacral plexus.

Tumor location and the degree of tissue invasion are key determinants of the likelihood of GTR (Fig. 23.8). For malignant peripheral nerve sheath tumors, rates vary from 20 to 95% for lesions with paraspinal versus extremity localization, respectively [96]. Unfortunately, only 40% of pediatric malignant peripheral nerve sheath tumors localize to the extremities [97]. In rhabdomyosarcoma the rate approximates 20%; in neuroblastoma, incidence is worthy of case report [98, 99]. As such, consideration of the feasibility of GTR, the systemic burden of disease, and the patient's physiological reserve should be considered prior to surgical referral. When clinically appropriate, adjuvant therapy prior to surgical resection may be elected in an effort to increase the likelihood of complete resection and decrease surgical morbidity [100].

23.8 Surgical Outcomes and Complications

When possible, gross total resection with subsequent resolution of pain and preservation or improvement of neurological function are the goals of surgical intervention. As can be expected, success is variable and dependent on pathology,

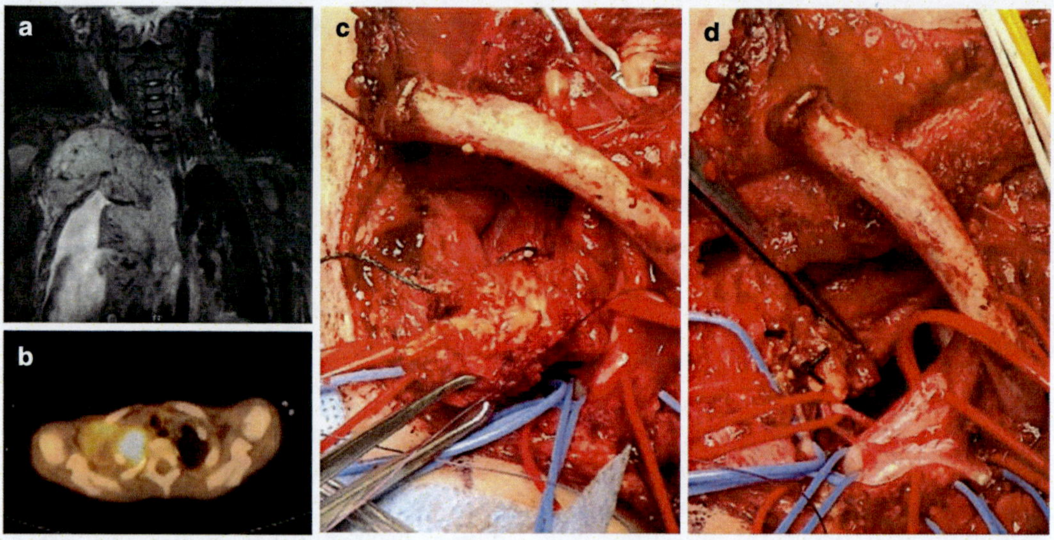

Fig. 23.8 Malignant atypical rhabdoid tumor in 2-year-old boy presenting with pain and progressive weakness of the right upper extremity and a palpable mass in the axilla and supraclavicular fossa. (**a**) Coronal STIR MRI demonstrating mass centered within the right axilla and right lung apex. (**b**) PET scan with evidence of increased uptake. (**c, d**) Supra- and infraclavicular approach to plexus tumor with clavicle mobilization by orthopedics

tumor location, duration of preoperative symptoms, and surgical technique.

23.8.1 Benign PNTs

23.8.1.1 Extent of Resection

In a review of a surgical series of 182 benign lesions in adults, Guha et al. found that GTR was achieved in 44.9% of neurofibromas as compared to 76.7% of schwannomas ($p < 0.001$). This difference persisted even when plexiform neurofibromas were excluded from consideration. Tumor location was shown to influence the extent of resection as extremity lesions were more likely to achieve GTR when compared to those in the brachial or lumbosacral plexus (OR 3.36, $p = 0.007$) [101]. As can be expected, GTR rates are typically decreased among patients receiving intraoperative neurophysiological monitoring [86].

23.8.1.2 Motor Function

In the series reviewed by Guha et al., all patients with a preoperative motor deficit exhibited stable to improved motor function postoperatively. New motor deficits in the immediate postoperative period were seen in 10.3% of schwannomas and 11.8% of neurofibromas; these were permanent in 5.2% and 8.8%, respectively. In their review of 361 benign PNSTs, Kim et al. mirrored these findings by demonstrating stable or improved motor function in 89% of schwannomas and 85% of solitary neurofibromas [102]. Levi et al., in turn, reported postoperative motor deficits in 8% of schwannomas and 5.9% of neurofibromas in a series of 121 adult and pediatric patients. Interestingly, tumor histopathology was not found to be a determinant of postoperative motor outcome. When considered in the context of grossly divergent GTR rates, this finding may reflect the authors' functionally driven surgical approach. In contrast, the duration of patients' preoperative symptoms was determined to be related to postoperative motor function; in fact, a duration of <6 months was associated with greater percent improvement [103].

23.8.1.3 Sensory Symptoms

Pre-existing sensory disturbances were stable to be improved in 97.2% of cases reviewed by Guha et al. New sensory disturbances were seen in the immediate postoperative period in 12.9% of schwannomas and 3.7% of neurofibromas; deficits were permanent in 7.5% and 0%, respectively. Generally, symptom duration of >6 months prior to surgical intervention was associated with lower rates of improvement [103].

23.8.1.4 Pain Outcomes

Guha et al. reported pain as a preoperative symptom in 57.9% of schwannoma and 75.5% of neurofibroma patients. For all patients, these symptoms were stable to improved postoperatively. New postoperative neuropathic pain was seen in four patients; symptoms were permanent in two. In a review of 119 surgical cases featuring adult and pediatric patients, Artico et al. provided further insight by detailing a rate of 50%, 22%, 15%, 7%, and 6% for resolved, improved, unchanged, worsened, and new pain, respectively [104]. Generally, duration of symptoms (greater than or less than 6 months) did not correlate with rates of improvement [103].

23.8.1.5 Recurrence Rates

Despite their reassuring histology, benign PNTs may recur locally. Reported recurrence rates range widely in the literature, with rates approximating 44% referenced for pediatric plexiform neurofibromas [102, 104, 105]. In the Guha et al. series, recurrence rates for schwannomas and neurofibromas were 5.3% and 8.2%, respectively. The most consistently identified predictor of recurrence in the literature, subtotal resection (STR), was associated with increased recurrence for all benign PNTs in this series (OR 13.16, $p = 0.007$). Interestingly, tumor location influenced the extent of resection in schwannomas but not neurofibromas. As schwannomas inherently grow extrinsic to their parent fascicles while neurofibromas are intertwined with multiple fascicles of origin, this difference may be ascribed to the fact that neurofibromas are less likely to be fully resected, regardless of their accessibility. Importantly, tumor histopathology has been shown to impact recurrence regardless of the extent of resection; specifically, NF type was significantly associated with recurrence: NF-1 for neurofibromas (OR 1.18, $p = 0.002$) and NF3 (schwannomatosis) for schwannomas (OR 4.29, $p = 0.048$).

23.8.2 Malignant PNTs

23.8.2.1 Malignant Peripheral Nerve Sheath Tumors

A diagnosis of MPNST is associated with an increased likelihood of worsened postoperative sensorimotor function. In fact, Levi et al. reported that 36.8% of patients in the surgical cohort had some type of functional deficit: 26.3% incidence of sensory deficits, a 21.1% incidence of motor deficits, and a 10.5% incidence of neurogenic pain syndromes. The pursuit of GTR and negative margins accounts for these deficits; unfortunately, GTR is significantly less likely for MPNSTs than their benign counterparts (OR 0.22, $p = 0.002$) [101]. The consequence to patient outcome is obvious. DeCou et al. found a significant difference in 2-year survival between pediatric patients in whom GTR was achieved (79%) and those with unresectable tumors (22%) [106]. Because tumor cells readily invade fascial planes, local recurrence and distant metastases are common. In a series of 205 patients with localized MPNSTs, Anghileri et al. found the cumulative incidence of local recurrence and distant metastasis to approximate 30% at 10 years [97]. As can be inferred, prognosis is poor. In a series of 167 children, Carli et al. reported a 5-year overall survival of 51% and 10-year overall survival of 37% [33].

Although limited by patient and tumor heterogeneity, retrospective reviews have identified additional negative prognostic factors: truncal location, tumor size (>5 cm), infiltrative growth pattern, younger age, high grade, S11b negativity, and p53 mutations [28, 32, 107–110]. Although NF-1 status has traditionally been associated with poorer prognosis, several studies, including a meta-analysis, have found no significant differences in overall survival [28, 97, 101, 111]. It has been suggested that unfavorable outcomes in NF-1 patients are related to the development of larger tumors rather than underlying biologic factors [97]. Resultantly, patients with NF-1 should be followed carefully so as to facilitate early detection of malignant lesions among the multitude of benign tumors.

While prospective, histology-driven trials to support their use are largely lacking, there is evidence to suggest that chemotherapy and radiation therapy (XRT) may be positive prognostic factors. Several studies have shown XRT to decrease local recurrence rates [97, 112]. Although radiation therapy has not been shown to affect rates of overall survival, its use is recommended by the Oncology Consensus Group [113]. Given the known propensity for radiation to trigger malignant transformation in neurofibromas, this recommendation should be applied with caution in the NF-1 population. Outcomes for chemotherapy, though rarely systematically reported, appear to be favorable in children and young adults—overall response rate of 45% and 11 patients whose disease was rendered resectable following therapy [33, 114]. Most experts currently recommend chemotherapy—either primary or adjuvant—for patients with the previously outlined high-risk features [115].

23.8.2.2 Neuroblastoma

Treatment strategies for neuroblastoma are tailored according to the predicted response to therapy and risk of relapse over a 40-year period. As a consequence of the biological and clinical heterogeneity of neuroblastomas, risk stratification and subsequent treatment determination rely on a variety of prognostic factors. These include clinical factors (tumor stage and age at diagnosis) as well as biological features—histology, DNA ploidy, cytogenetic factors (i.e., amplification of the MYCN oncogene and key chromosomal deletions or gains)—and serum tumor markers. (Table) Clinical outcomes for children with low- and intermediate-risk neuroblastoma have been excellent, achieving 90% long-term event-free survival rates. Unfortunately, high-risk neuroblastoma remains a challenge, with long-term survival rates for children currently under 50%.

Low- and Intermediate-Risk Neuroblastoma

Non-high-risk neuroblastoma is a heterogeneous group representing slightly more than half of newly diagnosed patients. For patients with localized and resectable disease, surgery alone is generally curative with chemotherapy functioning as an effective salvage for cases that relapse after resection [116, 117]. In a cohort of patients treated by surgical resection alone, the Children's Oncology Group P9641 study demonstrated a 5-year overall survival (OS) rate of 99% for INSS stage 1 and 96% for INSS 2A or 2B tumors [118]. Treatment for intermediate-risk neuroblastoma, in turn, is composed of multiagent chemotherapy followed by surgical resection. Baker et al. demonstrated an 88% event-free survival (EFS) rate of 88% and a 96% OS rate at 3 years with this approach [119].

High-Risk Neuroblastoma

The treatment algorithm for high-risk neuroblastoma includes four main stages: (1) induction chemotherapy, (2) local control, (3) consolidation, and (4) maintenance therapy. Patients' response to induction chemotherapy, as measured by semi-quantitative MIBG scoring systems, has been shown to be a key prognostic indicator [120]. Following four to six cycles of induction therapy, an attempt at local control is made with surgical resection. Importantly, several groups have found that it is surgical intervention, as opposed to the extent of resection, that is a positive prognostic factor for overall survival in this population [121, 122]. Data from a Children's Cancer Group study showed that, in stage 4 tumors, survival was comparable for those with and without complete resection; in fact, 5-year EFS rate was 25% and 30% for patients who achieved incomplete and complete resection, respectively ($p = 0.10$) [123]. Radiation therapy is an additional effector of local control. Utilized in the setting of residual disease post-induction chemotherapy and resection, XRT—administered subsequent to consolidation therapy with myeloablative chemotherapy and autologous stem cell rescue—helps achieve a local relapse rate of <10% [124].

23.8.2.3 Rhabdomyosarcoma

Among rhabdomyosarcoma patients, the extent of disease after resection is one of the most important prognostic factors [98, 125, 126]. Published outcome analyses have shown that a clear margin and no residual disease (Group I) are superior to microscopic margins (Group II) or gross residual disease (Group III); OS rates approximate 87%, 73%, and 59%, respectively. Not surprisingly, metastatic disease (Group IV) carries a 26% 5-year OS rate. Having been shown to positively influence local control and outcome, chemotherapy and XRT are key, albeit secondary, modalities in the rhabdomyosarcoma treatment algorithm.

23.9 Surgical Tricks of the Trade

- In the absence of high-risk clinical or imaging features, a biopsy procedure prior to definitive resection should be avoided as it carries a 2.7-fold higher risk of postoperative neurological deficits compared to definitive resection upfront [86].
- As a consequence of its safety profile and efficacy, intracapsular, interfascicular resection is the preferred surgical approach to benign PNTs [127].
- It is important to achieve adequate exposure of the proximal and distal aspects of the affected nerve prior to initiating tumor resection.
- In the context of benign lesions, safety and preservation of nerve fascicles should never be sacrificed in the pursuit of gross total resection.
- Intraoperative neurophysiologic monitoring decreases the risk of postoperative neurological deficits [86].

References

1. Harms D. Soft tissue sarcomas in the Kiel pediatric tumor registry. Curr Top Pathol. 1995;89:31–45.
2. Coffin CM, Dehner LP. Peripheral neurogenic tumors of the soft tissues in children and adolescents: a clinicopathologic study of 139 cases. Pediatr Pathol. 1989;9(4):387–407.
3. Kaatsch P. Epidemiology of childhood cancer. Cancer Treat Rev. 2010;36(4):277–85.
4. Young JL Jr, Ries LG, Silverberg E, Horm JW, Miller RW. Cancer incidence, survival, and mortality for children younger than age 15 years. Cancer. 1986;58(2 Suppl):598–602.
5. Keegan TH, Ries LA, Barr RD, et al. Comparison of cancer survival trends in the United States of adolescents and young adults with those in children and older adults. Cancer. 2016;122(7):1009–16.
6. Donner TR, Voorhies RM, Kline DG. Neural sheath tumors of major nerves. J Neurosurg. 1994;81(3):362–73.
7. Korf BR. Plexiform neurofibromas. Am J Med Genet. 1999;89(1):31–7.
8. Gabhane SK, Kotwal MN, Bobhate SK. Morphological spectrum of peripheral nerve sheath tumors: a series of 126 cases. Indian J Pathol Microbiol. 2009;52(1):29–33.
9. Ducatman BS, Scheithauer BW, Piepgras DG, Reiman HM, Ilstrup DM. Malignant peripheral nerve sheath tumors. A clinicopathologic study of 120 cases. Cancer. 1986;57(10):2006–21.
10. Sorensen SA, Mulvihill JJ, Nielsen A. Long-term follow-up of von Recklinghausen neurofibromatosis. Survival and malignant neoplasms. N Engl J Med. 1986;314(16):1010–5.
11. Rodriguez FJ, Stratakis CA, Evans DG. Genetic predisposition to peripheral nerve neoplasia: diagnostic criteria and pathogenesis of neurofibromatoses, carney complex, and related syndromes. Acta Neuropathol. 2012;123(3):349–67.
12. Gorlin RJ, Koutlas IG. Multiple schwannomas, multiple nevi, and multiple vaginal leiomyomas: a new dominant syndrome. Am J Med Genet. 1998;78(1):76–81.
13. Broehm C, Al-Ibraheemi A, Fritchie KJ. Pediatric non-vestibular schwannoma. Pediatr Dev Pathol. 2017;20(3):232–9.
14. Hornick JL, Fletcher CD. Soft tissue perineurioma: clinicopathologic analysis of 81 cases including those with atypical histologic features. Am J Surg Pathol. 2005;29(7):845–58.
15. Ferraresi S, Garozzo D, Bianchini E, Gasparotti R. Perineurioma of the sciatic nerve: a possible cause of idiopathic foot drop in children: report of 4 cases. J Neurosurg Pediatr. 2010;6(5):506–10.
16. Macarenco RS, Ellinger F, Oliveira AM. Perineurioma: a distinctive and underrecognized peripheral nerve sheath neoplasm. Arch Pathol Lab Med. 2007;131(4):625–36.
17. Wilson TJ, Howe BM, Stewart SA, Spinner RJ, Amrami KK. Clinicoradiological features of intraneural perineuriomas obviate the need for tissue diagnosis. J Neurosurg. 2018;129(4):1034–40.
18. Huang Y, Li H, Xiong Z, Chen R. Intraneural malignant perineurioma: a case report and review of literature. Int J Clin Exp Pathol. 2014;7(7):4503–7.
19. Pina-Oviedo S, Ortiz-Hidalgo C. The normal and neoplastic perineurium: a review. Adv Anat Pathol. 2008;15(3):147–64.
20. Lonergan GJ, Schwab CM, Suarez ES, Carlson CL. Neuroblastoma, ganglioneuroblastoma, and ganglioneuroma: radiologic-pathologic correlation. Radiographics. 2002;22(4):911–34.

21. Decarolis B, Simon T, Krug B, et al. Treatment and outcome of ganglioneuroma and ganglioneuroblastoma intermixed. BMC Cancer. 2016;16:542.
22. Boukovalas S, Rogers H, Boroumand N, Cole EL. Cellular neurothekeoma: a rare tumor with a common clinical presentation. Plast Reconstr Surg Glob Open. 2016;4(8):e1006.
23. Wilson AD, Rigby H, Orlando A. Atypical cellular neurothekeoma—a diagnosis to be aware of. J Plast Reconstr Aesthet Surg. 2008;61(2):186–8.
24. Stark AM, Buhl R, Hugo HH, Mehdorn HM. Malignant peripheral nerve sheath tumours—report of 8 cases and review of the literature. Acta Neurochir. 2001;143(4):357–63; discussion 363–354
25. Bates JE, Peterson CR, Dhakal S, Giampoli EJ, Constine LS. Malignant peripheral nerve sheath tumors (MPNST): a SEER analysis of incidence across the age spectrum and therapeutic interventions in the pediatric population. Pediatr Blood Cancer. 2014;61(11):1955–60.
26. Huang JH, Zaghloul K, Zager EL. Surgical management of brachial plexus region tumors. Surg Neurol. 2004;61(4):372–8.
27. Woodruff JM. Pathology of tumors of the peripheral nerve sheath in type 1 neurofibromatosis. Am J Med Genet. 1999;89(1):23–30.
28. Stucky CC, Johnson KN, Gray RJ, et al. Malignant peripheral nerve sheath tumors (MPNST): the Mayo Clinic experience. Ann Surg Oncol. 2012;19(3):878–85.
29. Wong WW, Hirose T, Scheithauer BW, Schild SE, Gunderson LL. Malignant peripheral nerve sheath tumor: analysis of treatment outcome. Int J Radiat Oncol Biol Phys. 1998;42(2):351–60.
30. Vauthey JN, Woodruff JM, Brennan MF. Extremity malignant peripheral nerve sheath tumors (neurogenic sarcomas): a 10-year experience. Ann Surg Oncol. 1995;2(2):126–31.
31. Amirian ES, Goodman JC, New P, Scheurer ME. Pediatric and adult malignant peripheral nerve sheath tumors: an analysis of data from the surveillance, epidemiology, and end results program. J Neurooncol. 2014;116(3):609–16.
32. Casanova M, Ferrari A, Spreafico F, et al. Malignant peripheral nerve sheath tumors in children: a single-institution twenty-year experience. J Pediatr Hematol Oncol. 1999;21(6):509–13.
33. Carli M, Ferrari A, Mattke A, et al. Pediatric malignant peripheral nerve sheath tumor: the Italian and German Soft Tissue Sarcoma Cooperative Group. J Clin Oncol. 2005;23(33):8422–30.
34. Rodriguez FJ, Folpe AL, Giannini C, Perry A. Pathology of peripheral nerve sheath tumors: diagnostic overview and update on selected diagnostic problems. Acta Neuropathol. 2012;123(3):295–319.
35. Guccion JG, Enzinger FM. Malignant schwannoma associated with von Recklinghausen's neurofibromatosis. Virchows Arch A Pathol Anat Histol. 1979;383(1):43–57.
36. Park JR, Eggert A, Caron H. Neuroblastoma: biology, prognosis, and treatment. Hematol Oncol Clin North Am. 2010;24(1):65–86.
37. Esiashvili N, Anderson C, Katzenstein HM. Neuroblastoma. Curr Probl Cancer. 2009;33(6):333–60.
38. Smith EI, Haase GM, Seeger RC, Brodeur GM. A surgical perspective on the current staging in neuroblastoma—the international neuroblastoma staging system proposal. J Pediatr Surg. 1989;24(4):386–90.
39. Darnell RB, Posner JB. Paraneoplastic syndromes involving the nervous system. N Engl J Med. 2003;349(16):1543–54.
40. Colon NC, Chung DH. Neuroblastoma. Adv Pediatr Infect Dis. 2011;58(1):297–311.
41. Han W, Wang HM. Refractory diarrhea: a paraneoplastic syndrome of neuroblastoma. World J Gastroenterol. 2015;21(25):7929–32.
42. Maris JM. Recent advances in neuroblastoma. N Engl J Med. 2010;362(23):2202–11.
43. Bleeker G, Tytgat GA, Adam JA, et al. 123I-MIBG scintigraphy and 18F-FDG-PET imaging for diagnosing neuroblastoma. Cochrane Database Syst Rev. 2015;9:CD009263.
44. Whittle SB, Smith V, Doherty E, Zhao S, McCarty S, Zage PE. Overview and recent advances in the treatment of neuroblastoma. Expert Rev Anticancer Ther. 2017;17(4):369–86.
45. Stasik CJ, Tawfik O. Malignant peripheral nerve sheath tumor with rhabdomyosarcomatous differentiation (malignant triton tumor). Arch Pathol Lab Med. 2006;130(12):1878–81.
46. Li G, Liu C, Liu Y, et al. Analysis of clinical features and prognosis of malignant triton tumor: a report of two cases and literature review. Oncol Lett. 2015;10(6):3551–6.
47. Cravioto H, Battista A. Clinical and ultrastructural study of painful neuroma. Neurosurgery. 1981;8(2):181–90.
48. Hanna SA, Catapano J, Borschel GH. Painful pediatric traumatic neuroma: surgical management and clinical outcomes. Childs Nerv Syst. 2016;32(7):1191–4.
49. Vernadakis AJ, Koch H, Mackinnon SE. Management of neuromas. Clin Plast Surg. 2003;30(2):247–68. vii
50. Krishnan KG, Pinzer T, Schackert G. Coverage of painful peripheral nerve neuromas with vascularized soft tissue: method and results. Neurosurgery. 2005;56(2 Suppl):369–78; discussion 369–378
51. Dumanian GA, Potter BK, Mioton LM, et al. Targeted muscle reinnervation treats neuroma and phantom pain in major limb amputees: a randomized clinical trial. Ann Surg. 2019;270(2):238–46.
52. Spinner RJ, Scheithauer BW, Amrami KK. The unifying articular (synovial) origin of intraneural ganglia: evolution-revelation-revolution. Neurosurgery. 2009;65(4 Suppl):A115–24.
53. Rendon D, Pescador D, Cano C, Blanco J. Intraneural ganglion cyst on the external popliteal nerve. BMJ Case Rep. 2014;2014

54. Kim DH, Murovic JA, Tiel RL, Moes G, Kline DG. A series of 146 peripheral non-neural sheath nerve tumors: 30-year experience at Louisiana State University Health Sciences Center. J Neurosurg. 2005;102(2):256–66.
55. Teles AR, Finger G, Schuster MN, Gobbato PL. Peripheral nerve lipoma: case report of an intraneural lipoma of the median nerve and literature review. Asian J Neurosurg. 2016;11(4):458.
56. Perez-Lopez C, Gutierrez M, Isla A. Inflammatory pseudotumor of the median nerve. Case report and review of the literature. J Neurosurg. 2001;95(1):124–8.
57. Mauermann ML, Scheithauer BW, Spinner RJ, et al. Inflammatory pseudotumor of nerve: clinicopathological characteristics and a potential therapy. J Peripher Nerv Syst. 2010;15(3):216–26.
58. Guedes F, Brown RS, Torrao-Junior FJL, Barbosa DAN, Ravanini GAG, Amorim RMP. Pediatric peripheral nerve tumors: clinical and surgical aspects. Childs Nerv Syst. 2019;35(12):2289–97.
59. Valeyrie-Allanore L, Ismaili N, Bastuji-Garin S, et al. Symptoms associated with malignancy of peripheral nerve sheath tumours: a retrospective study of 69 patients with neurofibromatosis 1. Br J Dermatol. 2005;153(1):79–82.
60. Ogose A, Hotta T, Morita T, et al. Tumors of peripheral nerves: correlation of symptoms, clinical signs, imaging features, and histologic diagnosis. Skeletal Radiol. 1999;28(4):183–8.
61. Ugarriza LF, Cabezudo JM, Ramirez JM, Lorenzana LM, Porras LF. Bilateral and symmetric C1-C2 dumbbell ganglioneuromas producing severe spinal cord compression. Surg Neurol. 2001;55(4):228–31.
62. Sughrue ME, Levine J, Barbaro NM. Pain as a symptom of peripheral nerve sheath tumors: clinical significance and future therapeutic directions. J Brachial Plex Peripher Nerve Inj. 2008;3:6.
63. Kakkar C, Shetty CM, Koteshwara P, Bajpai S. Telltale signs of peripheral neurogenic tumors on magnetic resonance imaging. Indian J Radiol Imaging. 2015;25(4):453–8.
64. Burt AM, Huang BK. Imaging review of lipomatous musculoskeletal lesions. SICOT J. 2017;3:34.
65. Panwar J, Mathew A, Thomas BP. Cystic lesions of peripheral nerves: are we missing the diagnosis of the intraneural ganglion cyst? World J Radiol. 2017;9(5):230–44.
66. Furniss D, Swan MC, Morritt DG, et al. A 10-year review of benign and malignant peripheral nerve sheath tumors in a single center: clinical and radiographic features can help to differentiate benign from malignant lesions. Plast Reconstr Surg. 2008;121(2):529–33.
67. Chhabra A, Soldatos T, Durand DJ, Carrino JA, McCarthy EF, Belzberg AJ. The role of magnetic resonance imaging in the diagnostic evaluation of malignant peripheral nerve sheath tumors. Indian J Cancer. 2011;48(3):328–34.
68. Wasa J, Nishida Y, Tsukushi S, et al. MRI features in the differentiation of malignant peripheral nerve sheath tumors and neurofibromas. AJR Am J Roentgenol. 2010;194(6):1568–74.
69. Bhargava R, Parham DM, Lasater OE, Chari RS, Chen G, Fletcher BD. MR imaging differentiation of benign and malignant peripheral nerve sheath tumors: use of the target sign. Pediatr Radiol. 1997;27(2):124–9.
70. Levine E, Huntrakoon M, Wetzel LH. Malignant nerve-sheath neoplasms in neurofibromatosis: distinction from benign tumors by using imaging techniques. AJR Am J Roentgenol. 1987;149(5):1059–64.
71. Matsumine A, Kusuzaki K, Nakamura T, et al. Differentiation between neurofibromas and malignant peripheral nerve sheath tumors in neurofibromatosis 1 evaluated by MRI. J Cancer Res Clin Oncol. 2009;135(7):891–900.
72. Broski SM, Johnson GB, Howe BM, et al. Evaluation of (18)F-FDG PET and MRI in differentiating benign and malignant peripheral nerve sheath tumors. Skeletal Radiol. 2016;45(8):1097–105.
73. Karsy M, Guan J, Ravindra VM, Stilwill S, Mahan MA. Diagnostic quality of magnetic resonance imaging interpretation for peripheral nerve sheath tumors: can malignancy be determined? J Neurol Surg A Cent Eur Neurosurg. 2016;77(6):495–504.
74. Demehri S, Belzberg A, Blakeley J, Fayad LM. Conventional and functional MR imaging of peripheral nerve sheath tumors: initial experience. AJNR Am J Neuroradiol. 2014;35(8):1615–20.
75. Ahlawat S, Blakeley JO, Langmead S, Belzberg AJ, Fayad LM. Current status and recommendations for imaging in neurofibromatosis type 1, neurofibromatosis type 2, and schwannomatosis. Skeletal Radiol. 2020;49(2):199–219.
76. Ahlawat S, Blakeley JO, Rodriguez FJ, Fayad LM. Imaging biomarkers for malignant peripheral nerve sheath tumors in neurofibromatosis type 1. Neurology. 2019;93(11):e1076–84.
77. Chhabra A, Thakkar RS, Andreisek G, et al. Anatomic MR imaging and functional diffusion tensor imaging of peripheral nerve tumors and tumorlike conditions. AJNR Am J Neuroradiol. 2013;34(4):802–7.
78. Schmidt M, Kasprian G, Amann G, Duscher D, Aszmann OC. Diffusion tensor tractography for the surgical management of peripheral nerve sheath tumors. Neurosurg Focus. 2015;39(3):E17.
79. Benz MR, Czernin J, Dry SM, et al. Quantitative F18-fluorodeoxyglucose positron emission tomography accurately characterizes peripheral nerve sheath tumors as malignant or benign. Cancer. 2010;116(2):451–8.
80. Ferner RE, Golding JF, Smith M, et al. [18F]2-fluoro-2-deoxy-D-glucose positron emission tomography (FDG PET) as a diagnostic tool for neurofibromatosis 1 (NF1) associated malignant peripheral nerve sheath tumours (MPNSTs): a long-term clinical study. Ann Oncol. 2008;19(2):390–4.

81. Solomon SB, Semih Dogan A, Nicol TL, Campbell JN, Pomper MG. Positron emission tomography in the detection and management of sarcomatous transformation in neurofibromatosis. Clin Nucl Med. 2001;26(6):525–8.
82. Cardona S, Schwarzbach M, Hinz U, et al. Evaluation of F18-deoxyglucose positron emission tomography (FDG-PET) to assess the nature of neurogenic tumours. Eur J Surg Oncol. 2003;29(6):536–41.
83. Khiewvan B, Macapinlac HA, Lev D, et al. The value of (1)(8)F-FDG PET/CT in the management of malignant peripheral nerve sheath tumors. Eur J Nucl Med Mol Imaging. 2014;41(9):1756–66.
84. Telleman JA, Stellingwerff MD, Brekelmans GJ, Visser LH. Nerve ultrasound in neurofibromatosis type 1: a follow-up study. Clin Neurophysiol. 2018;129(2):354–9.
85. Nguyen R, Jett K, Harris GJ, Cai W, Friedman JM, Mautner VF. Benign whole body tumor volume is a risk factor for malignant peripheral nerve sheath tumors in neurofibromatosis type 1. J Neurooncol. 2014;116(2):307–13.
86. Levi AD, Ross AL, Cuartas E, Qadir R, Temple HT. The surgical management of symptomatic peripheral nerve sheath tumors. Neurosurgery. 2010;66(4):833–40.
87. Pianta M, Chock E, Schlicht S, McCombe D. Accuracy and complications of CT-guided core needle biopsy of peripheral nerve sheath tumours. Skeletal Radiol. 2015;44(9):1341–9.
88. Mazal AT, Ashikyan O, Cheng J, Le LQ, Chhabra A. Diffusion-weighted imaging and diffusion tensor imaging as adjuncts to conventional MRI for the diagnosis and management of peripheral nerve sheath tumors: current perspectives and future directions. Eur Radiol. 2019;29(8):4123–32.
89. Huang JH, Simon SL, Nagpal S, Nelson PT, Zager EL. Management of patients with schwannomatosis: report of six cases and review of the literature. Surg Neurol. 2004;62(4):353–61; discussion 361
90. Huang JH, Johnson VE, Zager EL. Tumors of the peripheral nerves and plexuses. Curr Treat Options Neurol. 2006;8(4):299–308.
91. Huang JH, Zhang J, Zager EL. Diagnosis and treatment options for nerve sheath tumors. Expert Rev Neurother. 2005;5(4):515–23.
92. Ranalli NJ, Huang JH, Lee EB, Zhang PJ, Siegelman ES, Zager EL. Hemangiomas of the brachial plexus: a case series. Neurosurgery. 2009;65(4 Suppl):A181–8.
93. Stone JJ, Puffer RC, Spinner RJ. Interfascicular resection of benign peripheral nerve sheath tumors. JBJS Essent Surg Tech. 2019;9(2):e18.
94. Stone JJ, Spinner RJ. Go for the gold: a "plane" and simple technique for resecting benign peripheral nerve sheath tumors. Oper Neurosurg (Hagerstown). 2020;18(1):60–8.
95. Russell SM. Preserve the nerve: microsurgical resection of peripheral nerve sheath tumors. Neurosurgery. 2007;61(3 Suppl):113–7; discussion 117–118
96. Baehring JM, Betensky RA, Batchelor TT. Malignant peripheral nerve sheath tumor: the clinical spectrum and outcome of treatment. Neurology. 2003;61(5):696–8.
97. Anghileri M, Miceli R, Fiore M, et al. Malignant peripheral nerve sheath tumors: prognostic factors and survival in a series of patients treated at a single institution. Cancer. 2006;107(5):1065–74.
98. Leaphart C, Rodeberg D. Pediatric surgical oncology: management of rhabdomyosarcoma. Surg Oncol. 2007;16(3):173–85.
99. Giuliani S, Marachelian A, Franklin A, Shimada H, Grikscheit T. Forearm skeletal muscle neuroblastoma in a child: a rare primary location. J Pediatr Hematol Oncol. 2013;35(1):61–3.
100. Landy H, Feun L, Markoe A, et al. Extended remission of a recurrent median nerve malignant peripheral nerve sheath tumor after multimodal treatment. Case report. J Neurosurg. 2005;103(4):760–3.
101. Guha D, Davidson B, Nadi M, et al. Management of peripheral nerve sheath tumors: 17 years of experience at Toronto Western Hospital. J Neurosurg. 2018;128(4):1226–34.
102. Kim DH, Murovic JA, Tiel RL, Moes G, Kline DG. A series of 397 peripheral neural sheath tumors: 30-year experience at Louisiana State University Health Sciences Center. J Neurosurg. 2005;102(2):246–55.
103. Vetrano IG, Lucarella F, Dalolio M, et al. The importance of predicting factors in the surgical outcome of peripheral nerve sheath tumors. J Neurol Surg A Cent Eur Neurosurg. 2014;75(2):104–9.
104. Artico M, Cervoni L, Wierzbicki V, D'Andrea V, Nucci F. Benign neural sheath tumours of major nerves: characteristics in 119 surgical cases. Acta Neurochir. 1997;139(12):1108–16.
105. Requena L, Sangueza OP. Benign neoplasms with neural differentiation: a review. Am J Dermatopathol. 1995;17(1):75–96.
106. deCou JM, Rao BN, Parham DM, et al. Malignant peripheral nerve sheath tumors: the St. Jude Children's Research Hospital experience. Ann Surg Oncol. 1995;2(6):524–9.
107. An HY, Hong KT, Kang HJ, et al. Malignant peripheral nerve sheath tumor in children: a single-institute retrospective analysis. Pediatr Hematol Oncol. 2017;34(8):468–77.
108. Farid M, Demicco EG, Garcia R, et al. Malignant peripheral nerve sheath tumors. Oncologist. 2014;19(2):193–201.
109. Valentin T, Le Cesne A, Ray-Coquard I, et al. Management and prognosis of malignant peripheral nerve sheath tumors: the experience of the French Sarcoma Group (GSF-GETO). Eur J Cancer. 2016;56:77–84.
110. Zou C, Smith KD, Liu J, et al. Clinical, pathological, and molecular variables predictive of malignant peripheral nerve sheath tumor outcome. Ann Surg. 2009;249(6):1014–22.
111. Kolberg M, Holand M, Agesen TH, et al. Survival meta-analyses for >1800 malignant peripheral nerve

sheath tumor patients with and without neurofibromatosis type 1. Neuro Oncol. 2013;15(2):135–47.
112. Kahn J, Gillespie A, Tsokos M, et al. Radiation therapy in management of sporadic and neurofibromatosis type 1-associated malignant peripheral nerve sheath tumors. Front Oncol. 2014;4:324.
113. Ferner RE, Gutmann DH. International consensus statement on malignant peripheral nerve sheath tumors in neurofibromatosis. Cancer Res. 2002;62(5):1573–7.
114. Sordillo PP, Helson L, Hajdu SI, et al. Malignant schwannoma—clinical characteristics, survival, and response to therapy. Cancer. 1981;47(10):2503–9.
115. Grobmyer SR, Reith JD, Shahlaee A, Bush CH, Hochwald SN. Malignant peripheral nerve sheath tumor: molecular pathogenesis and current management considerations. J Surg Oncol. 2008;97(4):340–9.
116. Alvarado CS, London WB, Look AT, et al. Natural history and biology of stage A neuroblastoma: a Pediatric Oncology Group Study. J Pediatr Hematol Oncol. 2000;22(3):197–205.
117. De Bernardi B, Mosseri V, Rubie H, et al. Treatment of localised resectable neuroblastoma. Results of the LNESG1 study by the SIOP Europe Neuroblastoma Group. Br J Cancer. 2008;99(7):1027–33.
118. Strother DR, London WB, Schmidt ML, et al. Outcome after surgery alone or with restricted use of chemotherapy for patients with low-risk neuroblastoma: results of Children's Oncology Group study P9641. J Clin Oncol. 2012;30(15):1842–8.
119. Baker DL, Schmidt ML, Cohn SL, et al. Outcome after reduced chemotherapy for intermediate-risk neuroblastoma. N Engl J Med. 2010;363(14):1313–23.
120. Yanik GA, Parisi MT, Shulkin BL, et al. Semiquantitative mIBG scoring as a prognostic indicator in patients with stage 4 neuroblastoma: a report from the Children's Oncology Group. J Nucl Med. 2013;54(4):541–8.
121. Simon T, Haberle B, Hero B, von Schweinitz D, Berthold F. Role of surgery in the treatment of patients with stage 4 neuroblastoma age 18 months or older at diagnosis. J Clin Oncol. 2013;31(6):752–8.
122. Du L, Liu L, Zhang C, et al. Role of surgery in the treatment of patients with high-risk neuroblastoma who have a poor response to induction chemotherapy. J Pediatr Surg. 2014;49(4):528–33.
123. Adkins ES, Sawin R, Gerbing RB, London WB, Matthay KK, Haase GM. Efficacy of complete resection for high-risk neuroblastoma: a Children's Cancer Group study. J Pediatr Surg. 2004;39(6):931–6.
124. Modak S, Cheung NK. Neuroblastoma: therapeutic strategies for a clinical enigma. Cancer Treat Rev. 2010;36(4):307–17.
125. Meza JL, Anderson J, Pappo AS, Meyer WH, Children's Oncology Group. Analysis of prognostic factors in patients with nonmetastatic rhabdomyosarcoma treated on intergroup rhabdomyosarcoma studies III and IV: the Children's Oncology Group. J Clin Oncol. 2006;24(24):3844–51.
126. Stevens MC, Rey A, Bouvet N, et al. Treatment of nonmetastatic rhabdomyosarcoma in childhood and adolescence: third study of the International Society of Paediatric Oncology—SIOP malignant mesenchymal tumor 89. J Clin Oncol. 2005;23(12):2618–28.
127. Date R, Muramatsu K, Ihara K, Taguchi T. Advantages of intra-capsular micro-enucleation of schwannoma arising from extremities. Acta Neurochir. 2012;154(1):173–8; discussion 178

Part III

Peripheral Nerve Tumors in Genetic Diseases

24 Epidemiology of Genetic Diseases with Peripheral Nerve Tumors

Robert B. Kim and Mark A. Mahan

24.1 Introduction

Neoplasms arising from the peripheral nerve sheath may develop sporadically, but these peripheral nerve sheath tumors (PNSTs) are frequently associated with underlying genetic diseases. Depending on the genetic disease involved, there is a wide variability in the phenotypic manifestation of the PNST. For example, plexiform neurofibromas are disease defining for neurofibromatosis type 1, whereas disproportionate pain is a hallmark feature of schwannomatosis. Furthermore, PNSTs in association with certain genetic diseases have a greater risk of malignancy, which tends to have a poor prognosis and limited treatment options after metastasis. Therefore, greater efforts are being made to complete epidemiologic and genetic studies to better characterize these genetic diseases that predispose to PNST formation. In this chapter, we describe the epidemiology of genetic diseases that are associated with a high predisposition to peripheral nerve tumors; these include neurofibromatosis type 1 (NF1), neurofibromatosis type 2 (NF2), schwannomatosis, and rarely Carney complex (CNC) and multiple endocrine neoplasia type 2B (MEN 2B)—endocrinopathies with a tendency for peripheral nerve tumor development.

R. B. Kim · M. A. Mahan (✉)
Department of Neurosurgery, Clinical Neurosciences Center, University of Utah, Salt Lake City, UT, USA
e-mail: neuropubs@hsc.utah.edu

24.2 Neurofibromatosis 1

24.2.1 Overview

NF1 is an inherited, complex genetic disorder that afflicts approximately 1/2500–1/3000 individuals worldwide, regardless of sex, race, or ethnicity [1, 2]. The relatively high prevalence of NF1 is recognized by the National Institutes of Health (NIH), which has set forth specific diagnostic criteria. The NIH criteria indicate that the diagnosis for NF1 consists of specific features (Table 24.1) [3]. Its pattern of inheritance is autosomal dominant, in which a germline mutation in the *NF1* tumor suppressor gene on chromosome 17q results in loss of an important tumor suppressor protein, called neurofibromin. The loss of neurofibromin introduces dysregulation in the Ras proto-oncogenic pathway, ultimately leading to the development of benign and malignant tumors that affect the central and peripheral nervous systems [4]. Patients with NF1 develop a wide array of tumors, including PNSTs, optic and brainstem gliomas, astrocytomas, and glioblastoma. They can also develop non-nervous system tumors, particularly gastrointestinal stromal tumors, pheochromocytomas, breast cancers, and leukemias, among others.

F. Guedes et al. (eds.), *Diagnostic Assessment and Treatment of Peripheral Nerve Tumors*,
https://doi.org/10.1007/978-3-030-77633-6_24

Of all the known genetic disorders, NF1 patients have the highest predisposition to the development of PNSTs including neurofibromas, plexiform neurofibromas, and malignant peripheral nerve sheath tumors (MPNSTs) [5]. The penetrance of the disease reaches nearly 100% (5); however, there is extreme variability in phenotypical expression of NF1, making this an epidemiologically challenging disease to classify. The disease typically causes complications in the later stages of life, as the disease burden accumulates; this results in significant reduction in life expectancy, with the malignancy being the largest factor in reducing overall longevity in patients with NF1 [6].

Despite the known inheritance pattern of NF1, approximately 50% of affected individuals have sporadic mutations of the *NF1* gene [7]. Certain mutations lead to more devastating phenotypic features than others, which partly explain the disease's extreme variability. There is a subset of NF1 patients who harbor microdeletions of chromosome that result in the loss of the entire *NF1* locus and adjacent sequences. This subset comprises 5–10% of the total NF1 patients. These carriers of microdeletions demonstrate more severe phenotypic expression of the disease, characterized by earlier and more numerous distributions of neurofibromas and a higher incidence of MPNSTs [8, 9].

The risk factors for sporadic NF1 are unclear. Older paternal age has been implicated as a possible risk factor for sporadic NF1 [10, 11], as it has been historically associated with a number of autosomal dominant disorders such as achondroplasia [12], Marfan syndrome [13], and osteogenesis imperfecta [14]. Furthermore, some evidence specifically associates advanced paternal, but not maternal, age as a risk factor for the occurrence of sporadic NF1 [10]. Although these data show statistical association, the effect size is not large nor clearly causative.

Table 24.1 NIH-consensus NF1 diagnostic criteria

Two or more of the following:	
1.	Six or more café-au-lait spots >5 mm in diameter in children or >15 mm in individuals after puberty
2.	Two or more neurofibromas or one plexiform neurofibroma
3.	Axillary or inguinal freckling
4.	Optic pathway glioma
5.	Two or more Lisch nodules (iris hamartomas)
6.	Osseous lesions such as sphenoid dysplasia or thinning of long bones
7.	Any first-degree relative with NF1 by the above criteria

24.2.2 Peripheral Nerve Sheath Tumors in NF1

According to the World Health Organization (WHO) classification, the common benign PNSTs that develop in the setting of NF1 include those involving the skin, such as localized or diffuse cutaneous neurofibromas (Fig. 24.1), or those involving nerves, such as localized intraneural and plexiform neurofibromas [15].

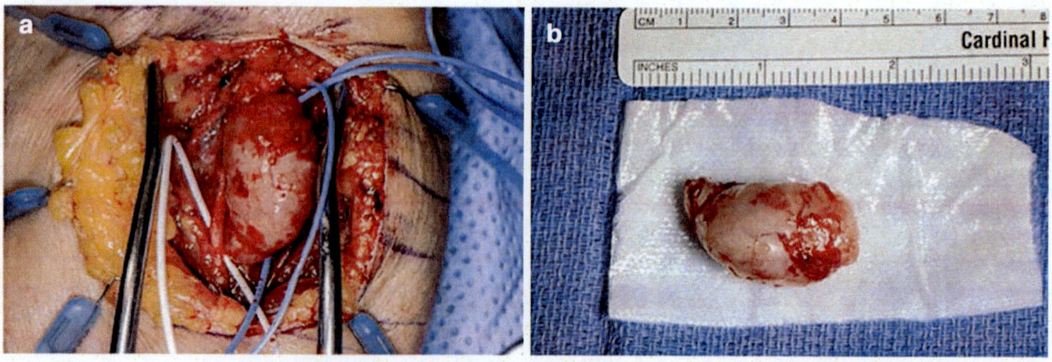

Fig. 24.1 Intraoperative photographs of a sporadic neurofibroma of the radial nerve at the level of supinator, presenting as finger drop. (Used with the permission of the Department of Neurosurgery, University of Utah). (**a**) Intraoperative photo. (**b**) Gross surgical specimen

Histologically, the cellular components of the cutaneous, intraneural, and plexiform neurofibromas are similar, containing neoplastic Schwann cells and non-neoplastic fibroblasts, mast cells, macrophages, endothelial cells, pericytes, and perineural cells [16–19]. Unlike cutaneous neurofibromas, which predominantly involve the skin and rarely internal organs, intraneural neurofibromas are found in peripheral nerve fascicles and even in a large nerve plexus [5]. Plexiform neurofibromas are a unique form of intraneural neurofibroma, which affect numerous or all fascicles of a nerve, producing massive enlargement of the nerve in a "cluster of grapes"-like appearance (Fig. 24.2). Plexiform neurofibromas are found in approximately 30–50% of individuals with NF1 and have been shown to enlarge most rapidly during the first decade of life (7). These tumors can be quite destructive as they can propagate into surrounding structures, including nerve roots and vertebral bony elements, causing severe pain and disability. Because plexiform neurofibromas affect the majority, if not all, of the nerve, complete surgical resection is impossible without removing the entirety of the nerve. Therefore, surgery is reserved for symptomatic or large tumors within the plexiform lesion. Moreover, plexiform neurofibromas are associated with an increased risk for the development of MPNSTs.

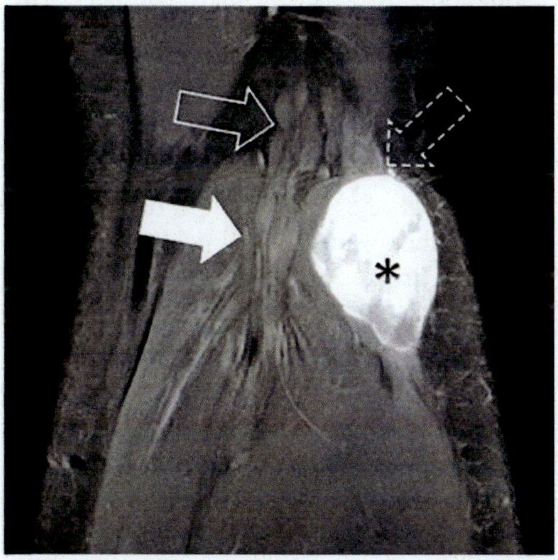

Fig. 24.2 Magnetic resonance imaging of the right knee obtained in a 14-year-old girl with NF1 showing a large 2.7 × 2.7 × 3.7 cm intraneural neurofibroma (asterisk) in association with a plexiform neurofibroma of the sciatic (open arrow), tibial (solid arrow), and common fibular nerves (dashed arrow). (Used with the permission of the Department of Neurosurgery, University of Utah)

MPNSTs, previously known as neurofibrosarcomas or neurogenic sarcomas, are high-grade Schwann cell-derived tumors with a high propensity for metastasis (Fig. 24.3). MPNSTs are the only primary cancer of peripheral nerves and are the leading cause of death in individuals with NF1 [20]. In the general population, they represent about 3–10% of all sarcomas, with a prevalence of 0.001% [21]; however, there is an astounding difference in their incidence (0.1%) and prevalence (8–13%) in individuals with NF1 [22]. Patients with microdeletions are at an even greater risk for the development of MPNSTs, with about 16–26% developing MPNSTs in their lifetime (9). MPNSTs can arise anywhere in the body, but there is a ~20-fold greater risk of malignant transformation in areas of existing plexiform neurofibroma [23]. However, cutaneous plexiform lesions are unlikely to be associated with MPNSTs, whereas it is the deeply located masses that are more commonly associated with MPNSTs [22]. Patients with NF1 tend to have MPNSTs diagnosed at an earlier age (median age at diagnosis of MPNST in NF1 patients was 26 years, compared with 62 years in patients with sporadic MPNST) and tend to have a worse survival rate (5-year survival from diagnosis was 21% for NF1 patients with MPNST, compared with 42% for sporadic cases of MPNST) [22].

24.3 Neurofibromatosis 2

24.3.1 Overview

NF2 is an autosomal dominant disorder that affects 1/33,000–1/40,000 births worldwide with an overall prevalence of 1 in 100,000 [24]. It is caused by mutations on the *NF2* tumor suppressor gene located on chromosome 22, and it is

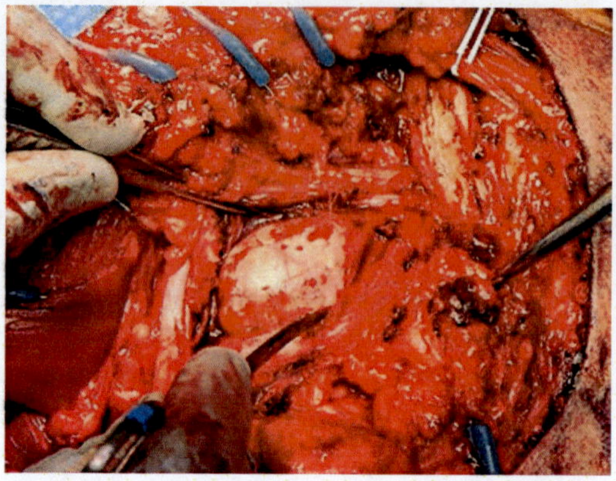

Fig. 24.3 Intraoperative photograph showing a malignant peripheral nerve sheath tumor associated with a plexiform neurofibroma involving the medial cord of the brachial plexus in a patient with NF1. (Used with the permission of the Department of Neurosurgery, University of Utah)

Table 24.2 Manchester criteria for NF2 (Evans et al. 1992)

a.	Bilateral vestibular schwannoma
OR	
b.	NF2 in first-degree relative PLUS unilateral vestibular schwannoma or any two of the following: neurofibroma, meningioma, glioma, schwannoma, and posterior subcapsular lens opacity
OR	
c.	Unilateral vestibular schwannoma PLUS any two of the following: neurofibroma, glioma, schwannoma, and posterior subcapsular lens opacity
OR	
d.	Two or more meningiomas PLUS unilateral vestibular schwannoma or any two of the following: neurofibroma, glioma, schwannoma, or cataract

estimated that over 50% of the mutations arise de novo [25]. The product of the *NF2 gene* is called Merlin or schwannomin. Merlin plays a critical role in contact-dependent inhibition [26]. Affected individuals are prone to a variety of central and peripheral nerve neoplasms, including vestibular schwannoma (usually bilateral), multiple meningiomas, ependymoma, as well as cutaneous (hairy pigmented plaque) and retinal hamartomas [27]. Thus, NF2 is a clinicopathologically and genetically distinct disease from NF1. A set of diagnostic criteria, named the Manchester criteria [25], define the diagnosis of NF2 (Table 24.2).

The penetrance of NF2 is nearly 100% by the age of 60 years [28]; however, there is a great deal of variability in how this disease manifests, which often determines the morbidity associated with the disease [29]. The average age at diagnosis of the first tumor is 18–24 years, with virtually all affected individuals developing bilateral vestibular schwannoma by age 30 [30]. A majority of adult patients with NF2 initially present with hearing loss, which often starts unilaterally and later progresses to involve bilateral hearing, as well as tinnitus and balance dysfunction [31]. In the pediatric population, however, the initial presentation usually does not involve cranial nerve VIII. Rather, a non-vestibulocochlear nerve tumor is the typical presentation, which includes intracranial meningiomas, spinal tumors, or cutaneous tumors [32]. Mononeuropathy that affects the oculomotor nerve, facial nerve, or hand or foot is also a common initial finding of pediatric-onset NF2.

Unlike those with NF1, however, individuals with NF2 develop cutaneous lesions (café-au-lait spots or cutaneous lesions) at a lesser degree, rendering less reliably the diagnosis of this disease by physical examination. In addition, NF2 mosaicism adds even more variability to the clinical manifestation such that patients may present with unilateral vestibular schwannoma with or without other NF2 phenotypes. NF2 mosaicism may occur sporadically in up to 30% of the patients [33, 34], thus warranting particular attention to follow up studies in patients without family history. The severity of the disease may be determined by the type of mutation affecting the *NF2* gene, in which nonsense or frameshift mutation results in a more severe phenotype compared with large deletions that result in complete loss of Merlin or retention of Merlin [35, 36].

24.3.2 Vestibular Schwannomas

The development of bilateral vestibular schwannomas is a hallmark of NF2. These are found in up to 95% of the adult NF2 patients [30, 37] and are usually associated with significant morbidity for the patients. Unlike sporadic vestibular schwannomas, which are typically unilateral and have predilection for the inferior vestibular nerve, NF2-associated vestibular schwannomas are usually bilateral (except NF2 mosaicism) and can affect the superior or inferior vestibular branches equally [38]. Bilateral vestibular schwannomas can arise de novo without any underlying NF2 mutation or mosaicism. In one series, up to 75% of the patients over the age of 50 years and up to 50% of the patients over the age of 70 years presented with bilateral vestibular schwannomas without any underlying mutations [39]. Hearing loss is frequent, and the degree of the hearing loss varies among affected individuals and even between the ears of an affected individual [40]. In addition, tumor size and tumor growth rate are not predictive of hearing loss [40]. Early surgical management of NF2-related vestibular schwannomas that are less than 3 cm in diameter has demonstrated a hearing preservation rate of 30–65% with relatively good facial nerve preservation of 75–92% [41]. Alternatively, stereotactic radiosurgery is also well-established as a viable treatment option, with hearing preservation up to 57% and facial nerve preservation up to 100% [42].

24.3.3 Peripheral Nerve Schwannomas

Schwannomas associated with NF2 can arise from other cranial nerves (III–VII, IX–XII) as well as spinal nerves and peripheral nerves. Upper cranial nerves are more commonly involved than lower cranial nerves, with up to 51% of patients having schwannomas in cranial nerves III, V, and VII [41, 43]. Spinal nerve root involvement is usually extensive, and multiple schwannomas are frequently found along the nerve roots. These account for almost 90% of the extramedullary spine tumors [43]. Peripheral nerve schwannomas can arise from virtually any peripheral nerve, and they usually manifest as nodular schwannomas that can cause peripheral neuropathies [30]. PNSTs may be found in up to 70% of the patients with NF2 [44].

24.3.4 Malignant Peripheral Nerve Sheath Tumor in NF2

Interestingly, NF2 does not seem to be a risk factor for the development of malignancy in peripheral nerve schwannomas. In one of the largest series of malignant peripheral nerve schwannomas, only one case was associated with presumed NF2 [45]. However, malignant transformation of vestibular schwannomas after radiosurgery has been reported [46].

24.4 Schwannomatosis

24.4.1 Overview

Schwannomatosis is another genetic syndrome with a high propensity toward the development of multiple schwannomas. Many of its clinical features overlap with NF2; thus it is characterized as a third form of neurofibromatosis. One distinctive feature of schwannomatosis is that it spares the vestibular nerve. Because of the similarities between schwannomatosis and NF2 and the lack of reliable genetic testing, the incidence and prevalence of schwannomatosis are not well established but are presumed to be similar to those of NF2 [47].

Pain and a palpable mass are common presenting symptoms and signs of schwannomatosis [48]. Germline mutations or deletions in *SMARCB1* (also called *hSNF5*, *INI1*, and *BAF47*), a tumor suppressor gene located on chromosome 22q, have been implicated as causes of schwannomatosis. Most cases are sporadic, although familial forms can have *SMARCB1* mutations in about 40–50% of cases [49]. This suggests that other loci may be involved in its tumorigenesis. Genetic analysis of the tumor specimen from patients with schwannomatosis revealed the presence of concomitant somatic mutation in *NF2* gene in addition to mutations in *SMARCB1*, suggesting the multiple-hit theory [50]. Pain out of proportion to tumor size or burden is a classic feature in schwannomatosis and may have a genetic relationship, especially to LZTR-1 mutation-associated schwannomatosis [51].

The diagnostic criteria have yet to be standardized for schwannomatosis because of its relatively recent characterization. Various diagnostic modalities have been proposed, including clinical, radiographic, and molecular characterization (Table 24.3) [52, 53]. Age appears to be a defining element, as most individuals with NF2 manifest with bilateral vestibular schwannoma by age 30 [30]. Therefore, the lack of bilateral (or unilateral in the case of NF2 mosaicism) vestibular schwannoma along with the presence of multiple biopsy-proven schwannomas after that age can effectively lead to the diagnosis of schwannomatosis.

There is a variant of schwannomatosis known as segmental schwannomatosis, which is diagnosed when schwannomas are restricted to one extremity. Segmental schwannomatosis was previously thought to be caused by genetic mosaicism, but segmental schwannomatosis may include germline mutations [54] and may be associated with subtle changes in the nerves of the limbs unaffected by schwannomas.

24.4.2 Peripheral Nerve Schwannomas

Schwannoma is the predominant tumor type for both NF2 and schwannomatosis; however, there are some clinical differences that distinguish the two. Schwannomas arising in association with schwannomatosis commonly involve the peripheral nerves, the spinal nerves, and rarely the trigeminal nerve (Figs. 24.4 and 24.5) [48]. NF2-associated schwannomas usually affect individuals in early childhood, whereas in schwannomatosis, the peak age at presentation is usually between the ages of 30 and 60 years [55]. The histologic features of the schwannoma are essentially identical between the two syndromes [25].

Table 24.3 Baser criteria for schwannomatosis (Baser et al.)

Definitive schwannomatosis	Possible schwannomatosis
Age >30 years AND ≥2 nondermal schwannomas, at least one with histologic confirmation	Age <30 or >45 years AND ≥2 nondermal schwannomas, at least one with histologic confirmation
Schwannoma (pathologically confirmed) AND first-degree relative with above criteria	Evidence of radiographic schwannoma AND first-degree relative with above criteria
Must not have NF2 criteria, NF2 first-degree relative, or NF2 germline mutation	Must not have NF2 criteria, NF2 first-degree relative, or NF2 germline mutation

24.4.3 Malignant Peripheral Nerve Sheath Tumor in Schwannomatosis

MPNSTs are usually associated with NF1, but they have been observed less frequently in other PNST predisposition syndromes. In a review by Evans et al. [22], three patients who were harboring schwannomatosis were also shown to have MPNSTs. Of interest, two of the patients had known family history of *SMARCB1* mutation.

24.5 Other Genetic Syndromes

24.5.1 Carney Complex

First described by Dr. J. Aidan Carney in 1985 as "the complex of myxomas, spotty pigmentation, and endocrine overactivity," CNC is a rare multiple neoplasia syndrome that also displays a high predisposition for peripheral nerve tumors [56]. It is inherited in an autosomal dominant pattern, with more than half of the cases being familial [57]. Because of its rarity, the incidence and prevalence of the disease are unknown, although in the largest series published to date, 63% of the patients were females and 37% were males [58]. To date, over 750 cases have been reported worldwide and compiled by the NIH–Mayo Clinic and Cochin Hospital in France [57, 59, 60].

CNC patients carry inactivating mutation in *PRKAR1A*, which is located on chromosome 17 and encodes the protein kinase A subunit that plays a critical role in cAMP signaling pathway

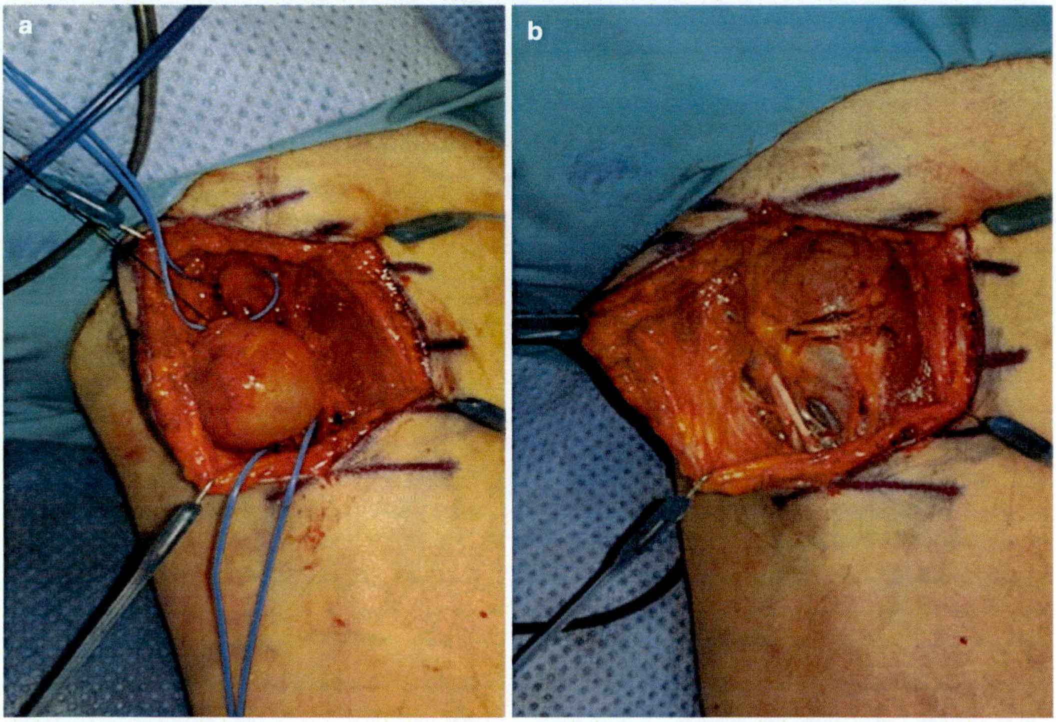

Fig. 24.4 Intraoperative photographs of a sporadic schwannoma of the proximal median nerve taken before (**a**) and after (**b**) resection. (Used with the permission of the Department of Neurosurgery, University of Utah)

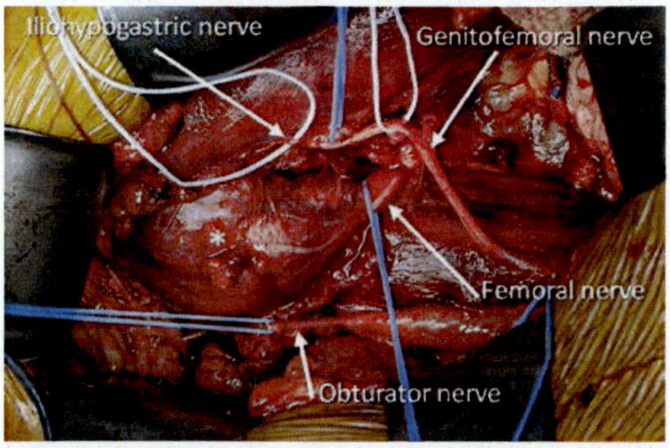

Fig. 24.5 Intraoperative photograph showing a sporadic schwannoma (asterisk) of the femoral nerve. The patient presented with quadriceps atrophy due to compression at the inguinal ligament. (Used with the permission of the Department of Neurosurgery, University of Utah)

[57]. Derangement of this molecular pathway leads to the development of multiple neoplasms, including myxoid neurofibromas and psammomatous melanocytic schwannomas [61]. Psammomatous melanocytic schwannoma most frequently involves the gastrointestinal tract and paraspinal sympathetic chain and is characterized by dark pigmentation (attributed by melanin) and calcifications [62]. Schwannomas found in CNC are histologically and molecularly distinct from those found in neurofibromatosis, such that psammomatous melanocytic schwannoma has a relatively high tendency for metastasis [63, 64].

24.5.2 Multiple Endocrine Neoplasia 2B

As the name implies, patients with MEN 2B have a high propensity for developing multiple neoplasms originating in various hormone-secreting organs, including medullary thyroid carcinoma, pheochromocytoma, and parathyroid hyperplasia. MEN 2B is also implicated in the development of certain peripheral nerve tumors such as mucosal neuromas and intestinal ganglioneuromatosis, originating from autonomic nervous system components [5], that are characterized by tortuous and abnormal enlargement of nerves and myenteric plexuses in the intestine, respectively.

MEN 2B is caused by activating mutations in the *RET* proto-oncogene located on chromosome 10, which encodes a membrane-bound tyrosine kinase that drives cellular proliferation. The incidence and prevalence of this disease are not well established because of its extreme rarity. It is estimated that MEN 2B has an incidence of about 1.4–2.6 per one million live births per year and prevalence of about 0.9–1.65 per million [65, 66].

24.6 Conclusion

Peripheral nerve tumors may arise de novo, by spontaneous mutations involving a variety of genetic syndromes; however, there is a strong association between inherited genetic syndrome and the development of peripheral nerve tumors. The neurofibromatosis group of diseases (NF1, NF2, schwannomatosis) is predominantly responsible for the majority of inherited peripheral nerve tumors. Rarely, certain neoplastic syndromes such as Carney complex or MEN 2B can also predispose individuals toward developing peripheral nerve tumors.

References

1. Evans DG, Howard E, Giblin C, et al. Birth incidence and prevalence of tumor-prone syndromes: estimates from a UK family genetic register service. Am J Med Genet A. 2010;152A(2):327–32.
2. Huson SM, Compston DA, Clark P, Harper PS. A genetic study of von Recklinghausen neurofibromatosis in south east Wales. I. Prevalence, fitness, mutation rate, and effect of parental transmission on severity. J Med Genet. 1989;26(11):704–11.
3. National Institutes of Health Consensus Development Conference statement: neurofibromatosis. Bethesda, Md., USA, July 13–15, 1987. Neurofibromatosis. 1988;1(3):172–178.
4. Cichowski K, Jacks T. NF1 tumor suppressor gene function: narrowing the GAP. Cell. 2001;104(4):593–604.
5. Rodriguez FJ, Stratakis CA, Evans DG. Genetic predisposition to peripheral nerve neoplasia: diagnostic criteria and pathogenesis of neurofibromatoses, Carney complex, and related syndromes. Acta Neuropathol. 2012;123(3):349–67.
6. Rasmussen SA, Yang Q, Friedman JM. Mortality in neurofibromatosis 1: an analysis using U.S. death certificates. Am J Hum Genet. 2001;68(5):1110–8.
7. Hirbe AC, Gutmann DH. Neurofibromatosis type 1: a multidisciplinary approach to care. Lancet Neurol. 2014;13(8):834–43.
8. Pasmant E, Sabbagh A, Spurlock G, et al. NF1 microdeletions in neurofibromatosis type 1: from genotype to phenotype. Hum Mutat. 2010;31(6):E1506–18.
9. De Raedt T, Brems H, Wolkenstein P, et al. Elevated risk for MPNST in NF1 microdeletion patients. Am J Hum Genet. 2003;72(5):1288–92.
10. Dubov T, Toledano-Alhadef H, Bokstein F, Constantini S, Ben-Shachar S. The effect of parental age on the presence of de novo mutations—lessons from neurofibromatosis type I. Mol Genet Genomic Med. 2016;4(4):480–6.
11. Snajderova M, Riccardi VM, Petrak B, et al. The importance of advanced parental age in the origin of neurofibromatosis type 1. Am J Med Genet A. 2012;158A(3):519–23.
12. Penrose LS. Parental age in acondroplasia and mongolism. Am J Hum Genet. 1957;9(3):167–9.
13. Murdoch JL, Walker BA, McKusick VA. Parental age effects on the occurrence of new mutations for the Marfan syndrome. Ann Hum Genet. 1972;35(3):331–6.
14. Carothers AD, McAllion SJ, Paterson CR. Risk of dominant mutation in older fathers: evidence from osteogenesis imperfecta. J Med Genet. 1986;23(3):227–30.
15. Louis DN, Ohgaki H, Wiestler OD, et al. The 2007 WHO classification of tumours of the central nervous system. Acta Neuropathol. 2007;114(2):97–109.
16. Wu M, Wallace MR, Muir D. Tumorigenic properties of neurofibromin-deficient Schwann cells in culture and as syngrafts in Nf1 knockout mice. J Neurosci Res. 2005;82(3):357–67.
17. Rutkowski JL, Wu K, Gutmann DH, Boyer PJ, Legius E. Genetic and cellular defects contributing to benign tumor formation in neurofibromatosis type 1. Hum Mol Genet. 2000;9(7):1059–66.
18. Le LQ, Parada LF. Tumor microenvironment and neurofibromatosis type I: connecting the GAPs. Oncogene. 2007;26(32):4609–16.
19. Yang FC, Ingram DA, Chen S, et al. Neurofibromin-deficient Schwann cells secrete a potent migratory stimulus for Nf1+/− mast cells. J Clin Invest. 2003;112(12):1851–61.
20. Zou C, Smith KD, Liu J, et al. Clinical, pathological, and molecular variables predictive of malignant peripheral nerve sheath tumor outcome. Ann Surg. 2009;249(6):1014–22.
21. Ducatman BS, Scheithauer BW, Piepgras DG, Reiman HM, Ilstrup DM. Malignant peripheral nerve sheath tumors. A clinicopathologic study of 120 cases. Cancer. 1986;57(10):2006–21.

22. Evans DG, Baser ME, McGaughran J, Sharif S, Howard E, Moran A. Malignant peripheral nerve sheath tumours in neurofibromatosis 1. J Med Genet. 2002;39(5):311–4.
23. Tucker T, Wolkenstein P, Revuz J, Zeller J, Friedman JM. Association between benign and malignant peripheral nerve sheath tumors in NF1. Neurology. 2005;65(2):205–11.
24. Evans DG, Huson SM, Donnai D, et al. A genetic study of type 2 neurofibromatosis in the United Kingdom. I. Prevalence, mutation rate, fitness, and confirmation of maternal transmission effect on severity. J Med Genet. 1992;29(12):841–6.
25. Kresak JL, Walsh M. Neurofibromatosis: a review of NF1, NF2, and Schwannomatosis. J Pediatr Genet. 2016;5(2):98–104.
26. Curto M, McClatchey AI. Nf2/Merlin: a coordinator of receptor signalling and intercellular contact. Br J Cancer. 2008;98(2):256–62.
27. Horvath A, Boikos S, Giatzakis C, et al. A genome-wide scan identifies mutations in the gene encoding phosphodiesterase 11A4 (PDE11A) in individuals with adrenocortical hyperplasia. Nat Genet. 2006;38(7):794–800.
28. Evans DG, Baser ME, O'Reilly B, et al. Management of the patient and family with neurofibromatosis 2: a consensus conference statement. Br J Neurosurg. 2005;19(1):5–12.
29. Evans DG, Moran A, King A, Saeed S, Gurusinghe N, Ramsden R. Incidence of vestibular schwannoma and neurofibromatosis 2 in the North West of England over a 10-year period: higher incidence than previously thought. Otol Neurotol. 2005;26(1):93–7.
30. Evans DG, Huson SM, Donnai D, et al. A clinical study of type 2 neurofibromatosis. Q J Med. 1992;84(304):603–18.
31. Evans DG, Sainio M, Baser ME. Neurofibromatosis type 2. J Med Genet. 2000;37(12):897–904.
32. Kanter WR, Eldridge R, Fabricant R, Allen JC, Koerber T. Central neurofibromatosis with bilateral acoustic neuroma: genetic, clinical and biochemical distinctions from peripheral neurofibromatosis. Neurology. 1980;30(8):851–9.
33. Kluwe L, Mautner V, Heinrich B, et al. Molecular study of frequency of mosaicism in neurofibromatosis 2 patients with bilateral vestibular schwannomas. J Med Genet. 2003;40(2):109–14.
34. Moyhuddin A, Baser ME, Watson C, et al. Somatic mosaicism in neurofibromatosis 2: prevalence and risk of disease transmission to offspring. J Med Genet. 2003;40(6):459–63.
35. Merel P, Hoang-Xuan K, Sanson M, et al. Screening for germ-line mutations in the NF2 gene. Genes Chromosomes Cancer. 1995;12(2):117–27.
36. Selvanathan SK, Shenton A, Ferner R, et al. Further genotype—phenotype correlations in neurofibromatosis 2. Clin Genet. 2010;77(2):163–70.
37. Parry DM, Eldridge R, Kaiser-Kupfer MI, Bouzas EA, Pikus A, Patronas N. Neurofibromatosis 2 (NF2): clinical characteristics of 63 affected individuals and clinical evidence for heterogeneity. Am J Med Genet. 1994;52(4):450–61.
38. Stivaros SM, Stemmer-Rachamimov AO, Alston R, et al. Multiple synchronous sites of origin of vestibular schwannomas in neurofibromatosis type 2. J Med Genet. 2015;52(8):557–62.
39. Evans DG, Freeman S, Gokhale C, et al. Bilateral vestibular schwannomas in older patients: NF2 or chance? J Med Genet. 2015;52(6):422–4.
40. Masuda A, Fisher LM, Oppenheimer ML, Iqbal Z, Slattery WH. Hearing changes after diagnosis in neurofibromatosis type 2. Otol Neurotol. 2004;25(2):150–4.
41. Samii M, Matthies C, Tatagiba M. Management of vestibular schwannomas (acoustic neuromas): auditory and facial nerve function after resection of 120 vestibular schwannomas in patients with neurofibromatosis 2. Neurosurgery. 1997;40(4):696–705; discussion 705–796.
42. Kida Y, Kobayashi T, Tanaka T, Mori Y. Radiosurgery for bilateral neurinomas associated with neurofibromatosis type 2. Surg Neurol. 2000;53(4):383–9; discussion 389–390.
43. Mautner VF, Lindenau M, Baser ME, et al. The neuroimaging and clinical spectrum of neurofibromatosis 2. Neurosurgery. 1996;38(5):880–5; discussion 885–886.
44. Hilton DA, Hanemann CO. Schwannomas and their pathogenesis. Brain Pathol. 2014;24(3):205–20.
45. Scheithauer BW, Erdogan S, Rodriguez FJ, Burger PC, Woodruff JM, Kros JM, et al. Malignant peripheral nerve sheath tumors of cranial nerves and intracranial contents: a clinicopathologic study of 17 cases. Am J Surg Pathol [Internet]. 2009;33(3).
46. Shin M, Ueki K, Kurita H, Kirino T. Malignant transformation of a vestibular schwannoma after gamma knife radiosurgery. Lancet. 2002;360(9329):309–10.
47. Antinheimo J, Sankila R, Carpen O, Pukkala E, Sainio M, Jaaskelainen J. Population-based analysis of sporadic and type 2 neurofibromatosis-associated meningiomas and schwannomas. Neurology. 2000;54(1):71–6.
48. Merker VL, Esparza S, Smith MJ, Stemmer-Rachamimov A, Plotkin SR. Clinical features of schwannomatosis: a retrospective analysis of 87 patients. Oncologist. 2012;17(10):1317–22.
49. Smith MJ, Wallace AJ, Bowers NL, Eaton H, Evans DG. SMARCB1 mutations in schwannomatosis and genotype correlations with rhabdoid tumors. Cancer Genet. 2014;207(9):373–8.
50. Sestini R, Bacci C, Provenzano A, Genuardi M, Papi L. Evidence of a four-hit mechanism involving SMARCB1 and NF2 in schwannomatosis-associated schwannomas. Hum Mutat. 2008;29(2):227–31.
51. Jordan JT, Smith MJ, Walker JA, et al. Pain correlates with germline mutation in schwannomatosis. Medicine (Baltimore). 2018;97(5):e9717.
52. Baser ME, Friedman JM, Joe H, et al. Empirical development of improved diagnostic criteria for neurofibromatosis 2. Genet Med. 2011;13(6):576–81.
53. MacCollin M, Chiocca EA, Evans DG, et al. Diagnostic criteria for schwannomatosis. Neurology. 2005;64(11):1838–45.

54. Farschtschi S, Mautner VF, Pham M, et al. Multifocal nerve lesions and LZTR1 germline mutations in segmental schwannomatosis. Ann Neurol. 2016;80(4):625–8.
55. Koontz NA, Wiens AL, Agarwal A, Hingtgen CM, Emerson RE, Mosier KM. Schwannomatosis: the overlooked neurofibromatosis? AJR Am J Roentgenol. 2013;200(6):W646–53.
56. Atherton DJ, Pitcher DW, Wells RS, MacDonald DM. A syndrome of various cutaneous pigmented lesions, myxoid neurofibromata and atrial myxoma: the NAME syndrome. Br J Dermatol. 1980;103(4):421–9.
57. Stratakis CA, Kirschner LS, Carney JA. Clinical and molecular features of the Carney complex: diagnostic criteria and recommendations for patient evaluation. J Clin Endocrinol Metab. 2001;86(9):4041–6.
58. Bertherat J, Horvath A, Groussin L, et al. Mutations in regulatory subunit type 1A of cyclic adenosine 5′-monophosphate-dependent protein kinase (PRKAR1A): phenotype analysis in 353 patients and 80 different genotypes. J Clin Endocrinol Metab. 2009;94(6):2085–91.
59. Espiard S, Bertherat J. Carney complex. Front Horm Res. 2013;41:50–62.
60. Boikos SA, Stratakis CA. Carney complex: the first 20 years. Curr Opin Oncol. 2007;19(1):24–9.
61. Carney JA. Psammomatous melanotic schwannoma. A distinctive, heritable tumor with special associations, including cardiac myxoma and the Cushing syndrome. Am J Surg Pathol. 1990;14(3):206–22.
62. Carney JA, Stratakis CA. Epithelioid blue nevus and psammomatous melanotic schwannoma: the unusual pigmented skin tumors of the Carney complex. Semin Diagn Pathol. 1998;15(3):216–24.
63. Cras P, Ceuterick-de Groote C, Van Vyve M, Vercruyssen A, Martin JJ. Malignant pigmented spinal nerve root schwannoma metastasizing in the brain and viscera. Clin Neuropathol. 1990;9(6):290–4.
64. Fu YS, Kaye GI, Lattes R. Primary malignant melanocytic tumors of the sympathetic ganglia, with an ultrastructural study of one. Cancer. 1975;36(6):2029–41.
65. Mathiesen JS, Kroustrup JP, Vestergaard P, et al. Incidence and prevalence of multiple endocrine neoplasia 2B in Denmark: a nationwide study. Endocr Relat Cancer. 2017;24(7):L39–42.
66. Znaczko A, Donnelly DE, Morrison PJ. Epidemiology, clinical features, and genetics of multiple endocrine neoplasia type 2B in a complete population. Oncologist. 2014;19(12):1284–6.

25 A General Introduction to Neurofibromatosis

Sumit Sinha, Nishant Yagnick, and Harsh Deora

25.1 Introduction

Neurofibromatosis (NFM) is a relatively common condition characterized by neurological and cutaneous lesions and present with a wide variety of clinical manifestations, which constitute a diagnostic and a therapeutic challenge. The term NFM comprises of at least four distinct sets of disorders (see below): neurofibromatosis 1 (NF1), neurofibromatosis 2 (NF2), segmental schwannoma, and schwannomatosis. All of them are genetically determined autosomal dominant disorders, each characterized by the presence of distinct nerve sheath tumors and other clinical features. This chapter will review the pathogenesis, diagnosis, and management of each of these forms of NFM.

25.2 Classification of NFM

Riccardi et al. classified NFM into eight types with peculiar clinical features and patterns of inheritance (Table 25.1) [1]. However, soon after it was proposed that NFM can be classified into five broad subtypes, based on clinical presentation and genetic implications for the patients: NF1, classical; NF2, acoustic; NF3, segmental; NF4, familial; and NF5, Noonan phenotype [2].

More recently, there have been at least four distinct types of NFM recognized, with the probability of other variant forms existing [3]:

1. Neurofibromatosis 1 (NF1)—also called as von Recklinghausen's disease or peripheral neurofibromatosis—is the most common form of NFM (85%). NF1 is an autosomal dominant disorder affecting 1 in 3500–5000 individuals. It is the most common single-gene disorder in humans. The genetic locus of NF1 has been localized to the long arm of chromosome 17. However, there is no positive family history in 35–50% of patients. These sporadic cases usually arise from (paternal) germ cell mutations.
2. Neurofibromatosis 2 (NF2)—or central neurofibromatosis—is also an autosomal dominant disorder and affects 1 in 40–50,000 individuals, with a prevalence of 1 in 2,10,000 in population. Sporadic gene mutations occur in 50% of cases. NF2 is characterized by the presence of bilateral schwannomas of the eighth cranial nerve, causing progressive hearing loss and the presence of multifocal meningiomas.
3. Segmental neurofibromatosis is characterized by café au lait macules dispersed in bands on

S. Sinha (✉)
Neurosurgery and Spine Services, Paras Hospital, Gurugram, Harayana, India

N. Yagnick
Paras Hospital, Gurugram, Harayana, India

H. Deora
Department of Neurosurgery, NIMHANS, Bangalore, India

F. Guedes et al. (eds.), *Diagnostic Assessment and Treatment of Peripheral Nerve Tumors*,
https://doi.org/10.1007/978-3-030-77633-6_25

Table 25.1 Riccardi classification of NFM

Type	Inheritance	Remarks
Neurofibromatosis (NF1)	AD	Café au lait spots, neurofibroma, Lisch nodules, axillary freckling, osseous and neurological involvement, and benign and malignant tumors
Acoustic (NF2)	AD	Bilateral acoustic neuromas, few café au lait spots, and neurofibromas
Mixed (NF3)	AD	Mixed NF1 and NF2
Variant (NF4)	Unknown	Variations of CNS tumors, café au lait spots, neurofibroma, and Lisch nodules
Segmental (NF5)	Non-inheritable	Segmental neurofibromas and café au lait spots
Familial (NF6)	Unknown	Café au lait spots
Late onset (NF7)	Unknown	After third decade-neurofibroma, few café au lait spots
Unspecified (NF8)	Unknown	Variable manifestations

the skin and limited to one or a few body segments.

4. Schwannomatosis is a condition sharing the presentation and phenotype with NF2, albeit with a distinct clinical and molecular signature, and presenting with multiple deep and intensely painful schwannomas.

25.3 Neurofibromatosis 1 (NF1)

NF1 was first described by Friedrich von Recklinghausen in 1882 [4]. Since then, there has been much genetic and clinical research on this multi-system, age-penetrating disorder with a predilection for the nervous system. It is also known as von Recklinghausen's disease or peripheral neurofibromatosis and characterized by the development of multiple neurofibromas of peripheral nerves. The incidence of NF1 is approximately 1 in 2500–3000 births [5]. The average life expectancy of patients with NF1 is 54 years, often due to associated malignancies [6].

25.3.1 Genetics of NF1

Neurofibromatosis is an autosomal dominant Mendelian disorder with complete penetrance. However, it can have variable expressivity in terms of the major manifestations and severity of the disease. This is exemplified by the microdeletion phenotype as it involves the entire NF1 gene vs the intragenic mutations. Another reason for this observation is that some of those genes co-deleted with NF1 exert an influence on the clinical manifestation of the disease in patients with NF1 microdeletions. Approximately 50% of the affected individuals don't have any affected parent and represent new mutations of the NF1 gene.

NF1 is inherited from parents in 50% of cases and is consequent to a spontaneous mutation in the remaining 50% [7, 8]. More than 1500 mutations have been identified in patients with NF1. Usually, NF1 is due to the loss of a function dominant mutation of NF1 gene (neurofibromin), which is a tumor suppressor gene located on chromosome 17q11.2. However, only a single "microdeletion" (equivalent to a loss of 1.5 MB), found in only 5–10% of cases, has been identified as a consistent prognostic indicator of the disease manifestation. Moreover, the wide spectrum of clinical pictures associated with the same mutation suggests that other factors determine the phenotype, yet their nature has not been identified [9–14].

The gene responsible for NF1 is more than 300 kb in size, located on chromosome 17, and includes 60 exons. All types of mutations are scattered throughout the gene, including nucleotide changes, insertion or deletions, splicing mutations, and whole gene mutations. A comprehensive genetic testing and direct sequencing for NF1 is able to detect the causative mutation in 95% of individuals fulfilling the diagnostic criterion and may be useful to confirm a diagnosis in an individual with only one clinical feature, especially in sporadically affected young children and for prenatal diagnosis.

25.3.2 Pathogenesis

The NF1 gene encodes for the "neurofibromin" protein which is a GTPase-activating protein (GAP) that promotes the conversion of Ras-GTP to Ras-GDP. The gene is involved with the control of response of the cells to growth stimuli [15]. Several pathways are known to be involved in the development of tumors associated with NF1. Loss of neurofibromin increases rat sarcoma viral oncogene homolog (RAS) activity, which causes unopposed cell growth and activation of downstream intermediates such as mitogen-activated protein kinase (MAPK) and the mammalian target of rapamycin (mTOR) pathways [16]. Neurofibromin is also involved in the regulation of cyclic adenosine monophosphate levels, which has been shown to affect the CNS, especially optic pathway glioma (OPG) formation [17–19].

The target cell for the mutations is Schwann cells in a neurofibroma and a melanocyte in café au lait macules. The neurofibroma contains a mixed population of fibroblasts, perineural cells, and mast cells. All of these cells proliferate due to the secretion of cytokines secreted by the mast cells. Some phenotypic characteristics, especially the cognitive deficits, are explained on the basis of haploinsufficiency.

The recognition of the role of Ras signaling pathway in the pathogenesis of NF1 has led to the development of ongoing preclinical trials of candidate therapies including Ras, downstream effectors of Ras, mTOR, cytokines, and angiogenesis factors.

25.3.3 Diagnostic Criterion

There are several diagnostic criteria developed to diagnose NF1, but the most commonly used one was developed by the Consensus Development Conference at the National Institutes of Health (NIH) in 1987 which concluded that the diagnosis of NF1 could be assigned to a person with two or more of the following criteria:

1. The presence of more than six café au lait spots measuring at least 15 mm in diameter in adults or five café au lait spots of 5 mm in children
2. Two or more neurofibromas of any type or at least one plexiform neurofibroma
3. Freckling in the axillary or inguinal region
4. Optic glioma
5. Two or more Lisch nodules (iris hamartomas)
6. A distinctive osseous lesion (sphenoid dysplasia or tibial pseudoarthrosis)
7. A first-degree relative with NF1 by the above criteria

While these criteria can be applied to adults, the same cannot be applied to children or at an early stage of the disease. This is because only about half of children with NF1 and no known family history of NF1 meet the NIH criteria for diagnosis by age 1 year. However, by 8 years of age, almost all cases will exhibit features of the same.

In case a child is born to a known NF parent, then they need only one criterion to fulfill the diagnosis, which is usually identified early in the form of cafe au lait spots, which develop in infancy in >95% of individuals with NF1. The young children with multiple café au lait spots and no other NF1 features whose parents do not show signs of NF1 on careful physical and ophthalmologic examination should be strongly suspected of having NF1 and followed clinically. A definite diagnosis of NF1 can be made in most of these children by age 4 years using the NIH criteria. The young children who present with six or more café au lait macules and freckling in axillary or inguinal regions but have no known family history of NF1 also meet the diagnostic criteria for NF1. However, the diagnoses of Legius syndrome or constitutional mismatch repair syndrome need to be considered in such cases, especially if no additional findings of NF1 develop with increasing age.

25.3.4 Clinical Manifestations

There seem to be two age peaks in the occurrence of severe clinical problems for NF1 patients: one from 5 to 10 years of age and the second from 36 to 50 years of age. At the second peak, 75% of the clinical problems are related to malignancy. There is extreme variability in features and complications of NF1 among affected individuals. Approximately one-third of patients with NF1 will suffer serious medical and cosmetic complications over their lifetime; the remaining two-thirds will have mild to moderate involvement.

NF1 can have varied manifestations, and the lifespan of these individuals is typically 15 years shorter than an average individual [20]. Apart from the increased risk of having neurofibromas, these patients can develop a plethora of other malignant and benign tumors which can contribute to an early demise and considerable morbidity. Although the peripheral nervous system is the focus of the disease in NF1, NF1-associated neoplasms can occur elsewhere in the body including the central nervous system, skin, the gastrointestinal tract, bone marrow, breast and soft tissues.

25.3.4.1 Neurofibromas

Neurofibromas (NF) are benign tumors arising from the Schwann cells and are a hallmark of NF1, present in all the patients older than 30 years. They may occur anywhere in the body, involving either a discrete length of an individual nerve or multiple nerve fascicles. They may appear typically on the skin surface or within the dermis and increase in number during puberty and pregnancy. Internal or deep NF may occur throughout the body including the periorbital, retroperitoneal, GI tract, and mediastinal locations or present with pain or neurological deficits, as are the spinal NF (Figs. 25.1 and 25.2). There are multiple types of neurofibromas that exist with a varying capacity to become malignant peripheral nerve sheath tumors. The WHO classification scheme defines five distinct neurofibroma subtypes (Table 25.2). The plexiform NF is pathognomonic of NF1, which grow along multiple fascicles or branch of a nerve.

The morbidity associated with plexiform NF is twofold. They can lead to cosmetic disfigurement, bony destruction, and pain and have 8–13% lifetime risk of malignant transformation

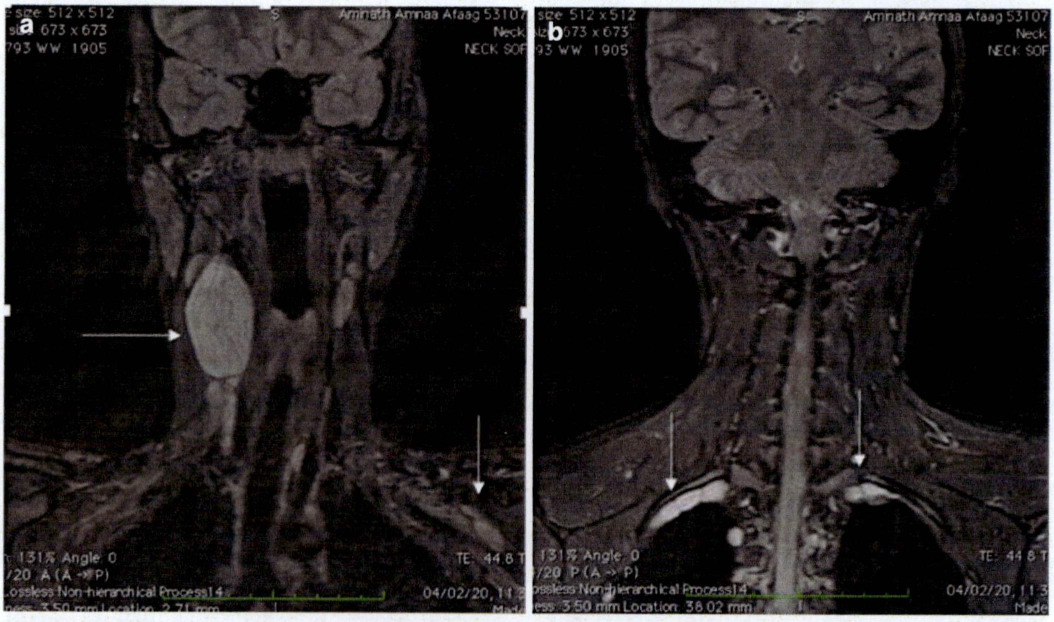

Fig. 25.1 (a) T2 weighted MRI coronal images showing hyperintense lesion involving the right carotid sheath/vagus nerve (white arrow); (b) T2 weighted MRI coronal images showing hyperintense lesion involving the bilateral intercostal nerves (white arrow)

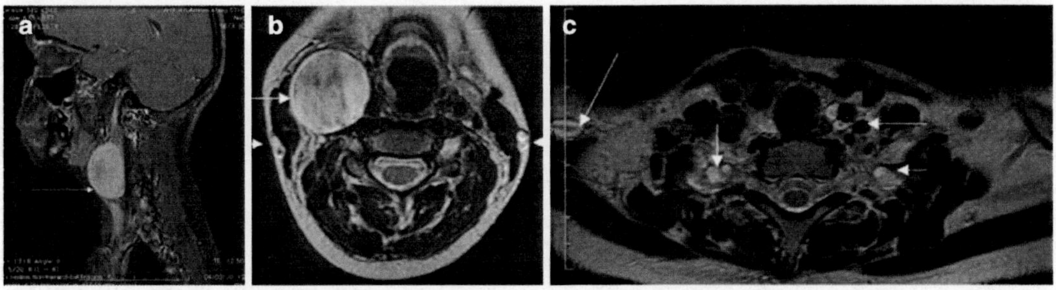

Fig. 25.2 (a) T1 weighted contrast-enhanced fat-suppressed sagittal images and (b) T2 weighted axial images showing a large enhancing and T2 hyperintense lesion involving the carotid sheath/vagus nerve (white arrows) (c) T2 weighted axial images in the same case showing other multiple subcutaneous and brachial plexus neurofibromas (white arrows)

Table 25.2 Types of Neurofibromas and their association with Neurofibromatosis

Type	Location	NF1 incidence	Malignant potential	Remarks
Localized cutaneous	Skin	10% NF1 90% sporadic	None	Most common, hidden under café au lait spots
Diffuse cutaneous	Skin	10% NF1 90% sporadic	Very low	Uncommon lesions that present as plaque-like lesions
Localized intraneural	Cranial, spinal, autonomic nerve plexus	Can be NF1 or sporadic	Intermediate	Second most common
Plexiform	Cranial, spinal, autonomic nerve plexus	Exclusively NF 1	Highest	Diagnostic of NF1
Massive soft tissue	Extremities, extensive soft tissue expansion with underlying large nerve	Exclusively NF 1	Intermediate	Less common called elephantiasis neuromatosa

into malignant peripheral nerve sheath tumor (MPNST).

25.3.4.2 CNS Tumors

In the central nervous system, astrocytoma is the most common manifestation. Gliomas can present throughout the CNS in patients with NF1. The relative risk of having a brain tumor is 100 times higher in children (<10 years) with NF1 than those without NF1. Most of these tumors are low-grade (WHO I–II grade) tumors. These patients also carry a chance of developing high-grade neoplasms like diffuse astrocytomas (WHO grade II–III) and glioblastomas (WHO grade IV), many of which occur in the brainstem. The Cancer Genome Atlas Research Network concluded that 18% of sporadic glioblastomas have a homozygous deletion or mutation of NF1 gene, underscoring the important role that NF1 loss plays in glioblastoma pathogenesis [21].

The patients develop optic pathway gliomas (OPG) during childhood or adolescence. NF1-associated optic gliomas can occur anywhere along the optic nerves, the optic chiasm, or the optic tracts and are found in ~15% of children with NF1 [22]. As the World Health Organization (WHO) grade I neoplasms (pilocytic astrocytomas), OPG typically follow a benign clinical course, involving optic nerve, chiasma, and/or hypothalamus. However, they can be clinically problematic as nearly half of NF1 patients with OPG develop moderate to severe visual impairment [23, 24]. Precocious puberty also occurs in a small fraction of NF1 patients whose OPG involve the optic chiasm and adjacent hypothalamus. OPG usually present before the age of 6 years with a loss of visual acuity, proptosis, or strabismus, but they may not become symptomatic until later in childhood or even in adulthood. Symptomatic OPG in NF1 are frequently stable and indolent for many years or are only very slowly progressive, and some of these tumors even regress spontaneously.

25.3.4.3 Café Au Lait Macules and Other Skin Manifestations

The café au lait spots occur in nearly all NF1 cases, and intertriginous freckling shall develop in 90% cases. By the age of 1 year, 99% of children with the diagnosis will have 6/>6 café au lait macules >5 mm. These spots are characteristically ovoid in shape with well-defined borders and usually about 1–3 cm in size. They are uniform in color, being a little darker than the background pigmentation of the individual (Fig. 25.3a, b). The pigmentation may also be irregular, with freckling or a more deeply pigmented smaller café au lait spot within a larger more typically colored lesion. The café au lait spots are flat and flush with the surrounding skin; however, if the skin of the lesion is raised or has an unusually soft or irregular texture in comparison to the surrounding skin, an underlying plexiform neurofibroma is more likely. The darker pigmentation of café au lait spots may be difficult to see in people with very dark skin, where the color of the lesions is similar to that of the rest of the skin. A Wood's light is useful in such cases to demonstrate the pigmented macules. Café au lait spots are not seen on the palms or soles in patients with NF1 but can occur almost anywhere else on the body. The size, number, and location of café au lait spots do not correlate with the severity of NF1 or the location of future neurofibromas.

The skin fold freckling appears first in the inguinal region and later in the axillae. This is often the next sign to appear, usually at 3–5 years of age. Only 40% will have freckling in infancy, while 90% of NF1 patients will have this by the age of 7 years. The freckles are frequent in sun-exposed areas and may also be seen diffusely over the trunk, proximal extremities, and neck in patients with NF1. Similar freckling is common in fair-skinned people who do not have NF1. However, patients with NF1 also develop freckles in areas where the skin rubs against the skin, i.e., in the axilla, groin, and under the breasts in women. These freckles look like any others; however, it is only their location that is unusual.

Other skin manifestations include juvenile xanthogranulomas which are small, tan, or orange-colored papules that may occur in clusters.

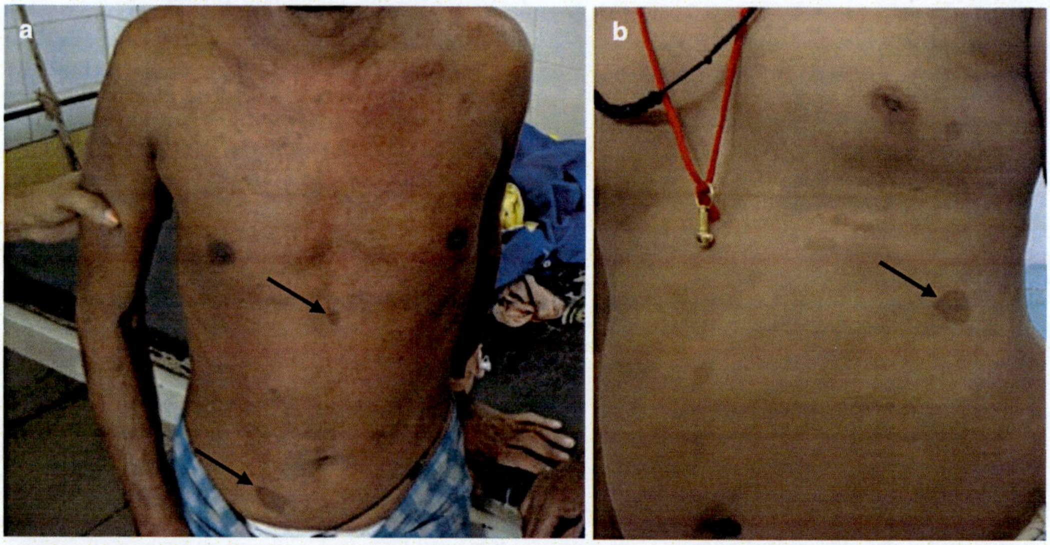

Fig. 25.3 (**a**, **b**) Photograph of patients with NF1 showing cafe au lait macules on the abdomen (black arrows)

Nevus anemicus is another such lesion which is an irregularly shaped macule, paler than the surrounding skin, and that does not get red when rubbed, as the skin surrounding it does.

25.3.4.4 Ocular Findings

Ocular manifestations include iris Lisch nodules. These are melanocytic hamartomas and are asymptomatic and highly specific for NF1. They are demonstrable in adults and half of the children <5 years with the help of a slit lamp [25]. Choroidal freckling cannot be seen on standard ophthalmologic examination but can be visualized by scanning laser ophthalmoscopy with infrared or near-infrared light, infrared reflectance imaging, or optical coherence tomography. Other infrequent ocular manifestations of NF1 include retinal vasoproliferative tumors and neovascular glaucoma [26, 27].

25.3.4.5 Neurological Manifestations

These can be divided as central and peripheral. NF1 patients have psychiatric and neuropsychological abnormalities with IQ scores which may be normal or slightly below normal. The learning disabilities have been reported in up to 80% of these children [28, 29]. This is more so in cases with microdeletion. Frank intellectual disability can be seen in 6–7% cases which is twice that of the general population. Further, nearly 40% of these children have attention-deficit/hyperactivity disorder, 30% have autism spectrum disorder [30], and many have visual-spatial deficits [31]. Deficits in visual-spatial performance, social competence, and attention are most commonly seen in people with NF1, but problems with motor function, executive function, memory, and language are also frequent. T2-weighted magnetic resonance imaging often identifies "unidentified bright objects" (UBOs) in the basal ganglia, thalamus, brainstem, cerebellum, or subcortical white matter of these children [32–34]. These UBOs, which have variously been interpreted as hamartomas [35], regions of abnormal myelination [36], heterotopias [37], or vacuolated myelin [38], are potentially related to the learning disabilities seen in children with NF1 [39]. UBOs can also be confused with the radiologic abnormalities associated with glioma.

Seizures are also more common than the general population which may be due to the presence of tumors or infarct [40]. Other central manifestations include sleep disturbances and headaches (migraines). The pain in association with plexiform neurofibromas is also common and must be distinguished from the pain that may be the first sign of transformation to a malignant peripheral nerve sheath tumor.

25.3.4.6 Malignant Peripheral Nerve Sheath Tumors (MPNSTs)

MPNSTs are aggressive spindle cell neoplasms derived from the Schwann cell lineage [41] with a 5-year survival of up to 60%. As a group, MPNSTs represent ~2 to 5% of all soft tissue sarcomas. However, MPNSTs are encountered in three very different clinical settings, which raise the question of whether there are distinct MPNST subtypes that arise via different pathogenic mechanisms. About 40–50% of MPNSTs arise in NF1 patients. MPNSTs are the most common malignancy encountered in NF1 patients, and the lifetime risk of developing an MPNST has been estimated at 5.9–10.3%. Another 40–47% of MPNSTs are sporadic, with the remaining 10–13% occurring at sites of previous radiation therapy. MPNST usually arise from a pre-existing plexiform NF. The signs of a malignant change are unexplained persistent pain, rapid growth, change in texture from soft to hard, and an increased uptake on FDG-PET scan.

25.3.4.7 Musculoskeletal Manifestations

The presence of skeletal abnormalities such as scoliosis, vertebral scalloping, unilateral sphenoid wing dysplasia, decreased bone mineral density, and tibial pseudoarthrosis has been found in nearly half of NF1 patients [42]. The serum 25-hydroxy vitamin D levels are reduced in individuals with a large number of dermal neurofibromas [43]. 25-Hydroxy vitamin D levels are inversely proportional to the burden of these tumors.

Osteopenia and osteoporosis are both more frequent in NF1 than in general population. The hypothesis is that there is a lower-than-expected serum 25-hydroxy vitamin D concentration, elevated serum parathyroid hormone levels, and evidence of increased bone resorption in patients with NF1. The neurofibromin gene plays a critical role in regulating the mesenchymal stem/progenitor cell differentiation into osteoblasts, affecting collagen synthesis and mineralization. The function of both osteoblasts and osteoclasts appears to be abnormal in NF1. Dysplasia can occur in long bones, most commonly in the tibia and fibula, which is infrequent but characteristic of NF1. This usually presents in infancy as unilateral anterolateral bowing of the lower leg, which is quite different from the common physiologic bowing seen in children when they begin to walk. Early recognition of tibial dysplasia permits bracing, which may prevent fracture. The initial radiographic changes consist of narrowing of the medullary canal with cortical thickening at the apex of the bowing. In contrast, sphenoid wing dysplasia can be incidental and can cause strabismus or even progressive pulsating enophthalmos.

Scoliosis can be seen in the dystrophic variety which occurs at a young age (6–8 years) and is characterized by an acute angle over a short segment of the spine and can be rapidly progressive. Non-dystrophic variety commonly presents with adolescent scoliosis and is not associated with vertebral anomalies.

Orbital dysplasia may occur due to the presence of a plexiform NF in trigeminal nerve.

25.3.4.8 Vascular Manifestations

Vascular abnormalities ranging from renal, coronary and cerebral artery stenosis to pulmonary stenosis, valvular malformations, and coarctation of the abdominal aorta occur in nearly 10% [44–47] and are some other factors contributing to mortality in these patients, particularly those who die before 30 years of age [48].

Hypertension and stroke are the most common manifestation of NF1 in the vascular system. Hypertension can be essential or associated with renal artery stenosis, coarctation of the aorta, or other vascular lesions associated with hypertension. A renovascular cause is often found in children with NF1 and hypertension. Stroke in young is a common manifestation with the involvement of both the brain and heart. Stenosis or ectasia of the cerebral and intracranial arteries are much more common in NF1 than the general population. Moyamoya disease is three times as common as the general population.

Cardiovascular abnormalities such as valvular pulmonic stenosis, congenital heart defects, or hypertrophic obstructive cardiomyopathy are more common in these cases. They can develop pulmonary hypertension in the adult age group which is often in association with parenchymal lung disease [49].

There is an increased risk of hemorrhagic and ischemic strokes in adult and pediatric population as compared to general population. The various associations include moyamoya angiopathy, cerebral aneurysm, and ectatic cerebral vessels.

25.3.4.9 Non-CNS Tumors

Apart from the involvement of the nervous system, patients with NF1 can also have systemic neoplasms. There is a 0.1–5.7% risk of NF1 patients developing pheochromocytomas, typically in the fifth decade of life [50–52].

The endocrine tumors of gastrointestinal tract (GIT) are also seen in NF1 with a predilection for periampullary region. The most common of these is a somatostatinoma. Gastric carcinoids are also associated with NF1, although this is a rare manifestation of the disorder [53]. NF1 patients are at increased risk (45-fold higher than that of the general population) for the development of gastrointestinal stromal tumors (GISTs) [54], with 60% of them occurring in the small intestine, whereas sporadic GISTs are most commonly gastric [55].

Young children with NF1 are prone to develop juvenile myelomonocytic leukemia, with boys being particularly susceptible to this malignancy

[56]. Glomus tumors, which are small benign but exquisitely painful tumors that develop at the end of digits, have also been suggested to be a feature of NF1 [57].

NF1 patients have a 20-fold increased risk for the development of embryonal rhabdomyosarcomas as compared with the general population [58–60]; this is, however, one of the less common manifestations of NF1, occurring in <1% of individuals with this disorder. Likewise, leiomyosarcomas and osteosarcomas occur rarely in NF1 but still at a rate higher than that of the general population [61]. The lifetime risk of developing breast cancer is found to be double in women with NF1, and the survival of NF1 patients with breast cancer is poorer than that of other breast cancer patients [62].

25.3.4.10 Other Manifestations

NF1 may present with dysmorphic features and overgrowth in childhood. Child overgrowth has been defined as any child with NF1 under the age of 18 years who has height and/or head circumference at least two standard deviations above the age- and sex-matched population. Facial dysmorphism is defined as having two or more of the following features: coarse face, flat occiput/brachycephaly, facial asymmetry, prominent forehead, frontal bossing, ptosis, down slanting deep-set eyes, eversion of the lateral eyelid, epicanthic folds, high and broad nasal bridge, bulbous nasal tip, large and low-set ears, malar hypoplasia, wide and prominent philtrum, micrognathia, small pointed chin, and low posterior hairline.

Macrocephaly and short stature are variably seen in NF1 cases [63–65].

25.3.5 Management

The management of NF1 consists of the following:

1. Surveillance
2. Surgery of progressive lesions
3. Genetic counseling

The important surveillance points depend upon the age of the patient. The presence of plexiform NF or orbital or long bone dysplasia should be sought for in the clinical examination in an infant suspected of having NF1. In children, besides plexiform NF, the presence of high blood pressure (due to renal artery stenosis), curved spine (due to scoliosis), and learning disability should be screened, as also the presence of optic glioma by performing an ophthalmological examination and assessment of growth and head circumference. The adults should be screened for the presence of NF, high blood pressure, neurological function (for the presence of hydrocephalus, optic glioma, spinal cord or peripheral nerve compression), and tumor growth for the possibility of MPNST.

The treatment of various lesions in NF1 depends upon their presentation and is summarized in Table 25.3. The development of newer therapies targeting MEK inhibitors and mTOR pathways is currently under research trials [66]. Anti-angiogenesis factors like bevacizumab have shown objective responses in vision testing in cases with refractory optic gliomas [67, 68].

The biopsy of the suspected tumors is not necessary as the imaging is diagnostic. Surgery is recommended for optic gliomas with deteriorating vision or proptosis.

Table 25.3 Treatment of various lesions in NF1

Dermal NF	Plastic surgery, CO_2 laser, electro-desiccation	To improve appearance or discomfort
Plexiform NF	Debulking	For cosmesis or neurological decompression. Complete removal not possible
Optic gliomas	Usually stable and do not require treatment. Surgery recommended for deteriorating vision or proptosis	Postoperative chemotherapy with carboplatin and vincristine. Five-year progression free survival is 70%
Learning disabilities	Neuropsychological assessment	
MPNST	Surgery and/radiation	

25.4 Neurofibromatosis 2 (NF2)

NF2, also known as bilateral acoustic neurofibromatosis or central neurofibromatosis, is a hereditary tumor syndrome characterized predominantly by the development of schwannomas, with meningiomas, ependymomas, and ocular abnormalities. Posterior subcapsular cataract is the only non-tumor manifestation.

NF2 is inherited in an autosomal dominant pattern with an estimated incidence of 1 in 25,000, a prevalence of 1 in 60,000, and penetrance of almost 100% [69]. Patients usually present around age 20, and prognostic considerations include age at diagnosis, meningioma status, and access to specialty medical centers. Over half of the cases are caused by de novo gene mutations in patients with no family history of the disease. The life expectancy of patients with NF2 is reduced as compared with unaffected individuals (69 vs 80 years) [70].

25.4.1 Genetics and Pathogenesis of NF2

The disease is caused by a germline mutation in the NF2 gene, which can be identified in 70–90% of affected individuals. NF2 was proven to be a genetically distinct entity from NF1, caused by abnormalities of a gene located on the q12 band of chromosome 22. This NF2 gene is composed of 17 exons spanning 110 kb and codes for the protein named "Merlin" (also known as schwannomin), which is a tumor suppressor protein impacting PI3 kinase/Akt, Raf/MEK/ERK, and mTOR signaling pathways. Merlin is named for its relationship to the moesin (membrane-organizing extension spike protein)—erzin (cytovillin)—radixin family of cytoskeleton-associated proteins, which suggests that it may be influential in communication between surface signaling and the cytoskeleton matrix.

The NF2 protein is a true tumor suppressor as biallelic loss results in tumor formation. Mutations in Merlin can be found in approximately 93% of patients with clinical evidence of NF2 and positive family history, in 90% of sporadic vestibular schwannoma and in 50–60% of sporadic meningiomas.

The phenotype of NF2 can have varying degrees of severity. Within an affected family, the natural history and phenotypic expression of NF2 are usually similar between its members. However, interfamily variations can be striking. The differences can be attributed to differing abnormalities within the NF2 gene. For instance, the most severe clinical manifestations have been associated with frameshift or nonsense mutations, which also happen to be the most common mutation types, in which the mutation causes truncated protein expression.

25.4.2 Diagnostic Criterion

NF2 is diagnosed using clinical criteria. There is a paucity of cutaneous stigmata in NF2, and cafe au lait macules are not a regular feature. Bilateral schwannomas of the superior vestibular branch of the eighth cranial nerve (vestibular schwannoma or acoustic neuroma) are pathognomonic for NF2. There have been several diagnostic criteria for NF2 as 41% of patients eventually proven to have NF2 do not have bilateral vestibular schwannomas at the initial time of presentation. These include the widely recognized Manchester criteria as well as additional NIH criteria as shown in Table 25.4.

Table 25.4 Diagnostic criteria of NF2

Main criteria	Additional criteria
Bilateral vestibular schwannomas	Unilateral vestibular schwannoma plus any two of the following: meningioma, glioma, schwannoma, or juvenile posterior lenticular opacities
First-degree relative with NF2 plus: 1. Unilateral vestibular schwannomas 2. Any two of the following: meningioma, glioma, schwannoma, or juvenile posterior lenticular opacities	At least two meningiomas plus: 1. Unilateral vestibular schwannoma 2. Any two of the following: glioma, neurofibroma, schwannoma, and cataract

25.4.3 Clinical Presentation

NF2 is known to have nervous system tumors including schwannomas followed by meningiomas and ependymomas (Fig. 25.4a–f). The patients can also have non-neoplastic ocular manifestations. The pathognomonic hallmark finding of bilateral vestibular schwannoma is found in >95% of NF2 patients.

25.4.3.1 Vestibular Schwannomas

These tumors arise from the superior division of the vestibular nerve and present with sensorineural hearing loss, tinnitus, and imbalance while walking (Fig. 25.5a–c). They histologically resemble sporadic tumors with the presence of alternating Antoni A and B bodies, Verocay bodies, and hyalinized blood vessels. However, in contrast to the sporadic schwannomas, the schwannomas in NF2 tend to be multifocal and multilobulated and invade the nerve fibers, rather than displacing them (as in sporadic NF) [71]. This accounts for the high recurrence rates for NF2 tumors as compared to sporadic tumors (44% vs 1.3%) with surgery or radiotherapy. The risk of malignant transformation after radiation is more in NF2 vestibular schwannomas as compared to sporadic ones [71].

25.4.3.2 Peripheral Schwannomas

Schwannomas of other cranial and peripheral nerves, especially paraspinal and cutaneous nerves, are encountered in up to 70% of patients with NF2 [72] (Fig. 25.6a–h). Symptoms attributable to peripheral schwannomas are most often pain, sensory loss, and weakness. These schwan-

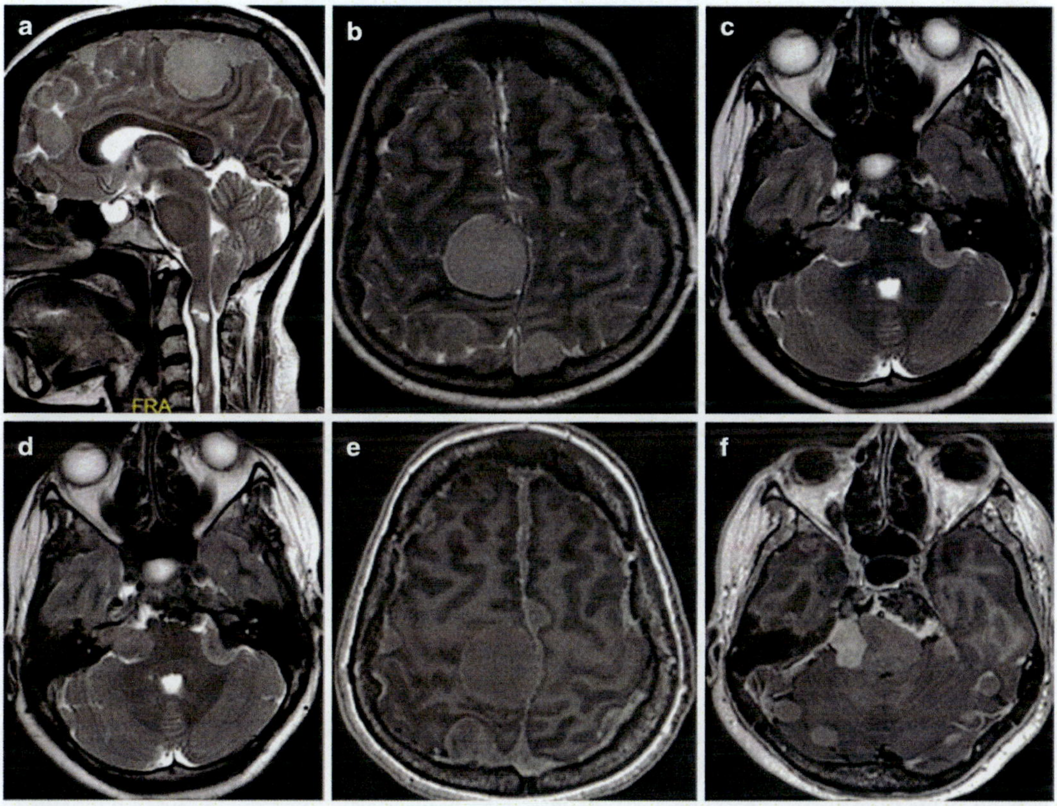

Fig. 25.4 (a–f) MRI of a patient with NF2 showing multiple meningiomas along the falx and bilateral acoustic neuroma

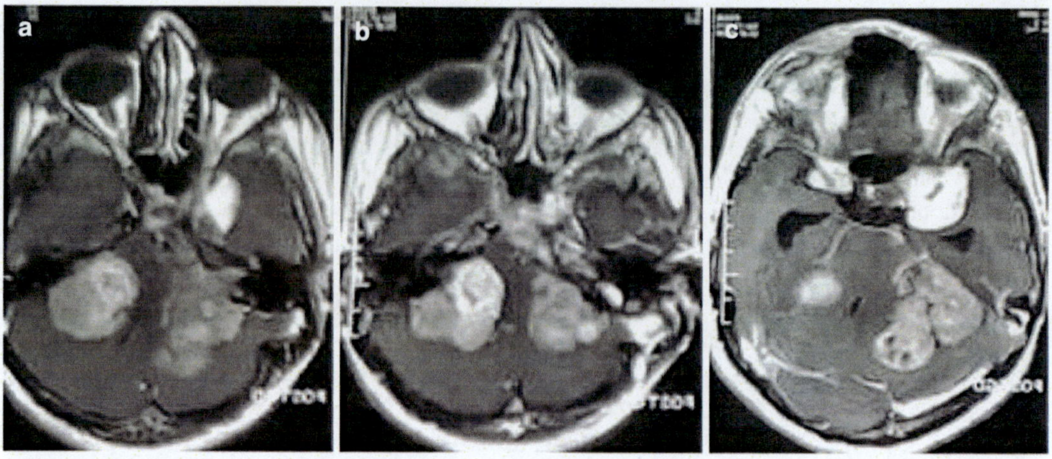

Fig. 25.5 (a–c) Contrast MRI of the brain of a patient with NF2 showing bilateral acoustic neuromas and left-side sphenoid wing meningioma and right-side optic nerve sheath meningioma

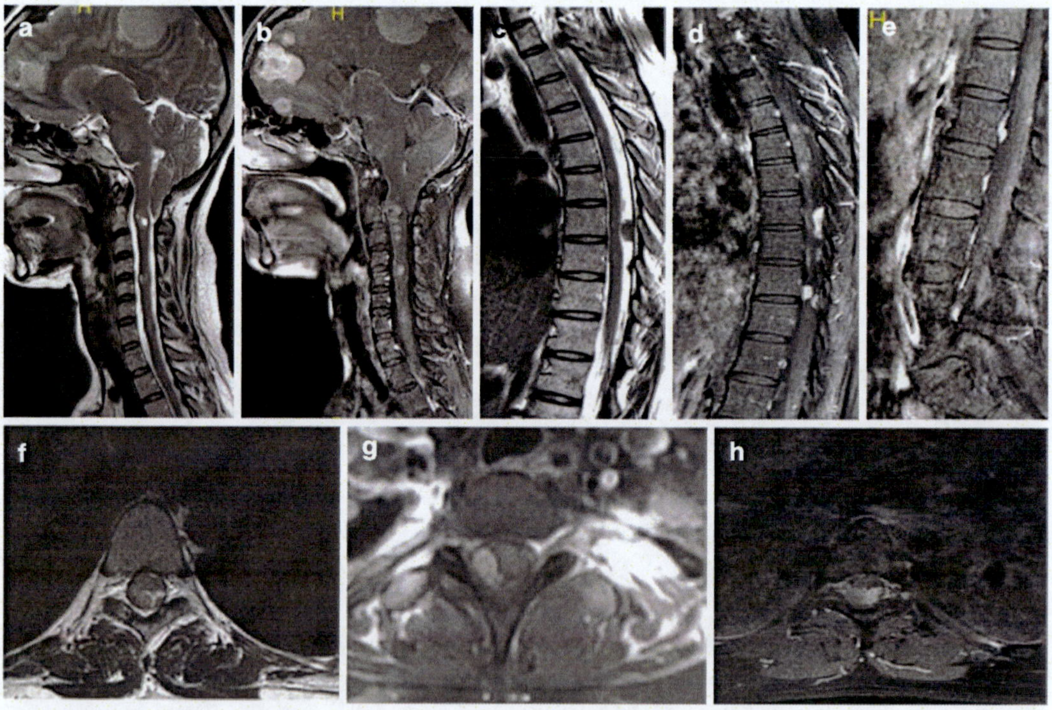

Fig. 25.6 (a–h) MRI of a patient with NF2 showing multiple intracranial (frontal convexity and falcine) meningiomas along with multiple intradural schwannomas

nomas also have a multifocal infiltration of the associated nerve as the NF2-associated vestibular schwannomas.

Small schwannomas are often found studded along the paraspinal nerve roots in NF2. These tumors are believed to be schwannoma precursors in these patients. The finding of a plexiform schwannoma confers a 10–50% chance that the patient has NF2. Plexiform schwannomas are most often cutaneous or subcutaneous with a predilection for the head and neck region. The schwannomas of NF2 are benign and rarely undergo malignant transformation in contrast to the neurofibromas of NF1.

25.4.3.3 Ependymomas

Intracranial ependymomas are not found in NF2. The spinal ependymomas are present in 50% of patients as intramedullary tumors. The intramedullary ependymomas in NF2 are most commonly found in cervical and cervico-medullary regions of the spinal cord (63–82%), followed by thoracic spine (36–44%), and present as multiple tumors in the form of a "string of pearl" appearance. These tumors are mostly asymptomatic and followed closely.

Ocular Manifestations:

These are found in a majority of NF2 patients in the form of posterior subcapsular lenticular opacities found in almost 80% of the patients. Other less common ocular findings include OPG, retinal hamartomas, epiretinal membranes, or schwannomas.

25.4.3.4 Meningiomas

These tumors are found at a younger age in NF2 than in the general population. About 20% of the children diagnosed with a meningioma will be found to have NF2. They are found in about 50% of patients with NF2 and are frequently multiple and intracranial. The intracranial meningiomas are most commonly found along the falx and convexity (70%) followed by skull base (25%) and intraventricular (3%). Spinal meningiomas also occur. The majority (>60%) of meningiomas in NF2 are stable and show no or little growth in the follow-up.

25.4.4 Management

The treatment strategy for NF2-associated tumors is different from sporadic tumors as the primary aim is to preserve the neurological function and quality of life.

The standard treatment of vestibular schwannomas is surgery, which is indicated for tumors with critical neural compression. However, a period of watchful waiting may be allowed in some patients with little or no neurologic dysfunction. In general, the schwannomas arising from other cranial nerves are slow-growing and are less symptomatic, and the surgical resection should be reserved for those with progressive neurological deficit or rapid tumor growth.

The radiation therapy is not encouraged in NF2-associated schwannomas because of the risk of malignant transformation, although the risk is absolutely low.

Several targeted therapies have been used in patients with NF2 and progressive vestibular schwannomas. The clinical trials with erlotinib (EGFR inhibitor) and lapatinib (EGFR/ErbB2 inhibitor) have been performed, although with low rates of radiologic response [73, 74]. A similar study with everolimus, an mTOR inhibitor, was associated with prolonged stable disease in NF2 patients with progressive vestibular schwannomas [75]. The treatment with anti-vascular endothelial growth factor, bevacizumab, has produced a durable hearing and radiologic response in patients with progressive vestibular schwannomas [76].

Surgery remains the standard treatment for progressive or symptomatic meningiomas or intramedullary ependymomas in NF2. The majority of these tumors have a benign histology and as such don't require radiation therapy after a good surgical excision.

25.5 Schwannomatosis

Schwannomatosis, as the name implies, is a syndrome characterized by the predisposition to development of multiple schwannomas (without concomitant involvement of the vestibular nerve) and much less commonly meningiomas (Fig. 25.7a–c). Schwannomatosis is distinct genetically from NF2; however, there is a considerable overlap in the phenotypes of these two syndromes. The true prevalence of schwannomatosis is difficult to assess given the clinical similarities to NF2 and lack of a reliable genetic test in all cases, though it is speculated to be about as common as NF2. Unlike the patients with NF1 with characteristic dermatologic manifestations and patients with NF2 with bilateral acoustic neuromas, the patients with schwannomatosis have non-specific symptoms that may delay the diagnosis.

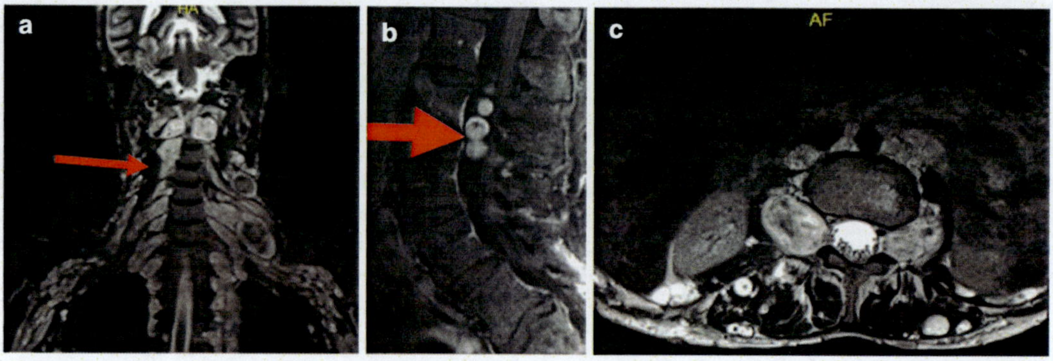

Fig. 25.7 (a–c) Cervical spine MRI of a patient with presumed schwannomatosis showing multiple cervical, mediastinal, and lumbar intra- and extra-dural schwannomas (red arrows). The patient did not have any evidence of vestibular schwannoma on brain MRI and had SMARCB1 positivity on genetic testing

25.5.1 Genetics and Pathogenesis of Schwannomatosis

Schwannomatosis is an autosomal dominant trait with incomplete penetrance, variable expression, and a high rate of mutation. Familial schwannomatosis accounts for 15% of the cases, while sporadic cases account for the rest 85%, with clinically unaffected parents. The germline mutations in the *SWI/SNF-related matrix-associated actin-dependent regulator of chromatin subfamily B member* (SMARCB1, also called hSNF5, INI1, BAF47) gene (located on chromosome 22q11.2, centromeric to the NF2 gene) have been found in 40–50% of families with familial schwannomatosis and in 10% of patients with sporadic schwannomatosis [77]. The SMARCB1 gene exerts its tumor suppressor function by regulating cell cycle, lineage-specific gene expression, and embryonic stem cell programming. The gene encodes for a protein involved in chromatin remodeling. It is also involved in the formation of rhabdoid and atypical teratoid tumors, and such tumors are found in some members of the families with schwannomatosis. The majority of the cases of schwannomatosis are caused by de novo mutations, though familial cases exist with an autosomal dominant inheritance pattern [78].

The mutations in the LZTR1 gene have also been identified fairly commonly in SMARCB1-negative schwannomatosis patients with NF2 loss in their tumors. The LZTR1 protein is involved in multiple cellular processes including regulation of chromatin and the cell cycle. The mutations in the second rhabdoid tumor locus, SMARCA4 (Brg1), which is also a component of SWI/SNF (AWItch/sucrose non-fermentable) complex, have also been reported in a small number of patients with schwannomatosis.

The clinical testing for both SMARCB1 and LZTR1 mutations is now available for schwannomatosis patients.

25.5.2 Clinical Presentation

Though schwannomas are common to both schwannomatosis and NF2, there are clinical differences [79]. The age at presentation for schwannomatosis peaks in adulthood, usually between the ages of 30 and 60 years, and often with chronic debilitating pain. In contrast, NF2 can be reliably diagnosed in early childhood and more commonly presents with neurological deficits [80]. Histologically, sporadic schwannomas and syndromic schwannomas are indistinguishable; however, similar to NF2, the schwannomas of schwannomatosis tend to have an intraneural growth pattern, peritumoral edema, myxoid change, and a mosaic INI1 staining pattern by immunohistochemistry [81].

25.5.3 Diagnostic Criteria

The diagnostic criteria incorporate both clinical and molecular markers. These are elaborated in Table 25.5.

The most common symptom is pain (46%), presence of a mass (27%), or both (11%). The schwannomas in schwannomatosis commonly affect the spine (74%) and peripheral nerves (89%), while cranial nerve schwannomas (mostly trigeminal) are uncommon (8%). Vestibular schwannomas are rare, and meningiomas occur in 5% of the schwannomatosis patients, with a special predilection for the falx. There is a phenotypic overlap between schwannomatosis and NF2, although bilateral acoustic neuromas have not been reported in schwannomatosis. The neurologic manifestations related to schwannomas are rare and occur often as a consequence of surgical excision of these lesions.

25.5.4 Management

Management of patients with schwannomatosis is symptom-based, and clinical observation is recommended for asymptomatic patients. The pain is the hallmark of this disorder and is the most challenging feature to treat. In cases of spinal cord compression or bothersome symptoms, surgery is performed to improve quality of life [82]. The major risk of the surgery is the iatrogenic damage to the nerve because of the growth within the myelin.

Table 25.5 Diagnostic criteria for schwannomatosis

Clinical criteria	Molecular criteria
At least two non-dermal biopsy-proven schwannomas + no radiographic evidence of bilateral vestibular schwannoma on MRI	Biopsy-proven schwannoma or meningioma + a germline mutation of SMARCB1 gene
One biopsy proven non-dermal schwannoma or intracranial meningioma + a first-degree relative with schwannomatosis	At least two biopsy-proven schwannomas or meningiomas harboring a shared SMARCB1 mutation and differing NF2 mutations

There has been a limited experience with radiation in the treatment of schwannomas related to schwannomatosis, and there have been reports of malignant transformation of schwannomas after the radiation treatment. Henceforth, most reserve the usage of radiation for enlarging schwannomas which cannot be treated with surgery. The role of chemotherapy in the treatment of painful schwannomas is unclear.

25.6 Conclusions

The NFM are a diverse set of conditions with a propensity for the development of nerve sheath tumors. These are classified as distinct tumor suppressor syndromes where loss of specific proteins due to mutations in tumor suppressor genes leads to dysregulation of pathways responsible for cell division and proliferation, thereby contributing to tumor formation at various sites in the body, including the central and peripheral nervous system. A multidisciplinary team effort with a deep understanding of the disorder and basic laboratory and clinical investigations with early implementation of the treatment can lead to excellent results. Genetic counseling is an important tool for the management of affected individuals and their families. Genetic testing is feasible and can identify patients with doubtful history and clinical manifestations.

Acknowledgments We thank the following for their contribution toward clinical photographs and MRI images for the manuscript: Dr. Nihar V Kathrani, Dr. Karthik Kulanthaivelu, Dr. Dattaraj Sawarkar, and Dr. Sunil Budappa.

References

1. Riccardi VM. Neurofibromatosis: clinical heterogeneity. Curr Probl Cancer. 1982;8:1–34.
2. Carey JC, Baty BJ, Johnson JP, Morrison T, Skolnik M, Kivlin J. The genetic aspects of neurofibromatosis. Ann N Y Acad Sci. 1986;486:45–6.
3. Stein DV, Crawford AH. Neurofibromatosis. Surgical management of spinal deformities.2009;211–231. https://doi.org/10.1016/b978-141603372-1.50018-4.

4. Von Recklinghausen F. Uber die multiple Fibrome der Haut und ihre Beziehung zu den multiplen Neuromen. Berlin: Hirschwald; 1882.
5. DeBella K, Szudek J, Friedman JM. Use of the national institutes of health criteria for diagnosis of neurofibromatosis 1 in children. Pediatrics. 2000;105(3 Pt 1):608–14.
6. Hirbe AC, Gutmann DH. Neurofibromatosis type 1: a multidisciplinary approach to care. Lancet Neurol. 2014;13(8):834–43.
7. Huson SM, Compston DAS, Harper PS. A genetic study of von Recklinghausen neurofibromatosis in South East Wales. 1—Prevalence, fitness, mutation rate, and effect of parental transmission on severity. J Med Genet. 1989;26:704–11.
8. Rasmussen A, Friedman JM. NF1 gene and neurofibromatosis 1. Am J Epidemiol. 2000;151:33–40.
9. Woodruff JM. Pathology of tumors of the peripheral nerve sheath in type 1 neurofibromatosis. Am J Med Genet. 1999;89:23–30.
10. Rodriguez FJ, Folpe AL, Giannini C, Perry A. Pathology of peripheral nerve sheath tumors: diagnostic overview and update on selected diagnostic problems. Acta Neuropathol. 2012;123:295–319.
11. Evans DG, Huson SM, Birch JM. Malignant peripheral nerve sheath tumors in inherited diseases. Clin Sarcoma Res. 2012;2:17.
12. King AA, Debaun MR, Riccardi VM, Gutmann DH. Malignant peripheral nerve sheath tumors in neurofibromatosis 1. Am J Med Genet. 2000;93:388–92.
13. Evans DG, Baser ME, McGaughran J, Sharif S, Howard E, Moran A. Malignant peripheral nerve sheath tumors in neurofibromatosis 1. J Med Genet. 2002;39:311–4.
14. Jadayel D, Fain P, Upadhyaya M, et al. Paternal origin of new mutations in von Recklinghausen neurofibromatosis. Nature. 1990;343:558–9.
15. Helfferich J, Nijmeijer R, Brouwer OF, et al. Neurofibromatosis type 1 associated low grade gliomas: a comparison with sporadic low grade gliomas. Crit Rev Oncol Hematol. 2016;104:30–41.
16. Brems H, Beert E, de Ravel T, et al. Mechanisms in the pathogenesis of malignant tumours in neurofibromatosis type 1. Lancet Oncol. 2009;10:508–15.
17. Rodriguez F, Stratakis CA, Evans DG. Genetic predisposition to peripheral nerve neoplasia: diagnostic criteria and pathogenesis of neurofibromatoses, Carney complex, and related syndromes. Acta Neuropathol. 2012;123:349–67.
18. Buchanan ME, Davis RL. A distinct set of Drosophila brain neurons required for neurofibromatosis type 1-dependant learning and memory. J Neurosci. 2010;30:10135–43.
19. Warrington NM, Gianino SM, Jackson E, et al. Cyclic AMP suppression is sufficient to induce gliomagenesis in a mouse model of neurofibromatosis-1. Cancer Res. 2010;70:5717–27.
20. Williams VC, Lucas J, Babcock MA, et al. Neurofibromatosis type 1 revisited. Pediatrics. 2009;123:124–33.
21. Cancer Genome Atlas Research Network. Comprehensive genomic characterization defines human glioblastoma genes and core pathways. Nature. 2008;455:1061–8.
22. Ferner RE, Huson SM, Thomas N, et al. Guidelines for the diagnosis and management of individuals with neurofibromatosis 1. J Med Genet. 2007;44:81–8.
23. Balcer LJ, Liu GT, Heller G, et al. Visual loss in children with neurofibromatosis type 1 and optic pathway gliomas: relation to tumor location by magnetic resonance imaging. Am J Ophthalmol. 2001;131:442–5.
24. Thiagalingam S, Flaherty M, Billson F, et al. Neurofibromatosis type 1 and optic pathway gliomas: follow-up of 54 patients. Ophthalmology. 2004;111:568–77.
25. Ragge NK, Falk RE, Cohen WE, Murphree AL. Images of Lisch nodules across the spectrum. Eye (Lond). 1993;7:95–101.
26. Hood CT, Janku L, Lowder CY, Singh AD. Retinal vasoproliferative tumor in association with neurofibromatosis type 1. J Pediatr Ophthalmol Strabismus. 2009;25:1–3.
27. Shields JA, Pellegrini M, Kaliki S, Mashayekhi A, Shields CL. Retinal vasoproliferative tumors in 6 patients with neurofibromatosis type 1. JAMA Ophthalmol. 2014;132:190–6.
28. Schwetye KE, Gutmann DH. Cognitive and behavioral problems in children with neurofibromatosis type 1: challenges and future directions. Expert Rev Neurother. 2014;14:1139–52.
29. Garozzo D. Peripheral nerve tumors in Neurofibromatosis 1: an overview of management and indications for surgical treatment in our experience. Neurol India. 2019;67:S38–44.
30. Garg S, Green J, Leadbitter K, et al. Neurofibromatosis type 1 and an autism spectrum disorder. Pediatrics. 2013;132:e1642–8.
31. Cutting LE, Levine TM. The cognitive profile of children with neurofibromatosis and reading disabilities. Child Neuropsychol. 2010;16:417–32.
32. Itoh T, Magnaldi S, White RM, et al. Neurofibromatosis type 1: the evolution of deep gray and white matter MR abnormalities. AJNR Am J Neuroradiol. 1994;15:1513–9.
33. Van Es S, North KN, McHugh K, et al. MRI findings in children with neurofibromatosis type 1: a prospective study. Pediatr Radiol. 1996;26:478–87.
34. Griffiths PD, Blaser S, Mukonoweshuro W, et al. Neurofibromatosis bright objects in children with neurofibromatosis type 1: a proliferative potential? Pediatrics. 1999;104:e49.
35. Braffman BH, Bilaniuk LT, Zimmerman RA. The central nervous system manifestations of the phakomatoses on MR. Radiol Clin North Am. 1988;26:773–800.
36. Smirniotopoulos JG, Murphy FM. The phakomatoses. AJNR Am J Neuroradiol. 1992;13:725–46.
37. Bognanno JR, Edwards MK, Lee TA, et al. Cranial MR imaging in neurofibromatosis. AJR Am J Roentgenol. 1988;151:381–8.

38. DiPaolo DP, Zimmerman RA, Rorke LB, et al. Neurofibromatosis type 1: pathologic substrate of high-signal-intensity foci in the brain. Radiology. 1995;195:721–4.
39. Torres Nupan MM, Velez Van Meerbeke A, Lopez Cabra CA, et al. Cognitive and behavioral disorders in children with neurofibromatosis type 1. Front Pediatr. 2017;5:227.
40. Brossier NM, Carroll SL. Genetically engineered mouse models shed new light on the pathogenesis of neurofibromatosis type I-related neoplasms of the peripheral nervous system. Brain Res Bull. 2012;88:58–71.
41. Pasmant E, Sabbagh A, Spurlock G, et al. NF1 microdeletions in neurofibromatosis type 1: from genotype to phenotype. Hum Mutat. 2010;31(6):E1506–18. https://doi.org/10.1002/humu.21271.
42. Elefteriou F, Kolanczyk M, Schindeler A, et al. Skeletal abnormalities in neurofibromatosis type 1: approaches to therapeutic options. Am J Med Genet A. 2009;149A:2327–38.
43. Lammert M, Friedman JM, Roth HJ, et al. Vitamin D deficiency associated with a number of neurofibromas in neurofibromatosis 1. J Med Genet. 2006;43:810–3.
44. Lin AE, Birch PH, Korf BR, et al. Cardiovascular malformations and other cardiovascular abnormalities in neurofibromatosis 1. Am J Med Genet. 2000;95:108–17.
45. Oderich GS, Sullivan TM, Bower TC, et al. Vascular abnormalities in patients with neurofibromatosis syndrome type I: clinical spectrum, management, and results. J Vasc Surg. 2007;46:475–84.
46. Rea D, Brandsema JF, Armstrong D, et al. Cerebral arteriopathy in children with neurofibromatosis type 1. Pediatrics. 2009;124:e476–83.
47. D'Arco F, D'Amico A, Caranci F, et al. Cerebrovascular stenosis in neurofibromatosis type 1 and utility of magnetic resonance angiography: our experience and literature review. Radiol Med. 2014;119:415–21.
48. Friedman JM, Arbiser J, Epstein JA, et al. Cardiovascular disease in neurofibromatosis 1: report of the NF1 cardiovascular task force. Genet Med. 2002;4:105–11.
49. Ennibi K, El Kassimi I, Asfalou I, Chaari J, Benyass A. Pulmonary hypertension and von Recklinghausen's disease: association and therapeutic difficulties. Pneumologia. 2015;64:55–7.
50. Bausch B, Koschker AC, Fassnacht M, et al. Comprehensive mutation scanning of NF1 in apparently sporadic cases of pheochromocytoma. J Clin Endocrinol Metab. 2006;91:3478–81.
51. Mannelli M, Castellano M, Schiavi F, et al.; Italian Pheochromocytoma/Paraganglioma Network. Clinically guided genetic screening in a large cohort of Italian patients with pheochromocytomas and/or functional or nonfunctional paragangliomas. J Clin Endocrinol Metab. 2009;94:1541–1547.
52. Eisenhofer G, Lenders JW, Timmers H, et al. Measurements of plasma methoxytyramine, normetanephrine, and metanephrine as discriminators of different hereditary forms of pheochromocytoma. Clin Chem. 2011;57:411–20.
53. Easton DF, Ponder MA, Huson SM, et al. An analysis of variation in expression of neurofibromatosis (NF) type 1 (NF1): evidence for modifying genes. Am J Hum Genet. 1993;53:305–13.
54. Barahona-Garrido J, Aguirre-Gutierrez R, Gutierrez-Manjarrez JI, et al. Association of GIST and somatostatinoma in a patient with type-1 neurofibromatosis: is there a common pathway? Am J Gastroenterol. 2009;104:797–9.
55. Miettinen M, Fetsch JF, Sobin LH, et al. Gastrointestinal stromal tumors in patients with neurofibromatosis 1: a clinicopathologic and molecular genetic study of 45 cases. Am J Surg Pathol. 2006;30:90–6.
56. Stiller CA, Chessells JM, Fitchett M. Neurofibromatosis, and childhood leukemia/lymphoma: a population-based UKCCSG study. Br J Cancer. 1994;70:969–72.
57. Brems H, Park C, Maertens O, et al. Glomus tumors in neurofibromatosis type 1: genetic, functional, and clinical evidence of a novel association. Cancer Res. 2009;69:7393–401.
58. McGaughran JM, Harris DI, Donnai D, et al. A clinical study of type 1 neurofibromatosis in northwest England. J Med Genet. 1999;36:197–203.
59. Patil S, Chamberlain RS. Neoplasms associated with germline and somatic NF1 gene mutations. Oncologist. 2012;17:101–16.
60. Crucis A, Richer W, Brugieres L, et al. Rhabdomyosarcomas in children with neurofibromatosis type I: a national historical cohort. Pediatr Blood Cancer. 2015;62:1733–8.
61. Afsar CU, Kara IO, Kozat BK, et al. Neurofibromatosis type 1, gastrointestinal stromal tumor, leiomyosarcoma, and osteosarcoma: four cases of rare tumors and a review of the literature. Crit Rev Oncol Hematol. 2013;86:191–9.
62. Uusitalo E, Kallionpaa RA, Kurki S, et al. Breast cancer in neurofibromatosis type 1: overrepresentation of unfavorable prognostic factors. Br J Cancer. 2017;116:211–7.
63. Clementi M, Milani S, Mammi I, et al. Neurofibromatosis type 1 growth charts. Am J Med Genet. 1999;87:317–23.
64. Szudek J, Birch P, Friedman JM. Growth charts for young children with neurofibromatosis 1 (NF1). Am J Med Genet. 2000;92:224–8.
65. Szudek J, Birch P, Friedman JM. Growth in North American white children with neurofibromatosis 1 (NF1). J Med Genet. 2000;37:933–8.
66. Avery RA, Fisher MJ, Liu GT. Optic pathway gliomas. J Neuroophthalmol. 2011;31:269–78.
67. Packer RJ, Jakacki R, Horn M, et al. Objective response of multiply recurrent low-grade gliomas to bevacizumab and irinotecan. Pediatr Blood Cancer. 2009;52:791–5.
68. Banerjee A, Jakacki RI, Onar-Thomas A, et al. A phase I trial of the MEK inhibitor selumetinib (AZD6244) in pediatric patients with recurrent or refractory low-

grade glioma: a Pediatric Brain Tumor Consortium (PBTC) study. Neuro Oncol. 2016;19:1135–44.
69. Friedman JM. Neurofibromatosis 1. 1998 [Updated 2019 Jun 6]. In: Adam MP, Ardinger HH, Pagon RA, et al., editors. GeneReviews® [Internet]. Seattle, : University of Washington; 1993–2020. https://www.ncbi.nlm.nih.gov/books/NBK1109/
70. Wilding A, Ingham SL, Lalloo F, et al. Life expectancy in hereditary cancer predisposing diseases: an observational study. J Med Genet. 2012;49(04):264–9.
71. Maniakas A, Saliba I. Neurofibromatosis type 2 vestibular schwannoma treatment: a review of the literature, trends, and outcomes. Otol Neurotol. 2014;35(5):889–94.
72. McCaughan JA, Holloway SM, Davidson R, et al. Further evidence of the increased risk for malignant peripheral nerve sheath tumor from a Scottish cohort of patients with neurofibromatosis type 1. J Med Genet. 2007;44:463–6.
73. Plotkin SR, Halpin C, McKenna MJ, Loeffler JS, Batchelor TT, Barker FG. Erlotininb for progressive vestibular schwannoma in neurofibromatosis 2 patients. Otol Neurotol. 2010;31(07):1135–14.
74. Karajannis MA, Legault G, Hagiwara M, et al. Phase II trial of lapatinib in adult an dpediatric patients with neurofibromatosis type 2 and progressive vestibular schwannomas. Neuro Oncol. 2012;14(09):1163–70.
75. Karajannis MA, Legault G, Hagiwara M, et al. Phase II study of everolimus in children and adults with neurofibromatosis type 2 and progressive vestibular schwannomas. Neuro Oncol. 2014;16(02):292–7.
76. Plotkin SR, Merker VL, Halpin C, et al. Bevacizumab for progressive vestibular schwannoma in neurofibromatosis type 2: a retrospective review of 31 patients. Otol Neurotol. 2012;33(06):1046–52.
77. Plotkin SR, Blakeley JO, Evans DG, et al. Update from the 2011 international schwannomatosis workshop: from genetics to diagnostic criteria. Am J Med Genet A. 2013;161A(03):405–16.
78. Longo JF, Weber SM, Turner-Ivey BP, Carroll SL. Recent advances in the diagnosis and pathogenesis of neurofibromatosis type 1 (NF1)-associated peripheral nervous system neoplasms. Adv Anat Pathol. 2018;25(5):353–68.
79. Trofatter JA, Mac Collin MM, Rutter JL, et al. A novelmoesin-, ezrin-, radixin-like gene is a candidate for the neurofibromatosis 2 tumor suppressor. Cell. 1993;72(5):791–800.
80. Rouleau GA, Merel P, Lutchman M, et al. Alteration in a new gene encoding a putative membrane-organizing protein causes neurofibromatosis type 2. Nature. 1993;363(6429):515–21.
81. Evans DG, Ramsden RT, Shenton A, et al. Mosaicism in neurofibromatosis type 2: an update of risk based on uni/bilaterality of vestibular schwannoma at presentation and sensitive mutation analysis including multiple ligation-dependent probe amplification. J Med Genet. 2007;44(7):424–8.
82. Kresak JL, Walsh M. Neurofibromatosis: a review of NF1, NF2, and Schwannomatosis. J Pediatr Genet. 2016;5(2):98–104. https://doi.org/10.1055/s-0036-1579766.

26 Genetic Aspects of Peripheral Nervous System Tumors

Marcela Ferrer, Patricia Ciavarelli, and Mariano Socolovsky

Tumors involving the peripheral nervous system (PNS) represent a heterogeneous population of neoplasms which include both benign and malignant forms. They are summarized in Table 26.1.

Benign peripheral nerve sheath tumors (BPNST) include schwannomas (the most common tumors arising from peripheral nerves), neurofibromas, and perineuriomas [2]. While schwannomas and perineuriomas are composed of uniform populations of Schwann cells and perineurial cells, respectively, neurofibromas consist of diverse cell types, including Schwann cells, fibroblasts, perineurial cells, and entrapped axons.

The advances in genetics with the developments in informatics and imaging allowed refining the classification of diseases, often with important prognostic and treatment implications [3].

M. Ferrer
Molecular Neuro-oncological Lab, Department of Genetics, Hospital de Clínicas, University of Buenos Aires School of Medicine, Buenos Aires, Argentina

P. Ciavarelli
Interdisciplinary Program on Neurofibromatosis, Hospital de Clínicas, University of Buenos Aires School of Medicine, Buenos Aires, Argentina

M. Socolovsky (✉)
WFNS Peripheral Nerve Surgery Committee, Peripheral Nerve & Brachial Plexus Surgery Program, Department of Neurosurgery, University of Buenos Aires School of Medicine, Buenos Aires, Argentina

In 2016, the World Health Organization (WHO) published an update of the 2007 fourth edition of the Classification of Tumors of the Nervous System [4, 5] based on (1) a combined phenotypic and genotypic classification and (2) the generation of "integrated" diagnoses. For the first time, molecular parameters were included. These more objective and more precisely defined entities will improve patient therapy and will facilitate the classification for clinical trials and epidemiological studies improving the quality of life of those patients suffering these lesions.

This fifth edition contains the codes of the third edition of the International Classification of Disease for Oncology (ICD-O), which closely corresponds to the histopathological classification with the aim of facilitating the epidemiological analyses of nervous system neoplasms [6].

For peripheral nervous system tumors (Table 26.1) [1, 7, 8], the major changes included in the 2016 WHO classification are the expansion and clarification of entities included in the section of nerve sheath tumors, with the addition of hybrid nerve sheath tumors and the separation of melanotic schwannoma from other schwannomas.

Benign neoplasms developing from the peripheral nervous system may arise in most cases sporadically, but they are also associated to specific inherited genetic disorders. The familial syndromes that predispose individuals to the development of tumors, often multiple, within

F. Guedes et al. (eds.), *Diagnostic Assessment and Treatment of Peripheral Nerve Tumors*,
https://doi.org/10.1007/978-3-030-77633-6_26

Table 26.1 The WHO classification of tumors of peripheral nervous system [1]

Name	ICDO	Behavior
Schwannoma	9560	0
Cellular schwannoma	9560	0
Plexiform schwannoma	9560	0
Melanotic schwannoma	9560	1
Neurofibroma	9540	0
Atypical neurofibroma	9540	0
Plexiform neurofibroma	9550	0
Perineurioma	9571	0
Hybrid nerve sheath tumor	9540	3
Malignant peripheral nerve sheath tumor		
Epithelioid MPNST	9540	3
MPNST with perineurial differentiation	9540	3

ICDO International Classification of Disease for Oncology (ICD-O 2013), Behavior 0 benign tumors; 1 unspecified, borderline, or uncertain; 2 carcinomas in situ and grade III intraepithelial neoplasia; and 3 malignant tumors

the PNS, are neurofibromatosis types 1 and 2, schwannomatosis, or Carney's complex [9] [10].

A tumor is any abnormal proliferation of cells, which may be either benign or malignant [11]. The continual unregulated proliferation of cells is the result of genetic and/or epigenetic alternations into two broad classes of genes, proto-oncogenes and tumor suppressor genes (TSGs). Proto-oncogenes are involved in pathways that promote cellular growth, and the mutated versions of these genes are known as oncogenes [12]. Tumor suppressors are the genes that protect cells from malignant alterations and are involved in DNA damage repair, inhibition of cell division, induction of apoptosis, and suppression of metastasis. Loss of TSG function is a common mechanism contributing to the development of tumors [13]. Most of the genes involved in the development of nervous system tumors are in fact tumor suppressors.

A wide spectrum of genetics and epigenetic aberrations are involved in the growth of malignant cells. Genetic alterations include mutations, genomic instability, loss of heterozygosity (LOH), and gene copy number variation (CNV). Epigenetics changes which regulate gene expression without altering the underlying nucleotide sequence involved histone modifications, DNA methylation, and loss of imprinting (LOI) [14].

In hereditary tumors, we can find constitutional alterations associated with somatic loss of function of wild-type alleles. In the corresponding sporadic tumors, biallelic somatic loss-of-function (LOF) mutations can be found.

Functional inactivation of TSGs is a common mechanism contributing to the development of cancer. Most of the TSGs follow the Knudson "two-hit" hypothesis [15] which postulated the recessive nature of loss-of-function mutations where both alleles of a TSG must be permanently inactivated by mutation and deletion or silenced by promoter methylation. However, there have been described other inactivation mechanisms of known TSGs that do not follow the classic Knudson two-hit hypothesis such as proteasomal degradation, abnormal cellular location, and transcriptional regulation [16].

In this chapter we attempt to summarize the genes and the knowledge of the underlying molecular mechanisms involved in the development of peripheral nerve system tumors. Excellent reviews are available covering clinical, histologic, and immunohistochemical aspects of these tumors [7, 8, 17–24]. Table 26.1 is a brief summary of inherited syndromes associated with neoplasms of peripheral nerve sheath.

26.1 Schwannomas

Most tumors of the human peripheral nervous system derive from Schwann cells or their precursors. Schwannomas are benign peripheral nerve sheath tumors (PNST) composed entirely of well-differentiated Schwann cells. Conventional, cellular, and plexiform variants can be found [5] and account for about 25–30% of spinal tumors [25]. Although they are benign, they cause many different morbidities. Ninety percent of them are sporadic, [26], but they are also associated with specific inherited genetic disorders: neurofibromatosis 2, schwannomatosis, and Carney complex.

Cellular variant: relatively uncommon [7, 8], lack malignant potential, and never metastasize.

Plexiform variant: usually occurs in superficial (cutaneous or subcutaneous) locations. There is a weak association (approximately 5% of the cases) with schwannoma predisposition syndromes such as NF2 and schwannomatosis.

The rare plexiform schwannomas that arise in deep anatomic locations may be difficult to distinguish from MPNST.

26.1.1 Genetic Profile

The common feature underlying formation of most conventional schwannomas, whether sporadic or syndromic, is the loss of merlin function, encoded by *NF2* gene, as a classical tumor suppressor which is inactivated according to Knudson's two-hit hypothesis [23, 27–29].

In sporadic tumors the biallelic somatic inactivation involve mainly frameshift variants (insertion or deletion involving a number of base pairs that is not a multiple of 3, which consequently disrupts the triplet reading frame of a DNA sequence) that results in truncated protein products followed by loss of the remaining wild-type allele on chromosome 22q [30]. Even though almost all sporadic schwannomas show loss of 22q, about 25% of all sporadic schwannomas do not harbor a *NF2* pathogenic [31].

SMARCB1 gene initially associated only with the familial and sporadic forms of schwannomatosis [32] may also play a role in the development of a small subset of sporadic schwannomas [33].

Schwannoma predisposition syndromes are neurofibromatosis 2 (NF2) (MIM #101000) and schwannomatosis (SWNTS) (MIM #162091) [23].

In neurofibromatosis 2, the pathogenic germline variants are (1) frameshift, (2) nonsense (genetic alteration that causes the premature termination of a protein), (3) splice-site variants (genetic alteration in the DNA sequence that occurs at the boundary of an exon and an intron and disrupt RNA splicing), or (4) small deletion followed by a second small genetic alteration or, more commonly, by loss of the remaining wild-type allele on chromosome 22 [34, 35].

In schwannomatosis, the mechanism of tumorigenesis is distinctive as it contemplates "four or more hits": the constitutional alteration of *SMARCB1* or *LZTR1* (one-hit) followed by loss of 22q wild-type allele (two-hit loss of wild-type *SMARCB1* or *LZTR1* and the loss of wild type *NF2*) and genetic mutation in the remaining wild-type *NF2* allele [36]. Figure 26.1 describes the models of tumorigenesis in schwannomatosis: basically concomitant mutational inactivation of two or more tumor suppressor genes.

There are some cases whose molecular mechanisms are unknown, those where there is loss of heterozygosity of chromosome 22 and no pathogenic variants can be demonstrated in either SMARCB1 or LZTR1. And also, those cases where no loss of chromosome 22 or pathogenic variants in the aforementioned genes is observed. In the first case, the underlying causes could be deep intronic pathogenic variants in SMARCB1or LZTR1 or pathogenic variants in some other gene on chromosome 22. In the second case, the predisposing gene could be localized on another chromosome.

26.1.2 Genes and Molecular Mechanisms

26.1.2.1 Gene NF2 (ID: 4771) Neurofibromin 2

The functional biallelic inactivation of the tumor suppressor gene *NF2* is a common feature underlying both inherited and sporadic forms of schwannoma, and pathogenic variants were found in approximately 60% of all schwannomas [30, 31]. However, about 25% of all sporadic schwannomas do not harbor a *NF2* pathogenic change [31].

The human *NF2* gene localized on chromosoma 22q12.2 spans 110 kb, comprises 17 exons, and encodes a protein named merlin or schwannomin [37, 38]. By alternative splicing it encodes two predominant protein isoforms and is ubiquitously expressed in all tissues during all periods of development [39].

Based on sequence homology (45–47%), schwannomin and merlin (for moesin, ezrin, radixin-like protein) are members of the band 4.1 superfamily (Fig. 26.1). Three widely expressed members of the family, ezrin, radixin, and moesin (ERM), are cytoskeleton-associated proteins that link cell surface glycoproteins to the actin cytoskeleton [40]. ERM proteins and Merlin, a 595 amino acid protein, have a highly conserved N-terminal domain (NTD/FERM domain), a central non-conserved α-helix region and a short-charged C-terminal domain (CTD) [38]. Merlin has the highest degree of amino acid identity across the FERM domain, a protein module of around 300 amino acids that is involved in localizing proteins to the plasma membrane and in mediating membrane–cytoskeleton and intercellular adhesion molecule interactions [41–43].

Merlin has two main isoforms arising from alternative splicing of exons 16 and 17. Merlin isoform 1 is a 595-residue protein that is derived from 16 constitutive exons, 1–15 and 17, and isoform 2 is a 590-residue protein that results from the alternatively spliced exon 16, replacing 16 terminal residues with 11 new residues (Fig. 26.1) [44]. It is generally accepted that the growth suppressor function of merlin is dependent on its ability to form a "close" (active) clamp conformation where the CTD binds to a site on the FERM domain [45]. The "open" (inactive) and "closed" (active) conformations are regulated by a physical intramolecular interaction between the N- and C-termini [46]. Although phosphorylation of serine 518 leads to an open conformation and to the inactivation of merlin-1 [47], merlin-2 which is shorter and couldn't have the "close" conformation inhibits cell growth [48]. Merlin functions both at the membrane and in the

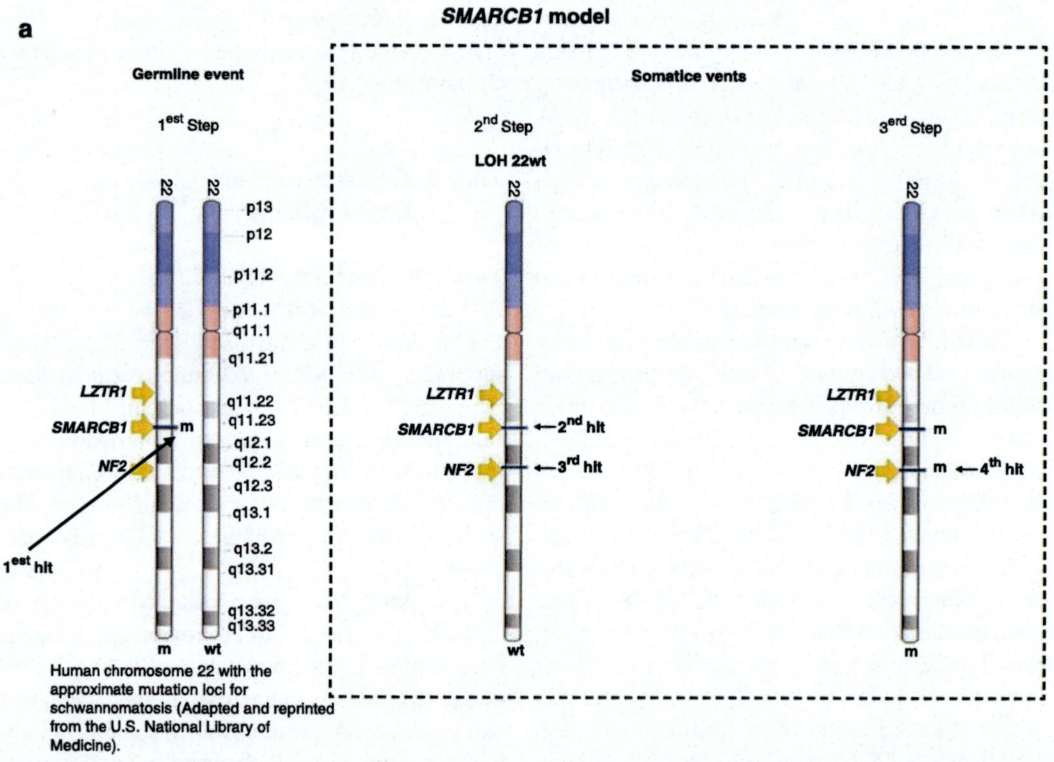

Fig. 26.1 Models of tumorigenesis in schwannomatosis: at least three tumor suppressor genes (TSGs) are involved in a complex mutational model. The first hit and step for both is the germinal mutation of *SMARCB1* (**a**) or *LZTR1* (**b**). In a second step, the allele of chromosome 22 carrying wild-type copies of genes is lost. For *SMARCB1* predisposition syndrome involves two hits (loss of *SMARCB1* and *NF2*); meanwhile for *LZTR1* predisposition schwannomatosis includes three hits (*LZTR1*, *SMARCB1*, and *NF2*). In the third step, a somatic mutation of *NF2* wild-type takes place, fourth hit for *SMARCB1* model and fifth hit for *LZTR1*

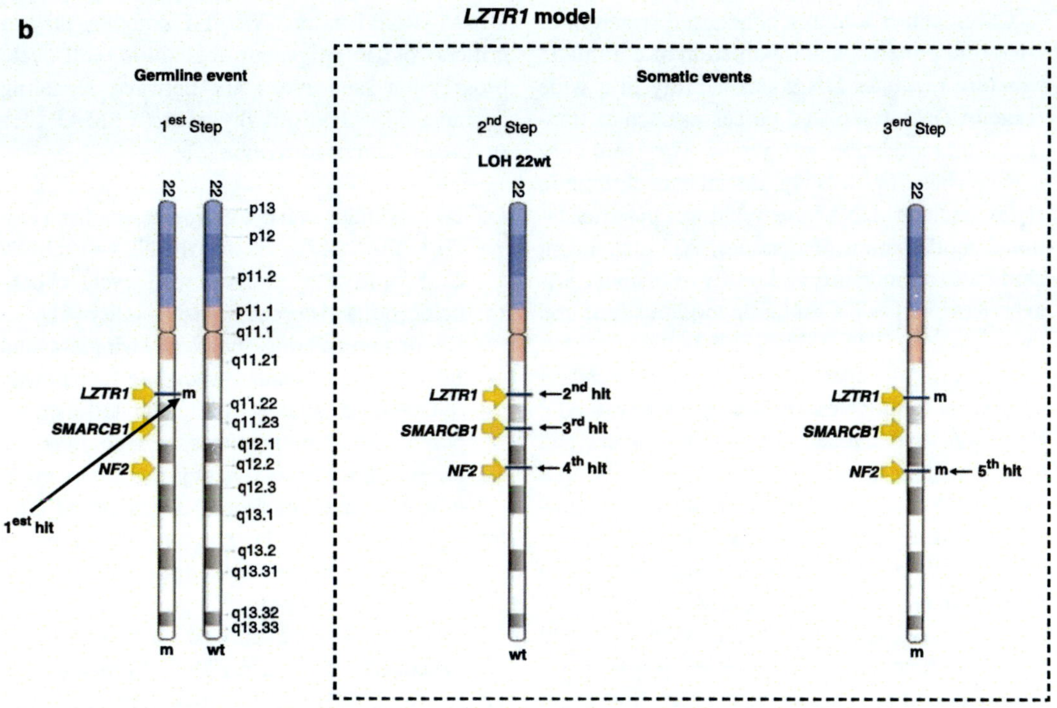

Fig. 26.1 (continued)

nucleus, while ERMs are mainly restricted to membranes and the cytoplasm [41]. Recently it has been found that the tumor suppression function of merlin is independent of its structural role [48]. The F2 subdomain of the merlin FERM domain and a domain defined by residues 532–579 near the C-terminal region of merlin are essential for inhibiting cell proliferation. The F1 subdomain is required for maintaining the cytoskeletal organization but not for inhibition of cell proliferation.

The only/unique member of the ERM's family that acts as tumor suppressor is merlin [44] and mediates its tumor suppressive effect by participating in multiple signaling pathways such as Rac–PAK and mTORC1 signaling, the EGFR–Ras–ERK pathway, and the PI3K–Akt pathway and FAK–Src signaling, Hippo signaling, and Wnt/β-catenin signaling [49]. In addition, recent studies have indicated that the closed form of merlin translocates to the nucleus to modify gene expression through inhibition of the E3 ubiquitin ligase CRL4DCAF1 [50].

26.1.2.2 Gene SMARCB1 (ID:6598) (SWI/SNF-Related, Matrix-Associated, Actin-Dependent Regulator of Chromatin, Subfamily b, Member 1), also Named INI1/ /SNF5/BAF47

It is one of the core subunit proteins in the SWI/SNF (SWItch/Sucrose Non-Fermentable) ATP-dependent chromatin remodeling complex encoded at chromosomal position 22q11.2 [51].

SMARCB1 gene comprises nine exons and spans approximately 50 kb, produces a 1.749-bp transcript variant 1 (NM_003073.3), and encodes isoform A. This isoform has been chosen as the canonical sequence, contains 385 amino acids (NP_003064.2), and has a molecular mass of 44 kDa. It is universally expressed in all normal mammalian nucleated cells [52]. The use of a cryptic splice donor site in exon 2 results in a SNF5/INI1 protein lacking a short peptide sequence in its N-terminal region (Isoform B, 376 amino acids, and 43 kDa).

Chromatin is a highly condensed structure of DNA and proteins, and modulation of chromatin structure regulates DNA accessibility in a wide range of DNA-templated processes such as transcription, replication, and repair. The regulatory mechanisms for defining distinctive chromatin states include DNA methylation, posttranslational modification of histones, ATP-dependent chromatin remodeling, and utility of histone variants (Kouzarides T. Chromatin modifications and their function. Cell. 2007;128:693–705).

The ATP-dependent chromatin remodeling complexes (remodelers) utilize the energy of ATP hydrolysis to modulate chromatin structure and are intimately associated with processes that require DNA access such as transcription, replication, and repair [53]. The SWI/SNF chromatin remodeling complex (an evolutionarily conserved family of remodelers) is a master regulator of developmental cell fate decisions and represents a novel link between epigenetic regulation and tumor suppression. The key target pathways have started to be characterized recently.

Mammalian SWI/SNF complexes comprise of 12–15 subunits (~2 MDa in size) and has been shown to play an essential role in many tissues and developmental processes, including vertebrate nervous system development [54]. In view of the large number of variant subunits, it has been estimated that several hundred versions of functional SWI/SNF complexes may exist [55].

Among different chromatin remodelers, SWI/SNF complexes are the more common chromatin remodeler dysregulated in human cancers and have shown to be collectively mutated in 20% of all human cancers [56].

SWI/SNF does not interact with one type of transcription factor, but rather it regulates the function of many diverse genes as well as the function of many signaling pathways suggesting a broad role for the complex of tumor suppression [57, 58].

The role of SMARCB1 within the complex is not completely understood. Loss of expression reflects biallelic inactivation, and these biallelic events may occur with or without a predisposing germline mutation [59].

SMARCB1 in the SWI/SNF complex plays a critical role in epigenetic regulation, cell cycle progression, and cross-talk between signaling cascades. Mechanisms by which SMARCB1 suppresses tumor formation are:

(a) By preventing cell cycle progression from G0/G1 to the S-phase via the p16INK4a-cyclinD/CDK4-pRb-E2F pathway cell cycle checkpoint [60] and chromosomal stability [61].
(b) By downregulating the Wnt (wingless and INT-1) canonical signaling pathway (β-catenin-dependent) [62]: secreted glycolipoproteins which regulates the amount of the transcriptional co-activator β-catenin by ubiquitination and proteasomal degradation [63].
(c) By inhibition of the Shh (sonic hedgehog) pathway blocking transcription of glioma-associated oncogene homologue (GLI) reducing downstream Hh pathway target genes (*GL1*, *GL2*, and *PTCH1*) [58, 64].
(d) By repressed EZH2 transcription, the catalytic subunit in polycomb repressive complex 2 (PRC2), a multi-subunit epigenetic protein complex that regulates gene expression by catalyzing trimethylation of histone H3 on lysine 27 [65].
(e) Other pathways involved in oncogenesis have been reported as targets of SMARCB1 as *c-MYC* (codes for a transcription factor) and *Aurora A* (a member of a family of mitotic serine/threonine kinases) [64].

26.1.2.3 Gene LZTR1 (ID:8216) (Leucine Zipper-Like Transcription Regulator 1)

Located at 22q11.21, it contains 21 exons and generates multiple alternatively spliced transcripts, with the longest ORF encoding an 840-residue protein, and is expressed ubiquitously and abundantly in human tissues [66]. It encodes a protein member of the functionally diverse BTB-kelch superfamily [67].

LZTR1 is a tumor suppressor gene found to be involved in the development of schwannomatosis [68]. Besides it has also been found to be involved in glioblastoma multiforme [69] and hepatocellular carcinoma [70], among many other cancers.

It is also implicated in Noonan syndrome (NS), a developmental syndrome that is part of the larger group of RASopathies characterized by mutations in components of the RAS-MAPK pathway [71], inherited in an autosomal dominant or recessive pattern [72, 73] and in the etiology of BEEC (bladder exstrophy–epispadias complex, which is a congenital malformation of the bladder and urethra) [74].

LZTR1 is an unusual BTB-kelch protein with distinctive structure organization, six-kelch repeats present in the N-terminus, and two BTB-BACK domains at the C-terminus, where the BTBII domain mediates localization of LZTR-1 to the Golgi complex (Fig. 26.1) [66].

Further LZTR1 may also be translocated to the nucleus as shown for another BBK family member [75] because it contains a bipartite nuclear localization signal (NLS) at the N-terminus and as also indicated by WoLF PSORT protein subcellular localization [68].

As there is a weak homology of LZTR-1 to certain known members of the basic leucine zipper-like family, it was first proposed to be a negative regulator of transcriptional factors [76], although its exclusive localization to the Golgi complex made this unlikely [66].

More recently, the molecular role of LZTR1 in cancers and Noonan syndrome was described. Protein ubiquitination, one of the most frequent post-translational modifications in eukaryotes [77], has a vital role controlling signaling pathways [78]. Also, it was shown that LZTR1, as other members of the BTB-kelch superfamily proteins [79], interacts with the Cullin3 (CUL3)-based E3 ubiquitin ligase complex [80, 81]. The RAS proteins polyubiquitinated by LZTR1 are directed to the proteasome and degraded via the ubiquitin-proteasome pathway resulting in reduced MAPK signaling [82]. LZTR1 loss in Schwann cells drives dedifferentiation and proliferation [81].

26.2 Melanotic Schwannoma

This is a rare, distinctive, and potentially malignant neoplasm [7, 8]. Two varieties have been described: non-psammomatous and psammomatous [1, 5], as about 50% of patients with psammomatous tumors have Carney complex (MIM 188830, 605244). This tumor shows frequent loss of *PRKAR1A* gene and appears to be genetically different from schwannomas based on gene expression analysis [23].

26.2.1 Genes and Molecular Mechanisms

Gene *PRKAR1A* (ID: 5573) (protein kinase cAMP-dependent type I regulatory subunit alpha) located at 17q24.2, it encodes the most widely expression of protein kinase A (PKA) and is a key component of the cAMP signaling pathway. Genomic region is approximately 21 kb. The longest transcript variant NM_212472.1 is composed of 11 exons; codon 1 is noncoding. It is a tumor suppressor gene and encodes a protein 384 amino acids organized in a dimerization/docking domain at the amino terminus, followed by a PKA inhibitor site, two tandem binding domains for cAMP at the carboxyl terminus (cAMP:A and cAMP:B), and a linker region that contains the main docking site for the C subunit [83].

26.3 Neurofibroma

Neurofibromas are benign peripheral nerve sheath tumors, composed of a variable mixture of Schwann, perineurial-like, and fibroblastic cells. They can arise sporadically or associated with neurofibromatosis type 1 (NF1) (OMIM #162200) (10%) [7, 8]. Germline heterozygous pathogenic variants in *NF1* gene are followed by somatic loss of the remaining wild-type allele in Schwann cells of NF1 patients, whereas somatic biallelic inactivation occurs in sporadic neurofibromas [84].

Atypical Variant

The genetic alterations described in neurofibromas with atypical features are loss of *CDKN2A/p16*, *p53*, *SMARCA2*, and others, especially on the 9p2 locus. These changes are also seen in MPNSTs, but not in typical neurofibromas [85, 86].

Plexiform Variant

Plexiform neurofibromas are pathognomonic of neurofibromatosis and have a significant risk of malignant transformation.

They are almost always associated with NF1, have a potential for malignant degeneration, and are a recognized precursor for MPNST in NF1 patients [7, 8].

26.3.1 Genes and Molecular Mechanisms

26.3.1.1 Gene *NF1* (ID:4763) (Neurofibromin 1)

The human NF1, located at chromosome 17q11.2, is one of the biggest genes in the human genome, spans approximately 350 kb of genomic DNA classified as a tumor suppressor gene, and comprises 58 exons [87, 88]. It encodes an mRNA of 11 to 13 kb and codes three alternatively spliced transcripts [89]. Also, the mRNA of NF1 may undergo RNA editing (CGA>UGA->Arg1306Term) resulting in premature translation termination. The unusual characteristic of NF1 gene is that it has three active genes called *OMGP* (164345) (oligodendrocyte myelin glycoprotein), *EVI2B* (158381), and *EVI2A* (158380) (ecotropic viral integration site) within the intron 35 but in opposite orientation (27b according to the previous numbering) [90, 91].

At least 11 NF1 pseudogenes have been identified in the human genome in 2q21.1 (NF1P8), 12q12 (NF1P12), 14q11.2 (NF1P4, NF1P7, NF1P11, NF1P10), 15q11.2 (NF1P1, NF1P2), 18p11.21 (NF1P5), 21q11.2 (NF1P3), and 22q11.1 (NF1P6). These can cause confusion in the mutation analysis of patients with NF1.

The most abundant form of NF1 mRNA is NM_000267.3 transcript of about 8.5 kb, which contains 57 exons and encodes neurofibromin isoform 2 (NP_000258.1), consisting of 2818 amino acids with a molecular weight of 280 kDa [92]. It is ubiquitously expressed but is enriched in neurons, Schwann cells, oligodendrocytes, and leukocytes [90].

Neurofibromin appears to be predominantly cytoplasmic, with different cell types displaying a variable subcellular localization, having a functional nuclear localization signal (NLS) in exon 43 [93].

Neurofibromin is a multifunctional protein with the ability to regulate several signal pathways associated with cell growth and proliferation. It belongs to a family of proteins known as Ras-GTPase-activating proteins which function as negative regulators for Ras proteins. It has a central domain of 250–400 amino acids and Gap-related domain (GRD) that binds to GTP-bound RAS, augment its intrinsic GTPase activity, and leads to RAS inactivation and to the inhibition of the RAS/MAPK signaling [94]. The aberrant function or decreased level of expression of genes that encode components or regulators of the Ras/MAPK pathway produces disorders collectively known as RASopathies [95].

26.4 Perineuroma

This is a rare benign neoplasm composed exclusively of perineurial cells, which develops in the dermis, subcutis, or deep soft tissue [96]. There are very few studies of genetic aberrations in these tumors, but both types, intraneural and soft tissue, have monosomy or deletion of the 22q11–22q13.1 bands [97].

Recently an association of perineuroma with NF1 [98] and NF2 has been reported [99, 100].

The sclerosing perineuroma variant has been associated with rearrangements or deletions 10q, with a cryptic deletion of the *NF2* gene, and with loss of the chromosome 13 [101–103].

26.5 Hybrid Nerve Sheath Tumor

These lesions are defined as tumors having combined characteristics of two benign nerve sheath tumors, either juxtaposed or intermixed [23]. The most common hybrid nerve sheath tumor is the hybrid perineurioma-schwannoma, typically without syndromic association. Hybrid neurofibroma-schwannomas are reported at increased frequency in NF2 and schwannomatosis patients, and there is evidence that hybrid perineurioma-neurofibroma is associated with NF1 [104].

26.6 Malignant Peripheral Nerve Sheath Tumor

MPNSTs account for ~5% of soft tissue sarcomas and are highly aggressive tumors that occur either sporadically, in the setting of neurofibromatosis type 1 (37–64%), or arise after irradiation (1%) [105].

One of the most challenging diagnoses in peripheral nerve tumors is MPNST, particularly in the sporadic setting.

Alterations in *NF1*, *CDKN2A/p16*, and *p53* were recurrently seen in MPNSTs as well as at some frequency in neurofibroma, with atypical feature spectrum, thereby being a presumably precursor of MPNST [23]. Recent studies showed inactivation of polycomb repressive complex 2 (PRC2) in a large subset of malignant peripheral nerve sheath tumors, due to loss-of-function mutations in PRC2 subunits EED or SUZ12 [106]. These co-occur with somatic mutations of *CDKN2A* and *NF1* and are associated with a distinct DNA methylation profile.

Polycomb repressive complex 2 (PRC2) is a multi-subunit epigenetic protein complex that maintain gene repression in part by modifying chromatin structure, through both physical compaction and covalent modification of histones in a tightly controlled spatial and temporal manner. Loss-of-function mutations in EED and SUZ12 result in PRC2 inactivation and subsequent loss of H3K27me3 in 34% to 73% of MPNST [21].

26.6.1 Epithelioid MPNST

Recently complete loss of SMARCB1/INI1 expression in 24 of 57 (42%) cases of sporadic epithelioid schwannomas [107] has been shown suggesting that SMARCB1/INI1 aberrations may play a role in the pathogenesis in a subset of these tumors.

26.6.2 MPNST with Perineural Differentiation

Perineurial MPNSTs are exceedingly uncommon, and in consequence there are scarcely descriptions of them. The few studies found in the literature only reported histologic and immunostaining features which are not enough to have a clear definition of them [108, 109] (Table 26.2).

Notes

1. NCBI: National Center for Biotechnology Information, a division of the National Library of Medicine, located on the campus of the US National Institutes of Health in Bethesda, MD, USA.
2. Gene ID is a stable ID for that particular locus in that organism, generates by Entrez Gene (NCBI's database for gene-specific information).
3. Sequence variants: DNA diagnostics critically depends on accurate and standardized description and sharing of the variants detected. Sequence variant nomenclature follows the recommendations of the Human Genome Variation Society (HGVS nomenclature). The HGVS nomenclature is authorized by the Human Genome Variation Society (HGVS), the Human Variome Project (HVP), and the HUman Genome Organisation (HUGO), web site, http://www.HGVS.org/varnomen
4. The terms "polymorphism" and "mutation" are no longer used because both terms have assumed imprecise meanings in coloquial use. Therefore, following recommendations HGVS currently only neutral terms are used such as "variant," "alteration," and "change."

Table 26.2 Genetic syndromic predisposition to peripheral nerve neoplasia

Syndrome	OMIM	Inheritance	Locus (from NCBI, GRCh38)	Protein and major functions	Nervous system manifestations	Other organ manifestations
Neurofibromatosis, type I; NF1 (NF, Peripheral type von Recklinghausen disease)	162200	AD	17q11.2	Neurofibromin: a GTPase-activating protein that is a negative regulator of Ras	Neurofibromas, MPNST, optic nerve glioma, pilocytic or diffuse astrocytomas	Café-au-lait macules, axillary, inguinal freckling, iris hamartomas (Lisch nodules), osseous lesions, pheochromocytoma, gastrointestinal stromal tumors, juvenile myelomonocytic leukemia
Neurofibromatosis, type II; NF2 (NF, central type Bilateral acoustic neurofibromatosis; BANF)	101000	AD	22q12.2	Merlin: mediates membrane–cytoskeleton and intercellular interactions; modify gene expression inhibiting E3 ubiquitin ligase (CRL4(DCAF1)	Bilateral vestibular schwannomas, nonvestibular schwannomas, meningioma, meningioangiomatosis, spinal ependymoma, glial microhamartomas, cerebral calcifications	Café-au-lait macules (rare), posterior lens opacities, retinal hamartomas, epiretinal membranes
Schwannomatosis 1; SWNTS1 (Neurilemmomatosis, congenital cutaneous)	162091	AD	22q11.23	INI1/SNF5/BAF47: subunit of Swi/Snf chromatin remodeling complex (epigenetic regulation)	Peripheral schwannomas, unilateral vestibular schwannomas, meningiomas	
Schwannomatosis 2; SWNTS2	615670	AD	22q11.21	LZTR1: Golgi-associated protein downregulates the MAPK signaling pathway by polyubiquitination of RAS proteins		
Carney complex, type 1; CNC1 (Name syndrome Lamb syndrome)	160980	AD	17q24.2	PRKAR1A: regulates cAMP signaling	Psammomatous melanotic schwannoma, somatotropic pituitary adenoma	Spotty pigmentation ("lentigines"), myxomas, epithelioid blue nevi, cardiac myxoma, pigmented nodular adrenocortical dysplasia, Sertoli cell tumor, thyroid carcinoma, osteochondromyxomas

OMIN (Online Mendelian Inheritance in Man), a comprehensive, authoritative compendium of all known human Mendelian disorders and over 15,000 genes, is freely available and updated daily. It focuses on the relationship between phenotype and genotype

References

1. Louis DN, Ohgaki K, Wiestler OD, Cavenee W, editors. World Health Organization Histological classification of tumours of the central nervous system. 4th ed. International Agency for Research on Cancer: Lyon; 2016.
2. Skovronsky DM, Oberholtzer JC. Pathologic classification of peripheral nerve tumors. Neurosurg Clin N Am. 2004;15:157–66.
3. Committee on a Framework for Developing a New Taxonomy of Disease, National Research Council. Toward precision medicine: building a knowledge network for biomedical research and a new taxonomy of disease. Washington, DC: National Academies Press; 2011.
4. Chhabda S, Carney O, D'Arco F, Jacques T, Mankad-Quant K. The 2016 World Health Organization classification of tumours of the central nervous system: what the paediatric neuroradiologist needs to know. Quant Imaging Med Surg. 2016;6(5):486–9.
5. Louis D, Perry A, Reifenberger G, von Deimling A, Figarella-Branger D, Cavenee W, Ohgaki H, Wiestler O, Kleihues P, Ellison D. The 2016 World Health Organization classification of tumors of the central nervous system: a summary. Acta Neuropathol. 2016;131:803–20.
6. ICDO. In: Fritz A, Percy C, Jack A, et al., editors. International classification of diseases for oncology. 3rd ed. Geneva: World Health Organization; 2000.
7. Rodriguez FJ, Folpe AL, Giannini C, Perry A. Pathology of peripheral nerve sheath tumors: diagnostic overview and update on selected diagnostic problems. Acta Neuropathol. 2012;123(3):295–319.
8. Rodriguez FJ, Stratakis CA, Evans DG. Genetic predisposition to peripheral nerve neoplasia: diagnostic criteria and pathogenesis of neurofibromatoses, Carney complex, and related syndromes. Acta Neuropathol. 2012;123(3):349–67.
9. Hilton D, Hanemann C. Schwannomas and their pathogenesis. Brain Pathol. 2014;24:205–20.
10. GeneReviews® (1993–2020) Adam MP, Ardinger HH, Pagon RA, and Wallace SE. Molecular Genetics: Bean LJH and Stephens K. Genetic Counseling Amemiya A. Seattle (WA): University of Washington, Seattle; 1993–2019. ISSN: 2372-0697: Friedman JM (updated June 2019) Neurofibromatosis 1; Evans DG (updated March 2018) Neurofibromatosis 2; Dhamija R, Plotkin S, Asthagiri A, Messiaen L, and Babovic-Vuksanovic D (updated March 2018) Schwannomatosis; Stratakis CA, and Raygada M (updated August 2018) Carney Complex.
11. Cooper GM, Hausman RE. The development and causes of cancer. The cell: a molecular approach. 3rd ed. Washington (DC): ASM Press; 2004; Sunderland (Massachusetts).
12. McDuff FK, Turner SD. Jailbreak: oncogene-induced senescence and its evasion. Cell Signal. 2011;23:6–13.
13. Sun W, Yang J. Functional mechanisms for human tumor suppressors. J Cancer. 2010;1:136–40.
14. Macaluso M, Paggi MG, Giordano A. Genetic and epi-genetic alterations as hallmarks of the intricate road to cancer. Oncogene. 2003;22:6472–8.
15. Knudson AG. Mutation and cancer: statistical study of retinoblastoma. Proc Natl Acad Sci U S A. 1971;68:820–3.
16. Wang LH, Wu CF, Rajasekaran N, Shin YK. Loss of tumor suppressor gene function in human cancer: an overview. Cell Physiol Biochem. 2018;51:2647–93.
17. Costales JR, Socolovsky M, Sánchez Lázaro JA, Álvarez García R, Costales DR. Peripheral nerve injuries in the pediatric population: a review of the litera-ture. Part III: peripheral nerve tumors in children. Childs Nerv Syst. 2019;35(1):47–5.
18. Garner HW, Wilke BK, Fritchie K, Bestic JM. Epithelioid schwannoma: imaging findings on radiographs, MRI, and ultrasound. Skeletal Radiol. 2019;48(11):1815–20.
19. Laskin WB, Fetsch JF, Lasota J, Miettinen M. Benign epithelioid peripheral nerve sheath tumors of the soft tissues: clinicopathologic spectrum of 33 cases. Am J Surg Pathol. 2005;29:39–51.
20. Le Guellec S. Nerve sheath tumours. Ann Pathol. 2015;35(1):54–70.
21. Martinez AP, Fritchie KJ. Update on peripheral nerve sheath tumors. Surg Pathol Clin. 2019;12(1):1–19.
22. McLaughlin CT, Kaffenberger BH, Gru AA. A hybrid tumor with schwannoma-perineurioma-neurofibroma morphology. J Cutan Pathol. 2015;42(11):911–3.
23. Meyer A, Billings SD. What's new in nerve sheath tumors. Virchows Arch. 2020;476(1):65–80.
24. Smith MJ, Bowers NL, Bulman M, Gokhale C, Wallace AJ, King AT, Lloyd SK, Rutherford SA, Hammerbeck-Ward CL, Freeman SR, Evans DG. Revisiting neurofibromatosis type 2 diagnostic criteria to exclude LZTR1-related schwannomatosis. Neurology. 2017;88:87–92.
25. Kleihues P, Cavenee WK, editors. Pathology and genetics of tumours of the nervous system. World Health Organization classification of tumours. Lyon: IARC Press; 2000.
26. Louis DN, Ohgaki H, Wiestler OD, Cavenee WK, Burger PC, Jouvet A, Scheithauer BW, Kleihues P. The 2007 WHO classification of tumours of the central nervous system. Acta Neuropathol. 2007;114(2):97–109.
27. Huynh DP, Mautner V, Baser ME, Stavrou D, Pulst SM. Immunohistochemical detection of schwannomin and neurofibromin in vestibular schwannomas, ependymomas and meningiomas. J Neuropathol Exp Neurol. 1997;56(4):382–90.
28. Jacoby LB, MacCollin M, Louls DN, Mohney T, Rublo M-P, Pulaski K, Trofatter JA, Kley N, Seizinger B, Ramesh V, Gusella JF. Exon scanning for mutation of the NF2 gene in schwannomas. Hum Mol Genet. 1994;3(3):413–9.
29. Sestini R, Bacci C, Provenzano A, Genuardi M, Papi L. Evidence of a four-hit mechanism involving

SMARCB1 and NF2 in schwannomatosis-associated schwannomas. Hum Mutat. 2008;29:227–31.
30. Jacoby LB, MacCollin M, Barone R, Ramesh V, Gusella JF. Frequency and distribution of NF2 mutations in schwannomas. Genes Chromosomes Cancer. 1996;17(1):45–55.
31. Agnihotri S, Jalali S, Wilson MR, Danesh A, Li M, Klironomos G, Krieger JR, Mansouri A, Khan O, Mamatjan Y, Landon-Brace N, Tung T, Dowar M, Li T, Bruce JP, Burrell KE, Tonge PD, Alamsahebpour A, Krischek B, Agarwalla PK, Bi WL, Dunn IF, Beroukhim R, Fehlings MG, Bril V, Pagnotta SM, Iavarone A, Pugh TJ, Aldape KD, Zadeh G. The genomic landscape of schwannoma. Nat Genet. 2016;48(11):1339–48.
32. Smith MJ, Wallace AJ, Bowers NL, Rustad CF, Woods CG, Leschziner GD, Ferner RE, Evans DG. SMARCB1 muta-tions in familial and sporadic schwannomatosis. Neurogenetics. 2012;13(2):141–5.
33. Paganini I, Capone GL, Vitte J, Sestini R, Putignano AL, Giovannini M, Papi L. Double somatic SMARCB1 and NF2 mutations in sporadic spinal schwannoma. J Neurooncol. 2018;137(1):33–8.
34. Ferrer M, Schulze A, Gonzalez S, Ferreiro V, Ciavarelli P, Otero J, Giliberto F, Basso A, Szijan I. Neurofibromatosis type 2: molecular and clinical analyses in Argentine sporadic and familial cases. Neurosci Lett. 2010;480(1):49–54.
35. Hadfield KD, Smith MJ, Urquhart JE, Wallace AJ, Bowers NL, King AT, Rutherford SA, Trump D, Newman WG, Evans DG. Rates of loss of heterozygosity and mitotic recombination in NF2 schwannomas, sporadic vestibular schwannomas and schwannomatosis schwannomas. Oncogene. 2010;29(47):6216–21.
36. Kehrer-Sawatzki H, Farschtschi S, Mautner VF, Cooper DN. The molecular pathogenesis of schwannomatosis, a paradigm for the co-involvement of multiple tumour suppressor genes in tumorigenesis. Hum Genet. 2017;136(2):129–48.
37. Rouleau GA, Merel P, Lutchman M, Sanson M, Zuc-man J, Marineau C, Hoang-Xuan K, Demczuk S, Desmaze C, Plougastel B, Pulst SM, Lenoir G, Bijls-ma E, Fashold R, Dumanski J, de Jong P, Parry D, Eldrige R, Aurias A, Delattre O, Thomas G. Alteration in a new gene encoding a putative membrane-organizing protein causes neuro-fibromatosis type 2. Nature. 1993;363(6429):515–21.
38. Trofatter JA, MacCollin MM, Rutter JL, Murrell JR, Duy-ao MP, Parry DM, Eldridge R, Kley N, Menon AG, Pulaski K, Haase VH, Ambrose CM, Munroe D, Bove C, Haines JL, Martuza RL, MacDonald ME, Seizinger BR, Short MP, Buckler AJ, Gusella JF. A novel moesin-ezrin-radixin-like gene is a candidate for the neurofibromatosis 2 tumor suppressor. Cell. 1993;72(5):791–800. Erratum 75(4):826.
39. Gutmann DH, Wright DE, Geist RT, Snider WD. Expression of the neurofibromatosis 2 (NF2) gene isoforms during rat embryonic development. Hum Mol Genet. 1995;4:471–8.
40. Tsukita S, Oishi K, Sato N, Sagara J, Kawai A, Tsu-kita S. ERM family members as molecular linkers between the cell surface glycoprotein CD44 and actin-based cytoskeletons. J Cell Biol. 1994;126:391–401.
41. Bretscher A, Edwards K, Fehon RG. ERM proteins and merlin: integrators at the cell cortex. Nat Rev Mol Cell Biol. 2002;3:586–99.
42. Louvet-Vallée S. ERM proteins: from cellular architecture to cell signaling. Biol Cell. 2000;92:305–16.
43. Neisch AL, Fehon RG. Ezrin, Radixin and Moesin: key regulators of membrane-cortex interactions and signaling. Curr Opin Cell Biol. 2011;23:377–82.
44. Gusella JF, Ramesh V, MacCollin M, Jacoby LB. Merlin: the neurofibromatosis 2 tumor suppressor. Biochim Biophys Acta. 1999;1423:M29–36.
45. Gautreau A, Louvard D, Arpin M. ERM pro-teins and NF2 tumor suppressor: the Yin and Yang of cortical actin organization and cell growth signal-ing. Curr Opin Cell Biol. 2002;14:104–9.
46. Meng JJ, Lowrie DJ, Sun H, Dorsey E, Pelton PD, Bashour AM, Groden J, Ratner N, Ip W. Interaction between two isoforms of the NF2 tumor suppressor protein, merlin, and between merlin and ezrin, suggests modulation of ERM proteins by merlin. J Neurosci Res. 2000;62:491–502.
47. Surace EI, Haipek CA, Gutmann DH. Ef-fect of merlin phosphorylation on neurofibromatosis 2 (NF2) gene function. Oncogene. 2004;23:580–7.
48. Lallemand D, Saint-Amaux AL, Giovannini M. Tumor-suppression functions of merlin are independent of its role as an organizer of the actin cytoskeleton in Schwann cells. J Cell Sci. 2009;122:4141–9.
49. Li W, Cooper J, Karajannis MA, Giancotti FG. Merlin: a tumour suppressor with functions at the cell cortex and in the nucleus. EMBO Rep. 2012;13(3):204–15.
50. Li W, You L, Cooper J, Schiavon G, Pepe-Caprio A, Zhou L, Ishii R, Giovannini M, Hanemann CO, Long SB, Erdjument-Bromage H, Zhou P, Tempst P, Giancotti FG. Merlin/NF2 suppresses tumorigenesis by inhibiting the E3 ubiquitin ligase CRL4(DCAF1) in the nucleus. Cell. 2010;140:477–90.
51. Roberts CW, Biegel JA. The role of SMARCB1/INI1 in development of rhabdoid tumor. Cancer Biol Ther. 2009;8:412–6.
52. Hollmann TJ, Hornick JL. INI1-deficient tumors: diagnostic features and molecular genetics. Am J Surg Pathol. 2011;35:e47–63.
53. Clapier CR, Iwasa J, Cairns BR, Peterson CL. Mechanisms of action and regulation of ATP-dependent chromatin-remodelling complexes. Nat Rev Mol Cell Biol. 2017;18:407–22.
54. Pulice JL, Kadoch C. Composition and function of mammalian SWI/SNF chromatin remodeling complexes in human disease. Cold Spring Harb Symp Quant Biol. 2016;81:53–60.
55. Mohrmann L, Verrijzer CP. Composition and functional specificity of SWI2/SNF2 class chromatin

remodeling complexes. Biochim Biophys Acta. 2005;1681:59–73.
56. Wang X, Haswell JR, Roberts CW. Molecular pathways: SWI/SNF (BAF) complexes are frequently mutated in cancer—mechanisms and potential therapeutic insights. Clin Cancer Res. 2014;20:21–7.
57. Kadoch C, Crabtree GR. Mammalian SWI/SNF chromatin remodeling complexes and cancer: mechanistic insights gained from human genomics. Sci Adv. 2015;1(5):e1500447.
58. Kohashi K, Oda Y. Oncogenic roles of SMARCB1/INI1 and its deficient tumors. Cancer Sci. 2017;108:547–52.
59. Agaimy A. The expanding family of SMARCB1(INI1)-deficient neoplasia: implications of phenotypic, biological, and molecular heterogeneity. Adv Anat Pathol. 2014;21:394–410.
60. Imbalzano AN, Jones SN. Snf5 tumor suppressor couples chromatin remodeling, checkpoint control, and chromosomal stability. Cancer Cell. 2005;7:294–5.
61. Vries RG, Bezrookove V, Zuijderduijn LM, Kia SK, Houweling A, Oruetxebarria I, Raap AK, Verrijzer CP. Cancer-associated mutations in chromatin remodeler hSNF5 promote chromosomal instability by compromising the mitotic checkpoint. Genes Dev. 2005;15:665–70.
62. Mora-Blanco EL, Mishina Y, Tillman EJ, Cho YJ, Thom CS, Pomeroy SL, Shao W, Roberts CW. Activation of β-catenin/TCF targets following loss of the tumor suppressor SNF5. Oncogene. 2014;33(7):933–8.
63. He X, Semenov M, Tamai K, Zeng X. LDL receptor-related proteins 5 and 6 in Wnt/beta-catenin signaling: arrows point the way. Development. 2004;131(8):1663–77.
64. Kim KH, Roberts CWM. Mechanisms by which SMARCB1 loss drives rhabdoid tumor growth. Cancer Genet. 2014;207:365–72.
65. Pasinia D, Di Croce L. Emerging roles for polycomb proteins in cancer. Curr Opin Genet Dev. 2016;36:50–8.
66. Nacak TG, Leptien K, Fellner D, Augustin HG, Kroll J. The BTB-kelch protein LZTR-1 is a novel Golgi protein that is degraded upon induction of apoptosis. J Biol Chem. 2006;281(8):5065–71.
67. Chen RH. Cullin 3 and its role in tumorigenesis. Adv Exp Med Biol. 2020;1217:187–210.
68. Piotrowski A, Xie J, Liu YF, Poplawski AB, Gomes AR, Madanecki P, Fu C, Crowley MR, Crossman DK, Armstrong L, Babovic-Vuksanovic D, Bergner A, Blakeley JO, Blu-menthal AL, Daniels MS, Feit H, Gardner K, Hurst S, Ko-belka C, Lee C, Nagy R, Rauen KA, Slopis JM, Suwannarat P, Westman JA, Zanko A, Korf BR, Messiaen LM. Germline loss-of-function mutations in LZTR1 predispose to an inherited disorder of multiple schwannomas. Nat Genet. 2014;46(2):182–7.
69. Frattini V, Trifonov V, Chan JM, Castano A, Lia M, Abate F, Keir ST, Ji AX, Zoppoli P, Niola F, Danussi C, Dolgalev I, Porrati P, Pellegatta S, Heguy A, Gupta G, Pisapia DJ, Canoll P, Bruce JN, McLendon RE, Yan H, Aldape K, Fi-nocchiaro G, Mikkelsen T, Privé GG, Bigner DD, Lasorella A, Rabadan R, Iavarone A. The integrated landscape of driver genomic alterations in glioblastoma. Nat Genet. 2013;45(10):1141–9.
70. Cancer Genome Atlas Research Network. Comprehensive and integrative genomic characterization of hepatocellular carcinoma. Cell. 2017;169:1327–1341.e23.
71. Tidyman WE, Rauen KA. The RASopathies: developmental syndromes of Ras/MAPK pathway dysregulation. Curr Opin Genet Dev. 2009;19:230–6.
72. Johnston JJ, van der Smagt JJ, Rosenfeld JA, Pagnamen-ta AT, Alswaid A, Baker EH, Blair E, Borck G, Brinkmann J, Craigen W, Dung VC, Emrick L, Everman DB, van Gas-sen PKL, Gulsuner S, Harr MH, Jain M, Kuechler A, Leppig KA, McDonald-McGinn DM, Can NTB, Peleg A, Roeder ER, Rogers RC, Sagi-Dain L, Sapp JC, Schäffer AA, Schanze D, Stewart H, Taylor JC, Verbeek NE, Walkiewicz MA, Zackai EH, Zweier C, Members of the Undiagnosed Diseases Network, Zenker M, Lee B, Biesecker GL. Autosomal recessive Noonan syndrome associated with biallelic LZTR1 variants. Genet Med. 2018;20:1175–85.
73. Yamamoto GL, Aguena M, Gos M, Hung C, Pilch J, Fahiminiya S, Abramowicz A, Cristian I, Buscarilli M, Naslavsky MS, Malaquias AC, Zatz M, Bodamer O, Majew-ski J, Jorge AAL, Pereira AC, Kim CA, Passos-Bueno MR, Bertola DR. Rare variants in SOS2 and LZTR1 are associated with Noonan syndrome. J Med Genet. 2015;52:413–21.
74. Lundin J, Markljung E, Baranowska Körberg I, Hofmeister W, Cao J, Nilsson D, Holmdahl G, Barker G, Anderberg M, Vukojević V, Lindstrand A, Nordenskjöld A. Further support linking the 22q11.2 microduplication to an in-creased risk of bladder exstrophy and highlighting LZTR1 as a candidate gene. Mol Genet Genomic Med. 2018;7(6):e666.
75. Lührig S, Kolb S, Mellies N, Nolte J. The novel BTB-kelch protein, KBTBD8, is located in the Golgi apparatus and translocates to the spindle apparatus during mitosis. Cell Div. 2013;8:3.
76. Kurahashi H, Akagi K, Inazawa J, Ohta T, Niikawa N, Kayatani F, Sano T, Okada S, Nishisho I. Isolation and characterization of a novel gene deleted in DiGeorge syndrome. Hum Mol Genet. 1995;4:541–9.
77. Wilhelm M, Schlegl J, Hahne H, Gholami AM, Lieberenz M, Savitski MM, Ziegler E, Butzmann L, Gessulat S, Marx H, Mathieson T, Lemeer S, Schnatbaum K, Reimer U, Wenschuh H, Mollenhauer M, Slotta-Huspenina J, Boese J-H, Bantscheff M, Gerstmair A, Faerber F, Kuster B. Mass-spectrometry-based draft of the human proteome. Nature. 2014;509:582–7.

78. Koepp DM, Harper JW, Elledge SJ. How the cyclin became a cyclin: regulated proteolysis in the cell cycle. Cell. 1999;97:431–4.
79. Geyer R, Wee S, Anderson S, Yates J, Wolf DA. BTB/POZ domain proteins are putative substrate adaptors for cullin 3 ubiquitin ligases. Mol Cell. 2003;12:783–90.
80. Bigenzahn JW, Collu GM, Kartnig F, Pieraks M, Vladimer GI, Heinz LX, Sedlyarov V, Schischlik F, Fauster A, Rebsamen M, Parapatics K, Blomen VA, Müller AC, Winter GE, Kralovics R, Brummelkamp TR, Mlodzik M, Superti-Furga G. LZTR1 is a regulator of RAS ubiquitination and signaling. Science. 2018;362:1171–7.
81. Steklov M, Pandolfi S, Baietti MF, Batiuk A, Carai P, Najm P, Zhang M, Jang H, Renzi F, Cai Y, Abbasi Asbagh L, Pas-tor T, De Troyer M, Simicek M, Radaelli E, Brems H, Legius E, Tavernier J, Gevaert K, Impens F, Messiaen L, Nussi-Nov R, Heymans S, Eyckerman S, Sablina AA. Mutations in LZTR1 drive human disease by dysregulating RAS ubiquitination. Science. 2018;362:1177–82.
82. Abe T, Umeki I, Kanno SI, Inoue SI, Niihori T, Aoki Y. LZTR1 facilitates polyubiquitination and degrada-tion of RAS-GTPases. Cell Death Differ. 2020;27:1023–35. https://doi.org/10.1038/s41418-019-0395-5.
83. Zawadzki KM, Taylor SS. cAMP-dependent protein kinase regulatory subunit type IIbeta: active site mutations define an isoform-specific network for allosteric signaling by cAMP. J Biol Chem. 2004;2279(8):7029–36.
84. Gutmann D, Aylsworth A, Carey JC, Korf B, Marks J, Pyeritz RE, Ru-benstein A, Viskochil D. The diagnostic evaluation and multidisciplinary management of neurofibromatosis 1 and neurofibromatosis 2. JAMA. 1997;278:51–7.
85. Beert E, Brems H, Daniëls B, de Wever I, van Calenbergh F, Schoenaers J, Debiec-Rychter M, Gevaert O, de Raedt T, van den Bruel A, de Ravel T, Cichowski K, Kluwe L, Mautner V, Sciot R, Legius E. Atypical neurofibromas in neurofibromatosis type 1 are premalignant tumors. Genes Chromosomes Cancer. 2011;50:1021–32.
86. Nielsen GP, Stemmer-Rachamimov AO, Ino Y, Moller MB, Rosenberg AE, Louis DN. Malignant transformation of neurofibromas in neurofibromatosis 1 is associated with CDKN2A/p16 inactivation. AmJ Pathol. 1999;155:1879–84.
87. HGNC (HUGO Gene Nomenclature Committee): standard reference for gene. https://www.genenames.org/index.html/
88. Trovo-Marqui AB, Tajara EH. Neurofibromin: a general outlook. Clin Genet. 2006;70:1–13.
89. Upadhyaya M, Cooper DN, editors. Neurofibromatosis type 1. Berlin: Springer; 2012.
90. Abramowicz A, Gos M. Neurofibromin in neurofibromatosis type 1 mutations in NF1gene as a cause of disease. Dev Period Med. 2014;18(3):297–306.
91. Xu G, O'Connell P, Viskochil D, Cawthon R, Robertson M, Culver M, Dunn D, Stevens J, Gesteland R, White R, Weiss R. The neurofibromatosis type 1 gene encodes a protein related to GAP. Cell. 1990;62:599–608.
92. Barron VA, Lou H. Alternative splicing of the neurofibromatosis type I pre-mRNA. Biosci Rep. 2012;32(2):131–8.
93. Vandenbroucke I, Van Oostveldt P, Coene E, De Paepe A, Messiaen L. Neurofibromin is actively transported to the nucleus. FEBS Lett. 2004;560(1–3):98–102.
94. Bos JL, Rehmann H, Wittinghofer A. GEFs and GAPs: critical elements in the control of small G proteins. Cell. 2007;129:865–77.
95. Rauen KA. The RASopathies. Annu Rev Genomics Hum Genet. 2013;14:355–69.
96. Theaker JM, Fletcher CDM. Epithelial membrane antigen expression by the perineurial cell: further studies of peripheral nerve lesions. Histopathology. 1989;14:581–92.
97. Emory TS, Scheithauer BW, Hirose T, Wood M, Onofrio BM, Jenkins RB. Intraneural perineurioma. A clonal neoplasm associated with abnormalities of chromosome 22. Am J Clin Pathol. 1995;103(6):696–704.
98. Ausmus GG, Piliang MP, Bergfeld WF, Goldblum JR. Soft-tissue perineurioma in a 20-year-old patient with neurofibromatosis type 1 (NF1): report of a case and review of the literature. J Cutan Pathol. 2007;34:726–30.
99. Macarenco RS, Ellinger F, Oliveira AM. Perineurioma. A dintinctive and underrecognized peripheral nerve sheath neoplasm. Arch Pathol Lab Med. 2007;131:625–36.
100. Pitchford CW, Schwartz HS, Atkinson JB, Cates JMM. Soft tissue perineurioma in a patient with neurofibromatosis type 2: a tumor not previously associated with the NF2 syndrome. Am J Surg Pathol. 2006;30:1624–9.
101. Brock JE, Perez-Atayde AR, Kozakewich HPW, Richkind KE, Fletcher JA, Vargas SO. Cytogenetic aberrations in perineurioma. Variation with subtype. Am J Surg Pathol. 2005;29:1164–9.
102. Mott RT, Goodman BK, Burchette JL, Cummings TJ. Loss of chromosome 13 in a case of soft tissue perineurioma. Clin Neuropathol. 2005;24:69–76.
103. Sciot R, Dal Cin P, Hagemeijer A, De Smet L, Van Damme B, Van den Berghe H. Cutaneous sclerosing perineurioma with cryptic NF2 gene deletion. Am J Surg Pathol. 1999;23:849–53.
104. Kacerovska D, Michal M, Kuroda N, Tanaka A, Sima R, Denisjuk N, Kreuzberg B, Ricarova R, Kazakov DV. Hybrid peripheral nerve sheath tumors, including a malignant variant in type 1 neurofibromatosis. Am J Dermatopathol. 2013;35:641–9.
105. Le Guellec S, Decouvelaere AV, Filleron T, et al. Malignant peripheral nerve sheath tumor is a challenging diagnosis. Am J Surg Pathol. 2016;40:896–908.

106. Lee W, Teckie S, Wiesner T, Ran L, Prieto Granada CN, Lin M, Zhu S, Cao Z, Liang Y, Sboner A, Tap WD, Fletcher JA, Huberman KH, Qin LX, Viale A, Singer S, Zheng D, Berger MF, Chen Y, Antonescu CR, Chi P. PRC2 is recurrently inactivated through EED or SUZ12 loss in malignant peripheral nerve sheath tumors. Nat Genet. 2014;46:1227–32.
107. Jo VY, Fletcher CDM. SMARCB1/INI1 loss in epithelioid schwannoma: a clinicopathologic and immunohistochemical study of 65 cases. Am J Surg Pathol. 2017;41(8):1013–22.
108. Hirose T, Scheithauer BW, Sano T. Perineurial malignant peripheral nerve sheath tumor (MPNST): a clinicopathologic, immunohisto-chemical, and ultrastructural study of seven cases. Am J Surg Pathol. 1998;22:1368–78.
109. Mitchell A, Scheithauer BW, Doyon J, Berthiaume MJ, Isler M. Malig-nant perineurioma (malignant peripheral nerve sheath tumor with perineural dif-ferentiation). Clin Neuropathol. 2012;31(6):424–9.

27 Clinical Management of NF1 and Indications for Surgery

Debora Garozzo

27.1 Introduction

Neurofibromatosis (NF) comprises the most well-known form of phakomatoses, a group of genetic syndromes involving structures arising from the embryonic ectoderm; NF manifests with involvement of the nervous system, soft tissues, skin, and bone. Several forms have been described, but the most statistically frequent types are neurofibromatosis 1 (also known as von Recklinghausen's disease) with an incidence of approximately 1 in 2600 to 3000 individuals and neurofibromatosis 2 (bilateral acoustic neurofibromatosis or central neurofibromatosis) whose birth rate has been calculated as less than 1 in 30,000 and schwannomatosis whose incidence is approximately 1 in 60,000 [1–4].

The involvement of the nervous system is typical in all three forms, yet NF2 is prevalently associated with central nervous system neoplasms, whereas NF1 and schwannomatosis mostly affect the peripheral nervous system.

NF1 is undoubtedly a challenging disorder. Although a remarkable percentage of individuals affected by this genetic condition may be completely asymptomatic or present minor issues, severe clinical phenotypes are often encountered (Fig. 27.1); NF1 manifestations are widespread and affect many of the body systems (Table 27.1). Therefore, complex cases may often raise a management conundrum, requiring dedicated professional skills and high expertise.

The numerous implications and high complexity often related to NF treatment have undoubtedly demonstrated that multidisciplinary referral centers are the only valid sites to monitor the development of the disorder; as it is well known, NF is age-penetrating, and lifetime follow-up is therefore necessary in these patients. Moreover, individuals affected by NF are highly predisposed to developing MPNSTs (malignant peripheral nerve sheath tumors), and specialist clinics represent the best possibility to enforce prevention strategies.

Unfortunately, the foundation of multidisciplinary referral centers is mostly a prerogative of high-income countries where a national healthcare system is present (e.g., the UK or Italy). In low-/middle-income countries or countries that mainly rely on private/insurance-provided healthcare, financial issues burden the possibility to offer thorough diagnostic assessment; consequently, patients are often undiagnosed or inappropriately treated. Moreover, the general perception of the disorder is not accurate; most patients tend to underestimate their issues, and non-specialized medical staff frequently offer false reassurances or downplay the risks.

D. Garozzo (✉)
WFNS Peripheral Nerve Surgery Committee, Department of Neurosurgery, Mediclinic Parkview Hospital, Dubai, UAE
e-mail: debora.garozzo@esns.ae

F. Guedes et al. (eds.), *Diagnostic Assessment and Treatment of Peripheral Nerve Tumors*,
https://doi.org/10.1007/978-3-030-77633-6_27

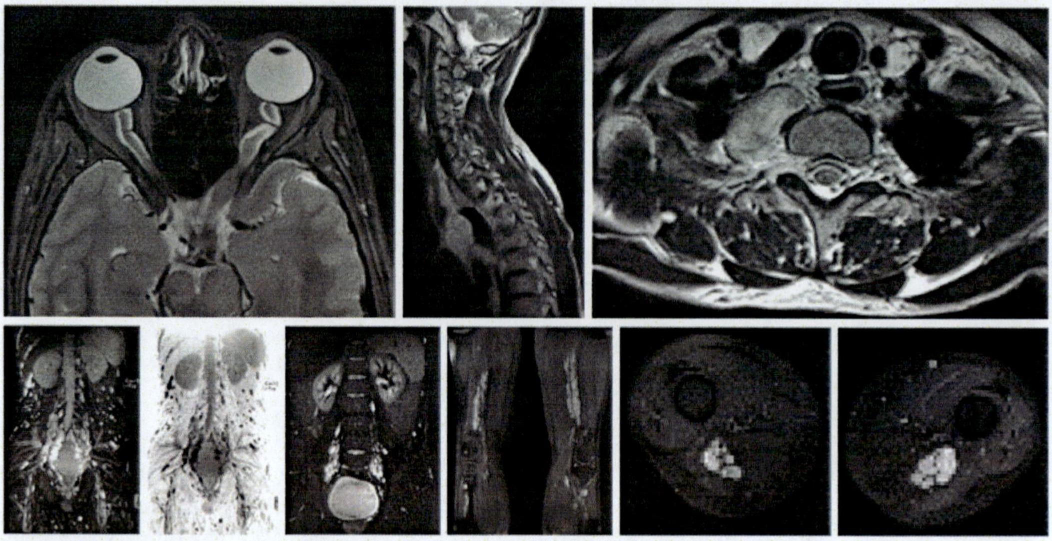

Fig. 27.1 De novo NF1 in a 19-year-old male patient: asymptomatic optic pathway glioma and multiple neurofibromas (including the plexiform variant). The patient was also diagnosed with autism

Table 27.1 Frequency and age of onset of major clinical manifestations in NF1

Clinical manifestation	Frequency	Age of onset
Café-au-lait spots	>99%	Birth to 12 years
Frecklings	85%	3 years to adolescence
Lisch nodules	90–95%	>3 years
Severe cognitive impairment	4–8%	Birth
Learning disability	30–60%	Birth
Cutaneous neurofibromas	>99%	>7 years (usually late adolescence)
Plexiform neurofibromas	27% (at physical examination) 50% (on diagnostic workup)	Birth to 18 years
MPNSTs	8–13% lifetime risk	5–75 years Average age at diagnosis is 26 years
Optic pathway gliomas	15% (only 5% symptomatic)	Birth to 7 years (up to 30 years)
Scoliosis	10%	Birth to 18 years
Epilepsy	6–7%	Lifelong
Renal artery stenosis	2%	Lifelong
Pheochromocytoma	2%	>10 years
Pseudoarthrosis of tibia	2%	Birth to 3 years
Cerebral gliomas	2–3%	Lifelong
Sphenoidal wing dysplasia	<1%	Congenital
Aqueduct stenosis	1.5%	Lifelong

In this chapter, we will illustrate some aspects related to the general management of NF patients; we will also focus on peripheral nerve tumors, although some specific aspects, such as plexiform tumors, prevention strategies for malignancy, and management of MPNSTs, will be the subject of the next two chapters.

27.2 The Role of Genetic Counseling

At present, diagnosis primarily relies on clinical grounds [5–8] (see Chap. 25). Genetic testing is usually indicated in selected cases only, such as patients that present an unusual phenotype or an incomplete clinical picture [6, 8].

On the other hand, genetic counseling prior to conception should be strongly advised for all NF1 patients to prevent cases related to inheritance. Although 50% of NF cases are consequent to new, spontaneous mutations (de novo mutations), inheritance certainly plays a major role as individuals affected by NF1 present a 50% risk of passing on the condition to their children. Albeit at present we cannot predict how severely the genetic condition manifests in offspring, the risk of having a severely affected child is reported to be about 1 in 12 when complications that cause lifelong morbidity or early mortality are considered [6].

Direct mutation testing of fetal DNA extracted from chorionic villous sampling or from amniocentesis and DNA markers in families with two or more affected individuals is presently available for prenatal testing [6, 8]. However, a rather low percentage of couples choose to undergo prenatal tests. Patients with mild manifestations usually underestimate or completely ignore that their offspring might develop severe NF-related morbidity. In our practice, we have met a lot of parents of children with severe disabilities that recollected they had not been concerned about this possibility, simply based on their personal experience; even if informed about the risk, they chose to rely on their "good luck" ("we thought that 50% of possibilities that our baby wouldn't be affected was a lot!"). On the other hand, even when parents are fully aware of the risk that their child might be severely affected, the inability to predict the risk discourages them from considering the option of prenatal assessment.

During the course of pregnancy, ultrasound and MRI imaging might provide some evidence (e.g., cardiac and cranial abnormalities) consistent with NF1 in a third-trimester fetus; however this prenatal assessment has a limited value for obvious reasons [8, 9].

A much better option to prevent heritable cases might be preimplantation of genetic diagnosis; NF1 diagnosis is ascertained using single cells from 3-day-old embryos, and those that do not carry the mutation are eventually implanted in the mother's womb [6, 8]. Preimplantation genetic diagnosis should be enforced especially in countries and communities where consanguineous marriages are customary; unions between two individuals related as second cousins or closer are estimated to be practiced by more than one billion of the current global population and may account for up to 50% of all marriages in North Africa, Middle East, and South-West Asia as well as in large migrant communities in high-income countries (e.g., Pakistani migrants in the UK) [10]. Consanguineous marriages largely contribute to the incidence of genetic disorders in these areas [10–13]. In the United Arab Emirates (UAE), where one of the salient features of the Emirati population is the preference for marriage to relatives (usually first cousins), consanguinity with a high level of inbreeding causes high frequency of genetic disorders, including neurofibromatosis [13].

In addition to preventing heritable cases, preimplantation genetic diagnosis certainly represents the best option from an emotional point of view; it does not challenge any religious or ethical beliefs and avoids psychological stress in those couples that might have to face the choice of therapeutic termination of pregnancy.

27.3 Assessment and General Management of NF Patients

Clinical diagnosis is based on the patient's family history and physical examination. The latter primarily relies on the National Institutes of Health (NIH) criteria [5] that usually appear in the following predictable order: café-au-lait spots, axillary freckling, Lisch nodules, and neurofibromas. The characteristic osseous lesions typically appear within the first year of life, and optic gliomas are usually diagnosed from 3 to 6 years. Apparently 97% of NF1 patients meet the NIH criteria by the age of 8 years, and all do so by the age of 20 years [6–8]. However, nowadays there is emerging evidence for the need for a revision of NIH criteria since they have proved inadequate in establishing a diagnosis at an early age; in de novo NF1, 50% of children younger than 2 years only fulfill a single NIH criterion, often leading to a delay in diagnosis. Therefore, many have suggested to add other cutaneous (juvenile xanthogranulomas and nevus anemicus) and extracutaneous clinical signs (e.g., choroidal nodules) [7].

After NF is clinically suspected, the patient should be referred to clinicians subspecializing in the diagnosis and treatment of this medical condition in order to provide a thorough estimation of the burden of the disease. When a child seems to be the first individual in their family to be affected by NF, parents should be also examined; even if it is well known that 50% of patients are due to de novo mutations, clinical assessment often reveals that one of the parents was indeed affected by the condition although asymptomatic, as often related to segmental/mosaic forms. Thus this might be a crucial piece of information especially if the couple is willing to have more children.

Since NF is an age-penetrating disorder, the mainstay of management is monitoring clinical manifestations that typically appear in predictable order (see Table 27.1) [6–8]. Initial assessment implies multidisciplinarity (Table 27.2); special attention should be given to detect possible visual impairments and learning disabilities that are particularly frequent in these little patients [6, 7, 14–16]. Unless a severe clinical picture is already revealed in early age, children may be then reassessed once a year. The years from the onset of puberty to mid- and late 20s represent the most vulnerable period of life for these patients, especially if they have been diagnosed with microdeletion (deletion of the whole NF1 gene) [17, 18]. Puberty often triggers the “explosion” of the disorder; initially estimated mild or uncomplicated clinical pictures may turn and develop severe manifestations. Neurofibromas often start to grow in late adolescence; moreover, malignant transformation from pre-existing benign lesions or onset of de novo MPNST is reported to usually occur at mid-20s [6–8, 17, 18].

Afterwards, follow-up should be based on disease severity. In adult individuals already diagnosed as severe forms, lifelong monitoring in an NF1 specialist clinic obviously follows the progression of their clinical manifestations. Adults with mild clinical pictures should receive comprehensive education on the possible, future complications in order to urge them to promptly seek medical advice if unusual symptoms develop (Table 27.3). In particular, information about the risk of malignant transformation and symptoms related to neurological complications (e.g., spinal cord compression) is of paramount importance; malignancy and tumor-related neurological complications are reported to be the two major causes of death in this population. It has been estimated that individuals with NF1 have a lifespan of approximately 15 years less than that seen in the general population [19–21].

Table 27.2 Assessment in children affected by NF1; follow-up should be regularly performed once a year

• Evaluation of cognitive development with focus on scholastic progress
• Ophthalmic evaluation including fundoscopy until age 7 years
• One baseline assessment of color vision and visual fields at the appropriate developmental age
• Measurement of head circumference
• Records of height and weight and attention to all signs related to delayed/precocious pubertal development
• General cardiovascular examination, including blood pressure
• Evaluation of the spine
• Dermatological evaluation
• Specialist assessment if evidence of specific symptoms

Table 27.3 Symptoms that should raise a red flag in NF patients

Onset of pain of unknown etiology
Onset of paresthesias and/or sensory motor deficits in the extremities
Neurofibromas that rapidly change in size and/or become painful
Onset or increased frequency of headaches
Impairment/loss of balance or coordination
Visual disturbances
Abnormal neurological examination
Sudden onset of hypertension
Regression of cognitive skills or loss of developmental milestones
Significant deviation from individual’s established pattern of growth

27.4 General Introduction to Peripheral Nerve Tumors in NF and Their Assessment

Neurofibromatosis 1 (NF1) is associated with peripheral nerve tumors (PNTs) in at least 30% of cases [6, 7, 18]. Manifesting in childhood, PNTs mostly grow during adolescence (their volume increases more rapidly than body weight over time), and new tumors appear at an annual rate equal to 0.6 [22]. Whereas in sporadic forms, PNTs are almost invariably symptomatic, their NF1 counterpart may often be clinically silent. This explains why, in addition to the superficial lesions detected on physical examination, deeply located lesions (e.g., pelvic or mediastinal masses) may be frequently revealed by diagnostic assessment. Although a remarkable percentage of these tumors present with slow growth and actually remain asymptomatic, clinically silent tumors may turn and cause the onset of pain and paresthesias along the extremities or, when deeply located, compression on surrounding structures (e.g., dyspnoea in mediastinal lesions). The occurrence of a pre-existing or a newly formed lesion along the course of a nerve that suddenly presents rapid growth, associated with excruciating pain and onset of progressive neurological deficits, is also a likely possibility and should raise a red flag for the possibility of malignant transformation [18].

In comparison with sporadic forms, it is noteworthy to emphasize that NF1 PNTs also present other peculiarities.

Whereas sporadic PNTs are usually benign forms with schwannomas as prevailing histotype, neurofibromas represent the hallmark in NF (Fig. 27.2); the schwannoma/neurofibroma ratio, equal to 9:1 in the general population, is reversed (1:9) in NF individuals [18].

In addition to the histological forms present in the general population, individuals affected by NF also harbor pathognomonic variants, the so-called plexiform tumors that will be further described in Chap. 28.

Concerning the high incidence of malignant forms, whereas sporadic MPNSTs are extremely uncommon (their incidence is estimated at 0.001%) [23], NF1 MPNSTs account for 50% of the overall cases; NF patients have a lifetime risk to develop MPNSTs between 8 and 13% or even higher in individuals with microdeletion [17, 18]. Moreover, when compared to sporadic forms, NF1 MPNSTs are characterized by earlier onset (20–30 years versus third to sixth decade) and poorer survival rate [23–25]. Chapter 29 is focused on NF MPNSTs and deals in detail with assessment, management, and prevention strategies.

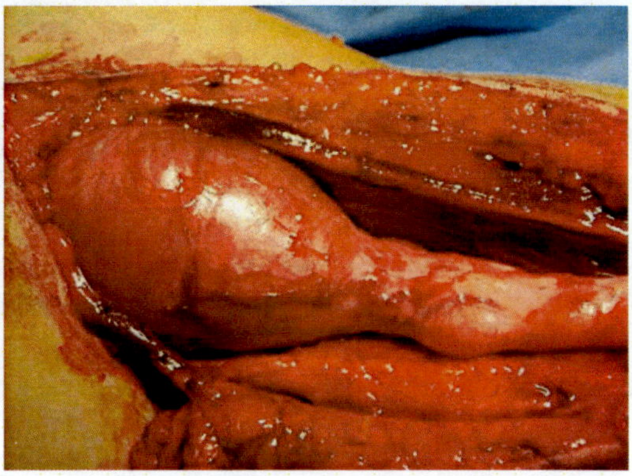

Fig. 27.2 Neurofibroma of the median nerve, note the rosary beads transformation of the nerve trunk

Concerning PNT's general diagnostic assessment, they are easily detected on clinical examination when superficial and of remarkable size. However, small lesions along the course of the nerves and deeply located, clinically silent tumors may be detected only by diagnostic workup. Ultrasound has been successfully utilized to detect both small-/medium-sized tumors along the limbs and deeply located masses, whose diagnostic workup is then completed with contrast MRI. Nevertheless we have more and more evidence that total body MRI should be the first-choice investigation to estimate the whole burden of tumors [25, 26].

MRI has a crucial role not only in revealing the presence of tumors, but it is also useful to identify the histological nature of the lesions. In addition to conventional (unenhanced T1, fluid-sensitive, contrast-enhanced T1-weighted sequences) MRI, the introduction of advanced MR imaging (DWI/apparent diffusion coefficient mapping, dynamic contrast-enhanced MR imaging) has increased the accuracy in ascertaining the histological nature of tumors, especially in detecting possible features of malignancy [27, 28]. However limitations are still present, especially related to the possibility of identifying atypical neurofibromatous neoplasms of uncertain biologic potential (ANNUBP) (see Chap. 29). In recent years the validity of fluoro-2-deoxy-D-glucose PET/CT (FDG-PET/CT) as the only imaging modality presently available to noninvasively identify ANNUBP and MPNSTs has been highlighted in the literature [18, 29, 30]. Yet FDG-PET/CT and diffusion MRI are helpful in the assessment of a presumed malignancy; they cannot confirm a diagnosis of a benign PNT or of a MPNST.

27.5 Indications for Surgery

After the initial assessment and estimation of the total burden of tumors, patients should be regularly followed up. General clinical examination and radiological assessment of deep lesions (that may be predisposed to malignant transformation especially when bulky) should be indicated once a year. Clear information about the clinical signs and symptoms suspicious for malignancy should be provided, urging patients to seek further consultation in case of changes in their clinical state in between follow-ups; individuals affected by NF often tend to be rather compliant toward their "lumps" and delay their treatment. Moreover they are often unwilling or hesitant when offered surgery.

Besides the reluctant attitude to accept surgery shown by patients themselves, it must be admitted that many physicians involved in the management of NF patients tend to be overconservative; for fear of neurological complications, they only advise surgical removal of symptomatic tumors and often discourage their patients from having surgery. Although the onset of postoperative neurological deficits cannot be completely ruled out, it must be emphasized that it is often a likely occurrence for procedures performed by surgeons with no background in peripheral nerve surgery otherwise excision of peripheral nerve tumors can be safely achieved in the hands of experts. Since it also constitutes a valid prevention strategy, a more aggressive surgical attitude should be advocated based on the evidence that in NF1 one-third of MPNSTs are consequent to malignant transformation of preexisting benign tumors (see Chap. 29).

On the other hand, NF individuals, especially those diagnosed as microdeletion, harbor a large number of tumors, and surgery cannot be indiscriminately advocated for all the neoplasms. Indications for surgery must be selective and appropriate; thorough clinical assessment and information provided by radiological workup must lead the physician in taking the ultimate decision and choosing between conservative management and surgical treatment.

Based on our 20-year experience, we recommend surgery in:

- Symptomatic tumors
- Lesions with radiological evidence of malignancy
- Bulky masses (diameter > 6 cm)

In symptomatic tumors, especially if sudden rapid growth, excruciating pain and onset of neurological deficits occur, surgery should be promptly offered, even when no preoperative confirmation of malignancy was evident.

Concerning surgical technique, removal of peripheral nerve tumors has been described in general terms in Chap. 10, whereas Chapters 28 and 29 include technical notes specifically related to excision of plexiform and malignant forms.

27.6 Conclusion

NF1 is related to a wide spectrum of phenotypes; although a large percentage of individuals affected by this genetic disorder are asymptomatic or present few issues, severe clinical manifestations are less than rare.

Due to the several implications and challenging complexity in NF treatment, multidisciplinary referral centers are the only valid tool to monitor and manage complex cases; specialist clinics are also essential to enforce prevention strategies. The role of NF associations in acting as reliable sources of information on the disorder should not be downplayed; they might prove extremely helpful in providing education and support to their affiliated patients and families.

Peripheral nerve tumors are frequently encountered in individuals affected by NF1. Since the occurrence of MPNSTs and neurological complications are the main causes of death in NF patients, the role of neurosurgeons and in particular those gifted with experience in peripheral nerve surgery is crucial and should be further emphasized. In experts' hands, surgical removal of peripheral nerve tumors may be safely achieved; it also represents the mainstay of prevention for MPNSTs.

References

1. Lammert M, Friedman JM, Kluwe L, Mautner VF. Prevalence of neurofibromatosis 1 in German children at elementary school enrollment. Arch Dermatol. 2005;141(1):71–4.
2. Evans DG, Howard E, Giblin C, Clancy T, Spencer H, Huson SM, Lalloo F. Birth incidence and prevalence of tumor-prone syndromes: estimates from a UK family genetic register service. Am J Med Genet A. 2010;152A(2):327–32. https://doi.org/10.1002/ajmg.a.33139.
3. Evans DG. Neurofibromatosis type 2 (NF2): a clinical and molecular review. Orphanet J Rare Dis. 2009;4:16. Published online 2009 Jun 19. https://doi.org/10.1186/1750-1172-4-16.
4. Evans DG. Schwannomatosis: a genetic and epidemiological study. J Neurol Neurosurg Psychiatry. 2018;89(11):1215–9.
5. National Institutes of Health Consensus Development Conference Statement: neurofibromatosis. Arch Neurol. 1988;45:575–578.
6. Ferner RE, Huson SM, Thomas N, Moss C, Willshaw H, Evans DG, Upadhyaya M, Towers R, Gleeson M, Steiger C, Kirby A. Guidelines for the diagnosis and management of individuals with neurofibromatosis 1. J Med Genet. 2007;44(2):81–8. Published online 2006 Nov 14. https://doi.org/10.1136/jmg.2006.045906.
7. Bergqvist C, Servy A, Valeyrie-Allanore L, et al. Neurofibromatosis 1 French national guidelines based on an extensive literature review since 1966. Orphanet J Rare Dis. 2020;15:37. https://doi.org/10.1186/s13023-020-1310-3.
8. Radtke HB, Sebold CD, Allison C, Haidle JL, Schneider G. Neurofibromatosis type 1 in genetic counseling practice: recommendations of the National Society of Genetic Counselors. J Genet Couns. 2007;16(4):387–407. Published online 2007 Jul 17. https://doi.org/10.1007/s10897-007-9101-8.
9. McEwing RL, Joelle R, Mohlo M, Bernard JP, Hillion Y, Ville Y. Prenatal diagnosis of neurofibromatosis type 1: sonographic and MRI findings. Prenat Diagn. 2006;26(12):1110–4.
10. Hamamy H. Consanguineous marriages. Preconcenception consultation in primary health care settings. J Community Genet. 2012;3(3):185–92.
11. Al Gazadi L, Hamamy H, Al Arrayad S. Genetic disorders in the Arab world. BMJ. 2006;33(7573):831–4.
12. Atibo-Tsiba PW. Mariage consaguin et morbi-mortalite', courte revue de la litterature a partir de une association exceptionelle: syndrome de Usher et neurofibromatose de von Reckligausen. Pan Afr Med J. 2016;23:29.
13. Al-Gazali L, Sztriha L, Dawodu A, Bakir M, et al. Patterns of central nervous system anomalies in a population with a high rate of consanguineous marriages. Clin Genet. 1999;55(2):95–102.
14. North KN, Riccardi VM, Samango-Sprouse C, Ferner R, Moore B, Legius E, Ratner N, Denckla MB. Cognitive function and academic performance in neurofibromatosis 1: consensus statement from the NF1 Cognitive Disorders Task Force. Neurology 1997;48:1121–7.
15. Ozonoff S. Cognitive impairment in neurofibromatosis 1. Am J Med Genet. 1999;89:45–52.
16. Hyman SL, Shores A, North KN. The nature and frequency of cognitive deficits in children with neurofibromatosis type 1. Neurology. 2005;11:1037–44.
17. De Raedt T, Brems H, Wolkenstein P, Vidaud D, Pilotti S, Perrone F, et al. Elevated risk for MPNST in NF1 microdeletion patients. Am J Hum Genet. 2003;72(5):1288–92. Epub 2003 Mar 26.
18. Garozzo D. Peripheral nerve tumors in neurofibromatosis 1: An overview on management and indications for surgical treatment in our experience. Neurol India. 2019;67. (Supplement):S38–S44.
19. Khosrotehrani K, Bastuji-Garin S, Riccardi VM, Birch P, Friedman JM, Wolkenstein P. Factors associated with mortality in neurofibromatosis, type 1. Am J Med Genet. 2005;132(1):49–53.
20. Rasmussen SA, Yang Q, Friedman JM. Mortality in neurofibromatosis 1: an analysis using U.S. death certificates. Am J Hum Genet. 2001;68(5):1110–8.
21. Zoller M, Rembeck B, Akesson HO, Angervall L. Life expectancy, mortality and prognostic factors in neurofibromatosis type 1: a twelve-year follow-up of an epidemiological study in Goteborg, Sweden. Acta Derm Venereol. 1995;75:136–40.
22. Nguyen R, Dombi E, Widemann BC, Solomon J, Fuensterer C, Kluwe L, et al. Growth dynamics of plexiform neurofibromas: a retrospective cohort study of 201 patients with neurofibromatosis 1. Orphanet J Rare Dis. 2012;7:75. https://doi.org/10.1186/1750-1172-7-75.

23. Sordillo PP, Helson L, Hajdu SI. Malignant schwannoma—clinical characteristics, survival, and response to therapy. Cancer. 1981;47:2503–9.
24. Evans DG, Huson SM, Birch JM. Malignant peripheral nerve sheath tumours in inherited diseases. Clin Sarcoma Res. 2012;2:17.
25. Evans DGR, Baser ME, et al. Malignant peripheral nerve sheath tumours in neurofibromatosis 1. J Med Genet. 2002;39:311–4.
26. Mautner VF, Asuagbor FA, Dombi E, Fünsterer C, Kluwe L, Wenzel R, Widemann BC, Jan M. Friedman assessment of benign tumor burden by whole-body MRI in patients with neurofibromatosis. Neuro Oncol. 2008;10(4):593–8. https://doi.org/10.1215/15228517-2008-011.
27. Ahlawat S, Fayad LM, Khan MS, Bredella MA, Harris GJ, Evans DG, Farschtschi S, Jacobs MA, Chhabra A, Salamon JM, Wenzel R, Mautner VF, Dombi E, Cai W, Plotkin SR, Blakeley JO, Whole Body MRI Committee for the REiNS International Collaboration; REiNS International Collaboration Members 2016. Current whole-body MRI applications in the neurofibromatoses: NF1, NF2, and schwannomatosis. Neurology. 2016;87(7 Suppl 1):S31–9. https://doi.org/10.1212/WNL.0000000000002929.
28. Demehri S, Belzberg A, Blakeley J, Fayad LM. Conventional and functional MR imaging of peripheral nerve sheath tumors: initial experience. Am J Neuroradiol. 35(8):1615–20. https://doi.org/10.3174/ajnr.A391.
29. Ferner RE, Golding JF, Smith M, et al. [18] 2-fluoro-2-deoxy-D-glucose positron emission tomography (FDG PET) as a diagnostic tool for neurofibromatosis 1 (NF1) associated malignant peripheral nerve sheath tumours (MPNSTs): a long term clinical study. Ann Oncol. 2008;19(2):390–4. Epub 2007 Oct 11
30. Toymassian D, Razab AR, London K. The role of [18F] FDG-Pet/CT in predicting malignant transformation of plexiform neurofibromas in neurofibromatosis -1. Int J Surg Oncol. 2016;2016:6162182. Published Online 2016 Dec 12.

28 Plexiform Tumors

Debora Garozzo

28.1 Histological and Clinical Peculiarities of Plexiform Tumors

Peripheral nerve tumors are a typical hallmark of neurofibromatosis. In addition to the benign and malignant histotypes found in the general population, this genetic disorder is associated with peculiar neoplastic variants, the so-called plexiform tumors [1–16]. The denomination "plexiform" (from the Latin *plectere*, meaning interweave) refers to their histological appearance similar to a network; they diffusely grow along the nerves and plexuses appearing as deforming, multinodular masses often involving connective tissue and skin folds.

Two histotypes of plexiform tumors have been identified: plexiform schwannomas (PSs) and plexiform neurofibromas (PNs). Depending on the form of neurofibromatosis they are associated with, each histotype presents peculiarities related to their incidence rate, distribution, and natural history.

Plexiform schwannomas (PSs) represent a rare variant of Schwann cell tumor that typically arises in superficial soft tissues with predilection for the head and neck region [4]. Initially described by Harkin et al. in 1978 [5], PSs are benign peripheral nerve sheath tumors composed of Schwann cells arranged in a plexiform pattern, presenting as single, soft to rubbery, movable, non-tender, and sometimes painful nodules ranging from 0.5 to 2.5 cm in diameter. On histopathological analysis, these tumors show multiple intradermal or subcutaneous nodules composed primarily of cellular Antoni type A regions with palisading nuclear and Verocay bodies. It is crucial to differentiate a plexiform schwannoma from a plexiform neurofibroma because the latter carries a significant risk of malignant transformation. Plexiform schwannomas can be distinguished by their greater cellularity, nuclear palisading (with or without Verocay bodies) and degenerative features, such as hyalinized blood vessels.

PSs are found in NF2 and schwannomatosis. They are generally solitary [6, 7], yet multiple tumors have been occasionally found in NF2 patients [8–14]. In both genetic disorders, they account for 5% of overall schwannomas.

Plexiform neurofibromas are histologically benign tumors that are made up of a variety of cell types including neuronal axons, Schwann cells, fibroblasts, mast cells, macrophages, perineural cells, and extracellular matrix materials such as collagen. The tumor originates from the central aspect of the nerve, and its progressive growth involves multiple fascicles; although the fascicles may be preserved, a diffusely enlarged,

D. Garozzo (✉)
WFNS Peripheral Nerve Surgery Committee,
Department of Neurosurgery,
Mediclinic Parkview Hospital, Dubai, UAE
e-mail: debora.garozzo@esns.ae

F. Guedes et al. (eds.), *Diagnostic Assessment and Treatment of Peripheral Nerve Tumors*,
https://doi.org/10.1007/978-3-030-77633-6_28

thickened, irregular, and tortuous nerve is produced. This tumoral growth pattern results in very peculiar morphologic appearance, classically compared to a "bag of warms" or "rosary beads" (Fig. 28.1) [1–3, 16].

Plexiform neurofibromas develop in individuals with neurofibromatosis 1 (NF1) [1–3, 16]. They can occur in any part of the body although they mostly arise in plexuses and nerves of large caliber (e.g., the sciatic nerve). Physical examination detects plexiform tumors in about 27% of NF1 patients; however, when patients are investigated with whole-body MRI, their incidence increases to 50% of NF1 patients due the detection of internal PNs (Fig. 28.2) [1, 16]. New tumors are infrequent in NF1 patients with PNs and unlikely in patients without PNs. Concerning clinical presentation, 55% of PNs in childhood seem to be symptomatic, whereas about 17% of superficial PNs, 38% of displacing PNs, and 64% of invasive PNs cause functional impairment [16]. The growth of these tumors varies greatly among patients, and its course over time has not been well delineated yet. Recent studies suggest that it is inversely correlated with age, at least in younger NF1 patients; children with NF1 and internal PNs are at risk for tumor growth [16]. Most PNs grow slowly or not at all, and some decrease in size. Some may become disfiguring (Fig. 28.3), disabling, or deadly via compression of vital structures or conversion to MPNST (malignant peripheral nerve sheath tumor) [1–3, 16]. Prevention and prompt detection of malignant transformation actually represent an absolute priority and a most demanding challenge in the management of these patients (see Chap. 29).

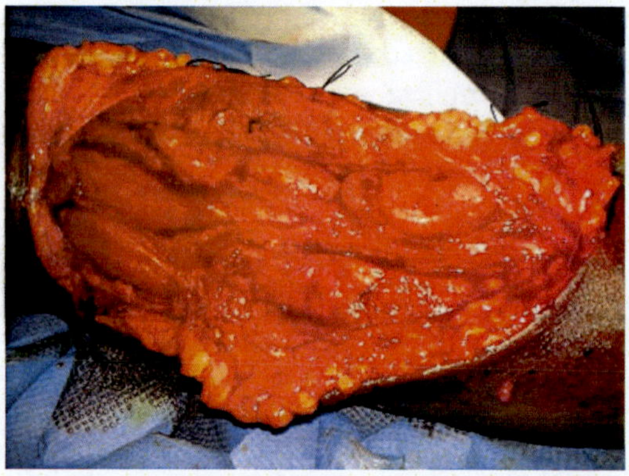

Fig. 28.1 Plexiform neurofibroma of the median nerve

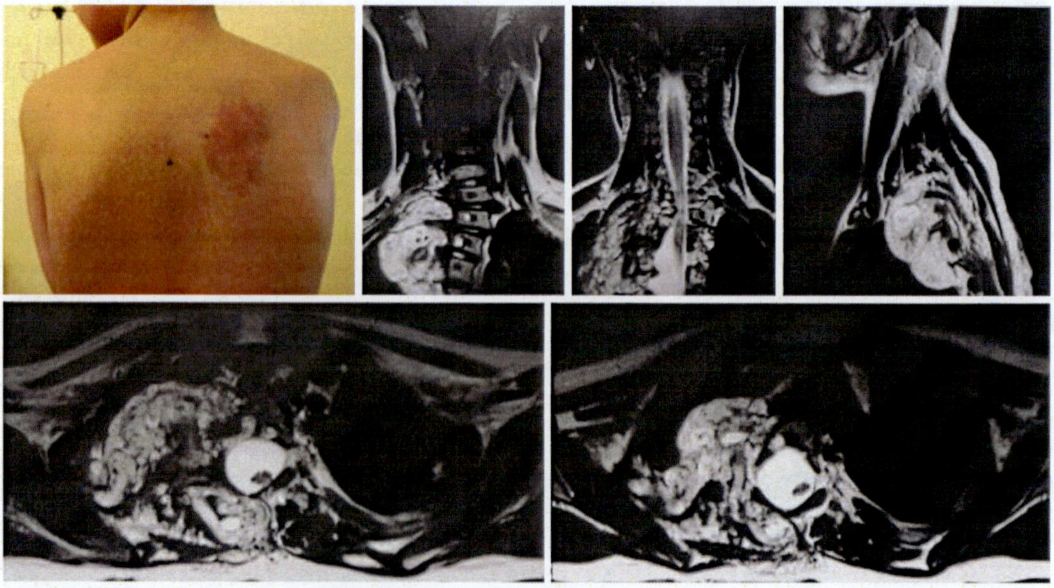

Fig. 28.2 Mediastinal plexiform neurofibroma

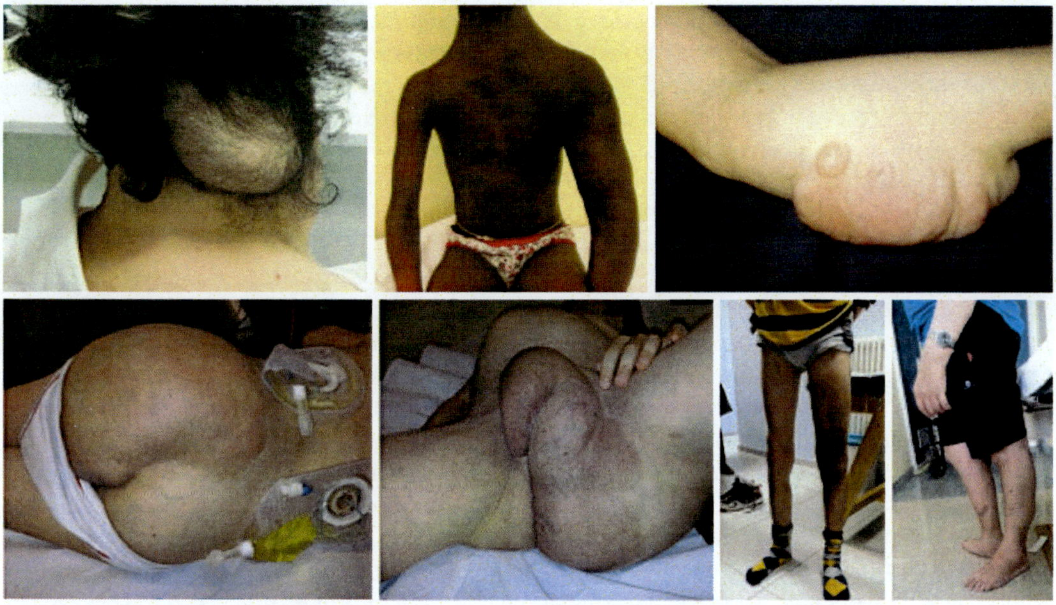

Fig. 28.3 Disfiguring plexiform neurofibromas

28.2 Medical Treatment

In recent years, research has focused on identifying drugs able to control or even reverse the ongoing growth of plexiform neurofibromas. Chemotherapeutic agents such as imatinib, tipifarnib, pirfenidone, sirolimus, or selumetinib [17–22] have been tested on cohorts of children and adults affected by NF. Some trial results were promising even reporting between 20 and 44% decrease in tumor volume in more than 70% patients over a 6-month period [17]. However, until present date, these trials have not provided unquestionable evidence of their effectiveness; patient cohorts are insufficient to warrant the treatment as beneficial [17–22]. Several trials are still ongoing, trying to gather further evidence on possibilities of medical control on plexiform neurofibromas growth, especially on tumors that are deemed inoperable.

Although many authors concluded that the drugs were rather well tolerated, in reality the percentage of serious adverse events (e.g., hypothyroidism, leukopenia, cardiac myopathy, ocular toxicity including retinal vein occlusion, retinal pigment epithelial detachment, and impaired vision) consequent to the administration of these agents is not negligible; for instance, in Killock's selumetinib trial on 50 children, toxicities resulted in dose reductions and treatment discontinuation in 28% and 10% of patients, respectively [17]. Moreover, grade 1 or 2 side effects of the treatment (e.g., nausea, vomiting, abdominal pain, diarrhea, fatigue, and frequent headaches) are extremely frequent and contribute to disruption of life quality, often prompting patients to request discontinuation of the drug. Additionally, the possible consequences of long-term administration in young patients are unknown and this concern should be also kept in mind when enrolling patients for these trials.

28.3 Remarks About Surgical Removal of Plexiform Tumors

Surgery still remains the current mainstay of treatment for these neoplasms. It can be undoubtedly challenging especially in disfiguring and/or deeply located lesions.

Regardless of the surgical approach used to expose the lesion, in tumors with disfiguring growth, removal should be performed planning more than one procedure, especially in children. When attempted in one single procedure, removal of bulky, widespread plexiform tumors is typically characterized by remarkable blood loss. Bleeding does not result from major feeders; these tumors behave like huge sponges soaked with blood, continuously dripping throughout the procedure. This apparently unremarkable yet continuous bleeding is extremely insidious; it may be underestimated and not timely compensated, until signs of severe acute anemia manifest during the procedure. This may result in severe postoperative complications, especially in children. Hence it is preferable to plan the surgery in stages; for instance, a plexiform tumor growing along the whole course of the sciatic nerve and its terminal branches might be removed in three stages.

Surgery is always performed under general anesthesia, and nerve stimulation rules out administration of paralytic agents. PNs appear as bulky, fusiform expansions of a nerve trunk; nerve fibers are dispersed amid the tumoral mass or have undergone neurofibromatous transformation. The surgeon must identify the functional fibers with the help of nerve stimulation in order to preserve them. Yet, due to the high percentage of nerve fibers affected by neurofibromatous transformation, radical removal is often not feasible and surgery just results in gross tumor debulking; radical excision would be achieved only at the expense of function.

Some of these tumors may actually be inoperable as the neurofibromatous growth involves all the nerve fascicles in such a way that radicality implies jeopardizing the function; unless the lesion has been clearly diagnosed as malignant or there are other major indications for radical removal, we believe function should never be sacrificed.

Regardless of accurate hemostasis, postoperative bleeding is persistent and may result in the formation of a progressively growing blood collection at the surgical site; subcutaneous drains should preferably be inserted and removed 2–3 days afterwards.

Another frequent complication is related to wound healing. In many cases, the skin overlying plexiform tumors is particularly thin (due to remarkable reduction of the dermal layer), and this affects the healing process; second intention healing is frequent in these cases. Preoperative consultation with a plastic surgeon and their involvement in the procedure may help for the prevention of such complication.

28.4 Recurrence After Surgical Removal of Plexiform Tumors

Since removal often just results in gross debulking, regrowth is likely. The postsurgical growth behavior of plexiform tumors has been followed up in a study published by Nguyen et al. in 2013 [23]; in their report the authors found that the median tumor progression was 0.6% change per year and 2.9% from baseline. Patients aged 21 years and younger had the highest progression rate; for every year of age, the mean growth rate decreased by −0.463 mean percent. With age as a continuous variable, age, the site of the tumor, and depth were the only factors associated with tumor progression. When surgery achieved radical removal, no relapse during observation (mean, 2.9 years; range, 1.1–5.8 years) was observed.

28.5 Conclusions

PNs are frequently encountered in NF1 patients. Since physical examination only detects superficial lesions, patients should be regularly screened with whole-body MRI to detect internal PNs. These tumors present a high risk to undergo malignant transformation; at present, no pharmaceutical trial has proved effective in arresting or reversing the growth of these tumors, and surgery remains the current mainstay of the treatment. In bulky widespread tumors, surgical removal should be performed in more than one procedure to prevent extensive bleeding, predisposing to complications related to severe ischemia. When preoperative examination reveals that the skin overlying the tumor is extremely thin, wound healing may be problematic; multidisciplinary management with involvement of a plastic surgeon may be helpful in preventing these complications.

Function should never be sacrificed to achieve radical removal unless there is clear evidence of malignancy or other major issues (e.g., compression of vital structures).

References

1. Garozzo D. Peripheral nerve tumors in neurofibromatosis 1: an overview on management and indications for surgical treatment in our experience. Neurol India. 2019;67(Supplement):S38–44.
2. Blakeley JO, Plotkin SR. Therapeutic advances for the tumors associated with neurofibromatosis type 1, type 2, and schwannomatosis. Neuro Oncol. 2016;18(5):624–38. Published online 2016 Feb 6.
3. Boyd KP, Korf BR, Theos A. Neurofibromatosis type 1. J Am Acad Dermatol. 2009;61(1):1–16. https://doi.org/10.1016/j.jaad.2008.12.051.
4. Berg JC, Scheithauer BW, Spinner RJ, Allen CM, Koutlas IG. Plexiform schwannoma: a clinicopathologic overview with emphasis on the head and neck region. Hum Pathol. 2008;39(5):633–40. https://doi.org/10.1016/j.humpath.2007.10.029.
5. Harkin JC, Arrinton HJ, Reed RJ. Benign plexiform schwannoma, a lesion distinct from plexiform neurofibroma [abstract]. J Neuropathol Exp Neurol. 1978;37:622.
6. Kao GF, Laskin WB, Olsen TG. Solitary cutaneous plexiform neurilemmoma (schwannoma): a clinicopathologic, immunohistochemical, and ultrastructural study of 11 cases. Mod Pathol. 1989;2:20–264.
7. Woodruff JM, Marshall ML, Godwin TA, Funkhouser JW, Thompson NJ, Erlandson RA. Plexiform (multinodular) schwannoma. A tumor simulating the plexiform neurofibroma. Am J Surg Pathol. 1983;7:691–7.
8. Sheikh S, Gomes M, Montgomery E. Multiple plexiform schwannomas in a patient with neurofibromatosis. J Thorac Cardiovasc Surg. 1998;115:240–2.
9. Lim HS, Jung J, Chung KY. Neurofibromatosis type 2 with multiple plexiform schwannomas. Int J Dermatol. 2004;43:336–40.
10. Ishida T, Kuroda M, Motoi T, Oka T, Imamura T, Machinami R. Phenotypic diversity of neurofibromatosis 2: association with plexiform schwannoma. Histopathology. 1998;32:264–70.
11. Reith JD, Goldblum JR. Multiple cutaneous plexiform schwannomas. Report of a case and review of the literature with particular reference to the association with types 1 and 2 neurofibromatosis and schwannomatosis. Arch Pathol Lab Med. 1996;120:399–401.
12. Val-Bernal JF, Figols J, Vazquez-Barquero A. Cutaneous plexiform schwannoma associated with neurofibromatosis type 2. Cancer. 1995;76:1181–6.
13. Miyakawa T, Kamada N, Kobayashi T, Hirano K, Fujii K, Sasahara Y, et al. Neurofibromatosis type 2 in an infant with multiple plexiform schwannomas as first symptom. J Dermatol. 2007;34:60–4.
14. Yeon KJ, Eun KJ, Hoon KY, Suck RY. Cutaneous plexiform schwannomas in a patient with neurofibromatosis type 2. Ann Dermatol. 2009;21(4):402–5. Published online 2009 Nov 30.
15. Shinde SV, Tyagi DK, Sawant HV, Puranik GV. Plexiform schwannoma in schwannomatosis. J Postgrad Med. 2009;55(3):206–7.
16. Nguyen R, Dombi E, Widemann BC, Solomon J, Fuensterer C, Kluwe L, Friedman JM, Mautner VF. Growth dynamics of plexiform neurofibromas: a retrospective cohort study of 201 patients with neurofibromatosis. Orphanet J Rare Dis. 2012;7:75. Published online 2012 Oct 4. https://doi.org/10.1186/1750-1172-7-75.
17. Killock D. Selumetinib benefits children with inoperable plexiform neurofibromas. Nat Rev Clin Oncol. 2020;17:273. https://doi.org/10.1038/s41571-020-0361-7.
18. Robertson KA, Nalepa G, Yang FC, Bowers DC, Ho CY, Hutchins GD, et al. Imatinib mesylate for plexiform neurofibromas in patients with neurofibromatosis type 1: a phase 2 trial. Lancet Oncol. 2012;13(12):1218–24. https://doi.org/10.1016/S1470-2045(12)70414-X. Epub 2012 Oct 23.
19. Widemann BC, Babovic-Vuksanovic D, Dombi E, Wolters PL, Goldman S, Martin S, et al. Phase II trial of pirfenidone in children and young adults with neurofibromatosis type 1 and progressive plexiform neurofibromas. Pediatr Blood Cancer. 2014;61(9):1598–602. https://doi.org/10.1002/pbc.25041. Epub 2014 Apr 22.
20. Widemann BC, Dombi E, Gillespie A, Wolters PL, Belasco J, Goldman S, et al. Phase 2 randomized, flexible crossover, double-blinded, placebo-controlled trial of the farnesyltransferase inhibitor tipifarnib in children and young adults with neurofibromatosis type 1 and progressive plexiform neurofibromas. Neuro Oncol. 2014;16(5):707–18. https://doi.org/10.1093/neuonc/nou004. Epub 2014 Feb 4
21. Weiss B, Widemann BC, Wolters P, Dombi E, Vinks A, Cantor A, et al. Sirolimus for progressive neurofibromatosis type 1-associated plexiform neurofibromas: a neurofibromatosis clinical trials consortium phase II study. Neuro Oncol. 2015;17(4):596–603. https://doi.org/10.1093/neuonc/nou235. Epub 2014 Oct 14
22. Weiss B, Widemann BC, Wolters P, Dombi E, Vinks AA, Cantor A, et al. Sirolimus for non-progressive NF1-associated plexiform neurofibromas: an NF clinical trials consortium phase II study. Pediatr Blood Cancer. 2014;61(6):982–6.
23. Nguyen R, Ibrahim C, Friedrich RE, Westphal M, Schuhmann M, Mautner VF. Growth behavior of plexiform neurofibromas after surgery. Genet Med. 2013;15(9):691–7. https://doi.org/10.1038/gim.2013.30. Epub 2013 Apr 18

29 Management of MPNST in Neurofibromatosis

Debora Garozzo, Zarina S. Ali, and Eric L. Zager

29.1 Epidemiology and Peculiarities of NF-Related MPNSTs

MPNSTs are aggressive soft tissue sarcomas associated with dismal clinical outcomes.

Historically, these tumors have been referred to as "malignant schwannomas," "neurogenic sarcomas," or "neurofibrosarcomas." These malignancies are rare, accounting for 5–10% of all soft tissue tumors. They are estimated to present an annual incidence of 1/1,000,000 individuals in the general population. Sporadic MPNSTs (sMPNTs) could be underestimated owing to the possible misclassification of other sarcomas. It is unquestionable that in individuals with neurofibromatosis type 1 (NF1), the risk of MPNST is dramatically increased with 50% of MPNSTs diagnosed in NF1 patients [1–3].

Although there is a general agreement on the higher incidence of MPNSTs in NF1 patients, until now their precise incidence is still controversial in the medical literature, ranging from 2–5% to 8–13% [1–8]. These statistical discrepancies might be due to inherent biases related to the population examined in these studies. There is an underrepresentation of elderly patients with this diagnosis reported in the literature, as they may not have been referred to tertiary centers historically. Similarly, many patients with minimal or no clinical manifestations often remain undiagnosed. Reports usually include a relatively low number of mildly affected patients with NF1, thus presenting a probable ascertainment bias toward more severely affected NF1 patients with MPNST. Consequently, a realistic calculation of the lifetime risk of MPNSTs in NF1 is unclear.

The association between a deletion of the whole *NF1* gene (microdeletion) and MPNSTs has been undeniably highlighted. Microdeletion (equivalent to a loss of 1.5 MB) is found in 5–10% of cases, and this subgroup of patients is characterized by a peculiar phenotype that easily identifies them on clinical examination (see Table 29.1). Microdeletion remarkably raises the lifetime risk of MPNSTs: this subgroup of patients has been estimated to have a 16–25% chance of developing malignancy [9–13]. Other factors that may be associated with a higher risk of developing MPNST in people with NF1 are the occurrence of neurofibromatous neuropathy, exposure to therapeutic radiation, previous occurrence of MPNST, or the occurrence of MPNST in a relative with NF1 [7, 14].

The higher incidence of MPNST is not the only hallmark of these malignant neoplasms in NF. Mean age at diagnosis of MPNST for NF1 patients is younger in comparison with the

D. Garozzo (✉)
WFNS Peripheral Nerve Surgery Committee, Department of Neurosurgery, Mediclinic Parkview Hospital, Dubai, UAE
e-mail: debora.garozzo@esns.ae

Z. S. Ali · E. L. Zager
Department of Neurosurgery, Perelman School of Medicine, University of Pennsylvania, Philadelphia, PA, USA

F. Guedes et al. (eds.), *Diagnostic Assessment and Treatment of Peripheral Nerve Tumors*,
https://doi.org/10.1007/978-3-030-77633-6_29

Table 29.1 Clinical features associated with microdeletion in NF1

Facial dysmorphism
Delayed cognitive development and/or learning disabilities
Attention-deficit/hyperactivity disorder
Cognitive impairment
Congenital heart disease
Hyperflexibility of joints
Large hands and feet
Muscular hypotonia (more evident in shoulders) or bone cysts
Childhood overgrowth
Higher number of peripheral nerve tumors

general population; NF-MPNSTs are usually detected in early or mid-20s, whereas sporadic MPNSTs (sMPNTs) usually manifest between the third and sixth decade [3, 7].

Clinical presentation may differ as well. Presenting signs in sMPNSTs are most commonly pain, a rapidly enlarging mass along the course of a nerve, usually associated with progressive neurological deficit. Although the clinical manifestations of NF-MPNSTs may present a similar course, a large percentage of these patients may develop malignancy in pre-existing tumors [1–3, 7, 13, 15, 16]. While most NF patients have benign neurofibromas and their plexiform variants, these tumors may frequently undergo malignant transformation. Indeed, pathological examination reveals coexisting benign neurofibroma in 81% of cases, suggestive of benign pre-existing tumor origin [1]. Malignant change has been estimated to occur in up to 38% of deeply located tumors (e.g., mediastinal or pelvic masses). These are often clinically silent. In addition, bulky neoplasms (diameter > 6 cm) seem to be highly predisposed to malignant transformation [1, 3, 7, 13].

Finally, when considering the prognostic role of a patient's NF1 status with regard to the MPNST treatment, outcomes seem to remain significantly poorer in NF-related patients in comparison with sporadic cases. Only one-third of patients are alive at a 5-year follow-up [3, 4, 6, 17, 18], although survival rates have recently been reported to improve, especially in females (46% versus 22%) [19]. The genetic factors underlying sMPNST and NF-MPNST differ, thus explaining the different natural course of the neoplasm in these two populations. It has also been suggested that the dismal outcome of MPNSTs in NF might be related to a delay in diagnosis and treatment in NF1 patients in comparison with non-NF1 patients. The presence of a rapidly growing mass, especially when painful and associated with progressive functional impairment, raises a red flag for the non-NF patient and prompts their medical attention, whereas NF1 patients may be complacent about the presence of their many and often clinically silent tumors and they are often unaware of the risk of developing malignancy [3, 13, 20].

29.2 Factors Triggering Malignant Transformation and the Role of Atypical Neurofibromas

The factors that trigger malignant transformation are still unrecognized. Mutation of both copies of the *NF1* gene has been demonstrated in MPNST, but this is a known feature of benign neurofibromas as well and therefore cannot be sufficient to explain the onset of malignant transformation. It is likely that additional genetic changes, such as loss of function of *p*53, may also contribute. Research has demonstrated epidermal growth factor receptor (EGF-R) expression and function in MPNST, including both primary tumors and cell lines. Since EGF-R expression is not characteristic of normal Schwann cells, these findings suggest that activation of EGF-R may be involved in the process of malignant change [21–23].

Prediction of malignant transformation in pre-existing tumors is clinically and histologically challenging. In recent years research has focused on a histologic subgroup of neurofibromas that seem to have a cardinal role in malignant change, the so-called "atypical neurofibromas." Morphologically and radiologically indistinguishable from purely benign forms, they present histologic features typical of malignancy and seem likely to be precursors for MPNSTs [24]. After a consensus meeting in October 2016, the histopathologic features and molecular mechanisms involved in the malignant transformation of neurofibromas were outlined. Nuclear atypia alone is generally insignificant. However, the detection of other findings such as atypia, loss of neurofibroma architecture, high cellularity and/or mitotic activity >1/50 but <3/10 high-power fields should raise a red flag for possible malignancy. At present, the term "atypical neurofibromatous neoplasms of uncertain biologic potential (ANNUBP)" for lesions displaying at least two of the above-mentioned features has been introduced in the current use. However, such tumors are diagnosed inconsistently as atypical neurofibroma or low-grade MPNST. Further investigation is necessary to highlight pathologic triggers in their evolution toward malignancy. Neurofibromas contain numerous S100 protein/SOX10-positive Schwann cells and CD34-positive fibroblasts. Both these components are reduced or absent in MPNST. Loss of p16/CDKN2A expression, elevated Ki67 labeling and extensive nuclear p53 positivity are also features of MPNST that can, to some degree, occur in ANNUBP. Some authors consider the complete loss of trimethylated histone 3 lysine 27 expression potentially more reliable, as it has been immunohistochemically detected in about half of MPNSTs [14, 24, 25].

Considering their role as MPNST precursors, identification of ANNUBP should be a priority in malignancy prevention. Many of these tumors are clinically silent and deeply located in the mediastinum or pelvis. It has been noted that patients that develop MPNSTs at a young age seem to present with a higher number of internal neurofibromas in comparison with the MPNST-free counterparts [26, 27]. Thus estimating the whole tumor burden in these patients is important as a possible marker of likelihood to develop malignancy. Whole-body MRI has proven to be a valid tool in screening these patients and to ascertain the presence of internal neurofibromas that cannot be identified on physical examination [27].

As initially mentioned ANNUBP are morphologically and radiologically indistinguishable from their fully benign counterparts. In recent years more and more research has highlighted the validity of fluoro-2-deoxy-D-glucose PET/CT (FDG-PET/CT) as the only imaging modality presently able to noninvasively identify ANNUBP. These neoplasms typically demonstrate avid uptake of the tracer (Fig. 29.1). In the studies reported in the literature, sensitivities ranged from 91 to 100% although specificity ranged from 72 to 95% depending on the different protocols applied to perform the investigation. In order to maximize its accuracy, early images should be taken at least 90 min after intravenous [^{18}F]-2-fluoro-2-deoxy-D-glucose is administered. Although no optimal SUV_{max} cut-off exists in the published literature, the use of SUV_{max} 3.5 as a cut-off was adopted by most trials [13, 28, 29]. Recent reports have identified low ADC values in DWI sequences of MRI as highly suggestive of malignancy [30].

29.3 Indications for Surgery and Key Principles in MPNST Removal

For fear of neurological complications, surgical removal of peripheral nerve tumors in NF patients is generally recommended for symptomatic tumors only. Yet, it can be safely performed by surgeons with experience and expertise in the field.

Based on the evidence that malignancy frequently occurs in pre-existing benign tumors, and given the above considerations about ANNUBP, the authors support the adoption of timely surgical intervention when appropriate. Prolonged conservative management in the presence of changing anatomic pathology or symptomatology has the potential to jeopardize the possibility to rescue the patient from the fatal prognosis associated with malignant transformation of disease. In our opinion, surgical intervention should be considered not only in symptomatic tumors but also for those lesions that, although clinically silent, present a high likelihood of undergoing malignant transformation.

Patients are often recommended to undergo a fine-needle aspiration or core biopsy. In our experience, there is a limited role for diagnostic biopsy. Needle biopsies often provide nondiag-

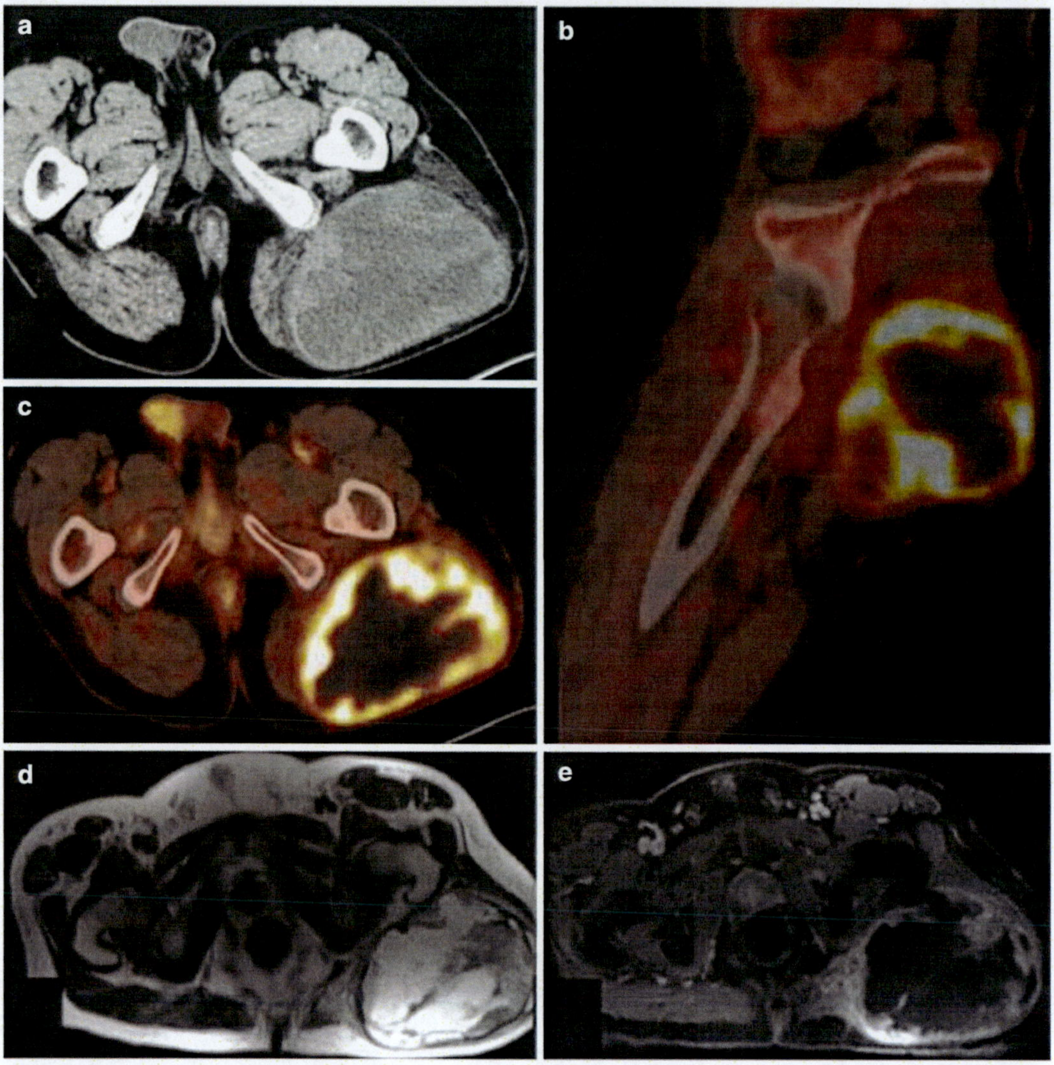

Fig. 29.1 Positron emission tomography (PET)/computed tomography (CT) and magnetic resonance imaging (MRI) appearance of malignant peripheral nerve sheath tumor (MPNST). A 42-year-old male with NF1 with a large left buttock MPNST. (**a**) Low-dose CT images revealed a large complex mass in the left buttocks measuring up to 15 cm with a hypodense center suggestive of central necrosis. (**b**) Axial PET/CT fused images demonstrate increased peripheral fluorodeoxyglucose (FDG) uptake in the lesion in keeping with viable tumor. There is no FDG uptake in the central hypodense regions in keeping with central necrosis. (**c**) Sagittal PET/CT fused image. (**d**) T2-weighted MRI demonstrates the heterogeneous appearance of the large left buttock MPNST. (**e**) Postcontrast T1 fat-saturated image demonstrates peripheral irregular enhancement corresponding to the viable FDG-avid regions with central nonenhancing necrotic region. (Reproduced with permission from Hong et al.: Malignant Peripheral Nerve Sheath Tumors. In: Manual of Peripheral Nerve Surgery, Thieme 2018)

nostic samples or sampling errors. Since malignant change may initially affect only a small portion of the tumoral mass in bulky lesions, biopsies may be misleading, providing false reassurance and downplaying the risk of malignancy [13, 31, 32]. Moreover needle biopsies have the potential to induce significant neuropathic pain syndrome and/or neurologic deficit due to fascicular disruption. If there is bleeding in association with the biopsy, the resultant scar formation may obscure surgical planes for subsequent tumor resection. It may be that MRI with DWI combined with FDG-PET/CT can direct the biopsy to the most metabolically active region to improve the diagnostic yield of needle biopsies. Some have advocated open biopsies for more reliable tissue sampling. The downside here is the likelihood of seeding tumor cells into surrounding tissue. It must also be noted that accomplished peripheral nerve surgeons may encounter few, if any, difficulties in removing tumors that are superficially located, with low risk of complications, offering these patients the option of radical resection of lesions that are proven to be malignant.

On the other hand, deeply located masses may require a multidisciplinary approach in order to provide the peripheral nerve surgeon access to the tumor.

It is not within the scope of this chapter to describe the surgical steps of peripheral nerve tumor removal, yet we will only include a few key remarks.

As we previously mentioned, in NF1 patients, MPNSTs may present two different patterns of clinical manifestation, clearly correlated with the morphological behavior of the neoplasm [13]. When MPNSTs are completely clinically silent or only responsible for pain/paresthesias without neurological deficits, their gross morphology is indistinguishable from benign forms. Often, these tumors appear well-encapsulated, respecting the nerve anatomy and its surrounding tissues. These tumors can be radically removed while preserving the nerve of origin and its function.

On the other hand, when tumors present at the onset with progressive neurological deficits, they tend to be infiltrative (Figs. 29.2 and 29.3). Grossly, they appear as an asymmetrical enlargement of the nerve trunk, often presenting adhesions to the surrounding structures. These tumors frequently have firm consistency and necrotic/hemorrhagic regions scattered on their surface (Fig. 29.4). The infiltrative behavior of these neoplasms is usually related to histological findings consistent with high-grade malignancy (Fig. 29.5). Since neural function has already been impaired by the destructive nature of the tumor, in these cases, the surgeon's priority is to radically remove the tumor and prevent local recurrences and metastatic spread. Resection of the neoplasm and its nerve of origin is mandatory, extending resection as distally as possible on each pole of the tumor in order to maximize local control of the infiltrative nerve disease. The margins of the resection may appear tumor-free under magnified vision at surgery; however, repetitive intraoperative biopsies are invaluable in ascertaining tumor-free boundaries. Surrounding soft tissues must be included in the resection in order to minimize the risk of local recurrence and metastatic spread.

Functional deficits can be compensated, in some cases, by distal nerve or tendon transfers during the same surgery [13, 32, 33]. Nerve graft reconstruction is usually not a feasible option in these cases, for several reasons. The tumor resection typically results in a long gap between the two nerve stumps, often longer than 10 cm. It is well known that excessive length of a nerve graft unfavorably impacts the functional outcome. Postoperative radiotherapy represents another impediment to regeneration through a nerve graft [13, 32]. In selected cases, distal nerve transfers can be performed distant from the irradiated area. Nerve transfers may provide functional restoration in several months; tendon transfers might be preferred in selected cases as the patient may regain function shortly after the procedure [33].

29.4 Post-surgical Treatment

Surgery is definitely the mainstay of treatment in MPNSTs [13, 32–34]. Concerning adjuvant therapy, radiotherapy has proved beneficial in limiting local recurrence [32–35]. Whenever available, hadrontherapy may be preferred as it may be more effective than conventional radiotherapy [36, 37]. Data concerning chemotherapy are controversial [32, 33, 38].

For many years, limb amputation or disarticulation has been included in the treatment of these tumors, and it is still advocated by some authors.

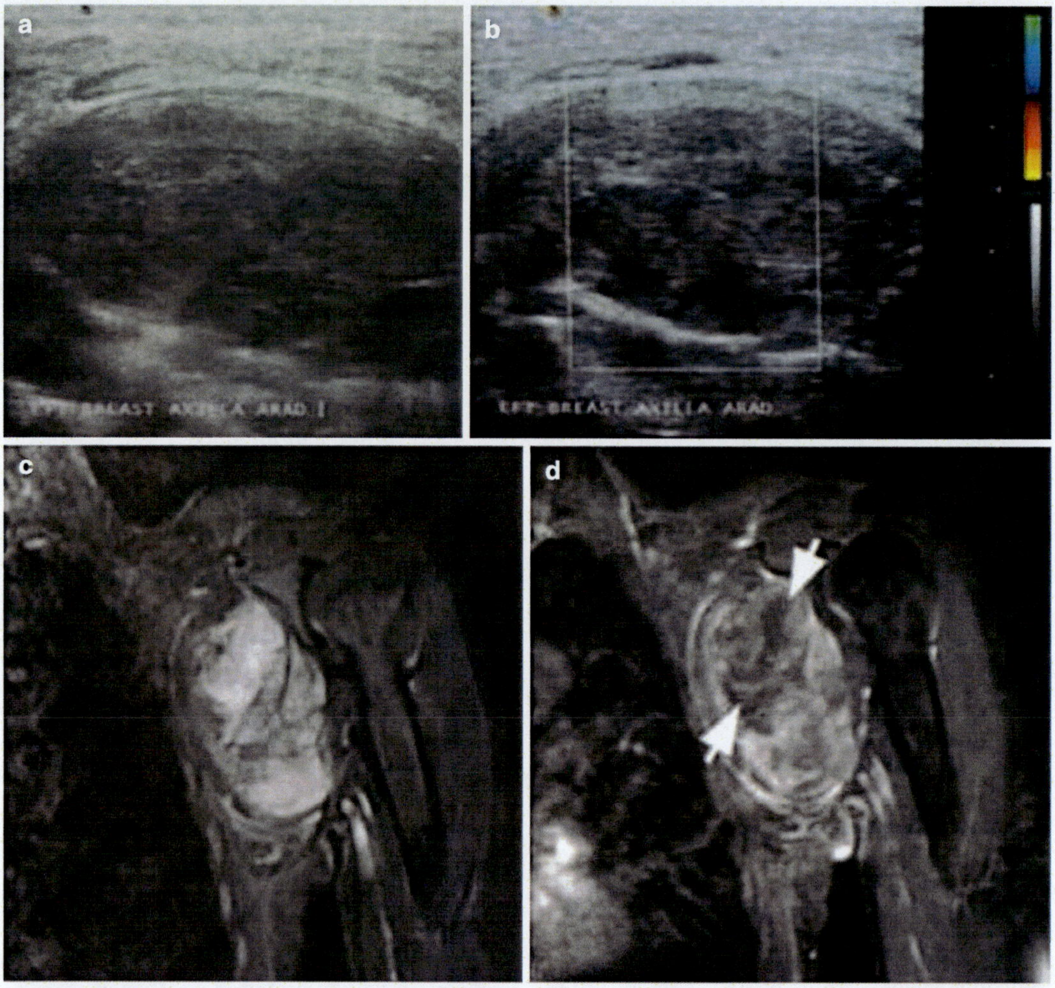

Fig. 29.2 Ultrasound and magnetic resonance imaging (MRI) appearance of an axillary malignant peripheral nerve sheath tumor (MPNST). A 38-year-old female presented with a left axillary mass and targeted ultrasound of the left axillary lesion was performed. Gray scale (**a**) and Doppler (**b**) ultrasound demonstrate a mildly heterogeneous hypoechoic circumscribed lesion with minimal internal vascularity. Subsequent ultrasound-guided biopsy revealed an MPNST. MRI of the axillary lesion was performed and STIR (short tau inversion recovery; [**c**]) sequence demonstrates an oval heterogeneous axillary lesion. Postcontrast T1 fat-saturation sequence (**d**) demonstrates heterogeneous peripheral dominant enhancement with central nonenhancing cystic and/or necrotic areas. (Reproduced with permission from Hong et al.: Malignant Peripheral Nerve Sheath Tumors. In: Manual of Peripheral Nerve Surgery, Thieme 2018)

In our opinion it should be abandoned in most cases. Amputation seems to be associated with a lower rate of local recurrence, yet it does not provide longer survival in comparison with limb-sparing procedures, and it has a devastating impact on quality of life [32, 33, 39, 40]. The rate of postoperative complications is high (up to 44% of cases), including a significant percentage of patients that are condemned to live with phantom limb pain (up to 85% of cases).

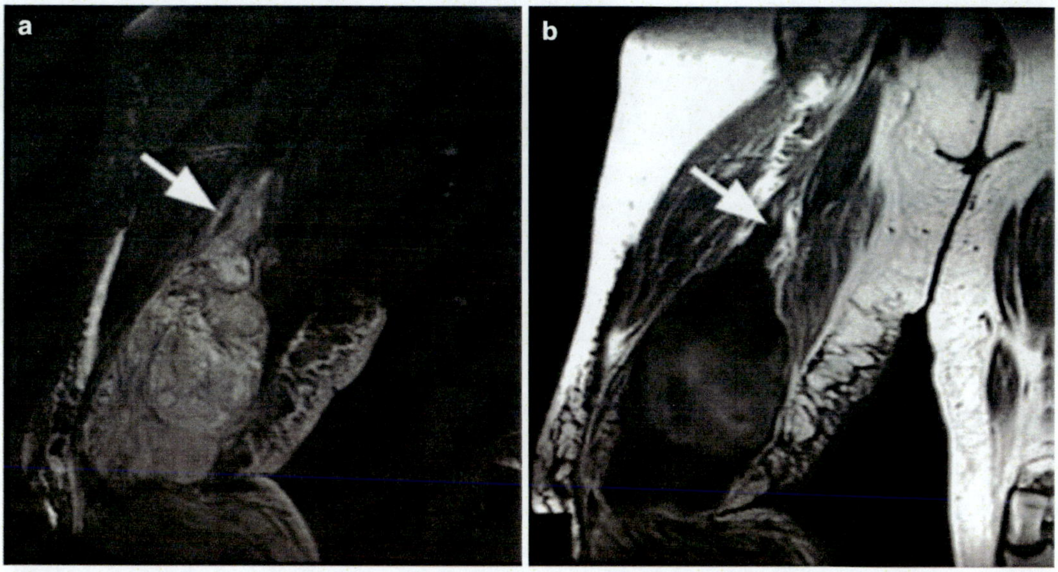

Fig. 29.3 Magnetic resonance imaging appearance of a right thigh malignant peripheral nerve sheath tumor with rhabdomyosarcoma, a "triton tumor," in a 33-year-old female with neurofibromatosis type 1. (**a**) Sagittal short tau inversion recovery (STIR) sequence demonstrates a large heterogeneous predominantly hyperintense lesion corresponding to the expected location of the sciatic nerve in the lower thigh. Peritumoral edema is seen at the proximal aspect of the lesion (white arrow). There is subcutaneous soft tissue edema in the lower thigh as well. (**b**) Sagittal T1 sequence demonstrates a predominantly hypointense lesion with areas of heterogeneity likely reflecting blood products/necrotic debris. A "tail sign" is seen at the proximal aspect of the lesion representing continuity with the sciatic nerve (white arrow). (Reproduced with permission from Hong et al.: Malignant Peripheral Nerve Sheath Tumors. In: Manual of Peripheral Nerve Surgery, Thieme 2018)

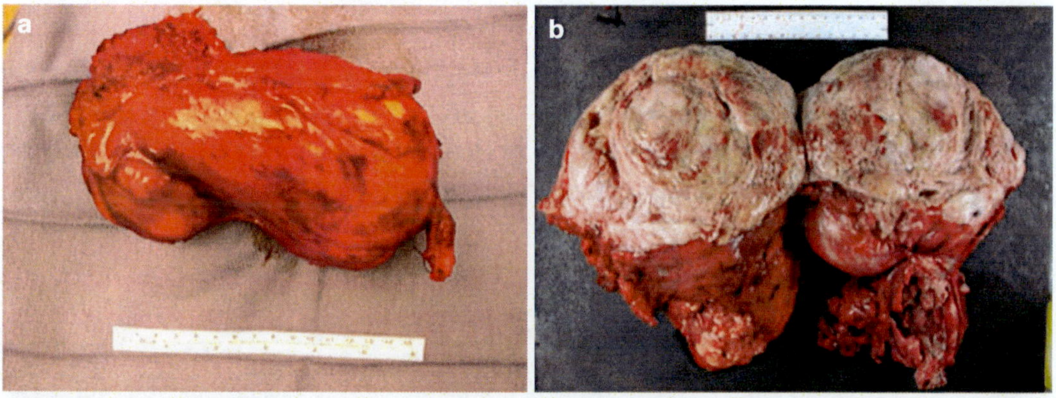

Fig. 29.4 Gross appearance of malignant peripheral nerve sheath tumor (MPNST). (**a**) Excised MPNST from femoral nerve. (**b**) Cut gross specimen. Note grayish, fleshy appearance and regions of necrosis. (Reproduced with permission from Hong et al.: Malignant Peripheral Nerve Sheath Tumors. In: Manual of Peripheral Nerve Surgery, Thieme 2018)

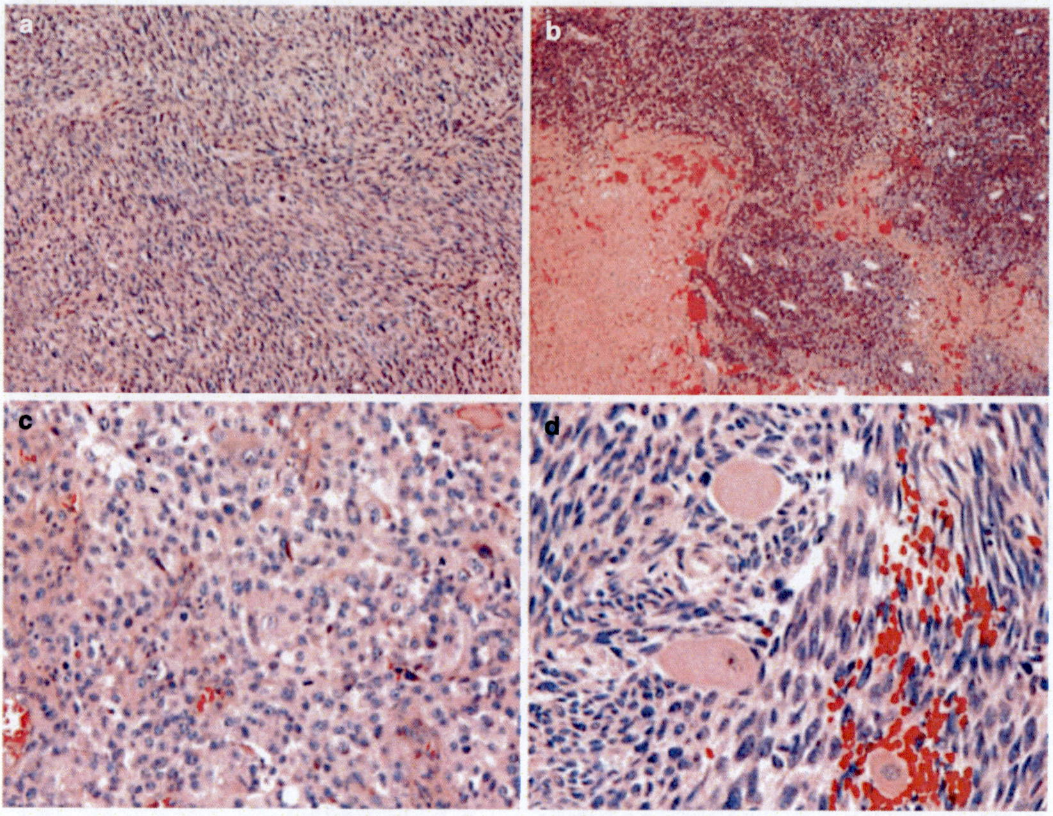

Fig. 29.5 Hematoxylin and eosin (H&E) staining of various malignant peripheral nerve sheath tumor (MPNST) subtypes. (**a**) Typical appearance of MPNST with spindle-shaped cells arranged in whorling and fascicular patterns at ×10 magnification. (**b**) Areas of geographic necrosis in a typical MPNST at ×5 magnification. (**c**) Epithelioid MPNST. Note the large, polygonal cells with central nuclei and prominent nucleoli at ×10 magnification. (**d**) Malignant triton tumor at ×20 magnification. Note the striated cells that appear similar to muscle fibers. (Reproduced with permission from Hong et al.: Malignant Peripheral Nerve Sheath Tumors. In: Manual of Peripheral Nerve Surgery, Thieme 2018)

29.5 Conclusions

MPNSTs rarely occur in the general population but frequently manifest in NF1 patients. Specifically, patients whose genetic screening detects a microdeletion seem to be remarkably predisposed to develop these malignant neoplasms. A worrisome feature of NF-related MPNSTs is the possibility that they may arise due to malignant transformation of pre-existing benign lesions, making prevention a major priority in the management of patients affected by this genetic disorder. At present, we have not identified all the factors associated with malignant change, and clearly further preclinical work is required to understand this pathophysiology. A histologic subgroup (ANNUBP) has been identified that are considered precursors of MPNSTs. At this time, surgical resection with wide margins is the mainstay of treatment. Multicenter clinical trials are needed to establish the roles for radiation therapy, chemotherapy, and immunotherapy.

References

1. Bruce R. Korf malignancy in neurofibromatosis type 1. Oncologist. 2000;5(6):477–85.
2. Ducatman BS, Scheithauer BW, Piepgras DG, Reiman HM, Ilstrup DM. Malignant peripheral nerve sheath tumors. A clinicopathologic study of 120 cases.

Cancer Res Treat. 2017;49(3):717–26. Published online 2016 Dec 1.
3. McCaughan JA, Holloway SM, Davidson R, Lam WW. Further evidence of the increased risk for malignant peripheral nerve sheath tumour from a Scottish cohort of patients with neurofibromatosis type 1. J Med Genet. 2007;44(7):463–6. Epub 2007 Feb 27
4. Hwang K, Hahn SM, Kim HS, Kim SK, Kim HS, Shin K-H, Suh CO, Lyu CJ, Han JW. Outcomes of treatment for malignant peripheral nerve sheath tumors: different clinical features associated with neurofibromatosis type 1. Cancer Res Treat. 1986;57(10):2006–21.
5. Evans DG, Huson SM, Birch JM. Malignant peripheral nerve sheath tumours in inherited diseases. Clin Sarcoma Res. 2012;2:17.
6. King AA, Debaun MR, Riccardi VM, Gutmann DH. Malignant peripheral nerve sheath tumors in neurofibromatosis 1. Am J Med Genet. 2000;93:388–92.
7. Evans DGR, Baser ME, et al. Malignant peripheral nerve sheath tumours in neurofibromatosis 1. J Med Genet. 2002;39:311–4.
8. Huson SM, Harper PS, Compston DA. Von Recklinghausen neurofibromatosis. A clinical and population study in south-east Wales. Brain. 1988;111:1355–81.
9. Pasmant E, Sabbagh A, Spurlock G, Laurendeau I, Grillo E, Hamel MJ, Martin L, et al. NF1 microdeletions in neurofibromatosis type 1: from genotype to phenotype. Hum Mutat. 2010;31(6):E1506–18. https://doi.org/10.1002/humu.21271.
10. De Raedt T, Brems H, Wolkenstein P, et al. Elevated risk for MPNST in NF1 microdeletion patients. Am J Hum Genet. 2003;72:1288–92.
11. De Raedt T, Maertens O, Chmara M, Brems H, Heyns I, Sciot R, et al. Somatic loss of wild type NF1 allele in neurofibromas: comparison of NF1 microdeletion and non-microdeletion patients. Genes Chromosomes Cancer. 2006;45(10):893–904.
12. Kehrer-Sawatzki H, Mautner VF, Cooper DN. Emerging genotype-phenotype relationships in patients with large NF1 deletions. Hum Genet. 2017;136(4):349–76. https://doi.org/10.1007/s00439-017-1766-y. Epub 2017 Feb 17
13. Garozzo D. Peripheral nerve tumors in neurofibromatosis 1: an overview on management and indications for surgical treatment in our experience. Neurol India. 2019;67(Supplement):S38–44.
14. Reilly KM, Kim AR, Blakely J, Ferner RE, Gutmann DH, Legius E, Miettinen MM, Randall RL, Ratner N, Jumbé NL, Bakker A, Viskochil D, Widemann BC, Stewart DR. Neurofibromatosis type 1–associated MPNST state of the science: outlining a research agenda for the future. J Natl Cancer Inst. 2017;109(8):djx124. https://doi.org/10.1093/jnci/djx124.
15. Ahlawat S, Blakeley J, Montgomery E, Subramaniam RM, Belzberg A, Fayad LM. Schwannoma in neurofibromatosis type 1: a pitfall for detecting malignancy by metabolic imaging. Skeletal Radiol. 2013;42(9):1317–22.
16. Broski SM, Johnson GB, Howe BM, Nathan MA, Wenger DE, Spinner RJ, Amrami KK. Evaluation of 18F-FDG PET and MRI in differentiating benign and malignant peripheral nerve sheath tumors. Skeletal Radiol. 2016;45(8):1097–105.
17. Vasconcelos RAT, Coscarelli PG, Alvarenga RP, Acioly MA. Malignant peripheral nerve sheath tumor with and without neurofibromatosis type 1. Arq Neuropsiquiatr. 2017;75(6):366–71.
18. Miao R, Wang H, Jacobson A, Lietz AP, Choy E, Raskin KA, Schwab JH, Deshpande V, Nielsen GP, DeLaney TF, Cote GM, Hornicek FJ, Chen YE. Radiation-induced and neurofibromatosis-associated malignant peripheral nerve sheath tumors (MPNST) have worse outcomes than sporadic MPNST. Radiother Oncol. 2019;137:61–70. https://doi.org/10.1016/j.radonc.2019.03.015. [Epub ahead of print]
19. Ingham S, Huson SM, Moran A, Wylie J, Leahy M, Evans DG. Malignant peripheral nerve sheath tumours in NF1: improved survival in women and in recent years. Eur J Cancer. 2011;47(18):2723–8.
20. Friedrich RE, Hartmann M, Mautner VF. Malignant peripheral nerve sheath tumors (MPNST) in NF1-affected children. Anticancer Res. 2007;27(4A):1957–60.
21. Legius E, Marchuk DA, Collins FS, et al. Somatic deletion of the neurofibromatosis type 1 gene in a neurofibrosarcoma supports a tumour suppressor gene hypothesis. Nat Genet. 1993;3:122–6.
22. Colman SD, Williams CA, Wallace MR. Benign neurofibromas in type 1 neurofibromatosis (NF1) show somatic deletions of the *NF1* gene. Nat Genet. 1995;11:90–2.
23. DeClue JE, Heffelfinger S, Benvenuto G, et al. Epidermal growth factor receptor expression in neurofibromatosis type 1-related tumors and NF1 animal models. J Clin Invest. 2000;105:1233–41.
24. Rodriguez FJ, Folpe AL, Giannini C, Perry A. Pathology of peripheral nerve sheath tumors: diagnostic overview and update on selected diagnostic problems. Acta Neuropathol. 2012;123(3):295–319.
25. Miettinen MM, Antonescu CR, Fletcher CDM, Kim A, Lazar AJ, Quezado MM, Reilly KM, Stemmer-Rachamimov A, Stewart DR, Viskochil D, Widemann B, Perry A. Histopathologic evaluation of atypical neurofibromatous tumors and their transformation into malignant peripheral nerve sheath tumor in patients with neurofibromatosis 1—a consensus overview. Hum Pathol. 2017;67:1–10. https://doi.org/10.1016/j.humpath.2017.05.010. Epub 2017 May 24
26. Tucker T, Wolkenstein P, Revuz J, Zeller J, Friedman JM. Association between benign and malignant peripheral nerve sheath tumors in NF1. Neurology. 2005;65(2):205–11.
27. Mautner VF, Asuagbor FA, Dombi E, Fünsterer C, Kluwe L, Wenzel R, Widemann BC, Friedman JM. Assessment of benign tumor burden by whole-body MRI in patients with neurofibromatosis 1. Neuro Oncol. 2008;10(4):593–8.

28. Tovmassian D, Razak MA, London K. The role of [^{18}F] FDG-PET/CT in predicting malignant transformation of plexiform neurofibromas in neurofibromatosis-1. Int J Surg Oncol. 2016;2016:6162182. Published online 2016 Dec 12.
29. Ferner RE, Golding JF, Smith M, Calonje E, Jan W, Sanjayanathan V, O'Doherty M. [18F]2-fluoro-2-deoxy-D-glucose positron emission tomography (FDG PET) as a diagnostic tool for neurofibromatosis 1 (NF1) associated malignant peripheral nerve sheath tumours (MPNSTs): a long-term clinical study. Ann Oncol. 2008;19(2):390–4. Epub 2007 Oct 11
30. Chhabra A, Thakkar RS, Andreisek G, Chalian M, Belzberg AJ, Blakeley J, Hoke A, Thawait GK, Eng J, Carrino JA. Anatomic MR imaging and functional diffusion tensor imaging of peripheral nerve tumors and tumorlike conditions. Am J Neuroradiol. 2013;34(4):802–7.
31. Bhat D, Socolovsky M, Singh V. Surgical dilemmas in the management of peripheral nerve tumors in neurofibromatosis 1. Neurol India. 2019;67(7):45–6.
32. Dorsi M, Belzberg A. Chapter 23. Peripheral nerve tumors of the extremities. In: Schmidek and Sweet, editors. Operative neurosurgical techniques. Elsevier; 2012. pp. 2319–2327.
33. Gortz O, Langer S, Uthoff D, Ring A, Strcker I, Tannapfel A, et al. Diagnosis, treatment and survival of 65 patients with malignant peripheral nerve sheath tumors. Anticancer Res. 2014;34:777–84.
34. Dunn GP, Spiliopoulos K, Plotkin SR, Hornicek FJ, Harmon DC, Delaney TF, et al. Role of resection of malignant peripheral nerve sheath tumors in patients with neurofibromatosis type 1. J Neurosurg. 2013;118(1):142–8. https://doi.org/10.3171/2012.9.JNS101610. Epub 2012 Oct 26.
35. Kahn J, Gillespie A, Tsokos M, Ondos J, Dombi E, Camphausen K, et al. Radiation therapy in management of sporadic and neurofibromatosis type 1-associated malignant peripheral nerve sheath tumors. Front Oncol. 2014;4:324. Published online 2014 Nov 17.
36. Keole S, Ashman JB, Daniels TB. Proton therapy for sarcomas. Cancer J. 2014;20(6):409–14.
37. Vitolo V, Fiore MR, Barcellini A, Vischioni B, Iannalfi A, Facoetti A, et al. Carbon ion radiotherapy in the management of the tumors of the peripheral nervous system. Anticancer Res. 2019;39:909–13.
38. Zehou O, Fabre E, Zelek L, Sbidian E, Ortonne N, Banu E, et al. Chemotherapy for the treatment of malignant peripheral nerve sheath tumors in neurofibromatosis 1: a 10-year institutional review. Orphanet J Rare Dis. 2013;8:127.
39. Williard WC, Collin C, Casper ES, Hajdu SI, Brennan MF. The changing role of amputation for soft tissue sarcoma of the extremity in adults. Surg Gynecol Obstet. 1992;175:389–96.
40. Daigeler A, Lehnhardt M, Khadra A, Hauser J, Steinstraesser L, Langer S, Goertz O, Steinau HU. Proximal major limb amputations—a retrospective analysis of 45 oncological cases. World J Surg Oncol. 2009;7:15. Published online 2009 Feb 9.

Check for updates

30 Schwannomatosis: Review of Diagnosis and Management

Zach Pennington, Daniel Lubelski, Ravi Medikonda, and Allan J. Belzberg

Abbreviations

GABA	γ-Aminobutyric acid
MRI	Magnetic resonance imaging
NF1	Neurofibromatosis type 1
NF2	Neurofibromatosis type 2
NSAID	Non-steroidal anti-inflammatory drug
VEGF	Vascular endothelial growth factor
WB-MRI	Whole-body MRI

30.1 Introduction and Epidemiology

Schwannomatosis is the least common form of neurofibromatosis and is characterized by formation of multiple non-cutaneous schwannomas without the presence of bilateral vestibular schwannomas [1]. Of the neurofibromatosis subtypes, neurofibromatosis type 1 (NF1 or von Recklinghausen's disease) accounts for approximately 96% of all cases, neurofibromatosis type 2 (NF2) for 3%, and schwannomatosis for the remaining 1% [2]. However, there is a lack of high-quality epidemiological evidence, and some suggest that the true incidence of schwannomatosis is similar to that of NF2 [3]. A population-based study from the United Kingdom documented a point prevalence of 1 in 126,315 persons and an incidence of 1 in every 68,956 live births [4]. In this same study, the mean age of diagnosis was 41.9 years (range 15–66), and the mean age at death was 76.9 (range 55–80), suggesting that schwannomatosis is associated with a later age of onset and better prognosis than the related NF2 [4]. Similar findings were made in an earlier Finnish study, which reported a median age of onset of 45 and an annual incidence of 0.06 per 100,000 person-years [5]. Some series have described a slightly higher disease burden among females [6]; however the Finnish study [5] and the International Schwannomatosis Registry (ISR) [7] suggest a weak predilection for males and no predilection for any specific race. Approximately one in three cases is classified as segmental schwannomatosis—defined by the presence of either multiple peripheral schwannomas in a single limb or multiple spinal schwannomas affecting ≤5 contiguous segments [6, 8, 9]. Lastly, though familial cases of schwannomatosis have been used for genetic investigations, they comprise only 13–25% of all cases [4, 10].

Z. Pennington · D. Lubelski · R. Medikonda
A. J. Belzberg (✉)
Department of Neurosurgery, Johns Hopkins University School of Medicine, Baltimore, MD, USA
e-mail: abelzbe1@jhmi.edu

F. Guedes et al. (eds.), *Diagnostic Assessment and Treatment of Peripheral Nerve Tumors*,
https://doi.org/10.1007/978-3-030-77633-6_30

30.2 Presenting Symptoms

In 75–85% of cases, newly diagnosed patients with schwannomatosis do not have a family history of the disease [3]. The majority of lesions localize to the neck, trunk, and extremities, with relative sparing of the autonomic nerves [3]. As the lesions grow, they generate symptoms e.g., neurologic disability, neuropathic pain, or locoregional organ dysfunction by compressing the affected nerve and surrounding structures. Because of the slow-growing nature of the lesions in this disease, the vast majority of which are WHO grade 1 lesions [5], it is common for patients to present after a symptom prodrome of 7 years or longer [6, 11]. When they do present, the most common presenting symptom is isolated neuropathic pain (29–46%), followed by discovery of an asymptomatic, palpable mass (17–27%) [6, 7, 12]. Additionally, 11–33% of patients will have both pain and a palpable mass on exam [6, 7, 12]. Neurological deficit is uncommon as a presenting feature [13, 14], being seen in only 20% of patients at the time of diagnosis and being the only presenting symptom in 4% of patients [7].

Given the nature of the disease, patients often have chronic symptoms, most frequently chronic pain, which affects up to three-quarters of patients with schwannomatosis [6, 7, 9, 12]. Schwannomas have been reported for all somatic nerves of the peripheral nervous system, including both the peripheral nerves (affected in 81–89% of patients) and spinal nerves (74%) [4, 6, 12]. Lesions in both the peripheral nerves and spinal roots are seen in roughly 55% of patients [4]. A systematic review by Chick and colleagues [11] focused on patients with sporadic schwannomatosis and found that on average patients had 4.6 peripheral nerve tumors and 2.6 spinal tumors; the mean number of peripheral nerve lesions was lower in those with spinal tumors however (2.7 vs 5.7). Interrogation of the peripheral nerve tumors demonstrated roughly equal involvement of the lower and upper limbs, with the most commonly involved nerves being the sciatic, ulnar, radial, and median nerves [11]. These data contrast with those previously published by Plotkin et al. [15], who performed whole-body MRI on 51 patients with familial or sporadic schwannomatosis and found the greatest burden of peripheral nerve schwannomas was within the legs. Both studies reinforce the relatively wide distribution Ṅof peripheral nerve lesions in this population. A contemporary study by the same group found that among spinal lesions, the most affected level is the lumbar spine (53%), though lesions are also commonly seen in the thoracic (35%) and cervical spine (23%) [6]. Multilevel involvement is seen in just over 40% of patients with at least one spinal schwannoma [6].

Overall, cranial nerve involvement is uncommon in schwannomatosis (8–11% of patients), and where it occurs, the trigeminal nerve is the most commonly affected [4, 6, 10]. Classically, schwannomatosis has been distinguished from NF2 by the absence of bilateral vestibular nerve involvement [8]. Case reports now exist describing unilateral vestibular nerve involvement in schwannomatosis patients [4, 16]. Additionally, the phenotype of segmental neurofibromatosis type 2 can be similar to that of schwannomatosis, making definitive diagnosis difficult. In such cases, genetic workup is crucial for definitive diagnosis and should include analysis of the NF2 and SMARCB1 genes in at least two anatomically distinct schwannomas. Schwannomatosis-related lesions will demonstrate a four-hit, three-step mutation pattern with biallelic inactivation of both the *NF2* and *SMARCB1* genes [17]. Along these lines, patients with schwannomatosis will show distinct *NF2* mutations in the different tumors, whereas patients with NF2 will have an identical NF2 mutation in all lesions [18].

30.3 Diagnostic Criteria

Formalized research diagnostic criteria for schwannomatosis were originally presented in 1996 by MacCollin and colleagues [19], who later refined them to give formalized clinical diagnostic criteria in 2005 [8]. The clinical criteria defined profiles for both "definite" and "possible" cases. "Definite" cases were defined as patients meeting one of two descriptions: (1) *sporadic variety*—age >30 years with two or more non-intradermal schwannomas (at least one histologically confirmed) and no vestibular tumor or (2) *familial variety*—patient has ≥1 histologically confirmed non-vestibular schwannoma and ≥1 first-degree relative meeting the criteria of description 1. “Possible” cases were split into three categories: (1) patients less than 30 years of age with ≥2 non-intradermal schwannomas (≥1 histologically confirmed) and without an *NF2* mutation or evidence of vestibular tumor on magnetic resonance imaging (MRI), (2) patients older than 45 with two or more non-intradermal schwannomas (at least one pathologically confirmed) and no symptoms of vestibulocochlear nerve dysfunction or *NF2* mutation, and (3) patients with at least one non-vestibular schwannoma and ≥1 first-degree relative meeting the criteria for “definite” schwannomatosis [8].

Since that time, the diagnostic criteria have been modified to incorporate the advances in genetic testing as well as to incorporate updates in the understanding of the pathology, including elimination of vestibular schwannoma and NF2 mutations as exclusion criteria. These latest criteria, published by an international cohort of experts, allow for diagnosis based upon clinical features alone or based upon a combination of clinical and genetic data (Table 30.1) [7].

30.4 Distinction from Neurofibromatosis Type 2

Clinically, schwannomatosis and NF2 share many phenotypic features, which can make their differentiation difficult. However, given the significantly poorer natural history of NF2 [4], differentiation of the two pathologies has prognostic significance. As recently summarized by Kehrer-Sawatzki et al. [10], borrowing from the work of MacCollin [20], Merker [6], and others, there are several phenotypic findings that can be used to distinguish schwannomatosis from NF2. Features unique to NF2 include the presence of bilateral vestibular schwannoma (90–95% of cases), ependymomas (18–58%), skin plaques/cutaneous lesions (41–48%), intradermal tumors (27%), retinal hamartomas (6–22%), epiretinal membranes (12–40%), and subcapsular cataracts (60–81%). Additionally, intracranial meningiomas (45–58% in NF2 vs 5% in schwannomatosis), unilateral vestibular schwannomas (18% of NF2 cases), non-vestibular cranial nerve schwannomas (24–51% vs 9–10%), and subcutaneous tumors (43–48% vs 23%) are all more common in NF2 than in schwannomatosis and should raise clinician suspicion for this disease entity. Schwannomas of the spine and peripheral nerves characterize both lesions, and their distribution cannot be used to reliably distinguish the

Table 30.1 Criteria for the diagnosis of schwannomatosis as published by the Johns Hopkins Comprehensive Neurofibromatosis Center [7]

Clinical diagnosis (Meets one of below)		**Combined clinical and genetic diagnosis** (Meets one of the below)	
• ≥2 non-intradermal schwannomas – ≥1 pathologically confirmed • No evidence of bilateral vestibular schwannoma on MRI	• ≥1 pathologically confirmed schwannoma or intracranial meningioma • ≥1 first-degree relative with schwannomatosis	• ≥2 tumors with 22q loss-of-heterozygosity and ≥2 distinct, somatic *NF2* mutations • ≥2 pathologically confirmed schwannomas or meningiomas	• Germline *SMARCB1* or *LZTR1* mutation • ≥1 pathologically confirmed schwannoma or meningioma
Exclusion criteria			
• Germline NF2 mutation • Schwannomas occur only in region of prior radiotherapy		• Meets diagnostic criteria for neurofibromatosis type 2 • First-degree relative with NF2	

LZTR1 leucine-zipper-like transcription regulator 1, *MRI* magnetic resonance imaging, *NF2* neurofibromatosis type 2, *SMARCB1* SWI/SNF-related matrix-associated actin-dependent regulator of chromatin subfamily B

two pathologies [10]. Ultimately, however, mutation analysis of *LZTR1*, *NF2*, and *SMARCB1* is the gold standard for distinguishing the two conditions.

30.5 Imaging and Workup

From the perspective of the neurosurgical clinical population, patients with schwannomatosis comprise only a small fraction of all patients who undergo operative management of schwannomas, estimated at 2–10% [5, 8, 21, 22]. Consequently, identification of a single meningioma or schwannoma does not necessarily merit an investigation for schwannomatosis. For this determination, the diagnostic criteria identified by the ISR [7] may be useful.

30.5.1 Imaging

Magnetic resonance imaging constitutes the gold standard of imaging in schwannomatosis and unless contraindicated should be used in all cases [1]. For those with contraindications, contrast-enhanced, high-resolution computed tomography is the next best option, though ultrasound can be considered for the evaluation of peripheral nerves. On MRI, suspicion of schwannomatosis should be raised by the presence of multiple, well-defined, round lesions extending along the length of peripheral nerves and within the spinal roots. The most common sites of involvement are the peripheral nerves (81–89%) followed by the spinal nerves (74%); cranial nerve involvement is rare [4, 6, 12]. Generally spinal lesions are found in one location, however they may affect multiple levels in one-third of cases [6]. Lesions of the peripheral nerve most commonly localize to the arms (46%) and legs (45%) but can implicate any peripheral nerve, including those of the head and neck (29%), chest (16%), pelvis (15%), and abdomen (9%) [6].

On CT, schwannomas appear as well-circumscribed masses that are hypo- to isodense relative to skeletal muscle with variable contrast enhancement. On MRI, lesions are low-to-intermediate intensity on T1-weighted sequences and high signal intensity on T2-weighted sequences and short-T1 inversion recovery (STIR) sequences [1]. MacCollin and colleagues [8] reported that lesions may have more homogeneous T2 signal hyperintensity relative to isolated, non-schwannomatosis-related lesions. Schwannomatosis-associated lesions demonstrate heterogeneous contrast enhancement, secondary to regions of cystic degeneration, which can be used to help distinguish them from neurofibromas [1]. In patients with multiple demonstrated schwannomas of the peripheral or spinal nerves, full radiological workup for schwannomatosis and other neurofibromatoses should be pursued, including contrast-enhancing sequences of the brain and spine. Brain imaging should include thin cuts (<3 mm) through the internal auditory canals to help differentiate schwannomatosis from NF2 [23]. Whole-body MRI (WB-MRI) can also be considered for diagnosis or the assessment of global disease burden [24] and is increasingly being used in clinical practice [23]. In a recent review on the imaging of patients with neurofibromatoses, Ahlawat and colleagues [23] recommended WB-MRI be performed using a 1.5- or 3-Tesla scanner and suggested the acquisition diffusion-weighted imaging, a fluid-sensitive sequence (T2 short tau inversion recovery), and an anatomic sequence (T1 volume-interpolated breath-hold examination). The authors argue that WB-MRI is indicated for the definitive diagnosis of schwannomatosis in those without a previous diagnosis. WB-MRI is also indicated for longitudinal surveillance of known peripheral nerve sheath tumors to determine the optimal time for intervention or to monitor progress while on treatment. Lastly, WB-MRI can be used to distinguish patients with segmental phenotypes from those with germline presentations.

30.5.2 Pathology

As indicated by the ISR criteria, pathological confirmation of a schwannoma is required to make the diagnosis of schwannomatosis. Schwannomas in this disease process are histologically very similar to sporadic schwannomas treated in patients without schwannomatosis. Consequently, while pathologic confirmation of one or more schwannomas is necessary to make the diagnosis, it is not sufficient. Similar to sporadic schwannomas, schwannomatosis-associated lesions are classically eccentric to the affected nerve and encapsulated by the epineurium. Neurofibromas, in contrast, classically lie centrally within the nerve and intercalate into the surrounding axons [1]. Schwannomas demonstrate two near-pathognomonic histological patterns, known as Antoni A and Antoni B. Respectively, these patterns are characterized by regions of high cellularity (Antoni A) and low cellularity (Antoni B) [6]. Antoni A regions are punctuated by Verocay bodies—regions of palisading, spindle-shaped nuclei interspaced with nuclear-free zones. Antoni B regions, which may reflect degeneration of Antoni A regions, are characterized by cystic degeneration and disorganized cellular matrix [1]. It has been suggested based upon small series that intra-tumoral myxoid changes, peritumoral edema, and an intraneural growth pattern are more common for schwannomatosis-related lesions [8]. However these features are not consistent across samples and should not be considered diagnostic.

30.6 Involvement of Genetics and Nonsurgical Specialties

Similar to patients with other neurofibromatoses, those with schwannomatosis benefit from multidisciplinary management. As previously described for neurofibromatosis 1 and 2 [25], a family history should be obtained, prioritizing first-degree relatives, to help distinguish sporadic from familial cases and identify other persons at risk. Consultation with genetic medicine should also be pursued to discuss family planning and the potential impact of the patient's disease on current and future offspring. Involvement of pain management is also crucial as medical management of chronic pain forms the core of treatment for patients with schwannomatosis, and many of these patients have extremely complex medication regimens, commonly including more than five agents of different classes [6]. Additionally, referral to a therapist or psychiatrist to discuss psychological comorbidity can be considered, as some case series have suggested that comorbid depression may be seen in nearly one in three patients with schwannomatosis [6]. Lastly, patients may benefit from referral to a support group composed of patients with schwannomatosis and other neurofibromatoses, such as those organized through the Children's Tumor Foundation.

30.7 Genetics

Hulsebos et al. provided the first description of the genetics of schwannomatosis in their report on a father-daughter pair with familial schwannomatosis [26]. Their report, along with other early data, suggested that schwannomatosis results from mutations in the SWI/SNF-related matrix-associated actin-dependent regulator of chromatin subfamily B (*SMARCB1*) [2, 12]. However, since that time, many patients meeting the clinical definition of schwannomatosis have been found to have *SMARCB1*-negative tumors. Some of these patients have been observed to have mutations in other genes, including leucine-zipper-like transcription regulator 1 (*LZTR1*) and *NF2*. The degree to which each of these mutations contributes to the clinical pathology is not clearly delineated, but emerging evidence suggests that their role may be different in familial and sporadic cases. Supporting this hypothesis includes population-based data documenting that mutations in *SMARCB1* are more common in patients with familial schwannomatosis, whereas *LZTR1* mutations are seen in similar proportions of familial and sporadic cases [4].

30.7.1 SMARCB1

Alternatively known as *INI1*, *BAF47*, or *hSNF5*, *SMARCB1* was the first gene described in the pathogenesis of schwannomatosis [26]. The gene sits on the long arm of chromosome 22 (22q11.2) and is found six megabases centromeric to the *NF2* gene, which may account for the similarity in clinical presentation between schwannomatosis and NF2 [2, 27]. The *SMARCB1* gene encodes a protein responsible for intracellular targeting of the SWI/SNF chromatin complex [10], an ATP-dependent protein complex that controls DNA structure through the movement of histone proteins [28–31]. The gene exhibits haplosufficiency, and patients require two inactivating mutations. Despite this, inheritance is autosomal dominant, likely secondary to recombination events between homologous chromosomes during mitosis. The index mutation in *SMARCB1* can occur in either germline or somatic cell lineages. In both cases, a similar event sequence is described, whereby homologous recombination leads to loss of heterozygosity in the mutant cell [28]. In germline mutations, this "first hit" occurs in germline cells and may be inherited, whereas for somatic mutations, the index mutation occurs in a somatic cell line [28]. In this latter group of patients—approximately 30% of those with schwannomatosis [8]—the patient is a genetic mosaic and is classified as having segmental schwannomatosis [12]. Though irrelevant to the overall pathogenesis, the segmental phenotype has potential therapeutic implications in that tumorigenesis is limited to a limb or ≤5 spinal segments, thereby reducing the portion of the body that requires monitoring [8, 9].

In contrast to many other disease-causing mutations, mutations in the genes implicated in schwannomatosis (i.e., *SMARCB1*) are embryonic lethal [32, 33], similar to what is seen with NF2 [34]. Consequently, biparental inheritance is not seen in schwannomatosis, though uniparental inheritance is seen in 10–20% of cases [5, 19]. Comparison of the disease-causing mutations in familial and sporadic cases has demonstrated the main distinction to be the prevalence of "non-truncating" mutations. Familial cases have been found to have higher proportions of "non-truncating"—ones that are missense or splice-site mutations; the exact therapeutic significance of this is unknown however [27].

30.7.2 LZTR1

The second gene commonly implicated in the pathogenesis of schwannomatosis is the *LZTR1* gene, which lies at position 22q11.23, roughly three megabases centromeric to *SMARCB1* [35]. In contrast to *SMARCB1*, the function of *LZTR1* is at present unknown [35]. However, like *SMARCB1*, mutations appear to be inherited in autosomal dominant fashion [35]. Mutations in this gene were first documented by Piotrowski and colleagues in 2014 [35] in a series of eight probands with either familial or sporadic schwannomatosis. Mutations in LZTR1 have subsequently been identified in other patients with schwannomatosis, and it is estimated that *LZTR1* mutations occur in roughly 29% of familial cases and 24% of sporadic cases [4].

Other mutations have been implicated in schwannomatosis, including *NF2*, which is seen in up to 8% of sporadic cases in population-based studies [4]. However, review of samples collected by the International Schwannomatosis Registry has suggested that *NF2* mutations may be far more common, occurring in 69% of tested patients [7]. Of note, *NF2* mutations in schwannomatosis occur only in somatic cell lineages and are thought to represent a "second hit," distinguishing them from the *NF2* mutations seen in neurofibromatosis type 2 [10]. Regrettably, over half of patients with sporadic disease and nearly a third of patients with familial disease have no identifiable pathogenic variant. Mutations in *COQ6*, which encodes a monooxygenase required for coenzyme Q10 (ubiquinone) biosynthesis, have been described in one family and posited as a locus that increases susceptibility to develop schwannomatosis; however the mechanisms by which it would do so are unclear [36]. Additionally, mutations in the TSC1, DDR1, CAST, ALPK2, TSC2, and TAB genes have been described in studies employing whole-exome sequencing [10]. The significance of these mutations is similarly unclear at present. Secondary to these gaps in current understanding, the genetics of schwannomatosis remain an area of ongoing investigation.

30.8 Pathogenesis

Based largely upon candidate gene studies and small clinical series, it is currently thought that schwannomatosis may develop through a multiple-hit mechanism involving at least two genes. In the most common mechanism, separate mutations in the two copies of SMARCB1 result in the loss of heterozygosity for the gene [10, 37]. The sites of original mutation appear to be at the 5′ or 3′ end of the SMARCB1 gene, in contrast to other tumors associated with SMARCB1, like rhabdoid tumors [10]. Consequently, the mutations are "non-truncating" and lead to the production of stable SMARCB1 transcripts coding for abnormal, truncated proteins, which have been identified on Western blot [10]. These proteins may retain partial functionality, in contrast to rhabdoid tumors, where nonsense mutations lead to complete loss of protein product [38]. Notably, mutant *SMARCB1* proteins in schwannomatosis retain the ability to inhibit cyclin D1, a key regulator of the cell cycle [38]. However, the proteins appear to be unstable and may be ineffective in helping to target the SWI/SNF complex to the proper chromatin regions.

After the mutations in SMARCB1, the second set of mutations are posited to occur in *NF2*, again with a single somatic cell mutation leading to loss of function through loss of heterozygosity [10]. This creates a four-hit/three-step process whereby schwannomas form in these patients: (1) initial *SMARCB1* mutation, (2) mutation in the second copy of the *SMARCB1* locus along with mutation of the *NF2* locus in a somatic cell line, and (3) loss of heterozygosity at the *NF2* locus through a mutation in the second copy [10]. A similar theoretical model is invoked in those with wild-type *SMARCB1* and mutant *LZTR1*, whereby the initial hit is in one of the *LZTR1* gene copies. A mutation in the second copy of the long arm of chromosome 22 then occurs, mutating both the second *LZTR1* copy and a copy of the *NF2* gene. As a fourth hit, the remaining *NF2* gene becomes mutated, resulting in loss of heterozygosity for both loci. However, as the *SMARCB1* gene lies between *LZTR1* and *NF2*, it is thought to be exceedingly unlikely for such a model to accurately explain tumorigenesis in these patients. Rather, it is posited that *LZTR1* mutant tumors are best described by a five-hit/three-step model, in which tumorigenesis occurs as described in the *LZTR1* model with the exception that one of the *SMARCB1* wild-type copies becomes mutated prior to the mutation in the *NF2* gene. In this model patient schwannoma cells are homozygous mutant for *LZTR1* and *NF2* but heterozygous for *SMARCB1*.

30.9 Management of Tumors and Symptoms

30.9.1 Medical Versus Surgical Management

Given the genetic predisposition to form new lesions in patients with schwannomatosis, symptomatic management forms the core of treatment [12]. First and foremost is control of chronic pain, which occurs at high rates among this clinical population [6]. Strategies for management of chronic pain include both pharmacologic [6] and non-pharmacologic therapies. With regard to pharmacotherapy, the γ-aminobutyric acid (GABA) analogs gabapentin and pregabalin are considered first-line agents, along with intermittent courses of short-acting opioids and nonsteroidal anti-inflammatory agents (NSAIDs) [39]. Where these agents fail or are unable to provide sufficient analgesia, other drug classes can be considered for the management of neuropathic pain, including anticonvulsants (e.g., topiramate, carbamazepine), serotonin-norepinephrine reuptake inhibitors (e.g., duloxetine), tricyclic antidepressants (e.g., amitriptyline), triptans (e.g., rizatriptan, zolmitriptan), and topical treatments (e.g., lidocaine patches) [39]. Large case series have demonstrated that patients with schwannomatosis require a median of three analgesic medications, most commonly gabapentin (44%), oxycodone (43%), and amitriptyline (37%) [6]. However, nearly one in ten may require more than ten medications as part of their pain regimen

[6]. Non-pharmacologic, non-operative management can be conducted in tandem with all of these pharmacologic therapies. These interventions include mindfulness-based stress reduction techniques, biofeedback, acupuncture, and hypnosis, and larger case series suggest that they may be underutilized [6].

Surgical management is generally reserved for those patients with tumors causing neurologic compromise, failed non-operative pain management, or which are rapidly expanding and concerning for possible dedifferentiation to a malignant peripheral nerve sheath tumor (MPNST) [1, 12]. Radiation therapy has been previously described for symptom management in other members of the neurofibromatosis syndrome family; however there is a theoretical risk of malignant transformation to MPNST [12]. For this reason, we recommend against the use of radiation for symptom management unless the lesion is enlarging on serial imaging and cannot be treated with surgery [40]. At present there is no clear role for chemotherapy [1].

30.9.2 Operative Intervention

Given the benign nature of the lesions in schwannomatosis [5], symptomatology and failure of medical management play key roles in determining surgical candidacy. Pain is by far the most common indication for surgical intervention, reported to be the primary indication in up to 80% of patients [6]. Unfortunately, a significant proportion of patients experience limited benefit with surgical intervention in this context, as nearly two in every five patients operated for pain have persistent local pain and over 25% experience no improvement in their pain [6]. Even for those who do experience post-operative relief, pain recurs in nearly three-quarters due to lesion recurrence or development of a new tumor.

Excision of schwannomas involving the cranial nerves has also been described [21] though it is less common than surgical intervention for spinal or peripheral nerve schwannomas. In their series of 14 patients with schwannomatosis, Gonzalvo et al. [21] reported excising cranial nerve schwannomas in five patients (5/6 lesions implicated the trigeminal nerve). Specific outcomes were only reported for one of these procedures, after which the patient experienced anesthesia dolorosa. Globally however, they reported good outcomes, identifying preservation of, or improvement in neurological function following excision for 30 of the 32 treated tumors in patients with familial schwannomatosis. They reported that only 2 of their 14 patients experienced tumor recurrence, suggesting that the post-operative natural history of schwannomatosis may differ from that of NF2, which is commonly characterized by local recurrence. However, a more recently published series by Alaidarous et al. [9] described outcomes in nine surgically treated patients with segmental schwannomatosis of the upper or lower limb. Tumor recurrence requiring repeated surgery was seen in five patients at a median follow-up of 3 years. Therefore, the natural course for surgically treated lesions remains unclear.

As suggested by the above series, the evidence for the surgical management of lesions in patients with schwannomatosis is limited. Given that schwannomatosis, like other neurofibromatoses, is characterized by tumor recurrence and multifocal disease, similar principles can be used to guide surgical intervention in both. For lesions of the peripheral nerves, this means that two mandatory principles must be adhered to (1) the use of microsurgical technique and (2) intraoperative electrical stimulation for functional nerve fiber mapping. For electrical stimulation, it has previously been recommended to use a threshold of 1 mA; if stimulation of a fascicle with this current produces a motor response, the fascicle is not taken [41]. Additionally, we recommend the use of intraoperative neuromonitoring as it has been shown to help reduce the risk of new post-operative neurological deficit [41].

The exact surgical approach employed is dictated by the lesion site and is beyond the scope of this chapter. However, in general we plan the surgical incision to allow access to the proximal and distal segments of the affected nerve. We also perform electrical stimulation prior to resection to map out the functional nerve fibers and find a silent/safe surgical corridor through which we can make the epineurium incision. Dissection proceeds eccentrically from the central tumor until the parent fascicle is isolated; depending on the size and location, intracapsular dissection and en bloc resection versus intralesional debulking may be used to facilitate excision [42]. The proximal and distal fascicle that enter and exit the tumor are then transected after complete mobilization of the lesion. Early identification of the entering or exiting fascicle can facilitate subsequent dissection. The goal of performing meticulous dissection is to achieve gross total resection with no or minimal damage to healthy fibers. We believe that the latter concern of prioritizing function preservation is especially important in schwannomatosis, as recurrence rates are likely higher than with sporadic lesions, and patients have a high risk of developing new, symptomatic lesions. However, where possible, gross total resection still remains the gold standard for both peripheral nerve [43–45] and spinal schwannomas [46, 47].

The major complication of surgery is iatrogenic nerve injury, as dissection involves manipulation of the affected nerve. For this reason, management by an experienced peripheral nerve surgeon is recommended [12]. One series examining operative outcomes of 40 spinal schwannoma resections in patients with schwannomatosis [6] found that nearly half of patients had persistent post-operative deficits, most commonly sensory (33%) or motor abnormalities (40%). In this same series, 145 peripheral nerve surgeries were performed, with 27% of treated patients having persistent post-operative deficits. Sensory abnormalities (17%) and motor weakness (7%) were again the most common.

30.9.3 Prognosis

As with other neurofibromatoses, schwannomatosis is a progressive condition, and patients develop additional lesions as time progresses. A recent systematic review found that patients with schwannomatosis develop nearly one new tumor each year [11]. Prognosis for the disease can then be described in terms of impact of survival and likelihood of symptom relief. With regard to the latter, prognosis is relatively poor as more than two-thirds of patients have been reported to experience chronic pain even after aggressive surgical and medical management [6]. Yet, unlike NF2, schwannomatosis has only minimal impact on life expectancy, with a mean age at death of 76.9 years relative to an average of 80.9 in the general population [4]. Unlike the other neurofibromatoses, the occurrence of malignant peripheral nerve sheath tumor in schwannomatosis is extremely rare [40].

30.10 Monitoring and Follow-Up

There is no uniformly accepted guideline for the management of patients with schwannomatosis. However, in a recent review, Evans and colleagues recommended that patients with schwannomatosis undergo baseline MRI imaging of the brain and spinal cord at the time of diagnosis for all patients [48]. In their view, the timing of follow-up should then be guided by the mutational profile of the patient. For those with *SMARCB1* mutations, they recommend repeat brain and spine MRI imaging every 2–3 years starting at the age of 10 [48]. By contrast, for patients with only *LZTR1*, they recommend delaying serial follow-up imaging until the age of 15–19 years. In the case of both *SMARCB1* mutant and *LZTR1* mutant patients who have clinical signs that can be correlated with their underlying disease, the authors offer that obtaining a whole body MRI might be reasonable [48].

For patients who meet the clinical diagnostic criteria of schwannomatosis, but who have not had mutational analysis, we recommend that genetic testing be pursued. Though of limited prognostic value in the context of clinically diagnosed disease, mutation identification can be used to assist with family planning and has the potential of influencing investigative therapies.

30.11 Future Directions

Relative to research on the other neurofibromatoses [49], research in schwannomatosis has been limited, likely due to a combination of the disease's rarity and relatively recent identification in the clinical literature. However, with the formation of multi-institutional, multinational collaborations, notably the International Schwannomatosis Registry, it appears more likely that breakthroughs in schwannomatosis may be seen in the near future. Subjects of research are likely to focus on the areas in which there are the greatest knowledge shortcomings, including the pathogenesis of these lesions and systemic therapies to halt or reverse the growth of schwannomas. A recently completed phase 2 trial (NCT01207687) looking at the use of the vascular endothelial growth factor (VEGF) antibody, bevacizumab, found it to be safe in patients with NF2 and to produce promising responses in radiographic tumor size and serum markers of disease burden [50]. Given the phenotypic similarities between schwannomatosis and NF2, it is possible that bevacizumab might also produce promising results in schwannomatosis [40, 51]. Additionally, trials are ongoing examining the therapeutic potential of the anti-nerve growth factor tanezumab (NCT04163419) as well as a vaccine of antigen-specific T cells modified ex vivo using immune-modified dendritic cells (NCT04085159).

30.12 Conclusions

Schwannomatosis is a rare hereditary syndrome characterized by the formation of multiple schwannomas in the peripheral nerves, spine, and cranial nerves. Relative to the other neurofibromatoses, schwannomatosis is poorly characterized and represents an opportunity for great therapeutic advancement. Current standard of care for these patients is medical management of chronic pain and operative excision of lesions in cases of refractory pain that is attributable to the schwannoma(s). Future directions include better definition of the underlying pathophysiology and identification of systemic agents capable of halting or reversing the disease course.

Disclosures Zach Pennington—None; Daniel Lubelski—None; Ravi Medikonda—None; Allan J. Belzberg—Consultant for Axogen and for AstraZeneca.

References

1. Koontz NA, Wiens AL, Agarwal A, Hingtgen CM, Emerson RE, Mosier KM. Schwannomatosis: the overlooked neurofibromatosis? Am J Roentgenol. 2013;200:W646–53.
2. Kresak J, Walsh M. Neurofibromatosis: a review of NF1, NF2, and Schwannomatosis. J Pediatr Genet. 2016;05:98–104.
3. Hilton DA, Hanemann CO. Schwannomas and their pathogenesis. Brain Pathol. 2014;24:205–20.
4. Evans DG, Bowers NL, Tobi S, et al. Schwannomatosis: a genetic and epidemiological study. J Neurol Neurosurg Psychiatry. 2018;89:1215–9.
5. Antinheimo J, Sankila R, Carpen O, Pukkala E, Sainio M, Jaaskelainen J. Population-based analysis of sporadic and type 2 neurofibromatosis-associated meningiomas and schwannomas. Neurology. 2000;54:71–6.
6. Merker VL, Esparza S, Smith MJ, Stemmer-Rachamimov A, Plotkin SR. Clinical features of Schwannomatosis: a retrospective analysis of 87 patients. Oncologist. 2012;17:1317–22.
7. Ostrow KL, Bergner AL, Blakeley J, et al. Creation of an international registry to support discovery in schwannomatosis. Am J Med Genet A. 2017;173:407–13.
8. MacCollin M, Chiocca EA, Evans DG, et al. Diagnostic criteria for schwannomatosis. Neurology. 2005;64:1838–45.
9. Alaidarous A, Parfait B, Ferkal S, Cohen J, Wolkenstein P, Mazereeuw-Hautier J. Segmental schwannomatosis: characteristics in 12 patients. Orphanet J Rare Dis. 2019;14:207.
10. Kehrer-Sawatzki H, Farschtschi S, Mautner V-F, Cooper DN. The molecular pathogenesis of schwannomatosis, a paradigm for the co-involvement of multiple tumour suppressor genes in tumorigenesis. Hum Genet. 2017;136:129–48.
11. Chick G, Victor J, Poujade T, Hollevoet N. Sporadic Schwannomatosis: a systematic review following the 2005 consensus statement. J Neurol Surg A Cent Eur Neurosurg. 2018;79:408–15.
12. Plotkin S, Wick A. Neurofibromatosis and Schwannomatosis. Semin Neurol. 2018;38:73–85.
13. Kwon NY, Oh H-M, Ko YJ. Multiple lower extremity mononeuropathies by segmental Schwannomatosis: a case report. Ann Rehabil Med. 2015;39:833–7.
14. Jia Y, Kraus JA, Reddy H, Groff M, Wong ET. Polyradiculopathies from Schwannomatosis. Open Neuroimaging J. 2011;5:9–13.

15. Plotkin SR, Bredella MA, Cai W, et al. Quantitative assessment of whole-body tumor burden in adult patients with neurofibromatosis. PLoS One. 2012;7:e35711.
16. Mehta GU, Feldman MJ, Wang H, Ding D, Chittiboina P. Unilateral vestibular schwannoma in a patient with schwannomatosis in the absence of LZTR1 mutation. J Neurosurg. 2016;125:1469–71.
17. Castellanos E, Bielsa I, Carrato C, et al. Segmental neurofibromatosis type 2: discriminating two hit from four hit in a patient presenting multiple schwannomas confined to one limb. BMC Med Genomics. 2015;8:2.
18. Leverkus M, Kluwe L, Roll E-M, Becker G, Brocker E-B, Mautner VF, Hamm H. Multiple unilateral schwannomas: segmental neurofibromatosis type 2 or schwannomatosis? Br J Dermatol. 2003;148:804–9.
19. MacCollin M, Woodfin W, Kronn D, Short MP. Schwannomatosis: a clinical and pathologic study. Neurology. 1996;46:1072–9.
20. MacCollin M, Willett C, Heinrich B, Jacoby LB, Acierno JS, Perry A, Louis DN. Familial schwannomatosis: exclusion of the NF2 locus as the germline event. Neurology. 2003;60:1968–74.
21. Gonzalvo A, Fowler A, Cook RJ, Little NS, Wheeler H, McDonald KL, Biggs MT. Schwannomatosis, sporadic schwannomatosis, and familial schwannomatosis: a surgical series with long-term follow-up. J Neurosurg. 2011;114:756–62.
22. Seppälä MT, Sainio MA, Haltia MJJ, Kinnunen JJ, Setälä KH, Jääskeläinen JE. Multiple schwannomas: schwannomatosis or neurofibromatosis type 2? J Neurosurg. 1998;89:36–41.
23. Ahlawat S, Blakeley JO, Langmead S, Belzberg AJ, Fayad LM. Current status and recommendations for imaging in neurofibromatosis type 1, neurofibromatosis type 2, and schwannomatosis. Skeletal Radiol. 2020;49:199–219.
24. Cai W, Kassarjian A, Bredella MA, Harris GJ, Yoshida H, Mautner VF, Wenzel R, Plotkin SR. Tumor burden in patients with Neurofibromatosis types 1 and 2 and Schwannomatosis: determination on whole-body MR images. Radiology. 2009;250:665–73.
25. Gutmann DH, Aylsworth A, Carey JC, Korf B, Marks J, Pyeritz RE, Rubenstein A, Viskochil D. The diagnostic evaluation and multidisciplinary management of neurofibromatosis 1 and neurofibromatosis 2. JAMA. 1997;278:51–7.
26. Hulsebos TJM, Plomp AS, Wolterman RA, Robanus-Maandag EC, Baas F, Wesseling P. Germline mutation of INI1/SMARCB1 in familial Schwannomatosis. Am J Hum Genet. 2007;80:805–10.
27. Smith MJ, Wallace AJ, Bowers NL, Rustad CF, Woods CG, Leschziner GD, Ferner RE, Evans DGR. Frequency of SMARCB1 mutations in familial and sporadic schwannomatosis. Neurogenetics. 2012;13:141–5.
28. Romero OA, Sanchez-Cespedes M. The SWI/SNF genetic blockade: effects in cell differentiation, cancer and developmental diseases. Oncogene. 2014;33:2681–9.
29. Dutta A, Sardiu M, Gogol M, Gilmore J, Zhang D, Florens L, Abmayr SM, Washburn MP, Workman JL. Composition and function of mutant Swi/Snf complexes. Cell Rep. 2017;18:2124–34.
30. Kadoch C, Crabtree GR. Mammalian SWI/SNF chromatin remodeling complexes and cancer: mechanistic insights gained from human genomics. Sci Adv. 2015;1:e1500447.
31. Wilson BG, Roberts CWM. SWI/SNF nucleosome remodellers and cancer. Nat Rev Cancer. 2011;11:481–92.
32. Guidi CJ, Sands AT, Zambrowicz BP, Turner TK, Demers DA, Webster W, Smith TW, Imbalzano AN, Jones SN. Disruption of Ini1 leads to peri-implantation lethality and tumorigenesis in mice. Mol Cell Biol. 2001;21:3598–603.
33. Steklov M, Pandolfi S, Baietti MF, et al. Mutations in LZTR1 drive human disease by dysregulating RAS ubiquitination. Science. 2018;362:1177–82.
34. Gutmann DH, Giovannini M. Mouse models of neurofibromatosis 1 and 2. Neoplasia. 2002;4:279–90.
35. Piotrowski A, Xie J, Liu YF, et al. Germline loss-of-function mutations in LZTR1 predispose to an inherited disorder of multiple schwannomas. Nat Genet. 2014;46:182–7.
36. Zhang K, Lin J-W, Wang J, et al. A germline missense mutation in COQ6 is associated with susceptibility to familial schwannomatosis. Genet Med. 2014;16:787–92.
37. Hadfield KD, Smith MJ, Urquhart JE, Wallace AJ, Bowers NL, King AT, Rutherford SA, Trump D, Newman WG, Evans DG. Rates of loss of heterozygosity and mitotic recombination in NF2 schwannomas, sporadic vestibular schwannomas and schwannomatosis schwannomas. Oncogene. 2010;29:6216–21.
38. Smith MJ, Walker JA, Shen Y, Stemmer-Rachamimov A, Gusella JF, Plotkin SR. Expression of SMARCB1 (INI1) mutations in familial schwannomatosis. Hum Mol Genet. 2012;21:5239–45.
39. Bellampalli SS, Khanna R. Towards a neurobiological understanding of pain in neurofibromatosis type 1: mechanisms and implications for treatment. Pain. 2019;160:1007–18.
40. Blakeley JO, Plotkin SR. Therapeutic advances for the tumors associated with neurofibromatosis type 1, type 2, and schwannomatosis. Neuro Oncol. 2016;18:624–38.
41. Levi AD, Ross AL, Cuartas E, Qadir R, Temple HT. The surgical management of symptomatic peripheral nerve sheath tumors. Neurosurgery. 2010;66:833–40.
42. Guha D, Davidson B, Nadi M, et al. Management of peripheral nerve sheath tumors: 17 years of experience at Toronto Western Hospital. J Neurosurg. 2018;128:1226–34.
43. Safaee MM, Lyon R, Barbaro NM, Chou D, Mummaneni PV, Weinstein PR, Chin CT, Tihan T, Ames CP. Neurological outcomes and surgical complications in 221 spinal nerve sheath tumors. J Neurosurg Spine. 2017;26:103–11.

44. Safaee M, Parsa AT, Barbaro NM, Chou D, Mummaneni PV, Weinstein PR, Tihan T, Ames CP. Association of tumor location, extent of resection, and neurofibromatosis status with clinical outcomes for 221 spinal nerve sheath tumors. Neurosurg Focus. 2015;39:E5.
45. Montano N, D'Alessandris QG, D'Ercole M, Lauretti L, Pallini R, Di Bonaventura R, La Rocca G, Bianchi F, Fernandez E. Tumors of the peripheral nervous system: analysis of prognostic factors in a series with long-term follow-up and review of the literature. J Neurosurg. 2016;125:363–71.
46. Fehlings MG, Nater A, Zamorano JJ, et al. Risk factors for recurrence of surgically treated conventional spinal schwannomas. Spine (Phila Pa 1976). 2016;41:390–8.
47. Pennington Z, Westbroek EM, Ahmed AK, Cottrill E, Lubelski D, Goodwin ML, Sciubba DM (2019) Surgical management of giant presacral schwannoma: systematic review of published cases and meta-analysis. J Neurosurg Spine: 1–12.
48. Evans DGR, Salvador H, Chang VY, Erez A, Voss SD, Druker H, Scott HS, Tabori U. Cancer and central nervous system tumor surveillance in pediatric Neurofibromatosis 2 and related disorders. Clin Cancer Res. 2017;23:e54–61.
49. Blakeley JO, Bakker A, Barker A, et al. The path forward: 2015 International Children's Tumor Foundation conference on neurofibromatosis type 1, type 2, and schwannomatosis. Am J Med Genet A. 2017;173:1714–21.
50. Blakeley JO, Ye X, Duda DG, et al. Efficacy and biomarker study of bevacizumab for hearing loss resulting from neurofibromatosis type 2–associated vestibular schwannomas. J Clin Oncol. 2016;34:1669–75.
51. Blakeley J, Schreck KC, Evans DG, Korf BR, Zagzag D, Karajannis MA, Bergner AL, Belzberg AJ. Clinical response to bevacizumab in schwannomatosis. Neurology. 2014;83:1986–7.